04/2017

Dear Tom!

Thank you very much for your excellent contribution.

Sincerely,

(signature)

Laparoscopic Liver, Pancreas, and Biliary Surgery

Laparoscopic Liver, Pancreas, and Biliary Surgery is an essential learning tool for all surgeons who manage patients considered for minimally invasive liver, pancreas, and biliary surgery.

Led by Claudius Conrad and Brice Gayet, pioneers in laparoscopic liver, pancreas, and biliary surgery, the authors have created a highly focused and multi-dimensional tool that takes the surgeon through the surgical procedures, one step at a time. Using a combination of text, illustrations, and high-definition videos, the authors explain and illustrate their excellence in surgical technique in a detailed and reproducible fashion.

The textbook contains contributions from world renowned experts and thought leaders in the field. They discuss key management concepts in the oncologic management of patients undergoing minimally invasive liver, pancreas, and biliary resections.

The accompanying comprehensive video atlas contains high-definition videos with a focus on true anatomic resections. The videos are supported by outstanding illustrations and 3D renderings of the relevant anatomy.

The authors expertly and logically demonstrate how to perform anatomic and non-anatomic liver, pancreas, and biliary resections. They cover patient and port positioning for laparoscopic and robotic approaches, detailed anatomy, and didactic breakdown of the operation. Including numerous surgical tips and tricks, and practical reviews for the management of patients with liver, pancreas, and biliary diseases before, during, and after operations the volume covers:

- Essential techniques (e.g. intraoperative ultrasound);
- Segmentectomies (I-VIII) and bisegmentectomies;
- Major hepatectomies, extended resections, and living donor liver transplantation;
- Pancreatectomies (e.g. Whipple) and Biliary resections;
- Advanced laparoscopic technologies and robotics.

This unparalleled resource will help a wide range of surgeons – including liver, pancreas, and biliary specialists, general surgeons, transplant surgeons, and surgical oncologists – to improve their surgical technique of both open and minimally invasive surgery.

Laparoscopic Liver, Pancreas, and Biliary Surgery

EDITED BY

Claudius Conrad MD, PhD

Department of Surgical Oncology
University of Texas MD Anderson Cancer Center
Houston, USA

Brice Gayet MD, PhD

Professor and Head, Medical and Surgical Department of Digestive Diseases
Institut Mutualiste Montsouris
Paris, France

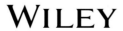

Library of Congress Cataloging-in-Publication Data

Names: Conrad, Claudius, editor. | Gayet, Brice, editor.
Title: Laparoscopic liver, pancreas, and biliary surgery /
  edited by Claudius Conrad, Brice Gayet.
Description: Chichester, West Sussex ; Hoboken, NJ : John Wiley & Sons Inc.,
  2017. | Includes bibliographical references and index.
Identifiers: LCCN 2015046826 | ISBN 9781118781173 (cloth)
Subjects: | MESH: Liver Diseases–surgery | Pancreatic Diseases–surgery |
  Biliary Tract Surgical Procedures | Laparoscopy
Classification: LCC RD546 | NLM WI 770 | DDC 617.5/56–dc23 LC record available
at http://lccn.loc.gov/2015046826

A catalogue record for this book is available from the British Library.

Wiley also publishes its books in a variety of electronic formats. Some content that appears in print may not be available in electronic books.

Cover design by Nao Kusuzaki; Cover Photo by Claudius Conrad

Set in 8.5/12pt MeridienLTStd by Thomson Digital, India
Printed and bound in Singapore by Markono Print Media Pte Ltd

1   2017

Contents

List of contributors

Anil K. Agarwal
Department of Gastrointestinal Surgery and Liver Transplant
Govind Ballabh Pant Hospital and Maulana Azad Medical
College, Delhi University
New Delhi, India

Thomas A. Aloia
Department of Surgical Oncology
University of Texas MD Anderson Cancer Center
Houston, TX, USA

Camerlo Antoine
Digestive Surgery Department
European Hospital of Marseilles, France

Kenichiro Araki
Department of General Surgical Science
Gunma University Graduate School of Medicine
Gunma, Japan

Horacio J. Asbun
Department of General Surgery
Mayo Clinic
Jacksonville, FL, USA

Adrian T. Billeter
Department of General, Visceral, and Transplantation Surgery
University of Heidelberg Hospital
Heidelberg, Germany

Markus W. Büchler
Department of General, Visceral, and Transplantation Surgery
University of Heidelberg Hospital
Heidelberg, Germany

Hop S. Tran Cao
Department of Surgery
Baylor College of Medicine
Houston, TX, USA

Jennifer Chan
Department of Medical Oncology
Dana-Farber Cancer Institute, Harvard Medical School
Boston, MA, USA

Pierre-Alain Clavien
Klinik für Viszeral- und Transplantationschirurgie
UniversitätsSpital Zürich
Zürich, Switzerland

Claudius Conrad
Department of Surgical Oncology
University of Texas MD Anderson Cancer Center
Houston, TX, USA

Danielle K. DePeralta
Division of Surgical Oncology
Harvard Medical School
Massachusetts General Hospital
Boston, MA, USA

David Fogelman
Department of Gastrointestinal Medical Oncology
University of Texas MD Anderson Cancer Center
Houston, Texas, TX, USA

Kathryn J. Fowler
Department of Radiology
Washington University School of Medicine
St Louis, MO, USA

David Fuks
Department of Digestive Diseases
Institut Mutualiste Montsouris
Paris, France

Matteo Fusaglia
ARTORG Center for Biomedical Engineering
Research
University of Bern
Bern, Switzerland

Kate Gavaghan
ARTORG Center for Biomedical Engineering
Research
University of Bern
Bern, Switzerland

Brice Gayet
Department of Digestive Diseases
Institut Mutualiste Montsouris
Paris, France

Vijaya N.R. Gottumukkala
Department of Anesthesiology and Perioperative Medicine
University of Texas MD Anderson Cancer Center
Houston, TX, USA

Claire Goumard
Department of Hepatobiliary Surgery and Liver Transplantation
Hôpital Pitié-Salpêtrière, Assistance Publique-Hôpitaux de Paris
Paris, France

Mahendran Govindasamy
Salem Gastro, Salem
Tamil Nadu, India

Ho-Seong Han
Department of Surgery
Seoul National University College of Medicine
Gyeonggi-do, Korea

Yasushi Hasegawa
Department of Surgery
Iwate Medical University School of Medicine
Morioka, Japan

Steven Y. Huang
Department of Interventional Radiology, Division of Diagnostic Imaging
University of Texas MD Anderson Cancer Center
Houston, TX, USA

William R. Jarnagin
Hepatopancreatobiliary Service, Department of Surgery
Memorial Sloan-Kettering Cancer Center,
New York, USA

Amit Javed
Department of Gastrointestinal Surgery and Liver Transplant
Govind Ballabh Pant Hospital and Maulana Azad Medical
College, Delhi University
New Delhi, India

Raja Kalayarasan
Department of Gastrointestinal Surgery and Liver Transplant
Govind Ballabh Pant Hospital and Maulana Azad Medical
College, Delhi University
New Delhi, India

Matthew H.G. Katz
Department of Surgical Oncology
University of Texas MD Anderson Cancer Center
Houston, TX, USA

Kimitaka Kogure
Institute for Molecular and Cellular Regulation
Gunma University
Gunma, Japan

Norihiro Kokudo
Hepatobiliary Pancreatic Surgery Division, Department
of Surgery
Graduate School of Medicine, University of Tokyo
Tokyo, Japan

David A. Kooby
Department of Surgery
Emory University School of Medicine
Atlanta, GA, USA

Universe Leung
Hepatopancreatobiliary Service, Department of Surgery
Memorial Sloan-Kettering Cancer Center
New York, USA

Keith D. Lillemoe
Division of Surgical Oncology
Harvard Medical School
Massachusetts General Hospital
Boston, MA, USA

Guy Maddern
University of Adelaide Discipline of Surgery
Queen Elizabeth Hospital
Woodville South, Australia

Masatoshi Makuuchi
Department of Hepato-Biliary-Pancreatic Surgery
Japanese Red Cross Medical Center,
Tokyo, Japan

Soeren Torge Mees
University of Adelaide, Discipline of Surgery
The Queen Elizabeth Hospital
Woodville South, Australia

Yoshihiro Mise
Hepatobiliary Pancreatic Surgery Division, Department of Surgery
Graduate School of Medicine, University of Tokyo
Tokyo, Japan

Beat Müller-Stich
Department of General, Visceral, and Transplantation Surgery
University of Heidelberg Hospital
Heidelberg, Germany

Hanno Niess
Department of General, Visceral, Transplantation, Vascular and
Thoracic Surgery
Hospital of the University of Munich
Munich, Germany

Takeo Nomi
Department of Surgery
Nara Medical University
Nara, Japan

Satoshi Ogiso
Department of Digestive Diseases
Institut Mutualiste Montsouris
Paris, France

Nicolas Paleari
Department of General Surgery
Mayo Clinic
Jacksonville, FL, USA

Matthias Peterhans
ARTORG Center for Biomedical Engineering
Research
University of Bern
Bern, Switzerland

Ruchir Puri
Department of General Surgery
Mayo Clinic
Jacksonville, FL, USA

Daniel Richard Rutz
Department of Surgery
Emory University School of Medicine
Atlanta, GA, USA

Yoshihiro Sakamoto
Hepatobiliary Pancreatic Surgery Division, Department of Surgery
Graduate School of Medicine, University of Tokyo
Tokyo, Japan

Olivier Scatton
Department of Hepatobiliary Surgery and Liver Transplantation
Hôpital Pitié-Salpêtrière, Assistance Publique-Hôpitaux de Paris
Paris, France

Hillary Shaw
Radia Inc., PS
Lynwood, WA, USA

Nairuthya Shivathirthan
Department of Surgical Gastroenterology
Apollo BGS Hospital
Mysore, India

John Stauffer
Department of General Surgery
Mayo Clinic
Jacksonville, FL, USA

Tadatoshi Takayama
Department of Digestive Surgery
Nihon University School of Medicine
Tokyo, Japan

Kenneth K. Tanabe
Division of Surgical Oncology
Harvard Medical School
Massachusetts General Hospital
Boston, MA, USA

Jean-Nicolas Vauthey
Department of Surgical Oncology
University of Texas MD Anderson Cancer Center
Houston, TX, USA

Go Wakabayashi
Department of Surgery
Ageo Central General Hospital
Ageo City, Japan

Michael J. Wallace
Department of Interventional Radiology, Division
of Diagnostic Imaging
University of Texas MD Anderson Cancer
Center
Houston, TX, USA

Stefan Weber
ARTORG Center for Biomedical Engineering Research
University of Bern
Bern, Switzerland

Jens Werner
Department of General, Visceral, Transplantation,
Vascular and Thoracic Surgery
Hospital of the University of Munich
Munich, Germany

Jonathan A. Wilks
Department of Anesthesiology and Perioperative
Medicine
University of Texas MD Anderson Cancer Center
Houston, TX, USA

Robert A. Wolff
Department of Gastrointestinal Medical Oncology
University of Texas MD Anderson Cancer Center
Houston, TX, USA

Jeff Siu-Wang Wong
United Christian Hospital
Hong Kong

Motoyo Yano
Department of Radiology
Washington University School of Medicine
St Louis, MO, USA

Foreword

It is with great pleasure that I write this foreword for the textbook and video atlas by Claudius Conrad and Brice Gayet on laparoscopic hepatopancreatobiliary (HPB) surgery. Claudius Conrad, who trained in my department at the Graduate School of Medicine, University of Tokyo, and Brice Gayet, who is a frequent guest-surgeon to Japan, have proved to me and the surgical community their excellent surgical skills in both open and laparoscopic surgery and their paramount concern for patient safety with their laparoscopic approach. Consequently, Claudius and Brice are very well equipped in creating this teaching material that promotes safe laparoscopic HPB surgery.

Today, almost all forms of hepatic resections have been performed via a laparoscopic approach, ranging from simple wedge resections to extended hepatectomies or resections with advanced vascular reconstruction. Brice Gayet and his team have certainly contributed significantly to its progress since its inception. Most studies that evaluate laparoscopic liver resection have shown comparable results to open resection in terms of operative blood loss, postoperative morbidity, and mortality. Many have demonstrated decreased postoperative pain, shorter hospital stays, and even lower costs. Preliminary oncological results, including resection margin status and long-term survival, are not inferior to open resection, although solid evidence proving equivalence is not available today as prospective and randomized studies are lacking. At least 40 studies (with more than 30 patients) on laparoscopic liver resection for malignancy have been reported although most of these were case series or case-control studies only. A larger series was first reported in 2002 while the majority of reports have been published since 2009. Therefore, reports on the long-term outcomes are not currently available.

As with open surgery, hepatocellular carcinoma and colorectal metastasis are the main indications for malignant tumor resection in laparoscopic surgery. However, in the earlier reports, a significant proportion of lesions resected laparoscopically were benign and this raises concerns as to whether these benign lesions were in fact resected because laparoscopy was readily available and not because their removal was deemed a necessity. It is important to recognize that laparoscopic surgery is merely a technique and its availability should not change the indication for resection. Further, the laparoscopic approach should not lead to shortcuts in terms of quality of oncological surgery provided.

Both Claudius and Brice have shown the importance of parenchyma-sparing liver surgery and how anatomical liver resection can indeed increase the safety of liver surgery. These important concepts can be successfully applied to laparoscopic surgery but do require a significant laparoscopic skill set. I am confident that this book and video atlas will allow a greater number of surgeons to successfully apply these concepts which will further the success of this field of laparoscopic surgery.

Progress in surgery is of the utmost importance and it is apparent to me that laparoscopic surgery will play a crucial role in HPB surgery in the near future. This informative textbook and atlas provides the community of HPB surgeons with what is laparoscopically feasible but it also clearly advocates the importance of operative and oncological safety. I am delighted to see this work by expert laparoscopic surgeons Claudius Conrad and Brice Gayet. I wholeheartedly endorse this book as a significant learning tool for surgeons who wish to attain valuable insights and to improve their laparoscopic skills in HPB surgery.

Congratulations on your great achievements, Claudius and Brice!

Professor Norihiro Kokudo
Department of Surgery
University of Tokyo Hospital
Tokyo, Japan

Foreword

As a "single-port, maximally invasive pancreatic surgeon," I have dreaded the day when laparoscopic pancreatic surgery would reach the point that these techniques would be available at all hospitals, provided by a wide variety of surgeons for every possible indication in almost every patient. I have been steadfast in my assumption that for these complex operations, especially with aggressive/invasive pancreatic malignancies, the wide exposure and an experienced surgeon using traditional open techniques would always be able to provide a "better" cancer operation, with superior short- and long-term outcomes, than "the new kids on the block" with either laparoscopic or robotic skills but limited experience in pancreatic surgery. I felt that even if high-volume centers with highly skilled surgical teams from around the world could report equivalent outcomes to open surgery, the rest of the surgical community would never catch up and I could play out the rest of my career as a "dinosaur" pancreatic surgeon with excellent outcomes but big incisions.

Then I met Brice Gayet and Claudius Conrad, and saw this well-written, this beautifully illustrated, this novel textbook and video atlas. I am realizing that the skills are now available in the surgical community and that there are teachers, such as Brice Gayet and Claudius Conrad, who can not only teach the techniques of minimally invasive pancreas surgery, but can build the confidence and determination of the next generation of pancreatic surgeons to push this field faster and further towards widespread application.

This textbook/atlas has clearly defined the laparoscopic technique for every common pancreatic surgical procedure and beautifully demonstrated the "tricks of the trade" in both the illustrations and video format. This book will be an essential for every institution developing a minimally invasive program in pancreatic surgery, as well as for those individuals training in surgical oncology, HPB surgery, and transplant surgery who hope to practice using the modern techniques for HPB surgery in the future.

In closing, it is likely too late for me, but for those early and midcareer pancreatic surgeons, be prepared, as it appears the "cows are out of the barn" with respect to minimally invasive pancreatic surgery and we are unlikely to corral the herd again with such a supportive and educational training tool such as this textbook/atlas.

Keith D. Lillemoe MD
Surgeon-in-Chief
Chief, Department of Surgery
Massachusetts General Hospital
W. Gerald Austen Professor of Surgery
Harvard Medical School
Boston, MA, USA

Foreword

Recent decades have seen tremendous progress in the treatment of patients with liver and pancreas diseases. The overarching theme of this progress is that treatment is becoming more tailored: less invasive when possible and more radical when necessary. This progress has been made possible in part by multidisciplinary innovations that support the work of the surgeon. For example, understanding of the mutational profile of the primary tumor and metastases not only allows for accurate prognostication but also enables surgeons to accurately determine which patients would benefit from undergoing extensive liver resections. Further, portal vein embolization via an interventional radiology approach has made portal vein ligation almost obsolete and allowed patients requiring major resection to be treated safely with hepatectomy. This minimal-access procedure has therefore enabled surgeons to perform more radical resections.

The community of minimally invasive hepatopancreatobiliary surgeons has also made significant strides towards reduce the morbidity of the surgery itself. Minimally invasive surgery for liver and pancreas diseases has progressed from a purely diagnostic procedure and minor resections of liver and pancreas to advanced procedures that include extended liver resections, pancreaticoduodenectomy, and vascular reconstructions. While diagnostic laparoscopy and minor laparoscopic liver and pancreas resections are practiced at many centers, advanced resections are limited to a select group of surgeons and a few institutions. The reason is that advanced skills in both hepatopancreatobiliary surgery and minimally invasive surgery are required to safely perform these advanced procedures. Mastery of both skills requires significant time investments in observerships, practice of laparoscopic technical skills, and creation of an infrastructure.

Brice Gayet and Claudius Conrad have created this important study material to facilitate learning these advanced procedures. In the video atlas, basic and advanced anatomic resections of liver and pancreas, many of which are challenging to master even via an open approach, are demonstrated in a didactically well-structured fashion. Three-dimensional renderings of the relevant liver anatomy, port positioning, and critical phases of the operation are depicted in wonderfully detailed images. The textbook provides the foundation in hepatopancreatobiliary oncology and the current data on minimally invasive hepatopancreatobiliary surgery necessary to set the illustrated video atlas in a conceptual framework. In the descriptions and the videos themselves we recognize the didactic skills of Claudius Conrad and Brice Gayet. The in-depth knowledge and technical skills demonstrated by Brice Gayet are not only rooted in his professorship of surgery but also in that of anatomy for many years.

I strongly recommend that everyone aspiring to master these skills use this work as a study guide on a routine basis. Mastery of the important theoretical concepts and internalization of the operative approaches presented in this work are needed for optimal outcomes. In addition, the excellent didactic set-up and the high-quality and beautiful operations presented in the video atlas make this work an excellent study tool for surgeons performing surgery via an open approach.

Congratulations to Brice Gayet and Claudius Conrad on this important study material that will facilitate mastery of the art of advanced minimally invasive hepato-pancreatobiliary surgery!

Jean-Nicolas Vauthey MD, FACS
Chief, Hepato-Pancreato-Biliary Section
Bessie McGoldrick Professor in Clinical Cancer Research
MD Anderson Cancer Center
Department of Surgical Oncology
MD Anderson Cancer Center
Houston, Texas

Preface

In the previous century, minimally invasive surgery was introduced to minimize trauma in gastrointestinal operations. After the first laparoscopic cholecystectomy, the indications for a laparoscopic approach increased significantly, particularly in colorectal surgery. Liver and pancreas surgery were initially thought to be unsuitable for laparoscopic techniques, due to the difficulties of safe mobilization and exposure. As a result, a significant number of experts in open hepaticopancreatobiliary surgery were reluctant to incorporate a laparoscopic approach into their practice and/or evaluate it in a randomized controlled trial.

Despite, and because of, significant advances in diagnostic, anesthesiological, and surgical technique that allowed for safer HPB surgery, these advances rarely became the bases for investigating how to make HPB surgery less invasive. This reluctance was rooted in the fear of losing the improvements the open HPB surgery community had achieved. Nevertheless, some expert centers reported on the feasibility and safety of laparoscopic HPB surgery and proved the benefits regarding reduced blood loss and pain, and improved recovery, compared to open liver surgery.

For open surgery, complete knowledge of HPB anatomy is essential. This is even more crucial when considering laparoscopic HPB surgery. For that reason, we have included two chapters on pancreas and liver anatomy by expert surgeons and anatomists from Japan, Drs Sakamoto and Takayama. These chapters will help to elucidate and safely reproduce the laparoscopic surgical techniques shown in the videos.

To date, two consensus conferences have been held on laparoscopic liver resections. One of the conclusions from the first consensus conference, held in 2009, was that laparoscopic resection of segments II and III should be considered the standard of care; the second conference in 2014 indicated that major resections were an innovative procedure, but still in an exploratory phase. An important conclusion by the consensus jury was

that a "major focused effort is necessary to determine what laparoscopic skills are required by trainees and HPB surgeons to successfully perform major laparoscopic liver resections." Claudius Conrad and I hope very much that this textbook and video atlas will help initiate or ease this learning curve.

The development of laparoscopy has also proved to be beneficial in pancreatic surgery, and laparoscopic distal pancreatectomy currently represents the standard of care. Other procedures, such as advanced enucleations, middle pancreatectomy or pancreatoduodenectomy, remain investigational. However, recent series on these advanced pancreatic procedures suggest that laparoscopy offers significant potential in reducing morbidity.

This atlas of minimally invasive HPB surgery has been designed as a high-quality, comprehensive didactic tool. A work of this magnitude could only be achieved by the input of experts from around the world who have extensive experience in treating HPB diseases and are established educators who have successfully mentored many young surgeons. In this atlas, we attempt to elucidate and provide an update on the surgical and perioperative management of HPB disorders from a laparoscopic point of view. Claudius Conrad and I have prepared the didactic videos for both trainees and specialized HPB surgeons in a comprehensive manner with an attempt to present the topics in an easy and understandable format.

What does the future hold for us? A state-of-the-art advancement, stereoscopic vision (3D), is the latest innovation that, in our experience, can significantly reduce both bleeding and operative time. As computer-assisted surgery in the operating room is implemented that includes not only robotics (co-manipulation, so-called cobot) but also cognitics (automated cognition), we can expect to see further improvement and progress in the safety and patient outcomes related to minimally invasive HPB procedures. Already today, patients' imaging studies are used for virtual 3D modeling and visualization of anatomical or pathological structures. In the future, the synthesis of these advances will allow us to create an augmented reality during surgery. The next step is likely the development of true robotic interfaces to improve safety and reduce operative time and automation of algorithms for a better understanding of operative scenarios and treatments.

The creation of this atlas was undoubtedly dependent on the support and enthusiasm of an expert team. Claudius Conrad and I wish to thank all the authors who agreed to participate in this educational work and share their vast experience. Finally, I would like to thank our editor and Claudius' editorial team at the University of Texas MD Anderson Cancer Center, Houston, Texas, USA.

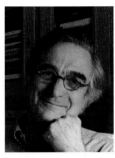

Brice Gayet
Paris

Preface

On résiste à l'invasion des armées; on ne résiste pas à l'invasion des idées . . .

Victor Hugo

We live in exciting times. Hepato-pancreato-biliary (HPB) surgery is forging ahead into new territory. Those of us who aim to pioneer the field must be mindful of not only how novel its frontiers are but also, and more importantly, how valuable and how to extend ourselves to reach them. Surgeons are aiming to minimize the trauma of surgery, with the hopes of lowering morbidity, lessening time spent in hospital, potentially returning patients earlier to chemotherapy, or even improving long-term outcomes.

Because of the complexity of advanced HPB surgery, it was previously thought not to lend itself to minimally invasive surgery, but my coeditor, Brice Gayet, and others have shown us through their creativity and innovative work that the time for considering less invasive HPB surgery has come. I am delighted to be part of a community of surgeons aiming to advance the field of minimally invasive HPB surgery through reducing its morbidity and improving outcomes. My surgical mentors in Germany, the United States, Japan, and France have enabled me to make a meaningful contribution to this community, and I am very thankful to them for this.

With all of the excitement over the possibilities of laparoscopic HPB surgery, we must not forget its overarching goal, which is to obtain the best possible short- and long-term outcome for our patients. Since most patients undergo HPB surgery for cancer, it is paramount

that oncological principles are observed if we are to ensure good outcomes. For that reason, it was important to me to ask international authorities in our field to contribute their expertise to this textbook and video atlas, since the best possible outcome can only be achieved if laparoscopic HPB surgery is put into the context of optimal oncological care. In addition to the contribution by these international experts, the camaraderie and the hard work of the international fellows at Institut Mutualiste Montsouris (IMM) were key in ensuring the success of this textbook and video atlas.

I hope very much that this textbook and video atlas will allow HPB surgeons to optimize outcome for their patients. I would like to thank Brice Gayet, our contributors, co-fellows at IMM, the editorial team, and, most importantly, my patients who have made this textbook and video atlas of laparoscopic hepato-pancreato-biliary surgery possible.

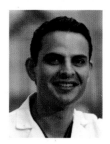

Claudius Conrad
Houston

Acknowledgments

We wish to thank the following people personally for their contributions to our inspiration and knowledge and other help in creating this book.

Dr Camerlo Antoine, Digestive Surgery Department, European Hospital of Marseilles, Marseilles, France.

Dr Kenichiro Araki, Division of Hepato-Biliary-Pancreatic Surgery, Department of General Surgical Science, Gunma University Graduate School of Medicine, Gunma, Japan.

Kristine K. Ash, Department of Surgical Oncology, University of Texas MD Anderson Cancer Center, Houston, USA.

Dr Mahendran Govindasamy, Salem Gastro, Salem, Tamil Nadu, India.

Nao Kusuzaki, Houston, USA.

Dr Takeo Nomi, Department of Surgery, Nara Medical University, Nara, Japan.

Dr Nairuthya Shivathirthan, Department of Surgical Gastroenterology, Apollo BGS Hospital, Mysore, India.

Storm Weaver PhD, Department of Surgical Oncology, University of Texas MD Anderson Cancer Center, Houston, USA.

Dr Jeff Siu-Wang Wong, United Christian Hospital, Hong Kong, China.

Dr Y Nancy You, Department of Surgical Oncology, University of Texas MD Anderson Cancer Center, Houston, USA.

Tom Bates, Angela Cohen, Pri Gibbons, Felicity Marsh, and Holly Regan-Jones at Wiley Blackwell.

About the companion website

This book is accompanied by a companion website:

www.wiley.com\go\conrad\liver-pancreas-biliary-laparoscopic-surgery

The website includes:

- videos, with transcription
- critical anatomy pictures
- port positioning
- important intraoperative pictures
- important points.

How to access the site:

- Find the redemption code on the inside front cover of this book and carefully scratch away the top coating of the label.
- Go to the companion website www.wiley.com\go\conrad\liver-pancreas-biliary-laparoscopic-surgery and follow the registration instructions.
- If you have purchased this title as an e-book, access to the companion website is available with proof of purchase within 90 days. Visit http://support.wiley.com to request a redemption code via the "Live Chat" or "Ask A Question" tabs.

PART I
Textbook

CHAPTER 1

The development of minimal access hepatopancreatobiliary surgery

Ruchir Puri, Nicolas Paleari, John Stauffer, and Horacio J. Asbun

Department of General Surgery, Mayo Clinic, Jacksonville, USA

EDITOR COMMENT

This wonderful chapter, which may spark the interest of surgeons beyond the field of HPB surgery, is an account of the challenges faced by the pioneers of minimally invasive HPB surgery, challenges of a scientific but also a social nature. Some of these pioneers' careers took an unfavorable turn because of their dedication to innovation. We owe these legends and also their families gratitude, not only for their ingenuity and the inquisitiveness from which the patients of minimally invasive HPB surgeons benefit in the operating room every day but also for taking on the societal challenge and risks to their career in order to drive innovation. The chapter also explores the available data on the development of modern laparoscopic and robotic liver, biliary, and pancreas surgery from its beginnings of limited resection to the advanced minimally invasive surgery that is practiced at many centers around the world today.

Keywords: advanced minimally invasive HPB surgery, history of minimally invasive HPB surgery

---

All truth passes through three stages:

- First it is ridiculed
- Second it is violently opposed
- Third it is accepted as self-evident

Arthur Schopenhauer

Hepatopancreatobiliary (HPB) operations are some of the most technically challenging procedures in surgery owing to the complex anatomy and proximity to vital structures. Over the years HPB procedures have excited, enthralled, and humbled surgeons all over the world. At the same time, the complexities of the disease processes have driven innovation not just in surgery but in medicine in general. The development of minimally invasive HPB surgery is synonymous with the development of laparoscopy and is perhaps the "holy grail" of laparoscopic surgery.

1.1 Beginnings

The term laparoscopy comes from "laparoskopie," which is derived from two Greek words: *laparo*, meaning "flank," and the verb *skopos*, meaning "to look or observe" [1]. The exploration of the human body through small or natural orifices dates back to the time of Hippocrates [2]. Hippocrates described the use of a primitive anoscope for the examination of hemorrhoids in 400 BC [2]. An Arab physician, Abulcasis, added a light source to the instrument for the

Laparoscopic Liver, Pancreas, and Biliary Surgery, First Edition.
Edited by Claudius Conrad and Brice Gayet.
© 2017 John Wiley & Sons, Ltd. Published 2017 by John Wiley & Sons, Ltd.

exploration of the cervix in AD 1000 [2,3]. Many centuries later, in 1585, Giulio Cesare Aranzi inspected the nasal cavity by reflecting a beam of light through water [2].

In 1805 Phillipp Bozzini examined the urethra using an instrument that consisted of a wax candlelit chamber inside a tube which reflected light from a concave mirror [2,3]. Bozzini called it the "lichtleiter," and it is considered the first real endoscope (Figure 1.1 and Figure 1.2) [2,3]. Using his lichtleiter, Bozzini managed to study the bladder directly, and his pioneering efforts laid the foundations of modern endoscopy.

Over the next century, Pierre Salomon Segalas and Antoine Jean Desormeaux from France refined Bozzini's lichtleiter and took the first steps in developing the modern cystoscope [2,3]. Desormeaux presented his idea to the Academy of Medicine in Paris, and for his efforts he is considered the "father of cystoscopy" [3]. Around the same time, over in the United States, John Fischer in Boston was using a similar instrument to perform vaginoscopies, and in Dublin, Ireland, Francis Cruise was performing endoscopies on the rectum [2].

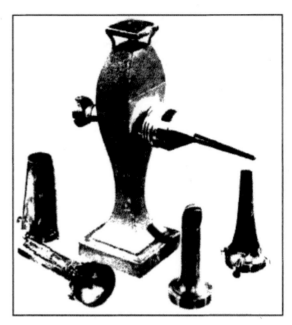

Figure 1.2 The lichtleiter (an original owned by the American College of Surgeons, Bush Collection). The 200th Anniversary of the First Endoscope: Phillip Bozzini (1773–1809).
Source: Morgenstern 2005 [4]. Reproduced with permission of Sage Publications.

In 1877 a urologist from Berlin, Maximilian Nitze, created what is considered the first modern endoscope using a platinum wire heated by electricity and encased in

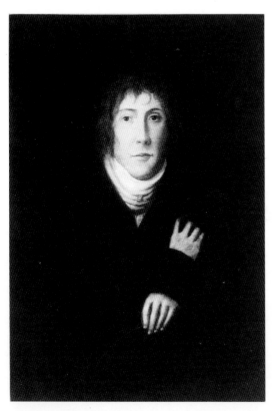

Figure 1.1 Self-portrait of a young Bozzini (ca. 1805).
Source: Frankfurt town archives.

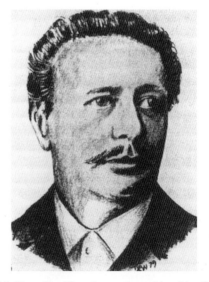

Figure 1.3 Maxmilian Nitze. Source: https://de.wikipedia.org/wiki/Datei:Max_Nitze_Urologe.jpg#file. Used under CC BY-SA 3.0 - http://creativecommons.org/licenses/by-sa/3.0/legalcode.

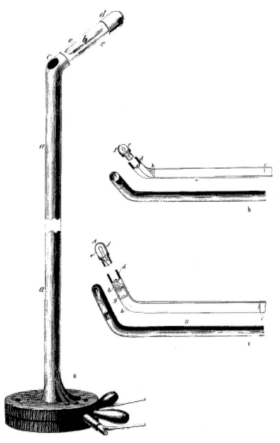

Figure 1.4 Nitze cystoscope of 1877. Source: Mouton 1998 [5]. Reproduced with permission of Springer.

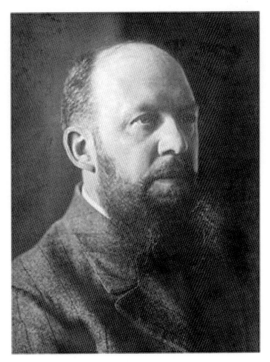

Figure 1.5 George Kelling. Source: https://en.wikipedia.org/wiki/Georg_Kelling#/media/File:Portrait_georg_kelling.jpg. Used under CC BY-SA 3.0 de - http://creativecommons.org/licenses/by-sa/3.0/de/deed.en.

a metal tube (Figure 1.3 and Figure 1.4) [2,3]. A few years later, in 1880, Thomas Edison invented the light bulb, which revolutionized the way endoscopies were performed [3,6]. While these innovations all made advances in laparoscopy possible, little else occurred in the field until the beginning of the twentieth century.

1.2 Advent of laparoscopy

George Kelling from Germany is credited with exploring the abdominal cavity using a scope after creating pneumoperitoneum in 1901 (Figure 1.5). Kelling was a surgeon and first performed laparoscopies on dogs; he called the procedure "coelioskope" [2,3,6,7] (Box 1.1). The technique involved injecting the canine's abdomen with oxygen filtered through sterile cotton and then using Nitze's cystoscope to inspect the abdominal contents. Kelling performed this procedure in humans, but his findings were not published [3]. Around the same time, a Swedish internist called Hans Christian Jakobaeus popularized the procedure in humans by using a colposcope with a mirror to assess the abdomen of a pregnant woman [7]. In 1911 Jakobaeus presented his work *Über Laparo- und Thorakoskopie* and later continued his work in thoracoscopy (Figure 1.6) [3,6,7,8]. Jakobaeus used trocars very similar to the ones used today and is also credited with coining the term "laparoscopy" [3]. Not too far away in Petrograd (modern-day St Petersburg), Dimitri Ott performed the same procedure and called it "ventroscopy" [6,7]. The first to use the laparoscopic technique in the United States was Bertram M. Bernheim in 1911 [9]. Bernheim was a surgeon at the Johns Hopkins University, and he called this procedure "organoscopy" [2,3,6–8,11].

Box 1.1 Different terms used historically

Coelioscope: George Kelling, 1901 (Germany)

Ventroscopy: Dimitri Ott, 1901 (Petrograd/St Petersburg)

Organoscopy: Bertram Berheim, 1911 (Johns Hopkins University)

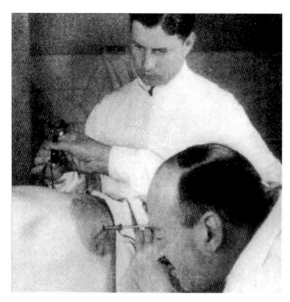

Figure 1.6 Hans Christian Jakobaeus MD, performing a thoracoscopy. Source: Braimbridge 1993 [10]. Reproduced with permission of Elsevier.

Bernheim, like many others at the time, had not heard of the work of Kelling and Jakobaeus.

Up to this point, all the procedures for exploring the abdominal cavity were performed with oxygen [3]. In 1924, Richard Zollikofer proposed that pneumoperitoneum be obtained using carbon dioxide. Carbon dioxide had two advantages: one was the rapid reabsorption of carbon dioxide by the peritoneal membrane and, unlike oxygen, it was noncombustible [3,6]. In 1929, Heinz Kalk, a German gastroenterologist, designed a new lens system with 135° vision and introduced the technique of "double trocar." This invention eventually led to more refinements and the introduction of instruments into the cavities [2,3,6,7]. Between 1929 and 1959, Kalk submitted many articles on diagnostic laparoscopy; he is considered the "father of modern laparoscopy" [3].

The first therapeutic intervention was carried out by the German physician Fervers, who performed the lysis of abdominal adhesions and a liver biopsy [3,6]. Another significant advancement in laparoscopy is credited to the Hungarian physician Janos Veress. In 1938, he created a retractable needle to create pneumoperitoneum. We are all familiar with the Veress needle, but interestingly, it was initially used for the treatment of tuberculosis with pneumothorax in the preantibiotic era [2,3,6,7]. This technique was not accepted by all surgeons as it was considered unsafe. This led, in 1974, to Chicago-based gynecologist

Harrith M. Hasson creating the open technique to access the abdominal cavity and achieve placement of the trocar that bears his name [2]. Raoul Palmer performed diagnostic laparoscopies in women and advised placing the patient in the Trendelenburg position for better visualization of the pelvis [2]. In addition, he was the first to control abdominal pressure during the procedure – two important aspects of modern laparoscopy [2].

In 1952, laparoscopic surgery underwent a revolution when French scientists M. Fourestier, A. Gladu, and J. Vulmiere created fiber-optics with cold light [3]. Two years later, scientists Lawrence Curtiss, Basil Hirschowitz, and Wilbur Peters did the same at the University of Michigan and brought cold light fiber-optics into practice in 1957. With improved visualization of the abdominal cavity, the advances in laparoscopy gained momentum [2].

Few surgeons have influenced the development of laparoscopic surgery more than the German gynecologist Kurt Semm. A pioneer in minimally invasive surgery, Semm developed a system of automatic insufflation in 1977. This consisted of a system of suction and irrigation, laparoscopic thermocoagulation, and the laparoscopic scissors as well as the "pelvitrainer" (Figure 1.7) used to teach laparoscopic techniques [2,3,6,7]. In 1981, Semm performed the first totally laparoscopic appendectomy [2,3,6,7]. The next significant milestone was the development of the high-resolution video camera in 1982 [2]. Since then the introduction of xenon/argon light sources and high-definition cameras has further improved visualization [2].

Despite the obvious potential advantages, skepticism regarding laparoscopic surgery remained prevalent because "big surgeons make big incisions" [3]. In 1985, the first

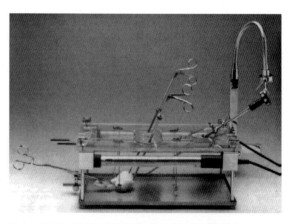

Figure 1.7 Kurt Semm's "pelvitrainer." Surgical training system with a novel approach. Source: Semm 1986 [12]. Reproduced with permission of Thieme.

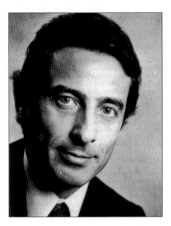

Figure 1.8 Erich Mühe. Source: Society of Laparoendoscopic Surgeons.

totally laparoscopic cholecystectomy using the Veress needle for access and the trocar called the "galloscope" was carried out by German surgeon Erich Mühe (Figure 1.8) during a two-hour-long intervention [5,11]. Mühe encountered significant criticism, and this great achievement was initially unrecognized [11]. Subsequently, in 1987, Philippe Mouret, a French gynecologist, performed the first laparoscopic cholecystectomy in France [2,3,6,13].

Over the years, continued refinements in techniques and instrumentation have enabled surgeons to push the envelope even further. In a short span of less than three decades, minimally invasive surgery has grown exponentially. What seemed like virtual reality in 1987 is now the new norm, and the laparoscopic approach has become the standard of care for many abdominal surgical procedures (Box 1.2).

Box 1.2 Important historical events in minimally invasive HPB surgery

1901: Kelling examines the abdominal cavity of the dog with a cystoscope

1911: Jakobaeus – first laparoscopic series in a human

1929: Kalk – oblique view, double trocar technique

1938: Veress – abdominal puncture needle

1970: Semm – automatic insufflation

1974: Hasson – open laparoscopy trocar

1986: TV camera adapted to optics

1987: First laparoscopic cholecystectomy by Mouret

1992: First laparoscopic liver resection by Gagner

1994: First laparoscopic pancreaticoduodenectomy by Gagner and Pomp

1.3 Laparoscopic hepatopancreatobiliary (HPB) surgery

1.3.1 Gallbladder surgery

As mentioned above, Mühe performed the first laparoscopic cholecystectomy in 1985 and was surprised by the patient's quick recovery [7,11]. He proclaimed "I can't believe it, the patient has bowel movements almost immediately after the surgery!" [11]. In 1986, Mühe presented his technique to the Congress of the German Surgical Society [11]. The audience was skeptical to say the least; Mühe's presentation received numerous negative comments, and his peers said that this was "Mickey Mouse surgery" or "small brains for small incisions" [11]. In 1988, Philippe Mouret from Lyon, France, presented a technique of laparoscopic cholecystectomy similar to that put forward by Mühe two years earlier [2,3,6,13]. Mouret also encountered criticism, this time from the French Surgical Society. This, however, inspired the French surgeons François Dubois (Paris) and Jacques Perissat (Bordeaux) to develop their technique for laparoscopic cholecystectomy independently in 1988 [13].

In 1988, the first laparoscopic cholecystectomy was performed in the United States by John Barry McKernan, a surgeon, and William Saye, a gynecologist [6,14]. Eddie J. Reddick and Douglas Olsen in Nashville collaborated with McKernan and Saye and started performing laparoscopic cholecystectomies regularly [14]. In April 1989, Professor Jacques Perissat was not allowed to present a laparoscopic cholecystectomy at SAGES! Nevertheless, he carried out his video presentation at a cabin near the SAGES auditorium, close to the men's restroom. Not surprisingly, this attracted a lot of attention [13]. This pivotal event marked the beginning of a revolution in laparoscopic surgery for general surgeons around the world [13]. Dubois subsequently published a series of 36 "celioscopic cholecystectomies" in *Annals of Surgery* [15]. The development and popularization of the technique of laparoscopic cholecystectomy practiced in the United States today are credited to Reddick and Olsen, who led the laparoscopic revolution in the continent [14].

It was quickly realized that the benefits of laparoscopic surgery centered on less postoperative pain, enabling better patient satisfaction and a quicker return to work. It seemed logical that the next set of innovations in laparoscopic surgery of the gallbladder be aimed at reducing the number and size of access points to the abdominal cavity. Schwenk *et al.* and Unger *et al.* evaluated patients who underwent laparoscopic cholecystectomy with 10 mm and 5 mm ports versus 5 mm and 2 mm ports. Both authors concluded that patients with smaller ports had less postoperative pain [16]. However, Bisgard found a significantly higher rate of conversion (38%) with mini-laparoscopy compared with standard laparoscopic trocars [17].

While the results of mini-laparoscopy were equivocal, in an effort to further reduce the number of ports, single-incision laparoscopic surgery (SILS) was born. This utilized a single 25 mm port with multiple trocars. The first SILS was performed in the late 1990s by Italian surgeon Fabrizio Bresadola and his team, who later published their experience after 100 cholecystectomies. They concluded that it is safe and feasible compared with traditional laparoscopic cholecystectomy but with better esthetic results [18]. Zehetner *et al.* and Pisanou *et al.* performed meta-analyses of studies comparing the single-port technique with the multiport laparoscopic technique and demonstrated that the only obvious advantage was improved cosmesis [19,20]. Further, reports of increased incidence of port site hernias with the single-port technique (1.2% versus 8.4%) have been published [21,22].

Another approach which had generated excitement was a NOTES (natural orifice transluminal endoscopic surgery) cholecystectomy performed transvaginally. Kalloo *et al.* were the first to describe the NOTES approach in 2004 [21]. The procedure can be cumbersome, and the main alleged advantage of this approach seems to be decreased postoperative pain. Even though feasible, the NOTES approach to laparoscopic cholecystectomy has failed to show definite advantage and has not gained widespread adoption. Introduction of the robotic platform in the 2000s further revolutionized laparoscopic surgery. Many surgeons now offer a robotic single-port cholecystectomy. Today, a distinct advantage of this approach is lacking, and it is safe to say that the conventional four-port cholecystectomy has stood the test of time and continues to be the gold standard.

Despite all the advantages demonstrated by laparoscopic cholecystectomy, an increased incidence of bile duct injury is still reported when compared with the incidence of the now historical open approach. Efforts to decrease that incidence are still evolving, and an important technical concept that has emerged is obtaining the "critical view of safety" prior to transecting the cystic duct (Figure 1.9). The premise behind this is that the cystic duct should be clearly identified, with the goal of avoiding injury to the common bile duct (CBD). This was originally proposed by Strasberg *et al.* in 1995 and is now accepted as the standard of care for the majority of cases [23]. Obtaining the critical view entails dissecting in Calot's triangle till the cystic plate is clearly visible and ensuring that two, and only two, structures enter the gallbladder: the cystic duct and artery [21]. Occasionally, this may not be possible, in which case a cholangiogram, an intraoperative ultrasound or a top–down technique may be beneficial.

1.3.2 Bile duct surgery
The laparoscopic exploration of the common bile duct has become an accepted procedure for the treatment of choledocholithiasis associated with cholecystolithiasis. The

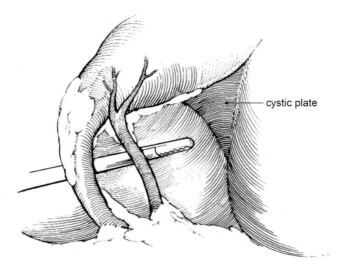

cystic plate

Figure 1.9 The critical view of safety. The triangle of Calot has been dissected free of fat and fibrous tissue, but the common bile duct has not been displayed. The base of the gallbladder has been dissected off the cystic plate and the cystic plate can be clearly seen. Two, and only two, structures enter the gallbladder and these can be seen circumferentially. Source: Strasberg 2010 [23]. Reproduced with permissions of Elsevier.

first exploration of the common bile duct was carried out by Dr Joseph Petelin [24] in 1989, and the first report of the exploration of the common bile duct was published in 1991 by Stoker *et al.* They described a series of five patients who underwent a laparoscopic exploration of the common bile duct with removal of gallstones and placement of a T-tube with satisfactory results [25]. In mid-1993 Petelin published his experience of the successful removal of gallstones in 83 of 86 patients who underwent exploration of the common bile duct [24]. Until then, the technique involved a laparoscopic choledochotomy and placement of a biliary drainage tube. Berci and Morgenstern described the laparoscopic transcystic common bile duct exploration in 1994 [26].

In 2003 Petelin *et al.* published their 12 years of experience in common bile duct explorations with encouraging results [27]. Dorman *et al.* presented their experience with 148 patients who underwent laparoscopic common bile duct exploration; gallstones were removed successfully in 143 cases and endoscopic retrograde pancreatography (ERCP) was conducted in the rest [28]. By the late 1990s, it became evident that transcystic exploration of

the common bile duct was technically feasible and ERCP could be used to treat residual lithiasis. As with many other minimally invasive procedures, traditional dogma was challenged when a laparoscopic common bile duct exploration was performed and the need for routine T-tube placement was questioned. Gurusamy *et al.* compared open bile drainage via a T-tube with primary closure and concluded that the use of a biliary T-tube prolonged both surgical time and hospital stay without any clear clinical benefit [29].

The laparoscopic approach has also been utilized for other biliary procedures including bilioenteric anastomoses, bile duct, and choledochal cyst excisions. The magnification afforded by the minimally invasive approach favors the complete excision of intrapancreatic choledochal cysts (Figure 1.10). Future interventions in surgery of the biliary tree will likely be centered around combined laparoendoscopic interventions in selected patients.

1.3.3 Pancreatic surgery
In Sanskrit, an ancient Indian language, the pancreas is called *agnyashay*, which is derived from *agni* meaning

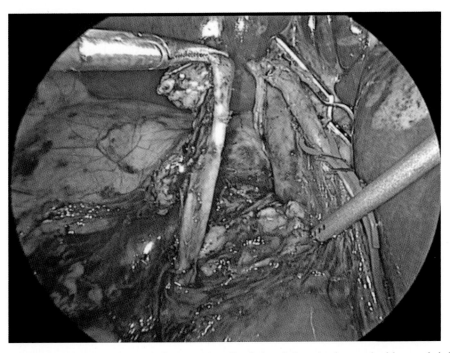

Figure 1.10 Laparosopic intrapancreatic choledochal cyst excision. The cholecochal cyst has been excised from cephalad to caudad with complete intrapancreatic dissection. A bulldog clamp is noted at the level of the bifurcation; the hepatic artery is surrounded by a vessel loop. Source: Horacio J. Asbun. Reproduced with permission.

"fire." It has been known since ancient times that the pancreas does not take too kindly to being disturbed. Anatomically, the pancreas is not easily accessible given its retroperitoneal location and proximity to vascular structures. Pancreatic resections have thus always been associated with significant morbidity and mortality. Initially, laparoscopy was utilized as a staging procedure in pancreatic malignant disease. However, with the evolution of new tools, refinements in technology, and increased surgeon experience, laparoscopic interventions on the pancreas seemed more plausible.

1.3.3.1 Laparoscopic pancreatic enucleation

So how do you approach an organ that does not like to be disturbed and makes most surgeons apprehensive? It seems intuitive that you do the least invasive surgery first. That is exactly what happened with the pancreas; enucleations of benign or malignant tumors were some of the first laparoscopic procedures performed. Gagner *et al.* and Tagaya *et al.* confirmed the feasibility and safety of this approach [30,31].

While feasible, the incidence of pancreatic fistula with a laparoscopic enucleation is high, as reported by Talamini *et al.* They found that the rate of pancreatic fistula in patients treated with laparoscopic pancreatic enucleation was 50% but only 12% in patients treated with laparoscopic pancreatectomy [32]. Fernandez Cruz *et al.*, in a different study, demonstrated a pancreatic fistula rate of 35% [33]. At present, it is felt that laparoscopic enucleation of pancreatic tumors is a feasible and safe technique but requires the surgeon to be cautious when selecting appropriate patients.

1.3.3.2 Laparoscopic distal pancreatectomy

Laparoscopic distal pancreatectomy is considered an advanced and difficult procedure by some. Soper *et al.* first described laparoscopic distal pancreatectomy in a porcine model [34]. Laparoscopic distal pancreatectomy in humans was initially performed simultaneously by Sussman and Cuschieri in 1994 for benign pathologies and subsequently by Gagner *et al.* [35–37]. European multicenter experience of laparoscopic distal pancreatectomies published by Marbut *et al.* established its efficacy [38].

Our group has described the "clockwise technique," with a 17.2% morbidity, 10.2% pancreatic fistula rate, and no mortality, confirming the benefit of a minimally invasive approach [39]. We subsequently published our experience of 172 patients; 90 patients underwent an open distal pancreatectomy and 82 underwent laparoscopy. We concluded that the benefits of laparoscopic surgery were based on less blood loss with less need for transfusions, shorter hospital stay, and less overall recovery time. The morbidity and mortality were similar in both groups, and oncologically there were no statistically significant differences [40].

While the laparoscopic approach proved to be efficacious for a variety of benign lesions, there was considerable debate regarding its role in the management of malignant disease. There were serious doubts related to the pancreatic margin, the retroperitoneal dissection, and the number of resected lymph nodes, as evidenced by the papers published by Merchant in 2009 [41] and Kubota [42]. However, Kooby *et al.* in 2010 published a multicenter study concluding that laparoscopic distal pancreatectomy compared with open resection has similar short- and long-term oncological outcomes [43]. Several meta-analyses confirmed that laparoscopic distal pancreatectomy had definite advantages over the open technique and presented no oncological compromise [44–46]. It is reasonable to conclude that, in experienced hands, the laparoscopic approach should be the procedure of choice for distal pancreatectomy even in patients with pancreatic cancer.

Another challenge in the development of laparoscopic distal pancreatectomy was the preservation of the spleen. Since Mallet *et al.* showed the important immunological role of the spleen in 1943, efforts to preserve it have intensified [47]. At present, there are two prevalent techniques. The first, described by Warshaw in 1997, requires division of the splenic artery and vein, leaving the spleen to be supplied by the gastroepiploic vessels and short gastric vessels [48]. The second technique, described by Kimura, allows the preservation of the splenic vessels joining the cross-collateral branches of both structures [49]. The Kimura technique demands greater laparoscopic skill and time in comparison to the Warshaw technique, which is faster but may increase the risk for the development of postoperative splenic abscesses and pain [48,59].

Robotic distal pancreatectomy has been developed over the last few years. The results compared with the laparoscopic approach appear to be mixed. Waters *et al.* showed that the robotic approach led to reduced hospital stay, lower cost, and a higher rate of splenic preservation with statistically significant differences [50]. Kang *et al.*, on the other hand, found the robotic approach to be more expensive with longer operative time but to have a higher success rate for splenic preservation [51]. Ergonomically, the robotic platform seems to have a clear advantage over conventional laparoscopy. While tactile feedback is lacking, a greater range of motion of the robot can potentially circumvent some of those challenges. It is evident that cost is an important determinant of the utility of robotically assisted laparoscopic surgery.

1.3.3.3 Laparoscopic pancreaticoduodenectomy

Open pancreaticoduodenectomy is considered one of the most difficult and challenging procedures. It is not surprising that the laparoscopic approach to a pancreaticoduodenectomy takes it to an even higher level of complexity. The first surgeons to perform a laparoscopic pancreaticoduodenectomy were Michel Gagner and Alfons Pomp in 1994 [52]. Gagner *et al.* in 1997 presented their initial series of 10 patients who underwent laparoscopic pancreaticoduodenectomy with a conversion rate of 40%. They reported significant morbidity for those completed laparoscopically with a mean hospital stay of 22.3 days. They concluded that laparoscopic pancreaticoduodenectomy did not offer any advantage over the open procedure and may increase morbidity.

However, other surgeons continued exploring this area [37]. Dulucq *et al.* presented their experience of 25 patients treated with laparoscopic pancreaticoduodenectomy where the mean hospital stay was 16.2 days, mortality rate 4.5%, morbidity 31.8%, and pancreatic fistula rate 4.5%. They concluded that laparoscopic pancreaticoduodenectomy is a difficult procedure to perform [53]. It was Palanivelu *et al.* who presented the first series which favored the laparoscopic approach. Forty-five patients underwent a laparoscopic pancreaticoduodenectomy with a mean hospital stay of 10.2 days, surgical time of 370 minutes, and an average of 13 lymph nodes harvested. There were no conversions, morbidity rate was 26.6%, mortality rate 2.2%, and median survival 49 months. They concluded that laparoscopic pancreaticoduodenectomy is safe and feasible in appropriately selected patients [54].

More recently, Nigri *et al.* published a meta-analysis comparing the minimally invasive versus the open approach to pancreaticoduodenectomy. They included 204 patients in the laparoscopic arm and 419 patients in the open arm. They reached the conclusion that there were no statistically significant differences in morbidity, mortality, pancreatic fistula, transfusion rate, oncological margin, resection of lymph

nodes, reoperation rate, or infection rate. The laparoscopic approach, however, revealed a statistically significant reduction in hospital stay and blood loss [55].

Our group published a study comparing 215 patients treated with open pancreaticoduodenectomy and 53 patients treated laparoscopically. In terms of morbidity, mortality, pancreatic fistula, rate of reoperation, and oncological outcomes there were no statistically significant differences. On the other hand, patients treated laparoscopically had a shorter hospital stay (eight days), only 1.1 days in the intensive care unit, longer surgery time, less blood loss, and a greater number of lymph nodes harvested (average of 23.4 nodes). All these variables represented a statistically significant difference [56].

The robotic approach to pancreaticoduodenectomy has also been introduced with significant success in experienced hands and offers the advantages demonstrated by the laparoscopic approach. Furthermore, the technique may facilitate its adoption by shortening the learning curve. The associated disadvantages are the cost involved, the need for two experienced surgeons for all procedures, and the fact that there has been no objective data demonstrating a clear benefit over the laparoscopic approach.

1.3.3.4 Laparoscopic duodenectomy with pancreatic preservation

Laparoscopic duodenectomy with pancreas preservation is a technique of choice for a variety of premalignant and benign duodenal lesions that are not amenable to endoscopic excision. In our opinion, this procedure holds significant promise as it allows pancreas preservation and obviates complications associated with resection of the head. This laparoscopic approach was first described by us in 2010 and 2011 [57–61]. The procedure can consist of a total duodenectomy (Figure 1.11) when the lesion involves the ampulla of Vater or a partial duodenectomy if the ampulla can be preserved. We have published a small series of patients who underwent a laparoscopic total duodenectomy with pancreas preservation. The outcomes were similar to pancreaticoduodenectomy with potentially better long-term results. Our unpublished data on 20 partial duodenectomies for non-ampullary neoplasms showed an operative time of 259 minutes and acceptable morbidity of 15%. The partial procedure does not require reimplantation of the biliary and pancreatic ducts and therefore is much simpler than the total duodenectomy.

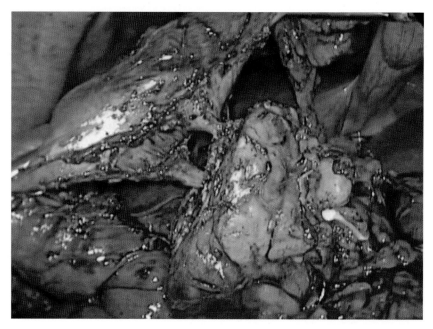

Figure 1.11 A laparoscopic pancreas-preserving total duodenectomy performed for a large ampullary adenoma in a patient with pancreas divisum. The duodenum has been completely separated for the pancreas except for the two ducts. Source: Horacio J. Asbun. Reproduced with permission.

1.3.4 Laparoscopic liver surgery

Laparoscopy for management of liver lesions was first introduced in the early 1990s. Gagner *et al.* performed the first reported laparoscopic liver resection in 1992 [62]. They reported a series of two patients who underwent nonanatomical laparoscopic liver resections for focal nodular hyperplasia and metastasis from colorectal cancer. Azagra *et al.* performed the first anatomical resection that consisted of a left segmentectomy in 1993 [63]. While laparoscopy has been widely accepted in general surgery, it faced many obstacles in the field of hepatic surgery. Several advances provided the impetus for laparoscopic liver resections, including improvements in imaging, anesthesia, and postoperative management, as well as greater experience in laparoscopy. The first laparoscopic liver resections to gain widespread acceptance were mostly wedge-type resections for benign lesions.

The minimally invasive approach includes the following techniques: pure laparoscopy, hand-assisted laparoscopy, and the hybrid approach in which the surgery begins with laparoscopy for mobilization of the liver and initial dissection followed by a small incision to complete the liver transection. Towards the late 1990s and beginning of 2000, more evidence favoring laparoscopic liver resections emerged. These resections were not just nonanatomical or segmentectomies but initial steps towards the acceptance of major laparoscopic hepatectomies. O'Rourke and Fielding published a small series of 12 patients in 2004 [64]. In 2009, Dagher *et al.* conducted a large multicenter study of six high-volume hepatobiliary surgery centers and recruited 210 patients treated with major laparoscopic liver resections; 43% of these were totally laparoscopic resections and 57% were laparoscopic hand-assisted technique. Complete resection (R0) was achieved in 111 patients. Specific morbidity was 8.1%, all-cause morbidity was 13.8%, and mortality rate was 1%. These results proved that the laparoscopic approach for major liver resections was feasible and safe in appropriately selected patients [65]. In the same year, Ito *et al.* compared the laparoscopic approach with the open approach. They presented 130 patients, of whom 52 were treated with laparoscopic surgery and 65 with open surgery. The conversion rate was 12 patients (18%) excluded from the laparoscopic group. The mortality rate and oncological results did not demonstrate significant differences, but the laparoscopic approach had fewer transfused patients, shorter hospital stay, less pain, fewer days to begin oral feeding, less overall morbidity, and a lower rate of incisional hernias, and all these differences were statistically significant. These findings allayed fears regarding the oncological efficacy of laparoscopic liver resections. Additionally, it was reported that the patients who underwent laparoscopic liver resections had a faster recovery and less intraoperative blood loss [66].

More recently, in 2010, Reddy *et al.* published the results of a meta-analysis comparing major liver resections performed laparoscopically with an open approach. This study included 1146 operations with laparoscopic approach and 1327 patients with open technique. The results were similar to Ito's [67]. In 2011, Machado *et al.* from Brazil published a new laparoscopic technique for major laparoscopic resections following the previously described open Glissonian approach. This technique was developed in 2008 for minor liver resections [68] and was subsequently described for a left hepatic lobectomy [69] and for a right hepatic lobectomy in 2011 [70].

Robot-assisted laparoscopic liver resections are being utilized to a greater degree. While the data are scarce at this time, there is some evidence supporting its use. Giulianotti *et al.* have published a small series of 24 patients who underwent a laparoscopic right hepatic lobectomy. The conversion rate was 4.2%, the mean surgery time was 337 minutes, and the average blood loss was 457 mL [71]. More recently, in 2013, Milone *et al.* published a meta-analysis of 72 patients who underwent robotic liver resections [72]. They concluded that the robotic approach is feasible albeit at a higher cost.

The most recent advances in liver resections include not just the surgical technique in itself; they involve improved planning of liver resections using computer-assisted 3D reconstructions. This was described in a recent publication by Mise *et al.* [73]. Using 3D technology, surgical planning includes the following steps: loading CT images into the software, reconstructing the liver anatomy (liver parenchyma, portal vein, hepatic veins, and tumors) in a 3D format, performing a virtual hepatectomy using the software (estimate the resection volume based on portal perfusion and venous congestion volume based on venous drainage), and finally, evaluating optimal procedures based on derived data. The practical application of navigation systems capable of transferring information for the preoperative planning of real-time surgeries could lead to safer and preplanned liver surgery. It is expected that in the near future there will be a major revolution in liver resection techniques with the improvement of 3D imaging, preoperative

planning, and intraoperative imaging superimposition for augmented-reality surgery [73].

1.4 Laparoscopic ultrasound in liver and pancreatic surgery

The idea of applying ultrasound for diagnostic purposes during surgery evolved in the early 1960s. Schlegel *et al.* [74] used ultrasound for the first time to find kidney stones, and then Knight and Newell reported the use of the same technique applied to the intraoperative search for stones in the common bile duct [75]. Over time, laparoscopic transducers similar to standard linear transducers have been introduced.

The first to report the use of laparoscopic ultrasound was Fukuda *et al.*, who in 1981 described diagnostic liver laparoscopies. With the rapid refinements in imaging technology such as computed tomography and magnetic resonance imaging, the use of ultrasound for the diagnosis of liver lesions has diminished [75]. However, the use of intraoperative ultrasound for locating liver and pancreatic lesions has gained popularity. It can be an invaluable tool in helping to localize lesions in the liver and pancreas and to define the anatomy of the hepatoduodenal ligament. For example, when a hepatoma is associated with liver cirrhosis, laparoscopic ultrasound helps in the detection of small lesions and in defining the relationship of large lesions to portal or hepatic vessels. This information may be crucial for operative planning [76]. Ultrasound is also useful to define the liver section in living donor hepatectomies [76]. The use of laparoscopic ultrasound has become routine for the localization of endocrine tumors of the pancreas, especially in the evaluation of the relationship with the pancreatic duct. The sensitivity for the localization of insulinomas is 83–100%, allowing the detection of insulinomas 3–5 mm in diameter [76].

1.5 Conclusion

The past century has been one of innovation in every sphere of human life, including surgery. From Theodor Billroth and William Steward Halstead to Emil Theodor Kocher, the list of innovators is endless. Our lives have been changed because of these brilliant minds. Few innovations in the last century, however, have had a more lasting impact on human civilization than laparoscopy. From humble beginnings, laparoscopy has spread globally and minimally invasive HPB surgery has been at the forefront of this revolution. We have proved beyond doubt that it is safe, effective, and oncologically sound and that for the majority of patients it leads to better outcomes. HPB surgeons around the world are constantly pushing the envelope and challenging conventional wisdom and surgical dogma. We live in exciting times, and as far as HPB surgery is concerned,

minimally invasive surgery is here to stay. It is becoming the standard of care for left-sided pancreatic resections as well as limited hepatic resections, and it is likely to become the standard of care for many other HPB procedures in the near future. However, caution and reassessment should be practiced on a regular basis when new advancements are introduced, keeping the interest of the patient at the forefront and as the guiding principle.

KEY POINTS

- The history of minimally invasive surgery in general and minimally invasive HPB surgery specifically is a history of scientific and social challenges.
- Laparoscopic pancreas, biliary, liver, and duodenal surgery has proved over time to be beneficial for patients.
- Significant future advances in the field of minimally invasive HPB surgery can be expected that include innovations in liver imaging, navigation-guided surgery, and augmented reality.

References

1 Meillet A, Ernout A. Dictionnaire Étymologique de la Langue Latine. Paris: Belles Lettres, 2001.
2 Shawn D, Holcomb III G. History of Minimally Invasive Surgery. Philadelphia: Saunders Elsevier, 2008.
3 Spaner S, Warnock G. A brief history of endoscopy, laparoscopy and laparoscopic surgery. J Laparendosc Adv Surg Techn 1997; 7(6):369–373.
4 Morgenstern L. The 200th anniversary of the first endoscope: Philipp Bozzini (1773–1809). Surg Innov 2005; 12(2):105–106.
5 Mouton WG, Bessell J, Maddern GJ. Looking back to the advent of modern endoscopy: 150th birthday of Maximillian Nitze. World J Surgery 1998; 22:1256–1258.
6 Harrel A, Heniford B. Minimally invasive abdominal surgery – lux et veritas past, present and future. Am J Surg 2005; 190 (2):239–243.
7 Himal H. Minimally invasive (laparoscopic) surgery. Surg Endosc 2002; 16:1647–1652.
8 Jakobaeus H. Über Laparo- und Thorakoskopie. In: Brauer L. (Hrsg) Beiträge zur Klinik der Tuberkulose und spezifischen Tuberkulose-Forschung Kabitzsch. Munchen Medizinisch Wochenschr 1910; 40.
9 Bernheim B. Organoscopy. Hunterian Laboratory of Experimental Medicine, Johns Hopkins University, 1915: 765–767.
10 Baimbridge MV. The history of thorascopic surgery. Ann. Thorac. Surg. 1993; 56:610–614.
11 Litynski G. Erich Mühe and the rejection of laparoscopic cholecystectomy (1985): a surgeon ahead of his time. J Soc Laparoendosc Surgeons 1998; 2:341–346.
12 Semm K. Pelvi-trainer, a training device in operative pelviscopy for teaching endoscopic ligation and suture techniques. Geburtshilfe Frauenheilkund 1986; 46:60–62.
13 Polychronidis A. Twenty years of laparoscopic cholecystectomy: Philippe Mouret – March 17, 1987. Profiles in Laparoscopy. J Soc Laparoendosc Surgeons 2008; 2:109–111.
14 Dubois F, Icard P, Berthelot G, Levard H. Coelioscopic cholecystectomy. Preliminary report of 36 cases. Ann Surg 1990; 211(1):60–62.
15 Asbun HJ. Rossi L. Techniques of laparoscopic cholecystectomy. Biliary tract injuries revisted. Surg Clin North Am 1994; 74(4):755–775.
16 Schwenk W, Neudecker J. Mall B, et al. Prospective randomized blinded trial of pulmonary function, pain, and cosmetic results after laparoscopic vs microlaparoscopic cholecystectomy. Surg Endosc 2000; 14:345–348.
17 Bisgaard T, Klarskov B, Trap R, et al. Pain after microlaparoscopic cholecystectomy: a randomized double-blind controlled study. Surg Endosc 2000; 14:340–344.
18 Bresadola F, Pasqualucci A, Donini A, et al. Elective transumbilical compared with standard laparoscopic cholecystectomy. Eur J Surg 1999l 165:29–34.
19 Pisanu A, Reccia I, Porceddu G, et al. Meta-analysis of prospective randomized studies comparing single-incision laparoscopic cholecystectomy (SILC) and conventional multiport laparoscopic cholecystectomy (CMLC). J Gastrointest Surg 2012; 16:1790–1801.
20 Zehetner J, Pelipad D, Darehzereshki A, et al. Single-access laparoscopic cholecystectomy versus classic laparoscopic cholecystectomy: a systematic review and meta-analysis of randomized controlled trials. Surg Laparosc Endosc Percutan Tech 2013; 23(3):235–243.
21 Kalloo AN, Singh VK, Jagannath SB, et al. Flexible transgastric peritoneoscopy: a novel approach to diagnostic and therapeutic interventions in the peritoneal cavity. Gastrointest Endosc 2004; 60(1):114–117.

22 Marks JM, Phillips MS, Tacchino R, *et al.* Single-incision laparoscopic cholecystectomy is associated with improved cosmesis scoring at the cost of significantly higher hernia rates: 1-year results of a prospective randomized, multicenter, single-blinded trial of traditional multiport laparoscopic cholecystectomy vs single-incision laparoscopic cholecystectomy. J Am Coll Surg 2013; 216:1037–1047.

23 Strasberg S, Brunt L. Rationale and use of the critical view of safety in laparoscopic cholecystectomy. J Am Coll Surg 2010; 211:132–137.

24 Petelin J. Clinical results of common bile duct exploration. Endosc Surg All Technol 1993; 1:125–129.

25 Stoker ME, Leveillee RJ, McCann JC Jr, Maini BS. Laparoscopic common bile duct exploration. J Laparoendosc Surg 1991; 1(5):287–293.

26 Berci G. Morgenstern L. Laparoscopic management of common bile duct stones. Surg Endosc 1994; 8:1168–1174.

27 Petelin J. Laparoscopic common bile duct exploration. Lessons learned from >12 years' experience. Surg Endosc 2003; 17:1705–1715.

28 Dorman JP, Franklin ME Jr, Glass JL. Laparoscopic common bile duct exploration by choledochotomy. An effective and efficient method of treatment of choledocholithiasis. Surg Endosc 1998; 12(7):926–928.

29 Gurusamy K, Koti R, Davidson B. T-tube drainage versus primary closure after open common bile duct exploration (review). Cochrane Database Syst Rev 2013; 6:CD005640.

30 Gagner M, Pomp A. Laparoscopic pancreatic resection: is it worthwhile? Gastrointest Surg 1997; 1(1):20.

31 Tagaya N, Kasama K, Suzuki N, *et al.* Laparoscopic resection of the pancreas and review of the literature. Surg Endosc 2003; 17(2):201–206.

32 Talamini MA, Moesinger R, Yeo CJ, *et al.* Cystadenomas of the pancreas: is enucleation an adequate operation? Ann Surg 1998; 227(6):896–903.

33 Fernandez-Cruz L, Cosa R, Blanco L, *et al.* Curative laparoscopic resection for pancreatic neoplasms: a critical analysis from a single institution. J Gastrointest Surg 2007; 11(12):1607–1621.

34 Soper NJ, Brunt LM, Dunnegan DL, *et al.* Laparoscopic distal pancreatectomy in the porcine model. Surg Endosc 1994; 8:57–60; discussion 60–61.

35 Sussman LA, Christie R, Whittle D. Laparoscopic excision of distal pancreas including insulinoma. Aust NZ J Surg 1996; 66(6):414–416.

36 Cuschieri A. Laparoscopic pancreatic resections. Semin Laparosc 1996; 3(1):15–20.

37 Gagner M, Pomp A. Laparoscopic pancreatic resection: is it worthwhile? Gastrointest Surg 1997; 1(1):20.

38 Mabrut J, Fernandez-Cruz L, Azagra S, *et al.* Laparoscopic pancreatic resection: results of a multicenter European study of 127 patients. Surgery 2005; 137:597–605.

39 Asbun HJ, Stauffer J. Laparoscopic approach to distal and subtotal pancreatectomy: a clockwise technique. Surg Endosc 2011; 25:2643–2649.

40 Asbun HJ, Stauffer J, Rosales-Velderrain A, *et al.* Comparison of open with laparoscopic distal pancreatectomy: a single institution's transition over a 7-year period. HPB 2013; 15:149–155.

41 Merchant M, Parikh A, Kooby D. Should all distal pancreatectomies be performed laparoscopically? Adv Surg 2009; 43:283–300.

42 Kubota K. Recent advances and limitations of surgical treatment for pancreatic cancer. World J Clin Oncol 2011; 2(5): 225–228.

43 Kooby DA, Hawkins WG, Schmidt CM, *et al.* A multicenter analysis of distal pancreatectomy for adenocarcinoma: is laparoscopic resection appropriate? J Am Coll Surg 2010; 210(5):779–787.

44 Jin T, Altaf K, Xiong JJ, *et al.* A systematic review and meta-analysis of studies comparing laparoscopic and open distal pancreatectomy. HPB 2012; 14:711–724.

45 Venkat R, Edil BH, Schulick RD, *et al.* Laparoscopic distal pancreatectomy is associated with significantly less overall morbidity compared to the open technique: a systematic review and meta-analysis. Ann Surg 2012; 255:1048–1059.

46 Tran Cao HS, Lopez N, Chang DC, *et al.* Improved perioperative outcomes with minimally invasive distal pancreatectomy: results from a population-based analysis. JAMA Surg 2014; 149:237–243.

47 Mallet GP, Vachon A. *Pancreatites Chroniques Gauches.* Paris: Masson, 1943.

48 Warshaw A. Conservation of the spleen with distal pancreatectomy. Arch Surg 1988; 123:550–553.

49 Kimura W, Inoue T, Futakawa N, *et al.* Spleen-preserving distal pancreatectomy with conservation of the splenic artery and vein. Surgery 1996; 120(5):885–890.

50 Waters J, Canal F, Wiebke E, *et al.* Robotic distal pancreatectomy: cost effective? Surgery 2010; 148(4):814–823.

51 Kang C, Lee D, Chi J, *et al.* Conventional laparoscopic and robot-assisted spleen-preserving pancreatectomy: does da Vinci have clinical advantages? Surg Endosc 2011; 25:2004–2009.

52 Gagner M, Pomp A. Laparoscopic pylorus-preserving pancreatoduodenectomy. Surg Endosc 1994; 8(5):408–410.

53 Dulucq J, Wintringer P, Stabilini C, *et al.* Are major laparoscopic pancreatic resections worthwhile? Surg Endosc 2005; 19:1028–1034.

54 Palanivelu C, Rajan P, Rangarajan M, *et al.* Evolution in techniques of laparoscopic pancreaticoduodenectomy: a decade long experience from a tertiary center. J Hepatobiliary Pancreat Surg 2009; 16:731–740.

55 Nigri G, Petrucciani N, La Torre M, *et al.* Duodenopancreatectomy: open or minimally invasive approach? surge, 2014; 12(4):227–234.

56 Asbun HJ, Stauffer J. Laparoscopic vs open pancreaticoduodenectomy: overall outcomes and severity of complications using the Accordion Severity Grading System. J Am Coll Surg 2012; 215(6):810–819.

57 Asbun HJ, Grewal M, Stauffer JA. Laparoscopic pancreas preserving duodenectomy. Presented at the 96th Annual Clinical Congress of the American College of Surgeons, Washington, DC, October 3–7, 2010.

58 Asbun HJ, Stauffer J, Bowers SP, Goldberg R, Parker M. Laparoscopic pancreas sparing partial duodenectomy (PSPD). Presented at the American College of Surgeons Annual Meeting, San Francisco, CA, October 2011.

59 Grewal MS, Fuchshuber P, Asbun HJ. Laparoscopic pancreas preserving total duodenectomy. In: American College of Surgeons Multimedia Atlas of Surgery. Vol. Pancreas Surgery. Woodbury, CT: Cine-Med, Inc., 2011.

60 Asbun HJ, Stauffer JA, Adkisson C, et al. Pancreas-sparing total duodenectomy for ampullary duodenal neoplasms. World J Surg 2012; 36:2461–2472.

61 Asbun HJ, Stauffer J, Raimondo M, et al. Laparoscopic partial sleeve duodenectomy (PSD) for nonampullary duodenal neoplasms. Pancreas J 2013; 42(13):461–466.

62 Gagner M, Rheault M, Dubuc J. Laparoscopic partial hepatectomy for liver tumor. Surg Endosc 1992; 6:99.

63 Azagra J, Goergen M, Gilbart E, Jacobs D. Laparoscopic anatomical (hepatic) left lateral segmentectomy – technical aspects. Surg Endosc 1996; 10(7):758–761.

64 O'Rourke N, Fielding G. Laparoscopic right hepatectomy: surgical technique. J Gastrointest Surg 2004; 8:213–216.

65 Dagher I, O'Rourke N, Geller D, et al. Laparoscopic major hepatectomy: an evolution in standard of care. Ann Surg 2009; 250(5):856–860.

66 Ito K, Ito H, D'Angelica M, et al. Laparoscopic versus open liver resection: a matched-pair case control study. Gastrointest Surg 2009; 13:2276–2283.

67 Reddy S, Tsung A, Geller D. Laparoscopic liver resection. World J Surg 2011; 35:1478–1486.

68 Machado MA, Herman P, Makdissi FF, et al. Intrahepatic Glissonian approach for anatomical resection of left liver segments. Langenbecks Arch Surg 2008; 393(6):1017.

69 Machado MA, Makdissi FF, Herman P, et al. Intrahepatic Glissonian approach for pure laparoscopic left hemihepatectomy. J Laparoendosc Adv Surg Tech 2010; 20(2):141–142.

70 Machado MA, Surjan RC, Makdissi FF. Video: intrahepatic Glissonian approach for pure laparoscopic right hemihepatectomy. Surg Endosc 2011; 3930–3933.

71 Giulianotti P, Sbrana F, Coratti A, et al. Totally robotic right hepatectomy – surgical. Arch Surg 2011; 146(7):844–850.

72 Milone L, Daskalaki D, Giulianotti P, et al. State of the art in robotic hepatobiliary surgery. World J Surg 2013; 37:2747–2755.

73 Mise Y, Tani K, Aoki T, et al. Virtual liver resection: computer-assisted operation planning using a three-dimensional liver representation. J Hepatobiliary Pancreat Sci 2013; 20:157–164.

74 Schlegel J, Diggdon P, Cuellar J. The use of ultrasound for localizing renal calculi. J Urol 1961; 86:367–369.

75 Knight P, Newell J. Operative use of ultrasonics in cholelithiasis. Lancet 1963; 11(1):1023–1025.

76 Bezzi M, Silecchia G, De Leo A, et al. Laparoscopic and intraoperative ultrasound. Eur J Radiol 1998; 27(suppl 2): S207–S214.

Videos 1–26 will be of interest to readers of this chapter.

Visit the companion website at:

www.wiley.com\go\conrad\liver-pancreas-biliary-laparoscopic-surgery

CHAPTER 2

Acquisition of specific laparoscopic skills for laparoscopic hepatopancreatobiliary surgery

Soeren Torge Mees and Guy Maddern

University of Adelaide, Discipline of Surgery, The Queen Elizabeth Hospital, Woodville South, Australia

---

EDITOR COMMENT

In this important chapter on skill acquisition for advanced laparoscopic surgery, Drs Mees and Maddern highlight the important steps required to safely learn complex laparoscopic HPB surgeries. Recognizing that the acquisition of laparoscopic HPB surgery skills represents a time-consuming and challenging process, the authors suggest a thoughtful step-wise approach. In addition to simulator and nonsimulator-based skill acquisition, they propose a multistep process to develop not only the surgical skills required but also a well-trained team capable of efficient teamwork. The authors expand on ergonomics as an important factor for optimal application of learned laparoscopic HPB skills. Further, they describe how a surgical mentor allows for a safe transition from training to practice. Finally, we agree very much with the authors that advanced laparoscopic procedures require constant training and advancement to maintain the required skill level.

Keywords: ergonomics, laparoscopic skill acquisition, simulations, team training

---

2.1 Introduction

Laparoscopic surgery has risen in popularity in recent years, and laparoscopic training now represents an important factor in the surgical curriculum. Training in laparoscopic surgery is crucial, because insufficient training and limited experience are associated with an increase in the number of technical errors, can compromise patient safety, and may lead to poorer clinical outcomes [1]. This has been illustrated by the early experience with laparoscopic cholecystectomy. The incidence of adverse outcomes attributable to cautery injury was increased during early adoption of the technique and steadily diminished as surgeons became more experienced in the special requirements of laparoscopic surgery [2,3]. Crucial factors that limit the performance of surgical trainees in laparoscopic surgery are a lack of complete understanding of the operative steps, deficiency in synchronized movement of the nondominant hand, and fatigue [4].

The loss of depth perception because of the two-dimensional image, limited haptic feedback from tissue, usage of instruments with restricted range of motion, a small working field, and the fulcrum effect make laparoscopic techniques difficult to acquire for trainees. These challenges demand a comprehensive approach [5–7]. For laparoscopic surgery education, a variety of training options exists, including training in the operating room, synthetic (inanimate) models, box trainers, virtual reality trainers, animal models (ex vivo animal tissue models or in vivo animal models), and human cadaver models.

In the past, laparoscopic skill training was largely conducted via the mentored approach, consisting primarily of one-on-one teaching in the operating room. Though this approach is still widely used, it represents a suboptimal training option owing to current time and budget limitations. The restrictions on surgeons' work hours, from both a legislative and productivity perspective, have reduced the number of hours during which trainees are available for teaching. They have also reduced the time during

---

Laparoscopic Liver, Pancreas, and Biliary Surgery, First Edition.
Edited by Claudius Conrad and Brice Gayet.
© 2017 John Wiley & Sons, Ltd. Published 2017 by John Wiley & Sons, Ltd.

which experienced surgeons are available to assist and teach trainees [8–10]. Additionally, the mentored approach of learning new skills on actual patients raises ethical and medico-legal concerns. These issues have resulted in the increasing use of simulations in the education of minimally invasive surgery.

Simulators have an advantage over in-theater training, in that they allow for repetitive practice without any time limitations. The training is performed in a safe environment and provides immediate performance feedback that facilitates learning. The use of simulators for teaching laparoscopic surgery skills has been shown to improve cognitive skills, technical knowledge, psychomotor skills, and surgical performance of the surgeons in the operating room, when compared with conventional mentored, in-theater, training [11,12]. A prospective, randomized, controlled trial evaluating laparoscopic trainers for basic laparoscopic skills acquisition showed that the combination of inanimate box training and virtual reality training results in better laparoscopic skill acquisition than either training method alone or no training at all [13]. These findings are supported by a prospective single-blinded, randomized trial showing that learning laparoscopic suturing on either a virtual reality simulator or a box trainer significantly decreased the learning curve. This study also indicates that, while virtual reality training is the more efficient training modality, box training is the more cost-effective option [14]. In a recently published randomized study using fresh cadaver models, positive learning results were also seen. Training using this model resulted in significantly improved basic laparoscopic skills with subsequent improved performance in virtual reality trainer tasks [15].

The maximum benefit of laparoscopic skills training will be achieved if a single task is practiced repeatedly, at least 30–35 times [13] rather than practicing a variety of skills at the same time [16]. Training over several days [17] with a systematic, interval training schedule has proven to be superior for laparoscopic skill acquisition, compared with training in a single day [18]. Considering the limitations on work hours, training can be offered outside regular work hours if trainees are seeking additional training [19]. In terms of maintaining the acquired skills, studies have shown that deterioration in skills occurs after several weeks without training. It is therefore recommended that training is ongoing and repetitive [20].

In spite of positive reports for simulators in surgical education, there are signficant limitations. These relate to the lack of realism, inability to simulate unusual anatomy, and lack of realistic operative stress in which the training occurs. Technical skills are only one aspect of successful surgery, and simulators rarely teach clinical judgment and acumen, skills which only develop with real experience.

In 2006, a systematic review evaluated the effectiveness of surgical simulation in comparison with other methods of surgical training [21]. The review showed that none of the methods of simulated training has yet been shown to be superior to other forms of surgical training. Thus, the main question remains unanswered: does simulator performance correlate with operative performance? Recent studies show evidence to support the increase in use of simulators as a core component in the training of a competent laparoscopic surgeon [6,11,22,23]. Further, evidence is now accumulating that simulation training can be transferred into the operating room itself [24]. Therefore, the acceptance of simulation-based training into surgical skill training programs is improving and plays an important role in many training programs for advanced laparoscopic procedures, such as liver or colorectal surgery [12,25].

2.2 What skills and/or requirements are needed for laparoscopic liver and pancreatic surgery?

2.2.1 Surgeon's requirements
Minimally invasive surgery confronts the surgeon with problems that do not exist in traditional/open surgery. In minimal invasive surgery, ergonomics plays an important role in optimal surgical performance in an extended operation. It deals especially with difficulties due to the field of view (2D view of 3D space), eye–hand coordination, limitation of surgeon movement because of port placement, and handling of (inadequate) laparoscopic instruments. Ergonomic factors that should be considered before a hepatopancreatobiliary (HPB) laparoscopic procedure include maximizing patient safety and chances for successful minimally invasive completion of the case, while minimizing physical strain on the operative team and increase in surgery time.

2.2.2 Ergonomic considerations
Laparoscopic HPB surgery requires the use of dedicated equipment, as well as the proper positioning of

equipment, and also of the patient and the surgical staff to maximize ergonomics. Thus, one of the first steps before starting a laparoscopic procedure should be communication between the surgeon(s), the nurses, and the anesthetist, in order to clarify what procedure will be done and what equipment is needed. This discussion can prevent unnecessary and time-consuming measures, such as repositioning maneuvers or lack of instruments.

The positioning of the patient depends on surgeon preference. Thus, the surgeon responsible for the operation should position the patient himself or herself to ensure that he or she can carry out the operation in the most comfortable and most ergonomically efficient way to maximize patient safety. For this, not only has the port positioning to be considered but also the position of the patient may need to be modified to ensure that ports can be placed in the optimal positions.

It is most important that the equipment is placed and subsequently adjusted to be in the "optimal position"; the position of the equipment, instruments, and operating table should allow a physiological posture for the surgeon, including a straight head (without rotation or extension of the cervical spine), shoulders in a physiological position with arms alongside the body, elbows bent to 70–90°, forearms in an horizontal or slightly descending axis, and hands pronated [26]. The thoracic and lumbar spine and legs should be in a neutral position without rotation, anterior or lateral flexion. Noncompliance with these principles can cause cervical aches and pain to the shoulders, forearms, and fingers and can even cause paresthesia or hypoesthesia of the thumb [27,28]. The "optimal position" requires that the equipment – especially all cable-based items, such as scope, electrosurgical devices, or insufflation and light source – is easily accessible for the operative personnel.

Ergonomics of optics are very important in laparoscopic surgery and should be considered prior to every operation. The surgeon should face the target organ and be in line with the lens and monitor. The monitor must therefore be placed in the surgeon–organ–monitor line and be at or lower than eye level to minimize fatigue and cervical ache. The center of the monitor should be placed 20° lower than the eyes, because the position naturally adopted by the eyes is 15–20° towards the ground when the cervical spine is in a neutral position [29]. This position corresponds to the resting position of the oculomotor muscles, and differing from this position puts these muscles at strain. In longer operations, surgeons tend to overextend their cervical

spine in order to return to this resting position. Therefore, the vertical position of the monitors should be adapted to each surgeon.

2.2.3 Port placement

Every procedure has its ideal port positioning, which may be changed according to patient anatomy, esthetic considerations or surgeon's preference. Therefore, it always constitutes a compromise, taking into account patient factors, target organ, and surgeon preference.

In HPB laparoscopic surgery, the optical port is often placed near the umbilicus, allowing for a favorable overview of the abdominal cavity. Nevertheless, this central and generally suitable position may be unsuitable for some patients. For example, the umbilicus of obese patients is more caudal, and positioning the port at the umbilicus will move the optic away from the operative target. Furthermore, patients with previous midline laparotomies usually have periumbilical adhesion and the port placement in midline or the umbilicus can be difficult and even dangerous. Some surgeons prefer optic ports and insert them off midline (e.g. Palmer's point, 3 cm below the left costal margin in the midclavicular line) to gain optimal access. Nevertheless, there are two important principles that should be adhered to in order to optimize the view and range of instruments: triangulation and sectoring.

The principle of triangulation means that (i) ports are positioned on an arc 20 cm from the target; (ii) the optical port centers the image and operating ports are located 5–7 cm on either side; and (iii) ports form an angle of 60–90° to the target [30,31]. Retracting ports are placed outside this triangulation zone, either laterally or at the superior portion of the arc, minimizing instrument conflict. This principle reproduces the set-up of open surgery, with a central visual field bordered on either side by the operative hands. However, the camera positioned between the hands of the surgeon may represent a potential conflict owing to instruments clashing with the camera.

The second principle is sectoring [31]. The optical port is placed laterally to the operating port. A minimal distance of 5–7 cm is necessary between two ports for the instruments to meet at such an angle that permits the performance of complex movements. The main advantage of sectoring is that it allows the surgeon to move freely, as the camera is away from the operative field and there is no physical contact between the surgeon and the camera holder.

In conclusion, both triangulation and sectoring are important principles, and the final position of the ports depends on the exact location of the target, which must be considered prior to port insertion, on patient anatomy, and ergonomics of the surgeon.

2.2.4 Institutional requirements

Laparoscopic HPB surgery is complex and requires advanced laparoscopic skills. In 2008, the Louisville Statement (International Position on Laparoscopic Liver Surgery) was published following a consensus conference of 45 experts in hepatobiliary surgery [32]. This consensus paper stated that liver surgeons "should be facile with laparoscopic suturing and other techniques of laparoscopic hemorrhage control, negating the need to convert. Additionally, major vascular injuries, although exceptional, may not allow time for conversion and require a surgeon with extensive laparoscopic training." The group of experts furthermore agreed that "laparoscopic liver surgery should be initiated only in centers in which the combined expertise in liver and laparoscopic surgery exists" in line with statements from other published work [33,34]. The recommendations of the Louisville Statement clarify that HPB surgery should be performed by experienced HPB surgeons in hospitals with experience in complex surgery. In our personal opinion, hospitals in which laparoscopic HPB surgery is performed need a 24-hour/7 days a week service of at least (i) an experienced HPB surgeon; (ii) an interventional radiologist (the latter two should be at least off-site on call and available for emergency interventions within 20 minutes); and (iii) an intensive care unit. In addition, team orientation and training, especially in the beginning of a HPB surgery program, are highly recommended for HPB surgery to optimize surgical results and patient safety [35].

2.2.5 Acquisition of skills

In the last decade, several studies have reported feasibility, safety, and favorable outcomes after laparoscopic liver [36–40] and pancreatic surgery [41–44]. Learning laparoscopic HPB surgery is feasible via the mentored approach in theater [45]; however, distinct learning curves have been demonstrated for these complex procedures [46–49], and the quantity of these procedures is generally limited because of a careful selection of adequate cases. Therefore, a systematic training program needs to be developed to enable surgical trainees to gain required laparoscopic HPB skills.

In general, surgeons who have already acquired advanced laparoscopic and traditional HPB skills might consider the pathway presented in Figure 2.1 as a practical guideline to start their training.

With progress in the field of simulation-based training, HPB-specific psychomotor skills can be gained on a surgical simulator [50]. For example, performing the Pringle's maneuver or a left lateral hepatectomy on a virtual reality trainer would represent appropriate exercises to start the training. Laparoscopic training on these simulators is highly recommended, but they are expensive and not universally available.

As a next step, surgeons should attend a laparoscopic training course to gain primary laparoscopic HPB skills. A multitude of courses are available worldwide, but they are of variable quality. A worthwhile course should provide lectures, debates, and discussions concerning anatomical variations and factors. Furthermore, the course should include in vivo training in an animal model to practice placement of ports, use of instruments, dissection/resection of organs, and how to deal with potential complications (Figure 2.2).

A training program for laparoscopic liver resections should include the following key steps.

1 Positioning of ports for the planned surgery.
2 Placement around the hepatoduodenal ligament for a safe Pringle's maneuver.
3 Dissection of hilar structures, portal vein, hepatic artery, and confluence of the hepatic ducts and common bile duct.
4 Left lobe procedures.
  – Left lobe mobilization.
  – Parenchymal transection devices:
    i Electrosurgical devices (e.g. Harmonic, Thunderbeat, LigaSure, bipolar forceps)
    ii Ultrasonic devices (e.g. cavitron ultrasonic surgical aspirator)
    iii Stapling
    iv Additional relevant techniques
5 Right lobe procedures.
  – Right lobe mobilization.
  – Right hepatectomy including dissection/stapling of hilar structures and right hepatic vein.

After attending a laparoscopic HPB training course, an observership in an institution with expertise in laparoscopic HPB surgery is highly recommended. Observing an experienced surgeon and his or her team performing this complex surgery gives excellent insights and provides a

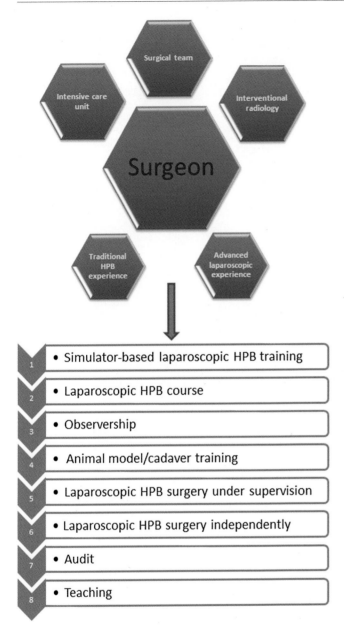

Figure 2.1 Pathway to acquiring laparoscopic HPB skills.

valuable opportunity to ask questions and evaluate differences in surgeon approach. The observer can follow the complete procedure, plan their own surgery in their mind, and discuss all major and minor issues around the laparoscopic surgery with the experienced team.

A recommended transition step between the observership and performing the first surgery on a patient is the consolidation of the acquired manual and theoretical skills in an animal model or human cadaver. The manual skills especially should be performed in a stress-free atmosphere with the opportunity to practice and perfect the surgical procedures. Additionally, learning to use high-energy devices such as diathermy, dissection or tissue handling, with the current simulators available, is still more efficient in an animal model compared with inanimate simulators.

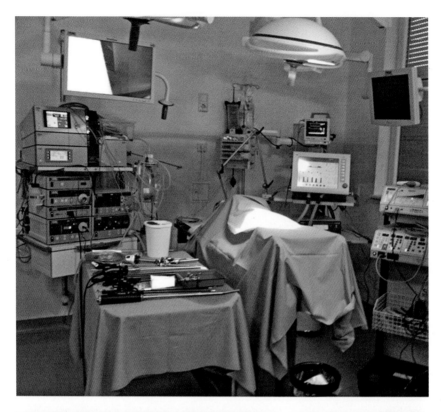

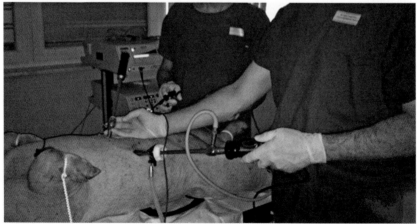

Figure 2.2 Exemplary presentation of an in vivo training set-up (pig model), including the use of modern electrosurgical devices and ultrasound dissector.

A number of different animal models have been widely used in laparoscopic training, but there are limitations to each of these models. In laparoscopic liver surgery, a variety of animal models have been described in the literature: rat [51] and canine [52,53] models have been advocated, but their major drawback is anatomical constraints, e.g. differences in size, number, and/or placement of liver lobes. Porcine models have been used extensively because of size and similar anatomy [54,55]. Sheep have also been used for liver resections because their anatomy is similar to humans [54,56]. For laparoscopic pancreas surgery, pancreaticoduodenectomies and distal pancreatectomies have been performed in porcine training models [57–59], although the porcine pancreas is less firm than the human pancreas.

Human cadavers have been used for many years to teach anatomy and are still considered a very effective approach for achieving important learning objectives in the field of anatomy [60–62]. In addition, cadaver training has been shown to be beneficial in the training program of general surgery [63,64], neurosurgery [65], vascular surgery [66], and trauma surgery residents [67].

Recently, frozen human cadavers have been used in laparoscopic skills training because of the close similarities to operative anatomical landmarks, consistency, handling of tissues, haptic feedback, and the use of gravity [68,69]. Additionally, patient positioning, port insertion, the use of instruments, and imitation of critical steps help to optimize the surgeon's training [70,71]. In this respect, hands-on training courses in colon, hernia, bariatric, and vascular surgery using Thiel human cadavers (a special method providing soft-fix embalmed cadavers) have been reported to be excellent models to teach advanced minimally invasive surgery [72]. For example, studies have demonstrated excellent learning results for laparoscopic nephrectomy using the Thiel human cadaver method [73] and have suggested that this training is superior to porcine models for urological laparoscopic training [74]. In terms of laparoscopic HPB surgery, cadavers have not been used for liver or pancreatic resection, but studies have shown evidence that in single-site laparoscopic cholecystectomy [75] and laparoscopic living donor procurement for liver transplantation such training is beneficial [76].

After training and consolidating surgical skills in an animal/cadaver model, it is advisable to perform the first laparoscopic HPB surgery on patients in the presence of a mentor or preceptor. The mentor, e.g. the surgeon from the observership, should be an experienced laparoscopic HPB surgeon who can supervise, support, and interact in this first laparoscopic case, if required. Mentorships have been shown to be helpful in medical training in general [77,78], and studies have demonstrated significant benefits in laparoscopic surgery training [79,80]. A mentored approach provides additional safety for the patient

and protects the surgeon-in-training. It also represents an opportunity to recognize learner-specific challenges and optimize the set-up. In our opinion, an ideal mentorship plan for training in this system may include four mentor-supervised resections on two consecutive days (two operations per day).

It is recommended that the trained surgeon starts their laparoscopic HPB surgery independently with less complex cases, such as a left lateral sectionectomy, and advances gradually. It should always be borne in mind that advanced minimally invasive HPB surgery is complex and requires teamwork. The entire team, including anesthetists, theater nurses, and surgical trainees, needs to be trained and prepared for these kinds of procedures and proficient to deal with potential complications.

It is important to establish the safety and effectiveness of new surgical procedures, and they should be monitored after their introduction. An audit of indications and outcomes is recommended to evaluate the surgical morbidity and mortality. Ideally, the audit should be performed by an external, experienced HPB surgeon in order to achieve an objective and nonbiased assessment. Furthermore, internal processes for the reporting of any adverse events from new procedures should be developed and external processes considered, e.g. participation in multicenter audits [81].

The final step in the process of training in laparoscopic HPB skills is teaching. It is time-consuming and difficult to gain proficiency in minimally invasive HPB surgery, and it is an obligation to transfer the acquired skills to other surgeons for the benefit of our patients.

2.3 Conclusion

Acquisition of laparoscopic HPB surgery skills represents a time-consuming and challenging process. The skills will be acquired in a multistep process, and these complex procedures demand a well-trained team and efficient teamwork to achieve success. Having a surgical mentor who will supervise the team performing their first procedures is highly recommended. Finally, it should be mentioned that these advanced laparoscopic procedures require constant training and advancement; therefore, skill acquisition in laparoscopic HPB surgery will require continuous re-education and refreshing and updating of knowledge on an ongoing basis.

KEY POINTS

• Laparoscopic HPB skill acquisition is time consuming but necessary to ensure patient safety during advanced laparoscopic HPB procedures.

• Simulator-based and nonsimulator-based training methods are effective in acquiring the necessary skills.

• A thought-out, step-wise process from skill acquisition to clinical application that may incorporate a mentor may be an effective way of applying the learned skill set.

• Team training should be incorporated in the skill acquisition process.

• Continuous learning and skill maintenance is necessary to perform advanced laparoscopic HPB surgeries at the highest level of proficiency.

References

1 Prystowsky JB. Are young surgeons competent to perform alimentary tract surgery? Arch Surg 2005; 140(5):495–500; discussion 500–492.

2 Barone JE, Lincer RM. Correction. A prospective analysis of 1518 laparoscopic cholecystectomies. N Engl J Med 1991; 325 (21):1517–1518.

3 Meyers WC. A prospective analysis of 1518 laparoscopic cholecystectomies. The Southern Surgeons Club. N Engl J Med 1991; 324(16):1073–1078.

4 Gupta R, Cathelineau X, Rozet F, Vallancien G. Feedback from operative performance to improve training program of laparoscopic radical prostatectomy. J Endourol 2004; 18(9): 836–839.

5 Gallagher AG, McClure N, McGuigan J, Ritchie K, Sheehy NP. An ergonomic analysis of the fulcrum effect in the acquisition of endoscopic skills. Endoscopy 1998; 30(7): 617–620.

6 Gurusamy K, Aggarwal R, Palanivelu L, Davidson BR. Systematic review of randomized controlled trials on the effectiveness of virtual reality training for laparoscopic surgery. Br J Surg 2008; 95(9):1088–1097.

7 Perkins N, Starkes JL, Lee TD, Hutchison C. Learning to use minimal access surgical instruments and 2-dimensional remote visual feedback. How difficult is the task for novices? Adv Health Sci Educ Theory Pract 2002; 7(2):117–131.

8 Antiel RM, Reed DA, van Arendonk KJ, *et al.* Effects of duty hour restrictions on core competencies, education, quality of life, and burnout among general surgery interns. JAMA Surg 2013; 148(5):448–455.

9 Pickersgill T. The European working time directive for doctors in training. BMJ 2001; 323(7324):1266.

10 1Schwartz SI, Galante J, Kaji A, *et al.* Effect of the 16-hour work limit on general surgery intern operative case volume. A multi-institutional study. JAMA Surg 2013; 148(9): 829–833.

11 Al-Kadi AS, Donnon T. Using simulation to improve the cognitive and psychomotor skills of novice students in advanced laparoscopic surgery. A meta-analysis. Medical Teacher 2013; 35(suppl 1):S47–55.

12 Palter VN, Grantcharov TP. Development and validation of a comprehensive curriculum to teach an advanced minimally invasive procedure. A randomized controlled trial. Ann Surg 2012; 256(1):25–32.

13 Madan AK, Frantzides CT. Prospective randomized controlled trial of laparoscopic trainers for basic laparoscopic skills acquisition. Surg Endosc 2007; 21(2):209–213.

14 Orzech N, Palter VN, Reznick RK, Aggarwal R, Grantcharov TP. A comparison of 2 ex vivo training curricula for advanced laparoscopic skills. A randomized controlled trial. Ann Surg 2012; 255(5):833–839.

15 Sharma M, Macafee D, Horgan AF. Basic laparoscopic skills training using fresh frozen cadaver. a randomized controlled trial. Am J Surg 2013; 206(1):23–31.

16 Kirk RM. Teaching the craft of operative surgery. Ann R Coll Surg Engl 1996; 78 (1 suppl):25–28.

17 Verdaasdonk EG, Stassen LP, van Wijk RP, Dankelman J. The influence of different training schedules on the learning of psychomotor skills for endoscopic surgery. Surg Endosc 2007; 21(2):214–219.

18 Gallagher AG, Jordan-Black JA, O'Sullivan GC. Prospective, randomized assessment of the acquisition, maintenance, and loss of laparoscopic skills. Ann Surg 2012; 256(2): 387–393.

19 Bonrath EM, Fritz M, Mees ST, *et al.* Laparoscopic simulation training. Does timing impact the quality of skills acquisition? Surg Endosc 2013; 27(3):888–894.

20 Bonrath EM, Weber BK, Fritz M, *et al.* Laparoscopic simulation training. Testing for skill acquisition and retention. Surgery 2012; 152(1):12–20.

21 Sutherland LM, Middleton PF, Anthony A, *et al.* Surgical simulation. a systematic review. Ann Surg 2006; 243(3): 291–300.

22 Gallagher AG, Seymour NE, Jordan-Black JA, Bunting BP, McGlade K, Satava RM. Prospective, randomized assessment of transfer of training (ToT) and transfer effectiveness ratio (TER) of virtual reality simulation training for laparoscopic skill acquisition. Ann Surg 2013; 257(6):1025–1031.

23 Diesen DL, Erhunmwunsee L, Bennett KM, *et al.* Effectiveness of laparoscopic computer simulator versus usage of box trainer for endoscopic surgery training of novices. J Surg Educ 2011; 68(4):282–289.

24 Sturm LP, Windsor JA, Cosman PH, Cregan P, Hewett PJ, Maddern GJ. A systematic review of skills transfer after surgical simulation training. Ann Surg 2008; 248(2):166–179.

25 Nugent E, Hseino H, Boyle E, *et al.* Assessment of the role of aptitude in the acquisition of advanced laparoscopic surgical skill sets. results from a virtual reality-based laparoscopic colectomy training programme. Int J Colorectal Dis 2012; 27(9):1207–1214.

26 Van't Hullenaar C, van Alphen M, Hendriks M, *et al.* Determination of the ideal posture for the surgeon during laparoscopic surgery. Presented at the SAGES Conference 2012, Session Number SS02 – Instrumentation/Ergonomics. Program number S010.

27 Berguer R, Rab GT, Abu-Ghaida H, Alarcon A, Chung J. A comparison of surgeons' posture during laparoscopic and open surgical procedures. Surg Endosc 1997; 11(2): 139–142.

28 Szeto GP, Cheng SW, Poon JT, Ting AC, Tsang RC, Ho P. Surgeons' static posture and movement repetitions in open and laparoscopic surgery. J Surg Res 2012; 172(1): e19–31.

29 Menozzi M, von Buol A, Krueger H, Miege C. Direction of gaze and comfort: discovering the relation for the ergonomic optimization of visual tasks. Ophthalm Physiol Opt 1994; 14(4): 393–399.

30 Trejo A, Jung MC, Oleynikov D, Hallbeck MS. Effect of handle design and target location on insertion and aim with a laparoscopic surgical tool. Appl Ergon 2007; 38(6): 745–753.

31 Garcia A, Mutter D, Henri M. Ergonomics. Available at: www.websurg.com/doi–ot02en321.htm (accessed 15 December 2015).

32 Buell JF, Cherqui D, Geller DA, *et al.* The international position on laparoscopic liver surgery. The Louisville Statement, 2008. Ann Surg 2009; 250(5):825–830.

33 Kluger MD, Vigano L, Barroso R, Cherqui D. The learning curve in laparoscopic major liver resection. J Hepatobiliary Pancreat Sci 2013; 20(2):131–136.

34 Pearce NW, Di Fabio F, Teng MJ, Syed S, Primrose JN, Abu Hilal M. Laparoscopic right hepatectomy: a challenging, but feasible, safe and efficient procedure. Am J Surg 2011; 202(5): e52–58.

35 Zheng B, Denk PM, Martinec DV, Gatta P, Whiteford MH, Swanstrom LL. Building an efficient surgical team using a bench model simulation: construct validity of the Legacy Inanimate System for Endoscopic Team Training (LISETT). Surg Endosc 2008; 22(4):930–937.

36 Abu Hilal M, Pearce NW. Laparoscopic left lateral liver sectionectomy: a safe, efficient, reproducible technique. Dig Surg 2008; 25(4):305–308.

37 Cai XJ, Wang YF, Liang YL, Yu H, Liang X. Laparoscopic left hemihepatectomy: a safety and feasibility study of 19 cases. Surg Endosc 2009; 23(11):2556–2562.

38 Martin RC, Scoggins CR, McMasters KM. Laparoscopic hepatic lobectomy: advantages of a minimally invasive approach. J Am Coll Surg 2010; 210(5):627–634, 634–626.

39 Rau HG, Buttler E, Meyer G, Schardey HM, Schildberg FW. Laparoscopic liver resection compared with conventional partial hepatectomy – a prospective analysis. Hepatogastroenterology 1998; 45(24):2333–2338.

40 Tsinberg M, Tellioglu G, Simpfendorfer CH, *et al.* Comparison of laparoscopic versus open liver tumor resection. a case-controlled study. Surg Endosc 2009; 23(4):847–853.

41 Choi SH, Hwang HK, Kang CM, Yoon CI, Lee WJ. Pylorus- and spleen-preserving total pancreatoduodenectomy with resection of both whole splenic vessels. feasibility and laparoscopic application to intraductal papillary mucin-producing tumors of the pancreas. Surg Endosc 2012; 26(7): 2072–2077.

42 Kim SC, Song KB, Jung YS, *et al.* Short-term clinical outcomes for 100 consecutive cases of laparoscopic pylorus-preserving pancreatoduodenectomy: improvement with surgical experience. Surg Endosc 2013; 27(1):95–103.

43 Kooby DA, Hawkins WG, Schmidt CM, *et al.* A multicenter analysis of distal pancreatectomy for adenocarcinoma: is laparoscopic resection appropriate? J Am Coll Surg 2010; 210(5):779–785, 786–777.

44 Song KB, Kim SC, Park JB, *et al.* Single-center experience of laparoscopic left pancreatic resection in 359 consecutive patients: changing the surgical paradigm of left pancreatic resection. Surg Endosc 2011; 25(10):3364–3372.

45 Hasegawa Y, Nitta H, Sasaki A, *et al.* Laparoscopic left lateral sectionectomy as a training procedure for surgeons learning laparoscopic hepatectomy. J Hepatobiliary Pancreat Sci 2013; 20(5):525–530.

46 Robinson SM, Hui KY, Amer A, Manas DM, White SA. Laparoscopic liver resection: is there a learning curve? Dig Surg 2012; 29(1):62–69.

47 Troisi RI, Montalti R, van Limmen JG, *et al.* Risk factors and management of conversions to an open approach in laparoscopic liver resection. analysis of 265 consecutive cases. HPB 2014; 16(1):75–82.

48 Vigano L, Laurent A, Tayar C, Tomatis M, Ponti A, Cherqui D. The learning curve in laparoscopic liver resection: improved feasibility and reproducibility. Ann Surg 2009; 250(5): 772–782.

49 Otsuka Y, Tsuchiya M, Maeda T, *et al.* Laparoscopic hepatectomy for liver tumors: proposals for standardization. J Hepatobiliary Pancreat Surg 2009; 16(6):720–725.

50 Strickland A, Fairhurst K, Lauder C, Hewett P, Maddern G. Development of an ex vivo simulated training model for laparoscopic liver resection. Surg Endosc 2011; 25(5): 1677–1682.

51 Krahenbuhl L, Feodorovici M, Renzulli P, Schafer M, Abou-Shady M, Baer HU. Laparoscopic partial hepatectomy in the rat: a new resectional technique. Dig Surg 1998; 15(2): 140–144.

52 Frezza EE, Wachtel MS. A proposed canine model of laparoscopic nonanatomic liver resection. J Laparoendosc Adv Surg Tech A 2006; 16(1):15–20.

53 Machado MA, Galvao FH, Pompeu E, Ribeiro C, Bacchella T, Machado MC. A canine model of laparoscopic segmental liver resection. J Laparoendosc Adv Surg Tech A 2004; 14(5): 325–328.

54 Eiriksson K, Fors D, Rubertsson S, Arvidsson D. Laparoscopic left lobe liver resection in a porcine model: a study of the efficacy and safety of different surgical techniques. Surg Endosc 2009; 23(5):1038–1042.

55 Consten EC, Dakin GF, Robertus JL, Bardaro S, Milone L, Gagner M. Perioperative outcome of laparoscopic left lateral liver resection is improved by using a bioabsorbable staple line reinforcement material in a porcine model. Surg Endosc 2008; 22(5):1188–1193.

56 Teh SH, Hunter JG, Sheppard BC. A suitable animal model for laparoscopic hepatic resection training. Surg Endosc 2007; 21(10):1738–1744.

57 Dorcaratto D, Burdio F, Fondevila D, et al. Laparoscopic distal pancreatectomy: feasibility study of radiofrequency-assisted transection in a porcine model. J Laparoendosc Adv Surg Tech A 2012; 22(3):242–248.

58 Jones DB, Wu JS, Soper NJ. Laparoscopic pancreaticoduodenectomy in the porcine model. Surg Endosc 1997; 11(4): 326–330.

59 Suzuki O, Hirano S, Yano T, et al. Laparoscopic pancreaticoduodenectomy is effective in a porcine model. Surg Endosc 2008; 22(11):2509–2513.

60 Azer SA, Eizenberg N. Do we need dissection in an integrated problem-based learning medical course? Perceptions of first- and second-year students. Surg Radiol Anat 2007; 29(2):173–180.

61 Chapman SJ, Hakeem AR, Marangoni G, Prasad KR. Anatomy in medical education. Perceptions of undergraduate medical students. Ann Anat 2013; 195(5):409–414.

62 Parker LM. Anatomical dissection: why are we cutting it out? Dissection in undergraduate teaching. ANZ J Surg 2002; 72(12):910–912.

63 Stefanidis D, Yonce TC, Green JM, Coker AP. Cadavers versus pigs. Which are better for procedural training of surgery residents outside the OR? Surgery 2013; 154(1):34–37.

64 Lewis CE, Peacock WJ, Tillou A, Hines OJ, Hiatt JR. A novel cadaver-based educational program in general surgery training. J Surg Educ 2012; 69(6):693–698.

65 Csokay A, Papp A, Imreh D, Czabajszky M, Valalik I, Antalfi B. Modelling pathology from autolog fresh cadaver organs as a novel concept in neurosurgical training. Acta Neurochir 2013; 155(10):1993–1995.

66 Duran C, Bismuth J, Mitchell E. A nationwide survey of vascular surgery trainees reveals trends in operative experience, confidence, and attitudes about simulation. J Vasc Surg 2013; 58(2):524–528.

67 Kuhls DA, Risucci DA, Bowyer MW, Luchette FA. Advanced surgical skills for exposure in trauma: a new surgical skills cadaver course for surgery residents and fellows. J Trauma Acute Care Surg 2013; 74(2):664–670.

68 Pattanshetti VM, Pattanshetti SV. Laparoscopic surgery on cadavers: a novel teaching tool for surgical residents. ANZ J Surg 2010; 80(10):676–678.

69 Udomsawaengsup S, Pattana-arun J, Tansatit T, et al. Minimally invasive surgery training in soft cadaver (MIST-SC). J Med Assoc Thailand 2005; 88 (suppl 4):S189–194.

70 Escobar PF, Kebria M, Falcone T. Evaluation of a novel single-port robotic platform in the cadaver model for the performance of various procedures in gynecologic oncology. Gynecol Oncol 2011; 120(3):380–384.

71 Wyles SM, Miskovic D, Ni Z, et al. Analysis of laboratory-based laparoscopic colorectal surgery workshops within the English National Training Programme. Surg Endosc 2011; 25(5): 1559–1566.

72 Giger U, Fresard I, Hafliger A, Bergmann M, Krahenbuhl L. Laparoscopic training on Thiel human cadavers: a model to teach advanced laparoscopic procedures. Surg Endosc 2008; 22(4):901–906.

73 Prasad Rai B, Tang B, Eisma R, Soames RW, Wen H, Nabi G. A qualitative assessment of human cadavers embalmed by Thiel's method used in laparoscopic training for renal resection. Anat Sci Educ 2012; 5(3):182–186.

74 Katz R, Hoznek A, Antiphon P, van Velthoven R, Delmas V, Abbou CC. Cadaveric versus porcine models in urological laparoscopic training. Urol Int 2003; 71(3):310–315.

75 Joseph RA, Salas NA, Donovan MA, Reardon PR, Bass BL, Dunkin BJ. Single-site laparoscopic (SSL) cholecystectomy in human cadavers using a novel percutaneous instrument platform and a magnetic anchoring and guidance system (MAGS): reestablishing the "critical view." Surg Endosc 2012; 26(1):149–153.

76 Pinto PA, Montgomery RA, Ryan B, et al. Laparoscopic procurement model for living donor liver transplantation. Clin Transplant 2003; 17(suppl 9):39–43.

77 Sambunjak D, Straus SE, Marusic A. Mentoring in academic medicine: a systematic review. JAMA 2006; 296(9): 1103–1115.

78 Levine WN, Braman JP, Gelberman RH, Black KP. Mentorship in orthopaedic surgery – road map to success for the mentor and the mentee. AOA critical issues. J Bone Joint Surg (Am) 2013; 95(9):e591–595.

79 Ho VP, Trencheva K, Stein SL, Milsom JW. Mentorship for participants in a laparoscopic colectomy course. Surg Endosc 2012; 26(3):722–726.

80 Broome JT, Solorzano CC. Impact of surgical mentorship on retroperitoneoscopic adrenalectomy with comparison to transperitoneal laparoscopic adrenalectomy. Am Surg 2013; 79(2):162–166.

81 Royal Australasian College of Surgeons. General Guidelines for Assessing, Approving & Introducing New Surgical Procedures into a Hospital or Health Service. Australian Safety and Efficacy Register of New Interventional Procedures – Surgical (ASERNIP-S) Research. Melbourne: RACS, 2008.

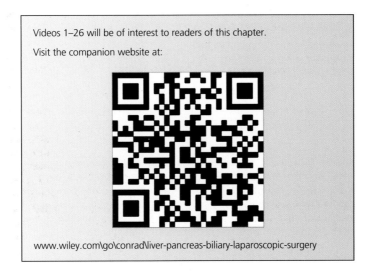

Videos 1–26 will be of interest to readers of this chapter.

Visit the companion website at:

www.wiley.com\go\conrad\liver-pancreas-biliary-laparoscopic-surgery

Optimal operating room set-up and equipment used in laparoscopic hepatopancreatobiliary surgery

Satoshi Ogiso,[1] Kenichiro Araki,[2] Brice Gayet,[1] and Claudius Conrad[3]

[1] *Department of Digestive Diseases, Institut Mutualiste Montsouris, Paris, France*
[2] *Department of General Surgical Science, Gunma University Graduate School of Medicine, Gunma, Japan*
[3] *Department of Surgical Oncology, University of Texas MD Anderson Cancer Center, Houston, USA*

EDITOR COMMENT

In this chapter, we describe the operating room set-up, equipment, and instrumentation needed to perform advanced laparoscopic HPB surgery. The operating room set-up should be optimized for ergonomics and team dynamics, as well as patient- and procedure-specific factors. A crucial aspect is an optimized eye–hand–target–monitor axis that may change during a case and therefore the operating room set-up may have to be altered. Here we discuss several energy device options which have advantages and disadvantages depending on the specific laparoscopic application. Further, when aiming to perform advanced laparoscopic HPB procedures, the surgeon must be practiced at laparoscopic suturing in order to be able to control bleeding. Because of the risk of significant hemorrhage, a laparoscopic vascular clamp should be a standard in a minimally invasive HPB surgery set. Various hemostatic agents are complementary to suturing and may assist in controlling bleeding. Considering the rapid technological developments, surgeons should maintain a continued interest in technological advances coming into practice in the field of minimally invasive HPB surgery.

Keywords: energy devices, ergonomics, hemostasis, instrumentation, operating room set-up, patient positioning, video display

3.1 Introduction

Complex laparoscopic HPB surgeries requiring precise dissection with minimal bleeding in a highly vascular area have become the standard of care in many centers today. These procedures are dependent not only on the specific skill set of the operative team but also on the advances in imaging, technique, and technology in minimally invasive surgery in general that have developed in the past several years. Proper knowledge of laparoscopic equipment and operating room (OR) set-up is essential in performing advanced laparoscopic HPB procedures safely. Specific technological knowledge will not only increase patient and staff safety but also enhance team performance, maximize chances to complete the laparoscopic HPB operation minimally invasively, and optimize patient outcome. This chapter discusses the optimal OR set-up and equipment used in advanced laparoscopic HPB surgery.

3.2 Operating room set-up

During a laparoscopic procedure, the operative field is visualized indirectly via a laparoscope connected to a camera that projects a two-dimensional (2D) image on a monitor. The procedure is completed somewhat remotely using various long instruments that accommodate the distance between target and the port in the abdominal wall. The "remoteness" created by the

---

Laparoscopic Liver, Pancreas, and Biliary Surgery, First Edition.
Edited by Claudius Conrad and Brice Gayet.

interfaces of laparoscopic imaging and longer instruments makes the relationship between surgeon and equipment an important factor in the surgeon's operative performance. Moreover, the "remoteness" of laparoscopic surgery is also an important factor in the surgeon's mental and physical well-being through the challenges related to ergonomics and 2D imagery. Optimization of this surgeon–equipment interface depends on multiple factors, including OR set-up, patient positioning, type of procedure performed, number of available monitors, and ability to reposition monitors. The optimal OR set-up adjusts for challenges specific to laparoscopic HPB surgery, such as monitor positioning above the patient for inline working during laparoscopic liver surgery, and picture-in-picture mode for intraoperative laparoscopic ultrasound. The ultimate goal for advanced laparoscopic HPB surgery is the creation of an optimal OR environment that enhances effectiveness and efficacy in the interaction between team members, equipment, and instruments while ergonomics as well as patient and team safety are ensured.

3.2.1 Optimal equipment positioning in the operating room

3.2.1.1 Monitor positioning

One of the key pieces of equipment for the accurate and effective completion of laparoscopic surgery is the monitor or bank of monitors that provide the visual field. Often, the monitor is positioned outside the sterile operating field, which may force the surgeon to work in one direction while viewing in another. Major deviations of working direction (hand–target axis) and view direction (eye–monitor axis) can disrupt proper spatial cognition and delicate control of instruments (Figure 3.1). In addition, such a suboptimal eye–hand–target–monitor axis imposes an uncomfortable and unnatural position of neck and spine, which impacts negatively on ergonomics and ultimately on surgical performance. Suboptimal ergonomics can lead to injuries and physical discomfort of neck, shoulders, and upper extremities. Monitor position above eye level can be particularly harmful. It may result in discomfort and fatigue of the lower back, neck, and shoulders, as well as extensive extraocular and ciliary muscle activity, causing eyestrain. Additionally, a monitor distance that is too close can cause excessive accommodation of eyes and convergent gaze by the extraocular musculature. A distance too far may result in staring and loss of resolution.

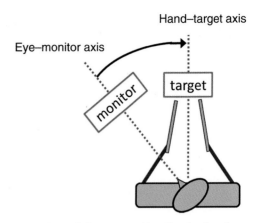

Figure 3.1 The angle between working direction (hand–target axis) and direction of view (eye–monitor axis) should be less than 15°.

The optimal angle between eye–monitor and hand–target axes for comfort, ergonomic safety, optimized procedural precision, and reduced operative time is less than 15°. Ideally, multiple monitors should be set in front of each surgeon in line with the hand–target axis and adjusted before, during, and after the procedure [1]. The optimal height of the monitor is just below eye level to allow a moderately declined viewing angle (preferably a downward direction of 15°) [1]. The optimal distance to the monitor depends on screen size and image resolution and has been reported to be between 80 cm and 120 cm for a 19-inch CRT monitor [1] (Figure 3.2, left). With newer and larger high-definition monitors, an optimal viewing distance would be further away. In the future, greater availability of three-dimensional (3D) cameras/monitors will facilitate the 3D motor movement required in laparoscopic surgery. Nevertheless, even with these advanced devices that reduce the fatigue from 2D image to 3D motor movement conversion, aspects of ergonomics and avoidance of motion sickness to optimize surgical performances apply.

3.2.1.2 Laparoscopic equipment

The equipment, cables, and tubing running from the equipment to the patient should not disrupt the eye–monitor or hand–target axis of the operating surgeon or block the view of the operating team members.

3.2.1.3 Dedicated minimally invasive surgery suite

Much of the laparoscopic equipment such as monitors, insufflators, light sources, video equipment, and

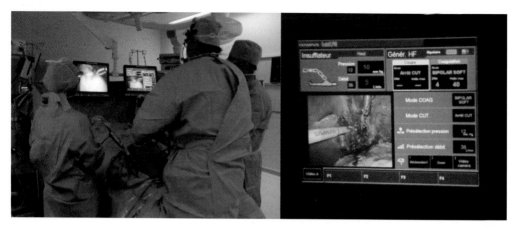

Figure 3.2 An IMM integrated operating room (ENDOALPHA OR, Olympus, Tokyo, Japan) has multiple ceiling-suspended monitors (*left*) and a centralized control system for equipment such as imaging system, insufflator, room light, and electrosurgery (*right*). A ceiling-suspended monitor is set in front of the operating surgeon in line with the hand–target axis and just below the eye height. ENDOBOY holds a laparoscopic retractor from the right side of the patient (*left*).

electrosurgery devices can be grouped together on one or multiple trolleys. These heavy trolleys take up space and clutter the floor with cables and tubing. This may pose a possible threat to the safety of patients and OR personnel. The room should be large enough to hold all the necessary equipment and to permit unencumbered transfer of the OR staff around tubing and equipment.

A number of ergonomic factors are different from open surgery before, during, and after laparoscopic HPB surgery. The establishment of an optimal OR environment for superior operating team performance depends on the needed and available equipment, especially the degree of freedom of the monitors. Unlike a monitor fixed on top of a trolley, a ceiling-suspended monitor can be positioned easily and independently from the rest of the laparoscopic equipment. The suspension system allows intraoperative repositioning, screen inclination for each monitor, and placement above the patient to optimize the important eye–hand–target–monitor axis for surgeon and assistant (see Figure 3.2, left).

The modern minimally invasive OR is equipped with centralized and simplified interfaces (see Figure 3.2, right) and permanently installed laparoscopic equipment that is operational on demand. The equipment, together with multiple high-definition flat-screen monitors, is attached to a ceiling-mounted suspension system to facilitate versatile positioning. Various cables (such as electric power supply and video transmission cables) are kept off the floor and within easy reach of the surgeon or OR staff.

Efficient design of such an OR improves overall operational efficiency and safety.

3.2.2 Patient positioning

Proper, stable positioning of the patient is a vital step in successful laparoscopic HPB surgery and critical for target organ exposure and optimal trocar placement. Arm and leg position should not disrupt the movement of the laparoscope or instruments, or the view of each surgeon on the monitors, and limbs should be positioned to prevent pressure injuries, such as ulnar or peroneal neuropathy. All bony prominences are given extra padding, and all patients should have cushioned arm covers as well as compression boots on their lower extremities to prevent formation of deep venous thrombus. A safety trap is placed on the chest to prevent the patient from sliding as the surgical bed tilts.

In laparoscopic HPB surgery, patients are generally placed in the low lithotomy or supine position with the legs abducted on straight leg boards (so-called French position) (Figure 3.3) and with both arms tucked alongside the body. Tucking the arms might minimize brachial plexus stretch and subsequent injury in case the patient slides in reversed Trendelenburg position. The operating surgeon stands between the legs, allowing for a straight eye–hand–target–monitor axis. Lumbar padding is added behind the right back when performing right hepatectomy, and patients are set in the left lateral position (Figure 3.4) when accessing the posterosuperior segments of the liver.

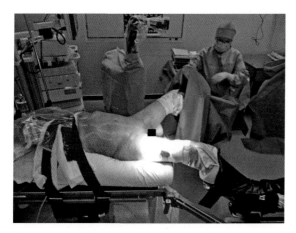

Figure 3.3 Low lithotomy position is often used in laparoscopic HPB surgery with both arms tucked alongside the body.

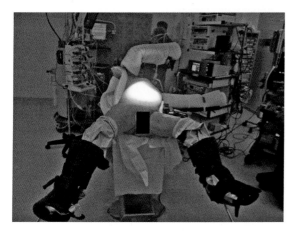

Figure 3.4 Patients are set in the left lateral position when accessing the posterosuperior segments of the liver with/without placing transdiaphragmatic trocars.

3.2.3 Staff positioning and fixed mounting devices

3.2.3.1 Operating surgeon

The operating surgeon should be positioned to work directly in front of the target organ, having the most direct access. The monitor for the operating surgeon is positioned to optimize the eye–hand–target–monitor axis. In many laparoscopic HPB procedures, the operating surgeon stands between the patient's legs, with some exceptions (e.g. transdiaphragmatic liver surgery).

3.2.3.2 Assisting surgeon and scrub nurse

The position of the assisting surgeons and scrub nurses should not disrupt the eye–hand–target–monitor axis of the operating surgeon. In order to avoid motion sickness, reduce fatigue, and optimize visualization, the assistant needs to provide a precise and stable laparoscopic image. To achieve this, the assistant surgeon who handles the laparoscope must be positioned in a comfortable and neutral posture to provide a stable image over a prolonged period of time. Constant small movements of the image lead to surgeon fatigue and motion sickness.

3.2.4 Laparoscope mounting devices

Several surgical robots capable of holding the laparoscope and altering its position in response to a surgeon's verbal command are available [2] (Figure 3.5, left). Such robotic devices consist of two main components: the voice- or motion-controlled computer interface and the motorized laparoscopic mounting arm. Some devices can store several presets of laparoscope position, allowing the surgeon to rapidly return the image

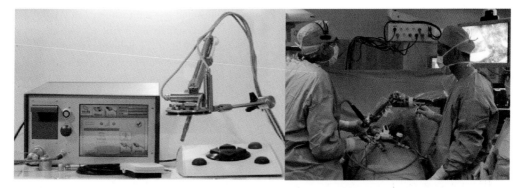

Figure 3.5 The Vision Kontrol endoscopY (VIKY) system (Endocontrol, Grenoble, France) consists of a display console, an autoclavable robotic camera holder, and a foot pedal (*left*). A robotic holder places the laparoscope just in front of the operating surgeon and between both instruments in the surgeon's hands (*right*).

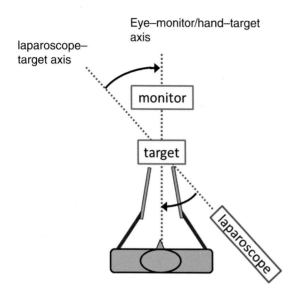

laparoscope–
target axis

Eye–monitor/hand–target
axis

monitor

target

laparoscope

Figure 3.6 The angle between the laparoscope–target axis and eye–monitor/hand–target axes should be minimized to avoid losing spatial orientation.

to a previous position. This can be particularly helpful during laparoscopic suturing: a first position is a close-up image, preferred when driving the needle through tissue, and a second position is a zoom-out when the knot is fashioned.

Ideally, a trocar for the laparoscope is placed between two working trocars of the operating surgeon. This set-up overlays the laparoscope–target axis to the eye–hand–target–monitor axes of the operating surgeon and facilitates optimal efficiency of the procedure. Extensive deviation of the laparoscope–target axis from the eye–hand–target–monitor axes can negatively impact the surgeon's spatial cognition – the so-called mirror image (see Figure 3.5, right; Figure 3.6). A robotic camera holder can decrease interference between the operating surgeon's hands/instruments as well as the assistant holding the camera, and it provides a surgeon with a controlled and stationary laparoscopic image.

3.2.5 Autostatic instrument stabilizer
Prolonged laparoscopic retraction in the same position (e.g. retraction of the liver during portal dissection) can effectively be accomplished by an autostatic instrument stabilizer such as ENDOBOY (ASFS Medic's, Niort, France) (see Figure 3.2, left), which has benefits similar

to the robotic camera holder. Stationary holding of a laparoscopic retractor is accomplished without interfering with the operating surgeon's movements. The autostatic retractor position can be manually altered with ease during the procedure, while being strong enough to retract large or heavy organs such as the liver over a prolonged period of time without perforating the liver capsule.

3.3 Imaging system

3.3.1 Standard laparoscope
Because the surgeon depends almost exclusively on the visual information provided through the imaging system, a high-quality image is vital in performing laparoscopic HPB procedures safely.

The laparoscope transmits light from an external light source through a bundle of glass fibers, illuminates the abdominal cavity, gathers images, and transmits them through a collection of rod lenses to digital imaging chips in a camera head. A 10 mm laparoscope is commonly used for its greater image quality and wider field of view compared with smaller caliber laparoscopes. Various diameters of laparoscope are available, ranging from 3 to 12 mm. Rigid, angled (0–120°) or flexible tip laparoscopes are chosen based on the type of procedure and surgeon preference. The laparoscope lens is prone to frequent fogging, especially early in the procedure before the lens warms up. This can significantly impede effective visualization. Warming the laparoscope using hot water, creating friction with a towel, and using anti-fog solutions or an electric warming device helps to reduce lens fogging.

A high-intensity light source and light cable are required for a sufficiently bright laparoscopic image. Light is transmitted from the light source, which is generally located off the operating field and reaches the scope through a fiber-optic light cable. The number of light fibers is a determinant factor for efficient light transmission. This means that broken fibers lead to light loss and persistently dark images. In those cases the cable should be replaced.

The video monitor receives electrical signals to synthesize optic images for the presentation of intra-abdominal images to the surgeon and OR staff. For a detailed image, the monitor should be high resolution at the same level as the charge-coupling device (CCD) tips and high

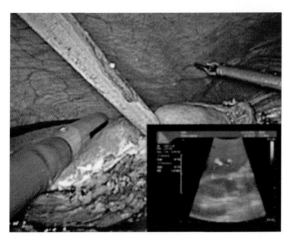

Figure 3.7 Laparoscopic and ultrasonographic images are simultaneously visualized in a single monitor using the picture-in-picture function.

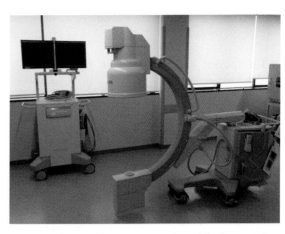

Figure 3.8 The portable C-arm system is used for fluoroscopic study in a variety of positions.

frequency (at least 100 MHz) to decrease sparkling artifacts. At least two monitors are required: one for the operating surgeon and the other for the assistant surgeon (see Figure 3.5). Ceiling-suspended multiple flat monitors are preferred to achieve the best monitor set-up and positioning. Some newer displaying systems have a picture-in-picture function, which enables the display of images from two different imaging devices at the same time: this is crucial when performing laparoscopic ultrasonography as it allows surgeons to visualize the laparoscopic and ultrasonographic images simultaneously in a single monitor (Figure 3.7). Through availability of the two images in the eye–hand–target–monitor axis, manipulation of the ultrasonic probe can be accomplished while analyzing the parenchymal transection plane and guiding a radiofrequency ablation probe or a biopsy needle. Further, equipment to record the procedure is important for transparency, furthering research on surgical technique or for self-assessment.

3.3.2 Imaging for bile duct stone

Intraoperative cholangiography is performed to detect bile duct stones and, in some centers, to decrease the risk of bile duct injury. Air cholangiograms can also be performed to detect possible biliary leakage after liver resection. The gallbladder or the cystic duct is cannulated to inject the radiographic contrast agent, and an image is obtained using a portable X-ray imaging system, referred to as a C-arm. The portable C-arm system encompasses an X-ray generator, image intensifier, viewing monitors, and workstation for image manipulation, and it is equipped with mechanisms to allow a variety of movements for maximum positional flexibility (Figure 3.8).

Once choledocholithiasis is suspected, the common bile duct is explored via transcystic or transcholedochal choledochoscopy. Common bile duct stones are extracted using a Dormia basket or Fogarty catheter. Newer choledochoscopes are flexible and equipped with irrigation, suction, and a working channel through which a catheter can be passed (Figure 3.9). The choledochoscope can be introduced through a 10 mm trocar placed under the right

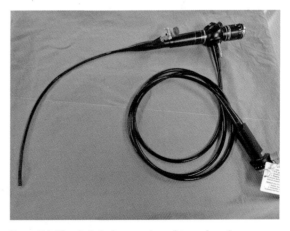

Figure 3.9 The choledochoscope is used to explore the common bile duct and extract bile duct stones.

costal margin, and images are transmitted to a monitor outside the surgical bed.

3.3.3 Special imaging devices

Laparoscopic ultrasound (Figure 3.10) is an essential device for HPB surgery to help surgeons understand patients' anatomy, detect additional or confirm known lesions, and ensure vascular flow. The mechanics and techniques for this device are discussed in detail in Chapter 15.

Indocyanine green (ICG) fluorescence technique offers real-time navigation for the localization of intrahepatic lesions, evaluation of the biliary tree, detection of biliary leakage, and visualization of the demarcation following portal pedicle occlusion (Figure 3.11). The technique necessitates a near-infrared probe and camera for providing light excitation and capturing of a luminescence signal. It has been used mainly in open surgery [3]. A laparoscopic probe for the ICG fluorescence technique is commercially available today and could become a vital tool for laparoscopic HPB surgeons.

Imaging systems (specialized laparoscope, camera head, and monitor) offering 3D images have been developed to overcome the difficulties of 2D images. Three-dimensional images allow depth perception and facilitate spatial navigation. The use of 3D imaging systems is not widespread yet, owing to their cost, the need for additional 3D glasses, head-up displays, 3D screens, and also because of so-called visually induced motion sickness caused by conflicting visual and physical motion and/or

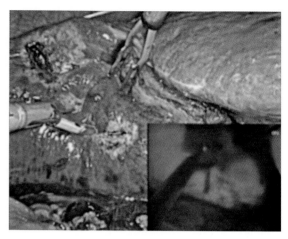

Figure 3.11 The transection border between segment V and VI is demonstrated using the ICG fluorescence technique. In the inset window, the ICG fluorescence image shows that the liver surface of segment VI is positively stained with ICG while that of segment V is negative for staining. This staining border is being incised using ultrasonic shears.

binocular stereopsis to fuse monocular vision into a single "normal" vision. Additionally, a significant proportion of surgeons lack the ability to see in 3D with the equipment available today. In these surgeons, motion sickness obviates the need for 3D cameras and displaying equipment. Overall, however, 3D vision for advanced laparoscopic HPB surgery has been shown to reduce both surgeon

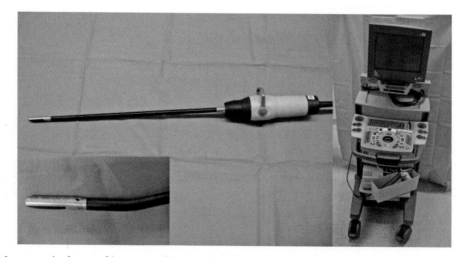

Figure 3.10 Laparoscopic ultrasound is an essential device to help surgeons understand the patient's anatomy, detect an intrahepatic lesion, and confirm vascular flow.

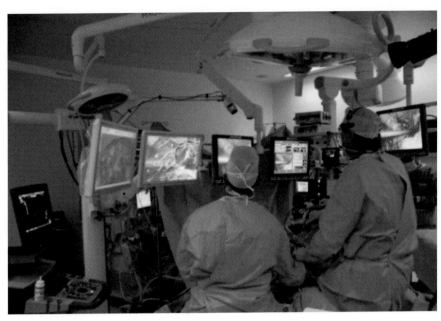

Figure 3.12 The operating surgeon refers to a total of four screens which display a virtual liver (in the leftmost screen), augmented reality (in the second left), laparoscopic view (in the second right), and centralized control system (in the rightmost).

fatigue and operative time. It is likely to become the standard display in the future.

Augmented reality technology has been developed using various modalities such as ultrasound, computed tomography, and magnetic resonance imaging and represents the next step towards more advanced surgical navigation (Figure 3.12). To date, however, no prototypes have provided the quality required for complex procedures such as laparoscopic liver and pancreatic resections, and there are several challenges. These include real-time deformation of reconstructed organ images (especially the liver) and precise image overlay of the laparoscopic image with high spatial resolution.

3.4 Abdominal entry and closure

A laparoscopic procedure begins with the establishment of pneumoperitoneum followed by the placement of several trocars through which the laparoscope and instruments are passed. Choice of the first trocar depends on the technique used to access the peritoneum. The closed technique by blind insertion of a Veress needle has been widely used to create laparoscopic entry and

pneumoperitoneum but the risk of major organ injury, including vascular injury, is well documented. An optically guided closed technique using a specialized trocar with a transparent tip (Figure 3.13) is often preferable for inserting the first trocar because of the increased safety afforded by direct visualization and quick entry to the abdominal cavity. Each layer of the abdominal wall can be seen with a 0° laparoscope in the optic trocar as it is being traversed. The open technique (Hasson method) is another choice with the benefit of a low risk for major complications but with the disadvantages of longer time and difficulty in obese patients.

Disposable and reusable trocars (Figure 3.14) are used today. Ten millimeter and 5 mm balloon-tipped blunt trocars (Figure 3.15) prevent accidental cannula withdrawal, which can be important especially when trocars are inserted through the diaphragm for operating on the posterosuperior liver. A trocar is preferably equipped with a separate insufflation route for clearing intra-abdominal smoke and steam produced by electrosurgical devices. Newer insufflation devices recirculate the gas insufflated into the abdomen to clear it of smoke, warm the gas, and provide a constant insufflation pressure.

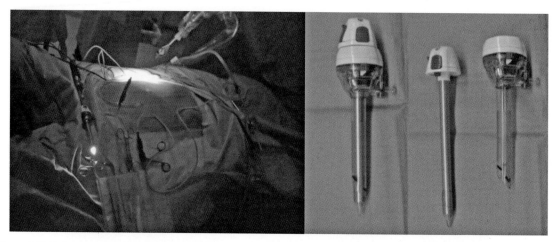

Figure 3.13 Before creating a laparoscopic entry with the optically guided closed technique, an optic trocar (*right*) is attached to the tip of a 0° laparoscope (*left*).

A wound protector (Figure 3.16, left) is used to decrease the risk of surgical site infection and obtain circumferential retraction during procedures via mini-laparotomy. Wound protectors combined with special covers or lids offer the additional benefit of giving access to a surgeon's hand or laparoscopic instruments while maintaining intra-abdominal pressure (see Figure 3.16, left, upper insets, and Figure 3.16, right). These devices enable a combination of pure laparoscopic with mini-laparotomy procedure

(hybrid technique) or hand-assisted procedure. They may also decrease the need for conversion to conventional open procedure, which allows maintenance of the benefits of the minimally invasive surgery. Even in patients with significant adhesions or bleeding that is challenging to control purely laparoscopically, hand access ports can facilitate completion of the procedure.

After removal of a 10 mm or greater trocar, the fascial defect should be closed with a suture to reduce the risk of

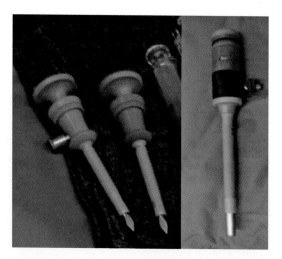

Figure 3.14 Reusable trocars in diameter of 5.5 mm (*left*) and 10.5 mm (*right*).

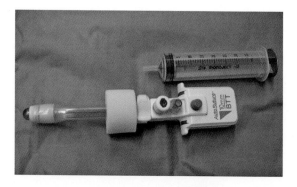

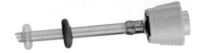

Figure 3.15 10 mm (Covidien, Dublin, Ireland) (*upper*) and 5 mm (Applied Medical, Rancho Santa Margarita, USA) (*lower*) balloon-tipped blunt trocars used to prevent an accidental cannula withdrawal.

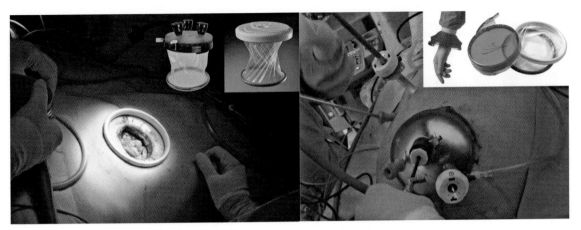

Figure 3.16 The use of a wound protector (*left*) decreases the risk of surgical site infection and provides circumferential retraction during a mini-laparotomic procedure. Alexis wound protector/retractor (*left*, right upper inset), Gelpoint advanced access platform (*left*, left upper inset), and Gelport laparoscopic system (*right*) are combined with the wound protector to provide single, triple or multiple laparoscopic and hand accesses (Applied Medical, Rancho Santa Margarita, USA).

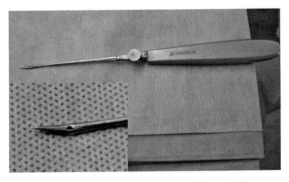

Figure 3.17 A Reverdin suture needle is used for a closing port site fascial defect. The sharp, notched tip passes through the fascia in one side of the trocar, holding a thread in its small window, and pulls through the fascia in the other side of the trocar, capturing the thread again.

developing a port site hernia. Fascial closure can be difficult under direct vision, especially in obese patients, and several specialized instruments for port site closure are available (Figure 3.17).

3.5 Energy devices

Prevention of bleeding and adequate hemostasis are essential during the laparoscopic procedure. Most devices used in open surgery have been modified for laparoscopic surgery.

3.5.1 Monopolar and bipolar electrocautery

Conventional electrosurgery and monopolar and bipolar cautery achieve tissue cutting and coagulating via the passage of high-frequency electrical current produced by an electrosurgical generator. During monopolar electrosurgery, electrical current passes through the tissue from an active electrode to a broad electrically indifferent plate which causes high current density and significant heat (up to 300 °C) with the risk of deeper injury [4]. In contrast to monopolar electrosurgery, with bipolar energy, the current flows back to a return electrode. Conventional electrosurgery remains the main laparoscopic modality thanks to its low cost and general availability.

Monopolar cautery can combine cutting and coagulating functions, and a wide variety of disposable and reusable laparoscopic instruments have a cautery attachment for monopolar current, including scissors and dissectors. In contrast, bipolar cautery has a higher hemostatic efficiency with no cutting ability and decreased risk of thermal injury to adjacent tissue. Modern electrosurgical generators have new or improved modes for high hemostatic efficiency using voltage-controlling technology, such as soft coagulation (e.g. ERBE, Tübingen, Germany) (Figure 3.18). Such modes contribute to the excellent usability of conventional electrosurgery, especially the bipolar technique, in complex HPB procedures [5].

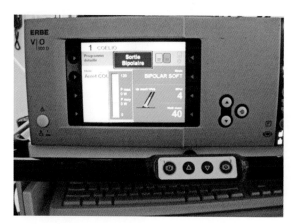

Figure 3.18 One of the new electrosurgical generators, VIO300D, has a soft coagulation mode with a high hemostatic efficiency.

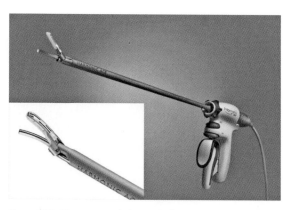

Figure 3.20 Shears type of ultrasonic device.

3.5.2 Advanced bipolar vessel sealing devices

Advanced bipolar sealing devices (e.g. LigaSure, Enseal) (Figure 3.19) combine bipolar current with optimized tissue apposition and compression to provide better vessel sealing capability while minimizing the risks associated with conventional electrosurgery [5]. Bipolar sealing technology has made laparoscopic suturing or clipping of vascular pedicles of up to 7 mm unnecessary in some cases. However, the need for an additional instrument for transection as well as the generally large size of the tip can potentially limit the use of bipolar sealing devices in tissue dissection.

3.5.3 Ultrasonic devices

Ultrasonic devices (e.g. SonoSurg, Harmonic ACE) (Figure 3.20) produce cutting and coagulating effects through

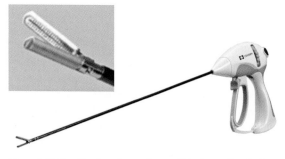

Figure 3.19 The LigaSure is an advanced bipolar sealing device and some types of LigaSure are equipped with scissors to transect tissue after sealing.

vibration of a piezoelectric crystal mounted at the tip (active blade) of the instrument. The Cavitron ultrasound surgical aspirator (e.g. CUSA Excel, SonoSurg) is widely used for liver parenchymal dissection through an open approach [6]. Liver parenchymal tissue is fragmented, irrigated, and aspirated away from the dissection field while preserving intrahepatic vessels and bile ducts. The shears-type ultrasonic devices offer less hemostatic ability when compared with bipolar sealing devices and are equipped with finer tips suitable for tissue dissection. The ultrasonic shears enable quick tissue transection concomitant with coagulation. Furthermore, the cavitation effect caused by an active blade can be utilized for dissecting liver parenchyma, similar to the CUSA device [7,8]. Nevertheless, inserting the active blade blindly into liver parenchyma for parenchymal transection carries the risk of inadvertent biliary or vascular injury and must be avoided by using a refined technique of parenchymal transection.

3.5.4 Combined bipolar sealing and ultrasonic devices

Today, devices have become available that allow for integration of both advanced bipolar sealing and ultrasonic technologies, which are delivered simultaneously through a single instrument (Thunderbeat, Olympus, Tokyo, Japan) (Figure 3.21). This integration provides the benefits of each individual energy device: the ability to rapidly cut tissue with ultrasonic shears and to create reliable vessel seals with bipolar sealing technology, which allows surgeons more secure hemostasis and fewer instrument exchanges [9]. When required, bipolar energy can be applied to seal the tissue without the cutting function being used.

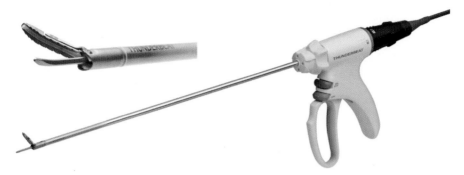

Figure 3.21 The Thunderbeat is the first integration of advanced bipolar sealing and ultrasonic technologies.

3.5.5 Radiofrequency ablation

Radiofrequency ablation (RFA) is often used to destroy small and deeply located intraparenchymal lesions while avoiding deep parenchymal resection and significant parenchymal volume loss. The RFA device generates a high-frequency alternating current to cause focal tissue destruction at the tip of the electrode, which is inserted through a trocar or directly through the abdominal wall and placed into the target lesion under the guidance of ultrasonography. The technique of precise targeting using laparoscopic ultrasonography guidance is relatively difficult. Nevertheless, it has an important role, especially in the management of bilobar, multiple or unresectable lesions, and in patients with impaired liver function [10]. The combination of direct visualization with ultrasonic guidance of target lesions during laparoscopic RFA has important benefits in certain cases over axial image-guided ablation techniques owing to the ability to directly inspect and screen the rest of the liver and the entire abdominal cavity.

3.5.6 Argon plasma coagulation

Argon plasma coagulation is used to create a coagulated tissue surface (mainly the transected liver surface) by passing electric current through a stream of ionized argon gas. High-flow infusion of argon gas can increase intra-abdominal pressure and has been reported as a risk factor for developing gas embolism in laparoscopic surgery [11]. For this reason, argon plasma coagulation should be used with caution, if at all, on visceral organs in laparoscopic surgery. A significant risk stems from injecting insoluble argon gas into an inadvertently opened hepatic vein during laparoscopic liver surgery with potentially fatal gas embolism.

3.6 Nonenergy devices

A significant number of specialized instruments are available for advanced laparoscopic HPB surgery with various features for a variety of preferences. Instruments frequently used in laparoscopic HPB surgery are discussed here.

3.6.1 Bipolar forceps

A bipolar forceps is an instrument with forceps properties but also the ability to deliver bipolar energy, as discussed in the previous section. Among the wide variety of bipolar forceps available in laparoscopic surgery, the one with wide and fenestrated tips (CEV 134, Medtronic MicroFrance, Dublin, Ireland) (Figure 3.22, upper) is most frequently used for HPB procedures. The tips open and close while keeping the jaws parallel to each other. Therefore, the closing pressure is equally distributed to the tissue between the tips. This mode of action works efficiently in tissue dissection, clamping of an

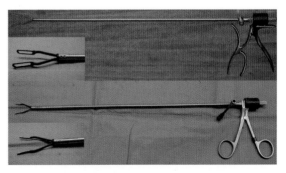

Figure 3.22 A laparoscopic bipolar forceps with wide and fenestrated tips and a newer handle (*upper*) and a bipolar forceps with thin liner tips (*lower*).

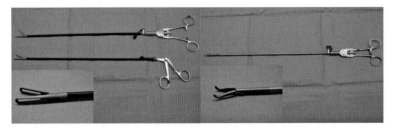

Figure 3.23 A laparoscopic grasping forceps with broad and flat tips (*left*) and serrated right angle forceps (*right*).

injured vessel, secure coagulation, and tissue retraction with atraumatic but high grasping force. Liver parenchyma can be transected similarly to the clamp crushing method [12]. For hemostasis of small vessels or fine structures, a bipolar forceps with nonfenestrated thin tips is more suitable (see Figure 3.22, lower).

3.6.2 Grasper

Grasping forceps are designed for tissue manipulation with or without a locking mechanism (ratchet). Toothed forceps are used to retract tissue with a lower risk of tissue slippage but higher application of force. Forceps with broad and flat tips are capable of more gentle grasping with lower pressure per square unit. Among these types of forceps, those with a lower grasping power are preferred because of their greater safety in preventing inadvertent tissue damage. Such graspers release the tissue between the tips spontaneously when external force is applied, which avoids serious damage to the tissue (Figure 3.23, left). Forceps with fine tips allow for handling of delicate tissue, and those with curved tips and pointed ends are used for tissue dissection and in developing a surgical plane (see Figure 3.23, right).

3.6.3 Retractor

A retractor should be strong enough to retract the large and heavy liver while not perforating the liver capsule in the process. For this purpose, most laparoscopic retractors have a mechanism to alter their configuration after being inserted into the abdominal cavity (e.g. articulating triangular retractor [Figure 3.24] and balloon retractor [Figure 3.25]), with the goal of increasing the contact area between the tissue and instrument and decreasing the pressure per unit area on the tissue. When retracting delicate tissue using a grasper or dissector, placing gauze between the tissue and forceps can help to increase friction for reliable retraction while decreasing the risk of tissue

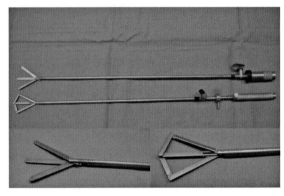

Figure 3.24 A laparoscopic retractor can alter the shape of tips from liner to triangular configuration.

injury. Gentle retraction to achieve the small working field is required for safe manipulation and decreases the risk of traction injury, particularly in a fragile steatotic liver. It is one of the advantages of laparoscopic surgery that even in a narrow working field, an excellent view is achieved and the procedure can be completed.

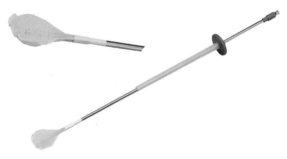

Figure 3.25 The Soft-wand balloon retractor (Gyrus ACMI, Maple Grove, USA) has an inflatable balloon covered with a mesh. The balloon is deployed through a trocar and inflated once inside the abdominal cavity to retract delicate tissue or organs such as the spleen and liver gently and effectively.

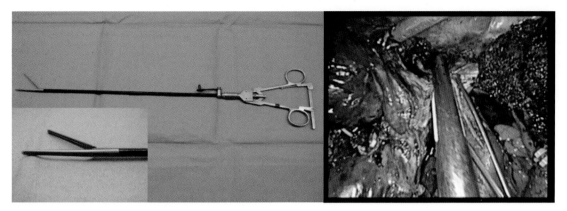

Figure 3.26 A laparoscopic vascular clamp with atraumatic tips of Debakey type (*left*) is used to manage bleeding and in case of inadvertent injury to large veins.

3.6.4 Vascular clamp

A vascular clamp is a forceps with atraumatic tips of Debakey forceps type (Figure 3.26, left). This is an essential instrument for laparoscopic HPB surgery because it can be crucial in controlling intraoperative bleeding. Once temporal hemostasis is achieved by clamping the vessel, the surgeon can reorganize the operative field, add ports, and find a way to obtain durable hemostasis. (e.g. coagulating, clipping, stapling, suturing or application of hemostatic agents). When dividing a major hepatic vein (left, right or middle hepatic vein), placing a vascular clamp within reach of the staple site (see Figure 3.26, right) to control bleeding from an inadvertent venous tear during stapling or malfunction of the stapler is recommended. Another use of the forceps is to temporarily occlude a portal pedicle to demarcate its feeding liver.

A vessel occlusion clamp (Bulldog clamp) is used to temporarily occlude vascular flow atraumatically for bleeding control or for vascular reconstruction (e.g. wedge resection of the portal vein). This endoscopic clamp is applied and removed intracorporeally using a special laparoscopic applicator.

3.6.5 Suction and irrigation

Suction is one of the instruments most frequently used during laparoscopic surgery. The instrument should be equipped with a mechanism to start and stop aspiration easily and quickly so that the surgeon avoids unnecessary aspiration of intra-abdominal gas to maintain pneumoperitoneum (Figure 3.27). Irrigation with water rather than normal saline can improve visualization of the operative field through lyzing of erythrocytes.

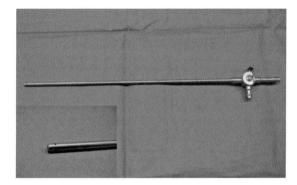

Figure 3.27 A suction instrument offers efficient aspiration of blood or body fluid while maintaining intra-abdominal pressure and pneumoperitoneum for organ exposure and hemostatic effect.

3.6.6 Needle holder and suture

Laparoscopic suturing is technically challenging but is an essential part of advanced HPB surgery. Suturing and ligation are performed during reconstructive procedures in laparoscopic HPB surgery (e.g. creation of gastrojejunal, hepaticojejunal or pancreatico-digestive tract anastomoses). However, it is also critical for the management of complications (e.g. closure of a bowel tear or a vascular injury) and may prevent conversion to open surgery in some cases. Safe management of complications during advanced HPB surgery or advanced reconstruction relies on mastering the challenge of intracorporeal suturing.

A variety of needle holder designs with several handle configurations is available, such as pistol, fingered or palm (Figure 3.28) grip, according to surgeon preference. Curved, straight, and grooved tips are available; the

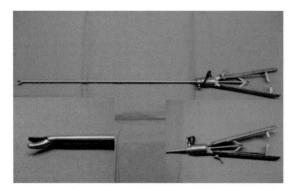

Figure 3.28 A needle holder with a palm grip.

grooved tip automatically orients the needle perpendicular to the needle holder, which facilitates the suturing process. JAiMY (EndoControl, Grenoble, France), a 5 mm motorized articulating laparoscopic needle holder (Figure 3.29), is designed to allow for greater flexibility of movement with increased degrees of freedom (flexion of the shaft and rotation of the jaw). Robotic systems have increased degrees of freedom of the arms and consequently enable more flexible instrumental movement which can facilitate creation of challenging anastomoses.

A pre-tied slip-knot prepared at the beginning of the case (Figure 3.30) saves time and effort in making the first knot intracorporeally, which is especially useful in achieving quick hemostasis in case of bleeding. Thus, several sets of needled sutures with a pre-tied knot can be prepared at the beginning of the case, as they are rapidly needed when hemorrhage occurs. Usually, a 20 cm suture equipped with nondetachable needle is used. A barbed suture is a

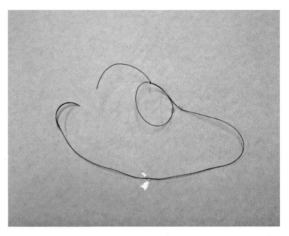

Figure 3.30 An extracorporeally pre-tied knot saves time and effort for making the first knot intracorporeally.

suture that does not require a knot at the end. The barbs on its surface penetrate the tissue and lock it into place, therefore eliminating the need for a knot. An Endoloop (Ethicon, New Jersey, USA) is a ready-to-use pretied ligation device with the disadvantage that only a limited number of suture types are available.

3.6.7 Surgical clip

Clips are used to occlude vessels or bile ducts prior to division to prevent bleeding or biliary leakage. Clips are made of titanium or polymer in a variety of clip sizes. Application of a clip to a vessel at a 90° angle with a sufficient length of vessel cuff can prevent clip slippage. Further, a polymer clip with a self-locking mechanism such as Hem-o-lok (Weck, Teleflex, Morrisville, USA) (Figure 3.31) is less likely to slip, and division can occur flush with the clip.

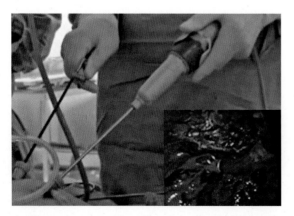

Figure 3.29 A motorized articulating laparoscopic needle holder.

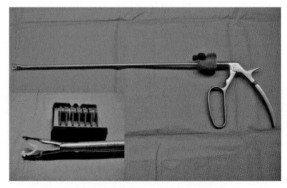

Figure 3.31 A polymer ligation clip with a self-locking mechanism is less likely to slip and seems to be more secure.

It is important to apply the proper clip size for the vessel diameter; applying a small clip to a thick vessel creates the risk of the clip opening because the force of the clip closing is increased beyond the design capacity of the clip. Applying too large a clip to too thin a vessel increases the risk of slippage as a result of low compression pressure. For the splenic artery, splenic vein, and other portal branches, 10 mm clips are generally applied.

Previously applied clips may interfere with the application of additional clips (e.g. clip on clip) or later stapling. A common problem in laparoscopic HPB surgery is clip slippage on small hepatic vein branches as the surgeon progresses further cranial with the caval dissection, accidentally knocking clips off the vessel. Therefore, some surgeons perform thermal sealing only on thin hepatic vein branches off the inferior vena cava.

3.7 Endoscopic stapler

Endoscopic linear staplers occupy an important position in laparoscopic HPB surgery. Secure hemostasis can be achieved or an anastomosis rapidly fashioned without the need for lengthy suturing (Figure 3.32). Linear staplers generate at least two rows (three rows in newer generation staplers) of staples on each side of the transected tissue. The staplers are loaded with disposable cartridges of various lengths (30–60 mm) containing staples of various heights (2.0–5.0 mm) for use in different tissue thicknesses. The major hepatic veins are commonly divided using a vascular load cartridge with staples of 2.0 or 2.5 mm in height which produce tissue compression to 0.75–1.0 mm. When dividing major hepatic veins at their origin, surgeons should be careful not to apply shear forces (especially pulling force) to the vessel during firing, to prevent vascular tears in a major hepatic vein or the inferior vena cava itself. Stabilization of the shaft of the stapler by an assistant can minimize shear forces during the stapling and division process. A thick portal pedicle and liver parenchyma (e.g. left lateral sectionectomy) can be divided using a cartridge with 2.5–3.5 mm staples. The pancreatic body and stomach can be transected using a cartridge with 3.5–4.8 mm staples. When using staples for dividing or anastomosing thick tissue, the tissue should be compressed between the jaws for more than 10 seconds to achieve proper tissue approximation for secure hemostasis or anastomosis.

Applying staples that are too long for thin tissue or too short for thick tissue carries a risk of bleeding as a result of insufficient tissue compression or tissue dehiscence due to improper interlock.

3.8 Tissue removal bag

A tissue bag is used for removal of specimens, to prevent spillage of tumor cells or infected tissue, and to decrease the risk of tumor implantation or surgical site infection.

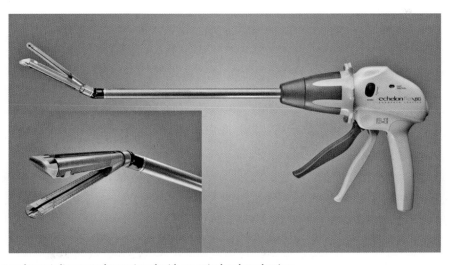

Figure 3.32 An endoscopic linear stapler equipped with an articulated mechanism.

The bag is inserted through a port site and removed through a suprapubic incision or enlarged port incision. Small specimens can be removed in the bag through a 12 mm port.

3.9 Hemostatic agent

In minimally invasive liver surgery, prevention of bleeding through meticulous dissection and pre-emptive identification of vascular structures are critical. However, once a vascular injury and consequent bleeding occur, local compression with gauze introduced into the abdominal cavity can allow the anesthesia team to prepare for further blood loss and bring devices for permanent hemostasis (bipolar cautery, vascular clamp, endoscopic clip or stapler) to the site without excessive blood loss. The adjunctive use of topical hemostatic agents promotes hemostasis and enhances coagulation.

Moderate bleeding can be stopped by applying Surgicel Fibrillar (Ethicon, New Jersey, USA) (oxidized regenerated cellulose) and compression to the bleeding site (Figure 3.33, left). Even if simple compression is not sufficient to completely stop bleeding, it may slow it down and allow the surgeon to remove blood from the operative field for a brighter video image and for further blood loss to occur without obstructing the view of the injury. Temporizing measures allow identification of the bleeding site and consideration of a strategy for definitive hemostasis.

TachoSil (Nycomed, Zurich, Switzerland), a biologically active agent, is composed of a collagen sponge coated with human fibrinogen and thrombin, and it can be used for achieving secure hemostasis (see Figure 3.33, right) [13]. Liquid fibrin sealant is also used to stop diffuse bleeding from the liver transection surface. However, when applying the fibrin sealant via a gas-charged applicator, development of air or gas embolism can be a concern [14].

When compression of the bleeding area with a sponge or laparoscopic instruments is insufficient, direct compression by the surgeon's hand via conversion to a hand-assisted or open approach must be performed. Nevertheless, rapid conversion during hepatic vein bleeding in a patient with low central venous pressure can lead to fatal air embolism. Therefore, a significant amount of preparation to prevent bleeding and, when it occurs, techniques to control it should be in place to avoid rapid conversion in the case of major hepatic vein bleeding. In complex liver resections, inflow occlusion by temporarily clamping the hepatoduodenal ligament (Pringle maneuver) is another useful option to decrease the amount of bleeding from the liver transection surface (Figure 3.34). The pneumoperitoneum itself, however, provides a form of Pringle maneuver, and recently surgeons have experimented with raising the pneumoperitoneal pressure to 21 mmHg and higher to provide some form of inflow control during minimally invasive liver surgery.

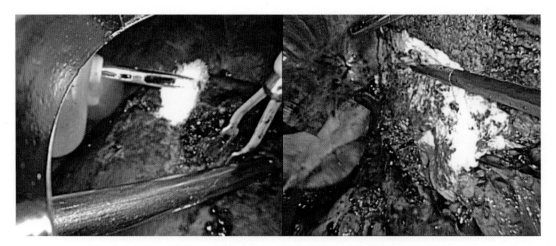

Figure 3.33 Surgicel (*left*) and TachoSil (*right*) are used to promote hemostasis and enhance coagulation.

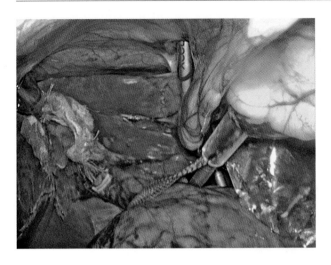

Figure 3.34 The hepatoduodenal ligament is taped for Pringle's maneuver in order to decrease the amount of bleeding during liver resection.

KEY POINTS

- Optimal positioning of laparoscopic monitors is essential to enhance procedural precision and speed as well as to reduce physical and mental stress on the surgical team. A dedicated minimally invasive surgery suite and special devices such as laparoscopic mounting devices and instrument stabilizers are helpful to maintain an optimal surgeon–equipment environment during advanced laparoscopic HPB procedures.

- Technological developments in imaging and electrosurgical devices greatly contribute to procedural safety and efficacy in laparoscopic HPB surgery. Up-to-date knowledge of new equipment and technologies is essential.

- Mastering laparoscopic suturing is a must for advanced minimally invasive HPB surgeons.

- Because of the possibility of significant blood loss during every laparoscopic HPB surgery, equipment, instruments, and agents for the management of intraoperative bleeding are crucial and should be prepared prior to commencing the case.

References

1 van Det MJ, Meijerink WJ, Hoff C, *et al.* Optimal ergonomics for laparoscopic surgery in minimally invasive surgery suites: a review and guidelines. Surg Endosc 2009; 23:1279–1285.

2 Gumbs AA, Crovari F, Vidal C, *et al.* Modified robotic light-weight endoscope (ViKY) validation in vivo in a porcine model. Surg Innov 2007; 14:261–264.

3 Ishizawa T, Zuker NB, Kokudo N, Gayet B. Positive and negative staining of hepatic segments by use of fluorescent imaging techniques during laparoscopic hepatectomy. Arch Surg 2012; 147:393–394.

4 Sutton PA, Awad S, Perkins AC, Lobo DN. Comparison of lateral thermal spread using monopolar and bipolar dia-thermy, the Harmonic Scalpel and the Ligasure. Br J Surg 2010; 97:428–433.

5 Hirokawa F, Hayashi M, Miyamoto Y, *et al.* A novel method using the VIO soft-coagulation system for liver resection. Surgery 2011; 149:438–444.

6 Scalzone R, Lopez-Ben S, Figueras J. How to transect the liver? A history lasting more than a century. Dig Surg 2012; 29:30–34.

7 Gayet B, Cavaliere D, Vibert E, *et al.* Totally laparoscopic right hepatectomy. Am J Surg 2007; 194:685–689.

8 Ishizawa T, Gumbs AA, Kokudo N, Gayet B. Laparoscopic segmentectomy of the liver: from segment I to VIII. Ann Surg 2012; 256:959–964.

9 Seehofer D, Mogl M, Boas-Knoop S, *et al.* Safety and efficacy of new integrated bipolar and ultrasonic scissors compared to conventional laparoscopic 5-mm sealing and cutting instruments. Surg Endosc 2012; 26:2541–2549.

10 De Jong KP, Wertenbroek MW. Liver resection combined with local ablation: where are the limits? Dig Surg 2011; 28:127–133.

11 Ikegami T, Shimada M, Imura S, *et al.* Argon gas embolism in the application of laparoscopic microwave coagulation therapy. J Hepatobiliary Pancreat Surg 2009; 16:394–398.

12 Takayama T, Makuuchi M, Kubota K, *et al.* Randomized comparison of ultrasonic vs clamp transection of the liver. Arch Surg 2001; 136:922–928.

13 Fischer L, Seiler CM, Broelsch CE, *et al.* Hemostatic efficacy of TachoSil in liver resection compared with argon beam coagulator treatment: an open, randomized, prospective, multicenter, parallel-group trial. Surgery 2011; 149:48–55.

14 Ebner FM, Paul A, Peters J, Hartmann M. Venous air embolism and intracardiac thrombus after pressurized fibrin glue during liver surgery. Br J Anaesth 2011; 106:180–182.

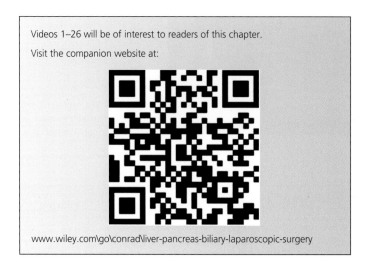

Videos 1–26 will be of interest to readers of this chapter.

Visit the companion website at:

www.wiley.com\go\conrad\liver-pancreas-biliary-laparoscopic-surgery

CHAPTER 4

Augmented reality for laparoscopic liver surgery

Kate Gavaghan, Matteo Fusaglia, Matthias Peterhans, and Stefan Weber

ARTORG Center for Biomedical Engineering Research, University of Bern, Bern, Switzerland

---

EDITOR COMMENT

This chapter is a glimpse into the future of advanced laparoscopic HPB surgery. The authors, expert engineers of augmented reality guidance solutions, describe the critical steps that lead to clinically applicable augmented reality. Augmented reality ultimately is the supplementation of a real-world view with aligned real-time computer-generated information. The challenges of this supplementation attributable to pre- or intraoperative data acquisition, creation of a selective augmented reality, image overlay, and tracking are shown. Issues specific to laparoscopic HPB surgery, such as liver deformation and display of depth information, are explained in detail. Further, the authors show how augmented reality has the potential to improve spatial understanding and the localization of underlying anatomy or tumors. Our own experience with augmented reality suggests that this chapter is important for those HPB surgeons who are looking to see where the field of advanced laparoscopic HPB surgery is headed.

Keywords: alignment, augmented reality, clinical application of augmented reality, image tracking, instrument tracking

---

4.1 Introduction

Despite its obvious benefits for patients, laparoscopic surgery presents multiple inherent challenges. The limited view of the two-dimensional (2D) laparoscopic image reduces depth perception and weakens spatial understanding, making localization of anatomy and prediction of surgical margins more difficult than in open surgery. Additionally, the lack of tactile feedback and the separation of visual feedback from the situs challenge the identification and manipulation of anatomical structures and greatly increase the required hand–eye coordination skills. Recent developments in high-resolution imaging and three-dimensional (3D) monitors have somewhat alleviated these problems but fail to provide a comprehensive solution.

In recent decades, advances in computing have resulted in an increase in the quality and quantity of information that needs to be processed during surgery. Advances in image processing techniques such as the fusion of multimodality imaging and structure segmentation have dramatically changed the way in which anatomy and target lesions are visualized; they have also changed the way in which surgeries are planned. The combination of medical image visualization techniques, preoperative planning, and surgical guidance has led to an increasing reliance on image guidance and computer assistance during a wide range of surgeries. While surgical guidance technologies were initially designed for use in surgeries on fixed anatomy such as neurosurgery, paranasal sinus surgery, and orthopedic surgery [1], solutions designed for soft tissue surgeries have recently become commercially available [2].

Surgeries can now be planned and visualized prior to surgery via 3D virtual representations of the patient anatomy and analyzed quantitatively using dedicated software. Measurements of volume, planning of resection margins, assessment of distances to anatomical structures, and functional parameters such as liver volumes can be evaluated preoperatively. This information can

---

Laparoscopic Liver, Pancreas, and Biliary Surgery, First Edition.
Edited by Claudius Conrad and Brice Gayet.
© 2017 John Wiley & Sons, Ltd. Published 2017 by John Wiley & Sons, Ltd.

then be used to determine surgical approaches that optimize clinical outcome and improve patient safety. Intraoperatively, stereotactic and image guidance technologies allow virtual surgical reality to be viewed interactively with precise capturing of surgical tools in 3D space. This information provides guidance beyond the mental representation traditionally relied on by surgeons.

Image guidance has the potential to alleviate many challenges currently facing laparoscopic surgeons. However, the display of increasing amounts of information in the operating room presents its own challenges. How shall we visualize information in a way that is useful, intuitive, and minimally distracting to the surgeon? Further, in laparoscopic surgery, where the surgeon relies on the operating monitor for visual input, the addition of new imaging information might draw the sight and attention away from potentially critical information being displayed via the traditional laparoscopic view (Figure 4.1).

Augmented reality (AR) enhances the surgeon's view by allowing additional information to be presented to the surgeon without the need for diversion of sight away from the patient. In this context, AR provides a useful solution to the fusion of multiple imaging sources, allowing laparoscopic surgery to benefit from the advantages of image guidance already offered in other surgical domains.

In this chapter, important concepts and principles of AR and image guidance for laparoscopic surgery are presented in detail. The purpose of AR and how it is achieved are discussed and recent live experiences with augmented reality laparoscopic hepatopancreatobiliary (HPB) surgery are reviewed. Finally, challenges pertaining to the realization of optimal AR solutions are described, along with a discussion of current research topics and a vision of the future role AR is likely to play in laparoscopic HBP surgery.

4.2 Augmented reality

Augmented reality is defined as the augmentation or supplementation of a real-world view with real-time computer-generated information that is registered to the real-world scene. AR gives the viewer an alternative perception of the depicted scene which encompasses real and virtual environments; this augments the classic view of the world and ensures additional feedback. Augmentation can utilize any sense; thus it can be delivered in the form of visual feedback, haptic feedback, or audial feedback. Historically, however, augmentation data have been displayed visually and, in the context of image-guided surgery, typically onto a monitor, using transparent layers or directly onto the patient surface using projection devices. Medical AR consists primarily of 3D reconstructions of physical objects (e.g. a virtual organ displayed onto the laparoscopic video stream) or textual or symbolic information (e.g. patient-specific information, geometric calculations or guidance for performing a particular procedure) overlaid at the same perspective as the scene of interest.

Three-dimensional anatomical representations allow structures of interest such as vessels and tumors to be viewed in an intuitive way, allowing the user to analyze

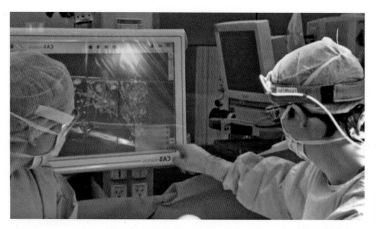
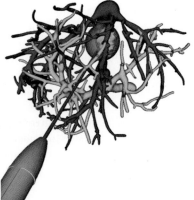

Figure 4.1 Surgical guidance data traditionally displayed on a monitor of other surgical domains are less suited to laparoscopic surgery because of the need for attention on a secondary monitor displaying laparoscopic images.

the preoperative information from different perspectives. This can reduce the mental effort required compared with classic computed tomography (CT) analysis. When used to augment the surgical view, the display also allows structures lying beneath the surface or out of the endoscopic field of view to be visualized, improving spatial awareness and aiding in structure localization. Augmented reality can also be used to overcome other challenges in laparoscopic surgery. For example, a surgeon might be able to compensate for the loss of depth perception with the laparoscopic image by overlaying computer-generated distance maps of specific structures of interest, or by sounding an alert when structures of interest are approached.

Using 3D anatomical reconstructions, surgical procedures can also be defined preoperatively in order to optimize surgical outcomes through, for instance, the maximization of preserved functional tissue or the removal of a sufficient resection margin. These plans can then be viewed interactively, relative to tool positions during procedures. Additionally, the display of anatomy or planned locations on the patient can aid in port placement or the labeling of structures and interactive task descriptions can be utilized as a powerful training tool during laparoscopic procedures.

The following sections present an overview of how these augmented views for laparoscopic surgery can be achieved and provide examples of their use during AR-guided laparoscopic procedures.

4.3 How is augmented reality achieved?

An augmented reality view of the surgical scene is composed of two primary components: the original or "real" view of the patient or surgical scene and an overlaid "virtual" scene. Optimally, the real view of the patient used in an augmented view would be the normal surgical view. Therefore, in laparoscopic surgery, the laparoscopic image projected by the operating camera is used. Based on this real scene, and using a virtual dataset, an augmented view is created. For example, virtual models of real anatomy, labels or interactive measurements can be created from medical imaging data. The next step is that the virtual data must be rendered at the same view as the real scene in order to align the two scenes. The alignment requires registration of the two datasets, and for automatic image alignment, calibration of the laparoscope in order to determine its view relative to its tracked position. Once aligned, the virtual data can be superimposed onto the real scene to create a single merged view. Finally, any dynamic components in the virtual scene must be tracked relative to the patient and updated in the virtual scene accordingly. The primary processes in the achievement of an augmented endoscopic view are depicted in Figure 4.2 and are discussed in more detail in the following sections.

4.3.1 Generation of virtual data

The virtual scene can be composed from a wide range of computer-generated data but is typically constructed from preoperative or intraoperative images. Such imagery often takes the form of virtual 3D reconstructions of anatomical structures of interest. While any 3D imaging modality providing sufficient contrast, resolution, and quality can be used for model construction, preoperative CT or magnetic resonance imaging (MRI) images are typically used.

Three-dimensional anatomical reconstructions can take one of two forms: a volume-rendered image or 3D surface models. While the former can be easily and automatically created by applying a color and opacity transfer function, 3D surface models provide an intuitive visualization of the patient anatomy and, through the definition of anatomical boundaries, allow for the automatic calculation of

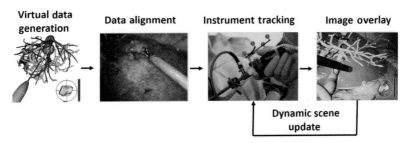

Figure 4.2 Overview of the primary steps required to create an augmented reality view.

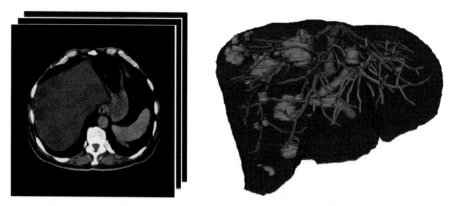

Figure 4.3 Three-dimensional anatomical surface models are created from the selection of anatomy in each image slice.

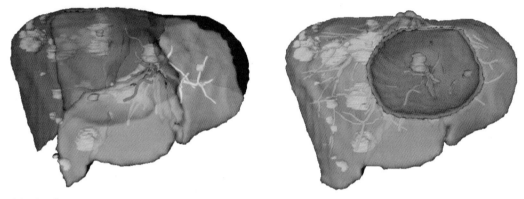

Figure 4.4 Virtual anatomical models of the liver, including organ surface, vascular structures, and tumors with liver segments and vascular supply (*left*) and the planned resection margin (*right*).

geometric parameters such as distances and volumes. Three-dimensional surface models of structures of interest, such as organ surfaces, vessels, and tumors, are created by identifying and separating the structures through each image slice in a process known as segmentation (Figure 4.3). Nevertheless, augmented reality is not restricted to anatomical models. Functional information such as liver segments and vascular supply can also be modeled from image data and included in the virtual scene. Additionally, surgical plans incorporating information such as safe resection margins can also be fitted onto generated 3D models and included in the augmented view for intra-operative guidance (Figure 4.4).

4.3.2 Data alignment

Accurately aligning the virtual scene with the real scene is the primary challenge pertaining to the creation of an augmented reality view during surgery. As the real view changes, or as objects of interest within the real scene change their position, the virtual scene must be updated, realigned, and displayed faster than the eye can detect.

The most basic method of data alignment consists of manually transforming images of the virtual scene such that features within the virtual model align to those in the laparoscopic image. This technique, as employed by Marescaux *et al.* [3], requires the preoperatively defined virtual scene to be manually resized and oriented on a monitor to the view of the laparoscopic image according to features visible in both views. Such a technique can be performed with basic technology and is unaffected by organ motion. However, the need for an operator dedicated to image alignment and suitable devices on which the alignment can be performed decreases the feasibility of such a technique. Additionally, the accuracy of this method is highly dependent on the user's ability to align the image correctly at a speed corresponding to the movement of the laparoscope.

Alternatively, data alignment can be performed automatically by employing an external position measurement system to track the position of the laparoscope and surgical instruments relative to the patient within a common coordinate system. Determining the position of the patient anatomy relative to the virtual model can be achieved via a process performed commonly in image-guided surgery known as "patient-to-image registration." The process can be performed at the commencement of the procedure and if necessary at intervals throughout the procedure (e.g. after significant organ movement). The process results in an adaption of the virtual scene (homogeneous transformation) to the coordinate systems of the patient. After registration, the transformation can be applied throughout the procedure to align virtual and real data within a single coordinate system. Registering the patient to the image via an external tracking system also allows the position of the tracked laparoscope and laparoscopic instruments to be registered and displayed within the virtual scene.

While alternative methods of patient-to-image registration exist [4], the majority of image guidance systems utilize a form of registration that determines the best fit transformation between the patient and the image data by minimizing the error between the locations of three or more corresponding features (Figure 4.5). Such features can consist of any object visible in both the real and virtual scenes. Often anatomical structures or landmarks such as the falciform ligament or the hepatic vein are used, but artificial objects positioned specifically for the registration process, known as fiducials, can also be utilized. While the latter are often more easily identified in image data, they can be difficult to place, and they are thus less effective in the registration of anatomy during HPB laparoscopic interventions.

The positions of features are typically selected in the virtual scene by the user via a touch screen or input device (e.g. a computer mouse), and the corresponding point on the patient is recorded by a position measurement system while the surgeon points at the location with a tracked laparoscopic instrument. From the corresponding point pairs, the registration transformation can be calculated using a least squares fitting algorithm.

While not indicative of the absolute accuracy, the use of a matching algorithm allows a measure of the alignment error to be expressed as the mean error between registered landmark sets (i.e. fiducial registration error – FRE). This value can be used as an indication of the level of accuracy of the registration and therefore indicates when a registration should be repeated.

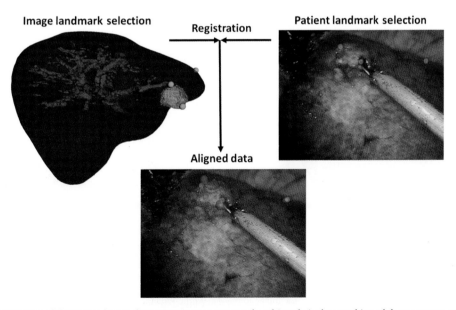

Figure 4.5 Registration of the image data to the patient is most commonly achieved via the matching of three or more corresponding features in both the real and virtual scenes in a process termed registration.

In order to provide better registration accuracy of moveable structures, virtual data may be generated from intraoperative imaging modalities, such as ultrasound, which then may be continuously registered to the real organ using internal landmarks such as vessel structures. This technique, described by Konishi *et al.* [5], is less commonly employed because of the difficulty of generating virtual registered data at sufficient quality and speed.

4.3.3 Laparoscope image calibration

Tracking the 3D position of the laparoscope facilitates automatic alignment of the data throughout the procedure. While the position measurement system can track the position and orientation (pose) of a marker attached to the laparoscope, the relation between the tracked pose and the view of the laparoscope camera must be determined via a calibration process. Calibration is achieved by using camera calibration techniques which, using captured images of a known pattern at a known position in space, determine the transformation between each laparoscopic image pixel and the real world [6]. Calibration is performed intraoperatively after the application of tracking markers and by using semiautomatic techniques; it can be performed in less than one minute (Figure 4.6).

Utilizing the tracked position of the laparoscope, the calibration of the laparoscope's pose and view, and the patient-to-image registration transformation, the preoperative 3D virtual model can be automatically rendered at the same point of view as the laparoscope and can subsequently be overlaid on the laparoscopic image (according to the transformation chain depicted in Figure 4.6). This method can adjust for movements of the laparoscope automatically at a speed greater than 20 Hz and does not require additional staff.

4.3.4 Instrument tracking

To maintain a correct alignment and correct representation of the surgical scene during the procedure, any dynamic component within the visualized scenes, be it anatomy, tools or the laparoscopic view itself, must be tracked in space (Figure 4.7). If the position of the virtual scene is not updated at the same speed as the real scene, a delay error effect known as lag is experienced in the augmented view. The real-time tracking of instruments is often accomplished, as in traditional image-guided surgery, via an optical or electromagnetic tracking system that monitors the positions of specific markers (optical) or sensor coils (electromagnetic) attached to the surgical instruments. An in-depth description of tracking techniques and technologies for image-guided procedures is outside the scope of this chapter. Readers are instead directed to the comprehensive overviews provided by Cleary and Peters and Konishi *et al.* [1,5]. Alternatively, objects can be tracked directly within image data by identifying their position using

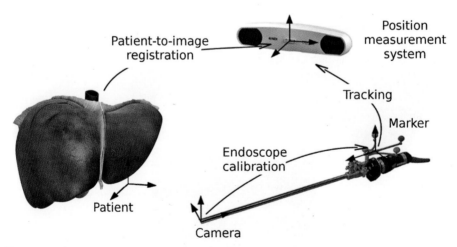

Figure 4.6 Calibration of a laparoscope. The relationship between the tracked marker and the laparoscopic images must be performed before a properly aligned AR view can be generated. Calibration is achieved by taking multiple images of a known pattern and determining the transformation from the image to the real world. Calibration devices such as this guide the calibration process and when combined with automatic calibration algorithms, allow calibration to be performed intraoperatively, quickly, and intuitively.

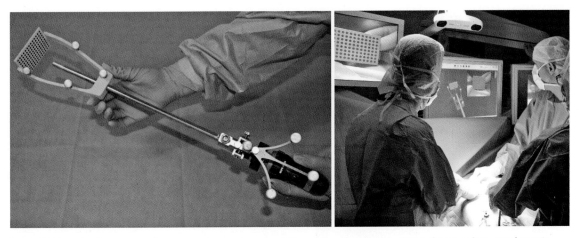

Figure 4.7 To maintain a correct alignment and correct representation of the surgical scene during the procedure, any dynamic components within the visualized scenes (e.g. anatomy, tools or the laparoscopic view itself) must be tracked in space.

image processing techniques. Although such techniques reduce the amount of external equipment required, the processing requirements increase significantly and tracking accuracy may be compromised.

4.3.5 Image overlay

Once the virtual scene is captured at the same view as the real patient, virtual data can be automatically merged with the real view. While virtual data promise to provide additional information to the operating surgeon, it is imperative that augmentation interferes minimally with the surgeon's laparoscopic view. Virtual data must possess sufficient contrast and clarity to be easily visible in the augmented view while not masking instruments or anatomy in the real patient view. Typically, virtual data are displayed in strong primary colors, in order to enhance contrast, while transparency is applied to ensure that information under the overlay can be seen. Additionally, functionality via a user interface that allows virtual models to be displayed or turned off ensures that augmentation is used only when needed.

Because of the introduction of an additional view in augmented reality, compared with the classic laparoscopic view, issues relating to visual depth perception or interference of laparoscopic instruments with the augmented view must be considered. This remains an unsolved challenge for developers of augmented reality systems (Figure 4.8). The created augmented laparoscopic image is most naturally displayed on a laparoscope monitor, although alternatives such as head-mounted

displays or projection directly onto the patient are possible. Direct projection onto the patient, while not requiring 3D models to be overlaid onto a 2D image, suffers from the parallax error which, owing to the projection of 3D virtual data onto a 2D viewing plane, causes the perception of the location of projected underlying anatomy to change with the viewing angle (see Figure 4.8). This effect is reduced for superficial anatomical structures and can be eliminated by deconstructing 3D information into 2D guidance information [7]. Anatomy or guidance can be projected onto the patient in a geometrically correct manner by employing a tracked projection device that can be calibrated using a method similar to that described for the calibration of a laparoscope [8].

4.4 Application of augmented reality for laparoscopic hepatopancreatobiliary surgery

The need to target underlying anatomical structures or lesions while preserving surrounding critical anatomical structures with few external navigation cues presents significant challenges in HPB surgery, particularly when liver surgery is performed by novice HPB surgeons. Visualization of the 3D surgical scene within a 2D laparoscopic image further increases the difficulty in determining target location and distance required for safe resection margins or anatomical structure preservation. These challenges

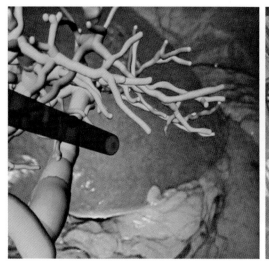 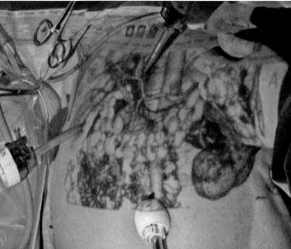

Figure 4.8 (*Left*) Endoscopic image overlay AR with virtual anatomical structures superimposed onto the endoscopic image and virtual tool model displayed within the virtual anatomy. (*Right*) Projection AR used with volume-rendered underlying anatomy displayed directly on the patient.

render HPB surgery an ideal candidate for AR visualization. Specifically, the resection of tumors buried within liver or pancreas parenchyma, located in tissue containing large vessels, may be significantly aided by the AR visualization of underlying anatomical structures, a surgical resection plane or distance information. Additionally, numerous HPB laparoscopic procedures require the mental representation of functional tissue regions such as liver segments. In such cases, the AR visualization of preoperatively determined segments can aid in anatomical understanding and reduce intraoperative cognitive workload.

Identified benefits of AR guidance for laparoscopic HPB surgery have led a number of groups to develop and clinically test AR systems. Although validation of the systems has been performed with only a small number of clinical cases, studies have proved the feasibility of the approaches and highlighted potential clinical applications. In this section, we review a number of AR systems that have been developed specifically for use in laparoscopic HPB surgery, demonstrating advantages and disadvantages of different AR approaches and exploring the breadth of clinical application within HPB laparoscopic surgery.

4.4.1 Head-mounted AR displays for laparoscopic surgery

In 2008, the concept of AR visualization for laparoscopic surgery was presented by Fuchs *et al.*, who described

direct visualization characteristics similar to those experienced during open surgery [9]. The development of a head-mounted display system for the visualization of a merged view of the real patient with synthetic images aimed at improving, first, the intuitiveness of the laparoscopic visualization and second, depth perception using cues superimposed on the laparoscopic image. Additionally, the head-mounted device widened the surgeon's range of view by displaying multiple laparoscopic imaging datasets. The proposed system suffered from delay in image generation and registration that was deemed unacceptable for clinical use. Despite these drawbacks, Fuchs *et al.* described the possible improvements in depth perception and field of view that could be achieved with AR for laparoscopic surgery. The group also proposed the use of registered preoperative images, surgical planning data, and intraoperative image data for the generation of a more comprehensive visualization of the operating field.

4.4.2 Laparoscopic image overlay AR for structure localization

A number of groups have attempted to overcome the problems of depth perception and spatial understanding experienced during laparoscopic HBP surgery by superimposing segmented anatomical models from imaging data onto the laparoscopic image. This technique enables underlying structures, normally hidden by overlying anatomy, to be visualized and localized. Using this method, pioneering work in the development and clinical use of an AR system for soft tissue laparoscopic procedures was conducted by Soler *et al.* [10]. By manually aligning preoperatively obtained semitransparent 3D models of tumors and vessels with intraoperative laparoscopic imaging, the authors reported more intuitive understanding of patient anatomy.

Similar AR viewing modalities were investigated by Konishi *et al.* [5]. They reported the use of a newly developed AR navigation system for laparoscopic surgery in which 3D ultrasound reconstructed models acquired by an operator and 3D models from preoperative CT were overlaid onto the laparoscopic view. The system was developed primarily for thoracic surgery but its evaluation during two liver procedures (radiofrequency thermal ablation for hepatoma and a partial hepatectomy) was also reported. In the two cases, the superimposition of ultrasound data increased understanding of spatial relationships between tumors and intrahepatic vessels, according to the authors.

The use of 3D reconstructed intraoperative ultrasound imaging, unlike models based on preoperative CT, allowed deformation and motion of the target organ to be incorporated into the virtual data. Registering the laparoscopic image to the intraoperative ultrasound data reduced discrepancies due to motion but required an additional electromagnetic tracking system in addition to the optical tracking system used for position detection of the laparoscope. The same group later continued with preoperative CT overlay, reporting six cases of pediatric laparoscopic splenectomy, specifically aiming at aiding understanding of anatomy in patients with anatomical anomalies. During a case of accessory spleen buried in fat tissue, the overlay helped with the localization of the splenic artery and vein and the pancreatic tail (Figure 4.9).

We report the use of an image guidance system for laparoscopic liver surgery during a portal vein ligation with in situ liver split procedure. An interactive view of the preoperative plan was displayed throughout the entire procedure on a touch monitor that enabled anatomy to be assessed from varying views (Figure 4.10). On a second monitor, an augmented view consisting of the laparoscopic image overlaid with 3D models of structures of interest, such as tumors, liver segments, and vascular structures, was displayed (Figure 4.11). Superimposed anatomical models suffered from a loss of depth perception relative to the laparoscopic image, and thus, to determine the relative position of deep-lying anatomy from the tool, a virtual model of the optically tracked instrument was included in the augmented view. Virtual

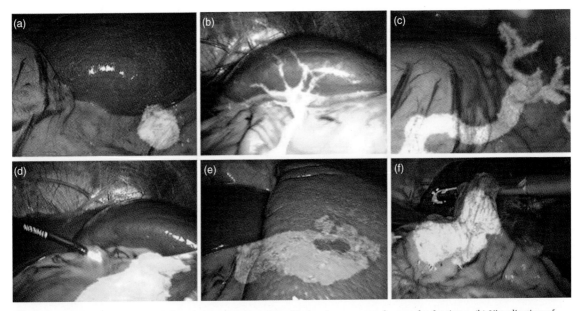

Figure 4.9 CT-based AR image-guided navigation. (a) Detection of isolated accessory spleen under fat tissue. (b) Visualization of splenic artery. (c) Visualization of splenic vein. (d) Visualization of pancreas. (e) Visualization of pancreas and vascular anatomy hidden under the large spleen. (f) Identification of pancreatic tail to protect it from injury during the stapling of the splenic vessels.

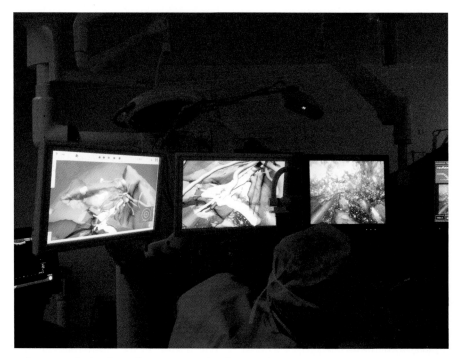

Figure 4.10 Virtual anatomy display alongside the augmented endoscopic display during a laparoscopic liver surgery.

anatomical models, segmented from preoperative CT images, were registered to the liver by selecting corresponding anatomical landmarks on the liver surface with the tracked tool. The laparoscope was calibrated prior to application using the automatic algorithm described in Fusaglia *et al.* [6]

This experience aimed to test the technological integration within a real-world surgical scenario and to evaluate a possible impact on the routine surgical workflow. The surgeons who evaluated the access to additional information noted benefits for anatomical structure and tumor localization. Based on this experiment, future

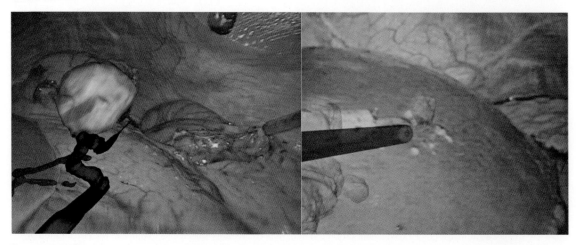

Figure 4.11 Endoscopic augmented view displayed during liver surgery with 3D models of vascular structures and tumor (*left*) and the virtual tool (*right*).

applications of our AR guidance system will include features that allow the display of distances from tracked tools to vascular structures, of liver segments, and encoding of depth information.

4.4.3 Console-integrated laparoscopic image overlay AR for robotic surgery

Advantages of robotic systems for minimally invasive surgery include a 3D view of the surgical field, instrument tremor reduction, better ergonomics, and the possibility of remote-controlled surgery. However, identification of deep structures and definition of spatial relationships are still a challenge. In order to compensate for these deficits, Buchs *et al.* reported the integration of the above described AR laparoscopic system with the da Vinci surgical console, and they employed this technology in two cases of hepatic lesion resection [11]. Patient-to-image registration was achieved by determining common anatomical landmarks between the virtual organ and the real liver, using the optically tracked robotic arm. Using two types of AR visualization (overlay of 3D anatomical models and a targeting guidance viewer), the operator was able to determine accurate surgical margins for tumor resections. The targeting guidance viewer, representing the real-time depth and lateral distance of a specific structure of interest (e.g. tumor) relative to the tip of a tracked instrument, provided depth information in a clear and measurable manner (Figure 4.12).

Although 3D models provide the general location of tumors, deconstructing position information into 2D guidance overcomes problems of depth perception, while enabling more accurate targeting. The author reported adequate resection margins and an increase in confidence during the resections.

4.4.4 Image overlay projection for structure localization and port placement

While AR for laparoscopic procedures finds its primary advantages in laparoscopic image overlay, projection-based overlay, in which virtual data are overlaid directly onto the patient's body, has also been investigated for use in laparoscopic procedures. For example, using a beamer attached over the operating table, Sugimoto *et al.* projected 3D reconstructed anatomy onto the patient's body during three cholecystectomies, two gastrectomies, and two colectomies [12] (Figure 4.13). By overlaying structures such as virtual cholangiography and surrounding vessels, they reported reduced operative times, reduced number of ports, and anticipation of structures such as the gallbladder and cystic ducts. A similar approach was reported by Volonté *et al.* [13]. The projection of computer-generated images allowed the adaptation of port placements (see Figure 4.6). Furthermore, the group suggested that projection of anatomical structures would assist inexperienced surgeons during port placement. While the image was only visually aligned to the patient without any formal registration and

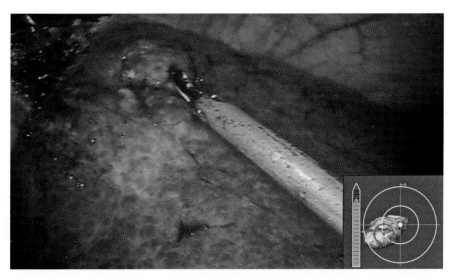

Figure 4.12 A targeting viewer superimposed onto the endoscopic image and displayed within the da Vinci console provides qualitative feedback regarding the relative position of the tool from a selected structure of interest such as the tumor shown here.

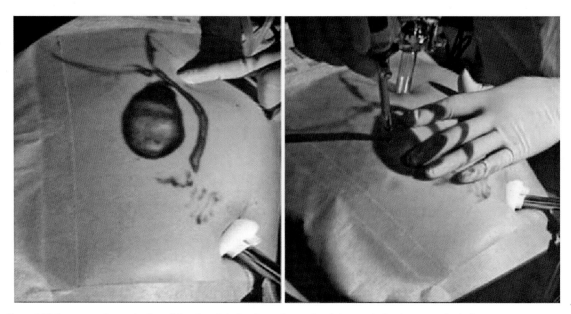

Figure 4.13 Image overlay projection of the virtual cholangiography on the abdomen during laparoscopic cholecystectomy.

tracking, incorporating registration and tracking methodologies such as those described for open liver surgery by Gavaghan *et al.* [8] would increase accuracy of the approach. As perception of the projection of underlying structures (especially deep-lying structures) is influenced by the angle of the viewer, the overlay of anatomy, without correction of viewing angle, can be used only as a relatively coarse guide. Alternatively, 2D rather than 3D surface projections of planned port positions could be projected onto the patient surface, allowing accurate AR guidance independent of viewer angle.

4.5 Challenges

Most reports on image guidance and AR for laparoscopic surgery have been positive, but AR technology and its application remain in their infancy. Initial clinical studies have highlighted possible usefulness, but they have also identified a number of challenges facing developers and users of AR technology. The two most prominent challenges, (i) organ movement and deformation, and (ii) effective visualization methods, are discussed below.

4.5.1 Organ motion and deformation
Obtaining an optimal alignment of the real and virtual scenes through registration, tracking, and image processing techniques remains one of the greatest challenges in the realization of AR in surgery. Any misalignment is considerably more evident and distracting in a merged scene than when additional data are displayed on a separate monitor. From a technological point of view, tracking of organ motion and deformation remains an unsolved challenge. Methods of nonrigid registration, typically based on the reconstruction of a 3D liver model from images of the organ surface, have been proposed, but technological limitations, such as computational power, result in inapplicability of these techniques in a real surgical scenario. Additionally, the relationship between surface deformation and the misplacement of internal structures is unknown.

Current image guidance systems for open liver surgery employ rigid registration techniques that function on the premise that registering a small local area of interest rigidly to preoperative data is sufficiently accurate. Studies support this hypothesis [14,15] and current research on registration of the liver is focusing on the possibility of increasing accuracy through the use of ultrasound imaging as the primary tool for registration. The use of tracked ultrasound allows for the creation of 3D volumes of the underlying vessels, which can then be used to align an internal volume of the liver with the surface models segmented from preoperative CT (Figure 4.14). The main advantage of this technique lies in the fact that

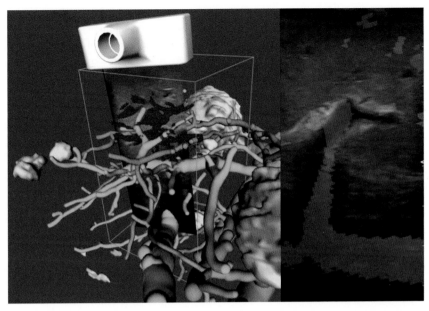

Figure 4.14 The guided acquisition of ultrasound images within a 3D volume allows vessels to be reconstructed and aligned to the preoperative CT surface models efficiently during surgery, improving registration accuracy in cases of organ deformation and movement. Source: Sugimoto *et al.* [12]. Reproduced with permission of Wiley.

detection of deeper structures ensures a more accurate alignment throughout the entire volume and allows the surgeon to repeat the alignment multiple times during the operation, thus adjusting for the deformation encountered during dissection. Such technology will be applied to laparoscopic liver surgery in the future, most likely utilizing electromagnetic tracking systems for position detection of the flexible ultrasound probe.

4.5.2 Visualization
Another fundamental challenge in the development and use of AR systems relates to data visualization. While AR eliminates the need for sight diversion, the display of additional information can potentially be misleading or disturbing during surgical procedures. Furthermore, depth encoding and visualization of deeper structures in a way that results in natural and coherent integration with the laparoscopic view has still not been addressed. Several different solutions have been proposed, such as the use of transparency and color depth coding or distance patterns [16], but few have found a place in a clinical scenario. Merging 3D surface models with a 2D laparoscopic image or projection of a 2D image onto the real-world 3D patient anatomy makes the achievement of realistic and understandable guidance challenging. For example, superimposition of a vascular structure onto the

laparoscopic image gives the perception of the structure floating in front of the image. The laparoscopic instrument is then visualized behind the superimposed structure in the laparoscopic image. Display of a virtual instrument allows the relationship of instrument with tissue to be visualized. However, the display of a 3D virtual instrument onto a real laparoscopic instrument can prove distracting (see Figure 4.8). For tasks in which contact between instrument and tissues is required, 2D guidance information such as that shown in Figure 4.12 may be more useful. Additionally, researchers are investigating the use of combined visual and audio feedback to overcome deficiencies experienced in purely visually augmented reality. For example, image overlay AR can be used to guide the surgeon's tool to the region of a structure, and sound can be used to indicate the distance from the tool to the structure as a structure of interest is approached.

4.6 The future of augmented reality for laparoscopic liver surgery

Despite the possible benefits of AR technologies for laparoscopic HPB procedures, quantitative clinical evaluations of their effectiveness are yet to be performed. To date, validation of AR systems for surgery has consisted primarily of feasibility studies conducted with a small number of clinical cases. Results are typically reported as subjective evaluations with little or no significant quantitative data. Evaluation of AR technologies in widespread and larger clinical trials would prove the advantages and disadvantages of the technology and aid in the development of existing systems. The general approach of AR for laparoscopic surgery has been successfully validated. Identifying applications for which AR can be most effective and developing dedicated systems for solving specific surgical challenges are the obvious next steps towards a successful integration of AR technologies into clinical routine.

Superimposed anatomical structures provide additional general information to the surgeon. Task-specific guidance, provided by image guidance systems in other surgical domains, such as needle guidance, resection margin calculations, distance or functional measurements, etc., has not been significantly explored for laparoscopic surgery. Therefore, AR applications that solve problems specific to laparoscopic surgeons must be developed. The development of features that aid in accomplishing specific tasks of laparoscopic HPB surgery may lead AR to transform from being something that is "nice to have" into an indispensable tool similar to image-guided systems in other surgical domains. The use of AR systems in laparoscopic surgeries as described in this chapter, although useful in some aspects of clinical practice, requires a significant amount of further research before the full potential of AR visualization can aid surgeons and ultimately patients.

From a technical perspective, AR technologies that provide optimal integration into the clinical workflow and a reliable level of accuracy are currently being investigated by a number of research groups. Devices and algorithms for automatic laparoscope calibration and methods of registration that more effectively address organ movement are currently being researched, and dedicated systems for AR guidance in laparoscopic liver surgery incorporating such functionalities are likely to become commercially available in the near future.

KEY POINTS

- Augmented reality is the supplementation of a real-world view with aligned real-time computer-generated information.

- Augmentation data can be created from preoperative or intraoperative images and can be superimposed onto laparoscopic images or projected directly onto the patient during HPB laparoscopic procedures.

- Augmented reality visualization for HPB laparoscopic surgery has the potential to improve spatial understanding and the localization of hidden underlying structures.

- Employing a position measurement system for instrument tracking allows augmented reality scenes to be updated in real time as the laparoscopic view changes.

- Challenges pertaining to the registration of deformable anatomy and to the display of depth information within augmentation data remain the primary focus for current research in laparoscopic augmented reality guidance solutions.

References

1 Cleary K, Peters TM. Image-guided interventions: technology review and clinical applications. Annu Rev Biomed Eng 2010; 12:119–142.

2 Peterhans M, Oliveira T, Banz V, Candinas D, Weber S. Computer-assisted liver surgery: clinical applications and technological trends. Crit Rev Biomed 2012:40:199–220.

3 Marescaux J, Rubino F, Arenas M, Mutter D, Soler L. Augmented-reality-assisted laparoscopic adrenalectomy. JAMA 2004; 292:2214–2215.

4 Peters TM. Image-guidance for surgical procedures. Phys Med Biol 2006; 51:R505–540.

5 Konishi K, Hashizume M, Nakamoto M, *et al.* Augmented reality navigation system for endoscopic surgery based on three-dimensional ultrasound and computed tomography: application to 20 clinical cases. Int Congr Ser 2005; 1281:537–542.

6 Fusaglia M, Gavaghan K, Beldi G, *et al.* Endoscopic image overlay for the targeting of hidden anatomy in laparoscopic visceral surgery. In: Augmented Environments for Computer-Assisted Interventions. Berlin: Springer, 2013.

7 Gavaghan K, Anderegg S, Peterhans M, Oliveira-Santos T, Weber S. Augmented reality image overlay projection for image guided open liver ablation of metastatic liver cancer. In: Augmented Environments for Computer-Assisted Interventions. Berlin: Springer, 2011, pp. 36–46.

8 Gavaghan K, Peterhans M, Oliveira-Santos T, Weber S. A portable image overlay projection device for computer-aided open liver surgery. IEEE Trans Biomed 2011; 58:1855–1864.

9 Fuchs H, State A, Yang H, *et al.* Optimizing a head-tracked stereo display system to guide hepatic tumor ablation. Stud Health Technol Inform 2008; 132:126–131.

10 Soler L, Nicolau S, Schmid J, *et al.* Virtual reality and augmented reality in digestive surgery. Presented at the Third IEEE and ACM International Symposium on Mixed and Augmented Reality, 2004, pp. 278–279.

11 Buchs N, Volonté F, Pugin F, *et al.* Augmented environments for the targeting of hepatic lesions during image-guided robotic liver surgery. J Surg Res 2013; 184(2):825–831.

12 Sugimoto M, Yasuda H, Koda K, *et al.* Image overlay navigation by markerless surface registration in gastrointestinal, hepatobiliary and pancreatic surgery. J Hepatobiliary Pancreat Sci 2010; 17:629–636.

13 Volonté, F, Pugin F, Bucher P, Sugimoto M, Ratib O, Morel P. Augmented reality and image overlay navigation with OsiriX in laparoscopic and robotic surgery: not only a matter of fashion. J Hepatobiliary Pancreat Sci 2011; 18: 506–509.

14 Schenk A, Zidowitz S, Bourquain H, *et al.* Clinical relevance of model based computer-assisted diagnosis and therapy. Proceedings of SPIE 6915, Medical Imaging 2008: Computer-Aided Diagnosis, 691502. doi: 10.1117/12.780270.

15 Peterhans M, Weber S. A navigation system for open liver surgery: design, workflow and first clinical applications. Int J Med Robotics Comput Assist Surg 2011; 7:7–16.

16 Hansen C, Wieferich J, Ritter F, Rieder C, Peitgen H. Illustrative visualization of 3D planning models for augmented reality in liver surgery. Int J Comput Assist Radiol Surg 2010; 2: 133–141.

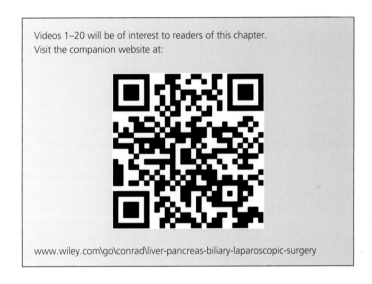

Videos 1–20 will be of interest to readers of this chapter. Visit the companion website at:

www.wiley.com\go\conrad\liver-pancreas-biliary-laparoscopic-surgery

CHAPTER 5

Imaging of hepatopancreatobiliary diseases

Motoyo Yano,[1] Hillary Shaw,[2] and Kathryn J. Fowler[1]

[1]Department of Radiology, Washington University School of Medicine, St Louis, USA
[2]Radia Inc., PS, Lynwood, USA

EDITOR COMMENT

In this important and practically written chapter, the authors detail important imaging modalities for HPB surgeons. The authors summarize the available imaging modalities and their complementary nature for the assessment of critical HPB lesions. Communication with the radiology team is crucial to determine the optimal imaging modality for each patient. This is especially true for minimally invasive HPB surgeons because of their greater reliance on imaging owing to reduced haptic feedback and the challenges of fully screening the liver with intraoperative ultrasound. MRI has the advantage of not using nephrotoxic contrast agents. Nevertheless, limitations for the use in patients with impaired renal function exist. Additional advantages of MRI are the ability to provide crucial information about lesion characteristics and underlying liver disease. Ultrasound is not only essential for intraoperative surgical planning; it is also an important screening modality for hepatocellular carcinoma in patients with chronic liver disease.

Keywords: computed tomography, focal liver lesions, imaging for hepatopancreatobiliary disease, imaging of liver disease, magnetic resonance imaging, nuclear imaging, ultrasound

---

5.1 Overview of available imaging modalities

There are various imaging modalities available for the evaluation of hepatopancreatobiliary (HPB) diseases, and each imaging modality has its strengths and weaknesses. Imaging modalities include ultrasound and Doppler, computed tomography (CT), magnetic resonance imaging (MRI), and nuclear medicine examinations. The best choice of imaging examination depends upon the clinical question, and examinations are often complementary. For example, if detailed anatomical information regarding the extent of vascular involvement by a pancreatic adenocarcinoma is desired, a CT or MRI would be the most appropriate imaging modality. On the other hand, the question of acute cholecystitis is best addressed with a right upper quadrant ultrasound. When the best choice of imaging is uncertain, consultation with the radiologist can help to develop a diagnostic plan (Table 5.1).

5.1.1 Ultrasound and Doppler

Ultrasound images are produced by the interaction of acoustic waves with tissues of varying densities. Acoustic waves propagate through tissues from the transducer applied to the patient, and the echoes that return to the transducer are processed into gray-scale images. Gray-scale images demonstrate structures in varying degrees of brightness, or echogenicity, based upon the degree to which the penetrated tissues attenuate the sound wave. Ultrasound can provide real-time anatomical information about the liver, bile ducts, and gallbladder. However, while ultrasound is ideal for assessing the liver, the pancreas can be difficult to evaluate because of the interposition of gas-containing bowel between the pancreas and abdominal wall; gas within the bowel impedes the transmission of acoustic waves. An advantage of ultrasound is the ability to assess vessels without the use of intravenous contrast. Doppler ultrasound generates color-scale images for evaluation of patency, flow direction, and flow velocity in

---

Laparoscopic Liver, Pancreas, and Biliary Surgery, First Edition.
Edited by Claudius Conrad and Brice Gayet.
© 2017 John Wiley & Sons, Ltd. Published 2017 by John Wiley & Sons, Ltd.

Table 5.1 Strengths and weaknesses of ultrasound, CT, and MRI.

Imaging modality	Strengths	Weaknesses
Ultrasound	Economical	Operator dependent
	Readily available	Limited spatial resolution and tissue characterization
	Doppler can assess vessel patency without need for intravenous contrast	Limitations due to obese body habitus
	No radiation	
Computed tomography	Widely available	Ionizing radiation
	Fast	Contrast media can be nephrotoxic
	Excellent spatial resolution	
	Multiphasic postcontrast imaging	
Magnetic resonance imaging	Excellent soft tissue contrast and characterization	Motion sensitive
		Not suitable for some patients (uncooperative, limited breath-holding, some implanted devices, claustrophobia)
	Multiphasic postcontrast imaging	Variable protocols and image quality between imaging centers
	No radiation	
	Contrast media not nephrotoxic	

vessels. Additional strengths of ultrasound include the lack of ionizing radiation, portability, low cost, and widespread availability [1].

There are some limitations to ultrasound. Image quality and detection of pathology are operator dependent (Figure 5.1). An ultrasound examination is a real-time interactive test during which the patient is asked to hold their breath and change position so that structures of interest can be optimally visualized. Ultrasound image quality may be limited by patient body habitus. Adipose tissue attenuates acoustic waves, limiting their ability to penetrate through the subcutaneous tissues of obese patients [2]. In the evaluation of the liver, hepatic steatosis also impedes the propagation of sound waves and makes detection of liver lesions more difficult [3]. Focal lesion detection in cirrhotic livers can also be more challenging as cirrhosis increases the echogenicity (brightness) and coarsens the echotexture of the liver [4].

Ultrasound in the intraoperative setting is crucial in the detection and localization of disease. It provides real-time high-resolution imaging which does not suffer from limitations of conventional sonography, such as large body habitus, since the transducer is placed directly on the organ/structure of interest [5]. For example, in the liver, lesions which were indeterminate preoperatively by CT or MRI can be further characterized by their sonographic features, with intraoperative ultrasound-guided biopsy for histological diagnosis. Intraoperative ultrasound not

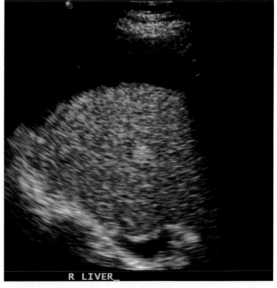

Figure 5.1 A 52-year-old man with ascites and cirrhosis secondary to hepatitis C. Annual screening ultrasound demonstrated increased echogenicity, coarsened echotexture, and surface nodularity consistent with cirrhosis. No lesions were initially identified by the sonographer. On further scanning by the radiologist, a hyperechoic liver lesion with a hypoechoic rim suspicious for hepatocellular carcinoma was identified in the dome of the liver on this transverse ultrasound image. This lesion demonstrated growth and features of hepatocellular carcinoma on follow-up MR examination (not shown).

infrequently identifies other unsuspected lesions in the liver [6]. Intraoperative ultrasound is similarly used in the identification of multifocal neuroendocrine tumors in the pancreas [7].

5.1.2 Computed tomography

Computed tomography examinations are commonplace and the modality is familiar to most physicians. Transaxial CT images are produced by attenuation of X-ray beams that rotate around the patient as the CT table advances the patient through the gantry in a single breath hold (new-generation scanners can acquire head-to-toe images in a matter of seconds). CT involves the use of ionizing radiation and frequently requires the use of iodinated intravenous contrast material to increase the sensitivity of the examination [8]. CT contrast agents can be nephrotoxic and generally should not be administered to patients in acute renal failure as there is an increased risk for contrast-induced nephrotoxicity [9]. In the setting of chronic renal failure, CT contrast can be administered and dialyzed. Patient reactions to CT contrast are commonly encountered and may necessitate either avoidance of contrast or premedication, depending on the severity of the reaction [10].

There are various CT imaging protocols which can be tailored to best answer a specific clinical question [11,12]. Variation in CT imaging technique is mostly related to phase of contrast for image acquisition, voltage, and section thickness [13]. Thin sections allow for improved multiplanar reconstructions of images acquired in the axial plane with minimal loss of resolution or blurring of the reconstructed image [14]. A routine contrast-enhanced abdomen CT is typically performed in the portal venous phase of contrast. For the purposes of assessing most HPB diseases, noncontrast CT is generally low yield, except to evaluate calcifications, to assess acute bleeding, or to evaluate enhancement in the setting of high attenuation material (such as hemorrhage or chemoembolization material). However, the precontrast phase is important and can help to identify areas of contrast enhancement amidst the high attenuation embolization material.

Evaluation of focal liver lesions should be performed with intravenous contrast using a dedicated liver protocol which consists of images acquired in the arterial, portal venous, and delayed phases [15]. The reason for these multiple phases of contrast in the liver relates to identification of classic enhancement patterns for distinguishing between lesions [16]. In the pancreas, lesion conspicuity is greatest in the late arterial phase (Figure 5.2). Additionally, thin section images are helpful for increased spatial resolution in pancreatic imaging to allow for detailed assessment of resectability [17,18]. The evaluation of the biliary tree is performed with both multiphase CT and thin section images [19]. Oral contrast is generally not necessary in the assessment of hepatopancreatobiliary disease; however, if there is concern for a duodenal mass or ampullary pathology, water administered by mouth while the patient is on the CT table can be helpful in distending the duodenum and improving visualization [20] (Table 5.2).

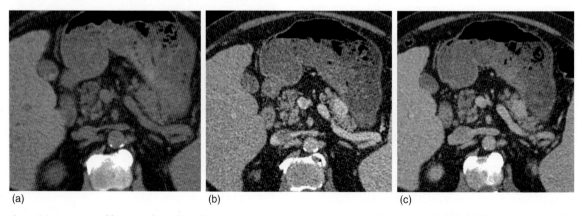

(a) (b) (c)

Figure 5.2 A 63-year-old man with incidentally discovered pancreatic lesion. Noncontrast (a), arterial (b), and venous (c) phases of the examination demonstrate arterially enhancing lesion in the pancreatic tail consistent with neuroendocrine tumor. Note the greater lesion conspicuity on the arterial phase images relative to the background normal pancreatic parenchyma.

Table 5.2 Phases of contrast used in typical CT protocols [11,15,21].

Region of interest		Non-con	Early art	Late art	Portal venous	Delayed
Abdomen					√	
Liver	Focal lesion characterization			√	√	√
	Post-TACE	√		√	√	
Bile ducts				√	√	
Pancreas		√		√	√	
Arteries		±	√			

TACE: transarterial chemoembolization; typically performed for hepatocellular carcinoma.

Non-con: noncontrast, prior to the infusion of intravenous contrast.

Early art: early arterial phase of contrast, approximately 25 sec after initiating contrast infusion. Bolus tracking is typically used with ROI placed in the descending aorta. This phase of contrast is helpful for arterial angiography (CT angiography).

Late art: late arterial phase which is approximately 35–45 sec after initiating contrast infusion. Usually results in enhancement of arteries and early opacification of the portal vein. This phase is adequate in assessing pertinent arterial vasculature.

Venous: this phase occurs approximately 60–80 sec after the start of contrast infusion.

Delayed: this phase refers to any phase of imaging beyond the venous phase, and the duration of delay is variable depending on the organ/structure of interest.

5.1.3 Magnetic resonance imaging

Magnetic resonance imaging utilizes magnetic fields and radiofrequency pulses to generate images that provide excellent soft tissue contrast [22]. MRI protocols are often customized to answer a specific clinical question. MR images can be obtained in any plane. While MRI entails no exposure to radiation, there is the possibility of tissue heating because of deposited energy. There are some patient populations, such as pregnant patients, in whom attempts are made to minimize sequences which in turn minimizes tissue heating (referred to as specific absorption rate – SAR) that occurs with MRI [23]. As with CT, postcontrast MR images are multiphasic, typically imaging during the late arterial, portal venous, equilibrium, and delayed phases. Some protocols which utilize contrast taken up by hepatocytes (hepatobiliary agents) call for delayed images, typically at one hour for gadobenate dimeglumine (Multihance) and 20–40 minutes for gadoxetic acid (Eovist).

Gadolinium intravenous contrast is required for full characterization of liver and pancreatic lesions. Gadolinium (in contrast to CT contrast media) is not nephrotoxic at clinically utilized doses and therefore will not have negative effects on glomerular filtration rate (GFR). While not nephrotoxic, gadolinium contrast agents have been linked to nephrogenic systemic fibrosis (NSF). NSF is a chronic, potentially fatal, systemic fibrosing disease highly associated with renal impairment and administration of gadolinium contrast [24]. The FDA has issued a black box warning against use of gadolinium contrast in the setting of severe renal disease. As a result, most imaging centers have enforced screening policies and GFR cut-off values which vary by institution. Pregnant patients are also generally imaged without gadolinium contrast, as gadolinium crosses the placenta and may remain indefinitely in the amniotic fluid, with unknown effects to the fetus [23].

Disadvantages of MRI include long exam times, approximately 30 minutes for an MRI of the abdomen, as well as the degradation of image quality by patient motion, both gross motion and inability to hold the breath. Some conditions such as severe ascites or large pleural effusions should be addressed prior to imaging to help improve the patient's ability to comply with breath-holding instructions.

Some patients may have contraindications to MR examination, such as presence of metallic shrapnel in the orbits or implantation of a non-MRI-compatible pacemaker/defibrillator. With the ever expanding list of new devices implanted in patients, dynamic online resources such as MRIsafety.com are valuable in determining the MR compatibility of devices [25].

5.1.4 Nuclear medicine

Nuclear medicine imaging differs from cross-sectional modalities in that these examinations provide metabolic and functional information, often fused with anatomical cross-sectional imaging. In nuclear scintigraphy examinations, the physiological uptake of intravenously administered radiopharmaceuticals is detected and imaged using a gamma camera. Many of these examinations require continuous patient imaging for greater than one hour and some examinations require patients to return for imaging at four hours and 24 hours, and even 48 hours after injection of radiopharmaceutical [26] (Table 5.3).

Cholescintigraphy is most often used in establishing the diagnosis of acute cholecystitis. While gallbladder sonography evaluates for secondary signs of gallbladder inflammation, hepatic iminodiacetic acid (HIDA) scans can determine functional obstruction of the cystic duct. The HIDA radiopharmaceutical is injected intravenously and is extracted by hepatocytes and excreted through the biliary system. In the setting of acute cholecystitis, there is obstruction of the cystic duct and the radiotracer fails to fill the gallbladder (Figure 5.3). Patients are required to be NPO for 3–4 hours prior to the exam, as a contracting gallbladder will prevent accumulation of tracer in the gallbladder. In patients who have been NPO for greater than 24 hours, a cholecystokinin (CCK) analogue is administered to contract and empty a full gallbladder,

which can prevent accumulation of radiotracer in the gallbladder. HIDA scans can also be performed for the evaluation of chronic acalculous cholecystitis in which gallbladder ejection fraction is compromised. Excretion of this agent can also be utilized to evaluate bile leak in the postoperative setting [27].

Some of the anatomical limitations of nuclear scintigraphy can be overcome with the simultaneous acquisition of CT images which allow for improved anatomical localization [26], such as the case with fluorodeoxyglucose (FDG) positron emission tomography (PET)/CT examinations. ^{18}F-FDG uptake occurs in metabolically active tissues, greater than background activity in many neoplasms and inflammatory conditions. Increased FDG uptake is seen with some hepatocellular carcinomas, cholangiocarcinomas, pancreatic adenocarcinomas, and many metastases to the liver. Some tumors, such as low-grade neuroendocrine tumors and mucinous adenocarcinomas from the gastrointestinal tract, are generally not FDG avid and cannot be detected with PET/CT [28]. Tumors that are less than 1 cm may also escape detection by PET/CT (Figure 5.4). False-positive results may be encountered secondary to local inflammatory reaction in the postoperative and postablation settings [28].

Heat-damaged red blood cell (RBC) scans will demonstrate uptake in splenic tissue. This exam is useful when accessory spleens and splenosis cause a diagnostic dilemma on CT and MRI. Depending on their location, these soft tissue deposits can be difficult to distinguish from neoplastic processes. A classic example is the identification

Table 5.3 Overview of common nuclear scintigraphy exams in HPB disease.

Nuclear scintigraphy exam	Common indications	Limitations
Cholescintigraphy (HIDA scan)	Acute cholecystitis Chronic acalculous cholecystitis Bile leak	False positives for acute cholecystitis with poor patient preparation
PET/CT	Detection of FDG-avid, hypermetabolic tumors and their distant metastases	Not all tumors are FDG avid FDG uptake by small lesions may not be detected Sensitivity of lesion detection may be limited in the postchemotherapy setting
Somatostatin receptor scintigraphy (octreoscan)	Neuroendocrine tumors (NETs) and their metastases	Not all NETs express the somatostatin receptor subtype 2 detected by octreoscan
Heat-damaged RBC	Identification of splenules, splenosis	

HIDA, hepatic iminodiacetic acid; HPB, hepatopancreatobiliary; FDG, fluorodeoxyglucose (^{18}F); PET/CT, positron emission tomography/computed tomography; RBC, red blood cell.

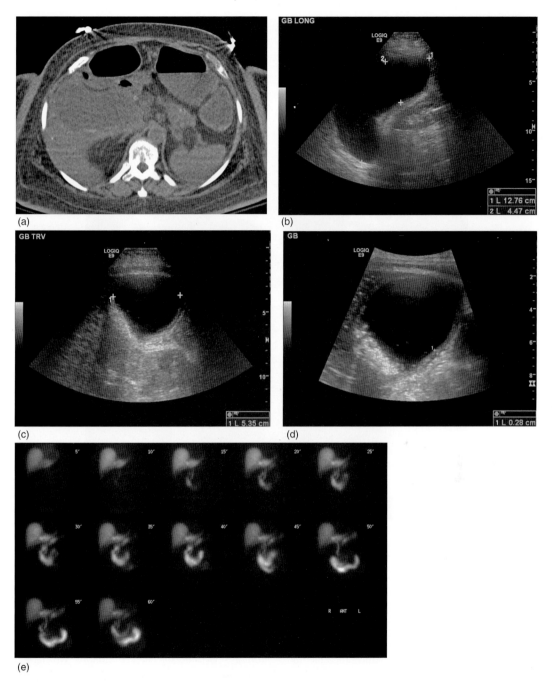

(a)

(b)

(c)

(d)

(e)

Figure 5.3 A 66-year-old woman with nausea, vomiting, and leukocytosis. Patient underwent noncontrast CT examination (a) in the emergency room, followed by right upper quadrant ultrasound, which both demonstrated gallbladder distention (b,c) and mild wall thickening (d). Sonographic Murphy's sign was negative. As a result of equivocal findings on ultrasound, patient underwent HIDA scan which failed to demonstrate radiotracer uptake within the gallbladder after one hour (e) and after administration of morphine (f). Failure to identify radiotracer uptake in the gallbladder is consistent with acute cholecystitis, in this case treated with cholecystostomy tube, as the patient was not a surgical candidate. For reference, a normal HIDA scan is shown, demonstrating tracer uptake in the gallbladder (g).

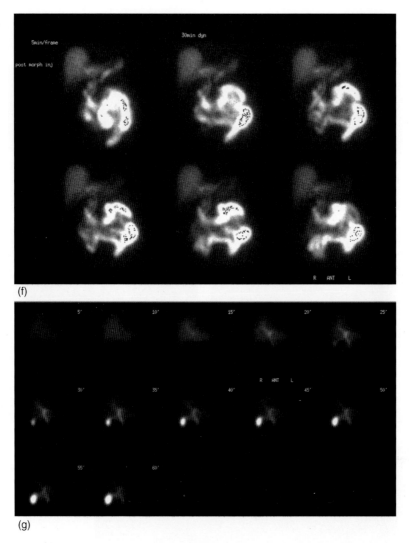

(f)

(g)

Figure 5.3 (*Continued*)

of a soft tissue nodule in the pancreatic tail prompting a differential diagnosis of a pancreatic neoplasm such as neuroendocrine tumor or an intrapancreatic splenule (Figure 5.5) [29]. Heat-damaged RBC scans are more sensitive and specific for splenic tissue than sulfur colloid scans, and they are the exam of choice [30,31] in this clinical scenario.

Somatostatin receptor scintigraphy utilizes ^{111}In-DTPA octreotide to detect tumors expressing somatostatin receptors. In HPB diseases, octreoscans are used in the detection of gastroenteropancreatic neuroendocrine tumors. Octreoscans detect tumors which express somatostatin receptor subtype 2, but not all neuroendocrine tumors express this subtype and therefore may fail to be detected [32,33]. Gallium 68-labeled somatostatin analogues for PET imaging, although less widely available, demonstrate greater lesion detection ability than somatostatin receptor scintigraphy [32].

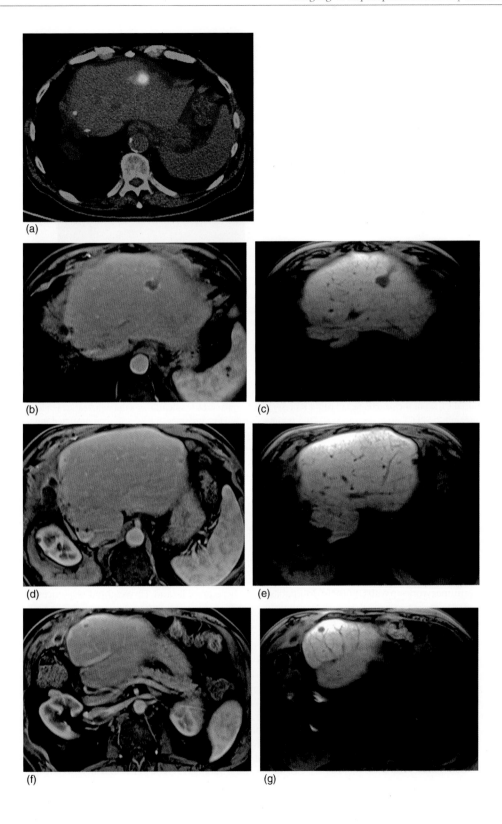

(a)

(b)   (c)

(d)   (e)

(f)   (g)

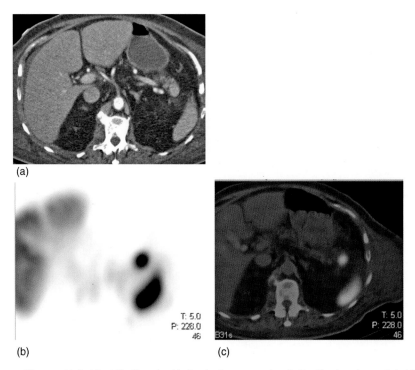

(a)

(b)   (c)

Figure 5.5 A 71-year-old man with incidentally discovered lesion in the pancreatic tail. Small enhancing nodule identified on contrast-enhanced CT (a) in the pancreatic tail could represent an intrapancreatic splenule or solid pancreatic neoplasm such as neuroendocrine tumor. SPECT (b) and fused SPECT/CT (c) images from a heat-damaged RBC scan demonstrated uptake within the nodule, diagnostic of intrapancreatic splenule.

5.2 Organ-specific imaging

5.2.1 Liver
5.2.1.1 Imaging options
Ultrasound is a useful screening modality, typically employed in the setting of hepatocellular carcinoma screening in at-risk patients with chronic liver disease. However, the imaging characteristics of focal lesions on US tend to be nonspecific, often requiring further work-up with CT or MRI. Multiphase contrast-enhanced CT [16] or MRI is the examination of choice for the characterization of focal liver lesions detected on ultrasound or portal venous phase CT [4,34].

5.2.1.2 MRI sequences, protocols, and contrast agents
Magnetic resonance imaging provides superior soft tissue contrast resolution and characterization of focal liver lesions [34,35]. While the large number of sequences can be intimidating to the nonradiologist, each MR sequence provides unique and complementary information about the tissue/lesion of interest. Generally speaking, there are T1- and T2-weighted sequences. T1-weighted images can provide information regarding fat content within the liver and also are the basis for postcontrast imaging. T2-weighted sequences are most useful for

Figure 5.4 A 75-year-old man with colon cancer status post resection developed colorectal metastases to the liver and underwent right hemihepatectomy. The postoperative course was complicated by abscess formation at the resection margin, with subsequent development of a fistula to the anterior abdominal wall (partially seen in (d) and (f)). On routine follow-up, the patient was found to have elevated carcinoembryonic antigen (CEA) levels, and PET/CT detected disease recurrence at the site of a previously ablated segment II lesion (a). Patient underwent Eovist-enhanced liver MRI the following week, with redemonstration of recurrence at the ablation site on arterial phase (b) and hepatobiliary phase (c) images. Note the linear hypointensity extending anteriorly from the lesion, representing the ablation tract. Eovist-enhanced MRI demonstrated two additional liver lesions, one in segment II measuring 12 mm (d,e) and a second in segment IVB measuring 14 mm (f,g). These surgically resected metastatic lesions were not detectable on PET/CT.

evaluation of fluid-containing structures such as cysts, bowel, biliary, and pancreatic ducts. MR sequences are packaged into MR protocols constructed to best characterize a lesion and answer a specific clinical question.

There are two basic types of gadolinium intravenous contrast agents available for MRI. They are classified by their biodistribution profiles into extracellular and hepatobiliary agents. Extracellular contrast agents are excreted through glomerular filtration while hepatobiliary agents have both renal and variable hepatobiliary excretion (5% for gadobenate dimeglumine [Multihance, Bracco Diagnostics] and 50% for gadoxetate disodium [Eovist, Bayer Healthcare Pharmaceuticals]) [36]. Standard gadolinium contrast agents are extracellular with enhancement of organs and lesions reflecting the biodistribution of contrast in the vascular and interstitial spaces. Enhancement patterns with these agents reflect differential vascularity of lesions relative to the hepatic parenchyma (tumors with neoangiogenesis tend to be hypervascular/hyperenhancing during the arterial phase relative to the liver). Enhancement of lesions with hepatobiliary agents reflects a combination of

the vascularity of lesions as well as differential uptake related to presence or absence of hepatocyte transporters. Eovist is taken up by a transporter expressed in normal hepatocytes but is not taken up by metastatic lesions, resulting in hypointense (dark) lesions on hepatobiliary phase images [37]. In contradistinction, focal nodular hyperplasia lesions express normal hepatocyte transporters and are iso- to hyperintense (similar to or brighter than) in comparison with the background liver on hepatobiliary phase images [38,39]. Use of a hepatobiliary contrast agent therefore may be advised when the differential diagnosis includes focal nodular hyperplasia.

5.2.1.3 Focal liver lesions

There are several benign liver lesions which have classic postcontrast imaging features on both CT and MRI [34]. Hemangiomas are the most common benign focal liver lesion. These lesions are classically described as demonstrating discontinuous, nodular, peripheral enhancement that gradually fills in on subsequent postcontrast phases (Figure 5.6). A characteristic feature of hemangiomas on MRI is

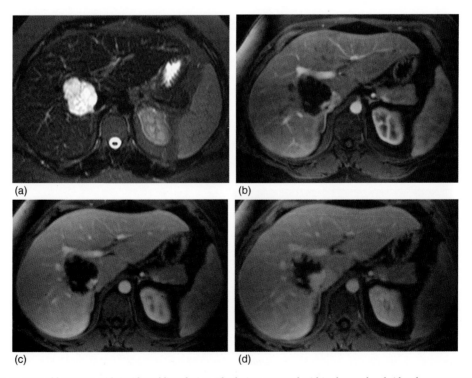

(a)   (b)

(c)   (d)

Figure 5.6 A 51-year-old woman with incidental liver lesion. The lesion centered within the caudate bridge demonstrates classic MR findings of hemangioma. On T2-weighted images (a), the mildly lobulated lesion is hyperintense. On T1 fat-saturated late arterial phase (b), the lesion is hypointense to liver and demonstrates discontinuous peripheral nodular enhancement, with progressive centripetal filling of contrast enhancement on the portal venous (c) and equilibrium (d) phase images.

"light bulb" bright T2 signal intensity. This can be a discriminating feature when compared with other lesions, like metastases, that show only intermediate T2 signal intensity. Focal nodular hyperplasia (FNH) is another benign lesion that has a characteristic appearance on MR and CT. Because FNH contains normal hepatocytes, it can be easily and confidently diagnosed with use of hepatobiliary contrast agents, such as Multihance and Eovist, because they retain contrast (appear bright) on the hepatobiliary phase images (Figure 5.7). Hepatocellular adenomas have variable

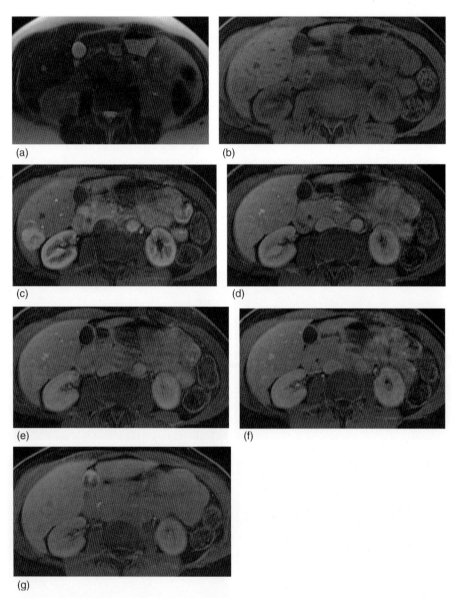

(a)

(b)

(c)

(d)

(e)

(f)

(g)

Figure 5.7 A 52-year-old woman with history of melanoma found to have a liver lesion on outside hospital CT exam. MRI of the liver demonstrates lesion in segment VI of the liver. This lesion is minimally hyperintense on T2 HASTE (a), hypointense on precontrast fat-saturated T1 sequences (b), demonstrates moderate arterial enhancement (c) which equilibrates on the portal venous (d) and equilibrium phase (e) images, without evidence of washout. The lesion demonstrates central enhancement on the five-minute delayed images (f), while the remainder of the lesion remains isointense to liver. This isointensity persists into the one-hour delayed images (g). These findings are classic for focal nodular hyperplasia.

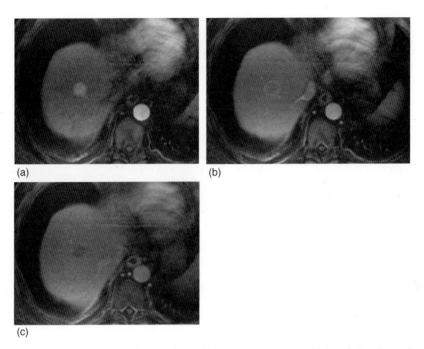

Figure 5.8 A 70-year-old man with alcoholic cirrhosis and portal hypertension presents with liver lesion detected on outside hospital imaging. MRI demonstrates liver lesion meeting imaging criteria for hepatocellular carcinoma. The round lesion within segment VIII demonstrates arterial enhancement (a), enhancing pseudocapsule on the portal venous phase (b) and washout on equilibrium phase (c) images.

appearance on MR and CT and may contain blood products from prior hemorrhage [40]. On MRI, these lesions may demonstrate intracellular lipid which is detectable on gradient echo in-phase and opposed-phase images. Hepatocellular adenomas can be suggested by imaging in the appropriate clinical context; however, the imaging appearance is not pathognomonic and follow-up or biopsy confirmation is often required.

Malignant liver lesions such as hepatocellular carcinoma, cholangiocarcinoma, and metastases can also be characterized by MR and CT. The most important discriminating feature for liver lesions is the enhancement pattern that they display. Hepatocellular carcinomas (HCC) usually occur in the setting of chronic liver disease and demonstrate arterial enhancement, washout, and delayed enhancing "capsule" (Figure 5.8) [41]. HCC may also demonstrate vascular invasion and tumor thrombus (Figure 5.9). Intrahepatic mass-forming cholangiocarcinomas demonstrate continuous peripheral enhancement and central delayed contrast enhancement, and they may show a peripheral thin rim of washout on delayed postcontrast images (Figure 5.10). These lesions are often associated with intrahepatic biliary duct dilatation when they occur centrally. They may

demonstrate capsular retraction when they occur in the periphery of the liver [42]. Metastases have variable appearances, often depending on the site of tumor origin [43]. Generally speaking, most metastases, including colorectal [44] (Figure 5.11; see also Figure 5.4) and pancreatic [45] adenocarcinomas, are hypovascular (enhance less than the background parenchyma). Metastases from primaries such as neuroendocrine tumor are hypervascular (enhance brighter than the background liver during the arterial phase) [46] (Table 5.4).

5.2.1.4 Diffuse liver disease

Diffuse liver disease, while not a surgical entity, is important in the presurgical planning of patients with focal liver lesions. Hepatic steatosis is commonly encountered and can be diagnosed by ultrasound, CT or MRI [47]. On ultrasound, there will be diffusely increased echogenicity of the liver when compared with the adjacent right kidney [3]. On CT, this manifests as diffusely low attenuation of the liver, diagnosed on noncontrast images when the liver is 10 Hounsfield units lower than the spleen [47].

Magnetic resonance imaging can quantitatively characterize steatosis and iron deposition. In-phase and

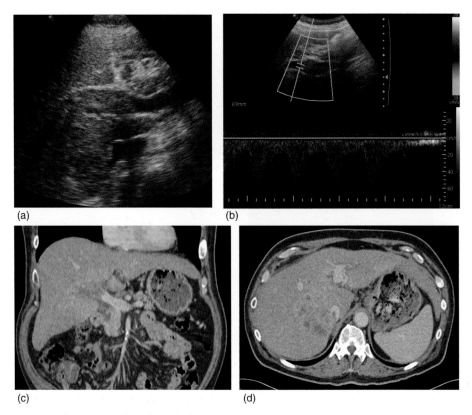

(a) (b)

(c) (d)

Figure 5.9 A 56-year-old man presenting with abdominal distension and pain was found to have an echogenic expansile mass in the main portal vein. Grayscale image of the right portal vein (a) demonstrates echogenic thrombus expanding the vein, contiguous with an ill-defined mass in the right hemiliver. Doppler interrogation of the portal venous waveform (b) fails to demonstrate normal portal venous flow but instead demonstrates arterial signal secondary to vascularized tumor thrombus. Correlative oblique coronal contrast-enhanced CT image (c) demonstrates infiltrative tumor thrombus within the main and right portal vein. Axial CT image (d) demonstrates contiguous infiltrative tumor in the right hemiliver, with tumor thrombus also invading the IVC.

opposed-phase gradient echo sequences take advantage of chemical shift artifact of fat and water protons. When the liver becomes darker on the opposed-phase images when compared with the in-phase images, this is referred to as "dropout" and indicates intravoxel lipid as seen with diffuse hepatic steatosis [48,49] (Figure 5.12). The degree of dropout can be quantified as a fat fraction or percentage of steatosis that has been shown to correlate with pathology [48]. Other diffuse processes that involve the liver, such as hemosiderosis, can also be detected. In contrast to dropout of hepatic steatosis, if the liver becomes darker on the in-phase image compared with the opposed-phase image, this reflects iron deposition in the liver [50] (Figure 5.13). The liver may also demonstrate abnormally increased T2 signal intensity (appear brighter) and show diffusion restriction in the setting of hepatitis and fibrosis.

5.2.2 Biliary

Several imaging modalities are available in the diagnostic work-up of biliary tract diseases, some of which are invasive. Noninvasive imaging modalities include CT, MRI with magnetic resonance cholangiopancreatography (MRCP), ultrasound, and cholescintigraphy. Invasive modalities include endoscopic retrograde cholangiopancreatography (ERCP) and percutaneous transhepatic cholangiography (PTC). These examinations are often complementary in the work-up of various biliary conditions (Table 5.5).

Intrahepatic biliary duct dilatation is readily detectable on US, CT, and MRCP/MRI. MRCP depicts the biliary tree in a noninvasive fashion (Figure 5.14) and has been shown to be superior to ultrasound in the detection of common bile duct stones [51,52]. It is useful in the evaluation of both benign and malignant entities of the biliary system, including biliary

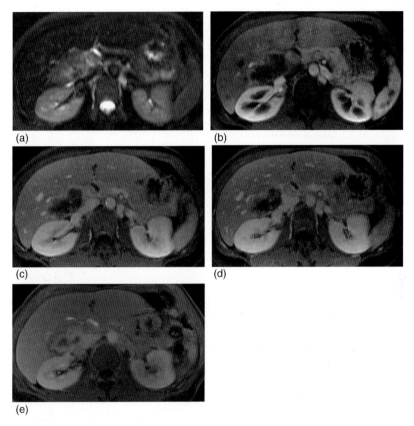

Figure 5.10 A 49-year-old woman with no significant past medical history presented with a several-month history of right upper quadrant discomfort. MRI was performed for further evaluation and demonstrated a large lobulated mass centered within the caudate bridge. This mass was T2 hyperintense (a) and demonstrated mild arterial enhancement (b), mostly in the periphery which demonstrates progressive centripetal enhancement on portal venous (c) and five-minute delayed (d) images. On the one-hour delayed images (e), the lesion demonstrates a thin rim of peripheral washout, a feature seen with cholangiocarcinoma and metastatic adenocarcinoma. Biopsy of the liver lesion demonstrated intrahepatic cholangiocarcinoma.

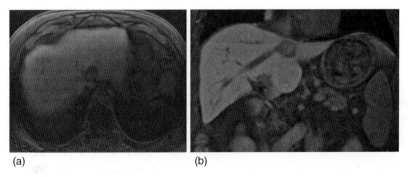

Figure 5.11 A 54-year-old man with previously resected colorectal cancer presents with new liver lesions. Liver MRI performed with Eovist contrast in the hepatobiliary phase (20 minutes post contrast) demonstrated two hypointense liver lesions, the larger of the two shown in the axial (a) and coronal (b) planes within segment II of the liver, abutting the left (a) and middle hepatic veins (b), as well as the IVC. Although surgical resection of the two liver lesions was planned, intraoperative evaluation revealed peritoneal implants, not visible on MR, consistent with metastatic disease. On palpation and intraoperative ultrasound, multiple other liver lesions suspicious for metastases were discovered and the planned surgery was aborted.

Table 5.4 Classic imaging appearance of select focal liver lesions.

Liver lesion	Contrast enhancement	Other findings
Hemangioma	Peripheral nodular contrast enhancement with centripetal fill-in of enhancement with time	T2 hyperintense ("light bulb" bright)
Focal nodular hyperplasia (FNH)	Early, avid arterial enhancement Isointense (stealthy) on later contrast phases Retention of hepatobiliary contrast agent	Isointense (stealthy) on T2 Central scar may enhance on delayed images
Hepatocellular adenoma	Variable	Typically T2 hyperintense May contain lipid May contain blood products
Hepatocellular carcinoma	Arterial enhancement with washout and delayed "capsule" appearance	Typically mild T2 hyperintensity May contain lipid May show vascular invasion
Intrahepatic cholangiocarcinoma	Peripheral arterial enhancement with gradual centripetal enhancement and peripheral rim of contrast "washout"	Typically mild T2 hyperintensity Capsular retraction Intrahepatic biliary duct dilatation

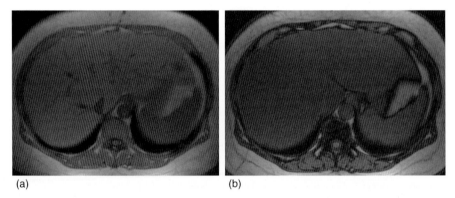

(a) (b)

Figure 5.12 A 49-year-old woman with diffuse hepatic steatosis. Gradient echo in-phase (a) and opposed-phase (b) MR images show decrease in liver signal intensity on the opposed-phase images compared with the in-phase images, consistent with diffuse hepatic steatosis.

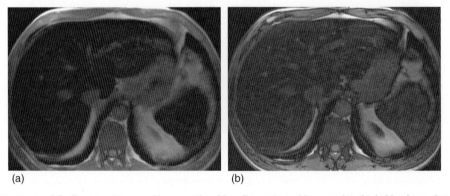

(a) (b)

Figure 5.13 MR images of the liver in a 41-year-old man with sickle cell anemia and history of multiple blood transfusions demonstrate greater loss of signal within the liver, spleen, and to a lesser extent the bone marrow on gradient echo in-phase (a) compared with opposed-phase (b) images consistent with iron deposition in the reticuloendothelial system in the setting of secondary hemosiderosis.

Table 5.5 Comparison of imaging modalities in the evaluation of biliary disease.

Imaging modality	Noninvasive	Strengths	Weaknesses
Computed tomography	√	Readily available Great spatial resolution/anatomical detail Intrahepatic and extrahepatic ductal dilatation well seen Radiodense cholelithiasis and choledocholithiasis may be seen	Cannot detect radiolucent biliary stones Not as sensitive as MRCP for subtle stricturing
Ultrasound	√	Assessment of sonographic Murphy's sign Identification of acute cholecystitis Identification of cholelithiasis and choledocholithiasis	Limitations by body habitus Distal CBD and much of pancreas can be difficult to visualize owing to bowel gas
MRI/MRCP	√	Comprehensive evaluation of biliary disease Strictures, masses, choledocholithiasis well evaluated Assessment of biliary tract in postbiliary-enteric anastomosis patients Eovist can be used to produce enhanced biliary imaging and assessment of bile leak	Eovist uptake and excretion may be impaired in setting of severe cholestasis or liver dysfunction
Cholescintigraphy	√	Assessment of physiology Detection of cystic duct obstruction in acute cholecystitis Detection of bile leak	Poor anatomical detail
ERCP		Detailed evaluation of biliary tree Potential for therapeutic intervention (balloon sweep/dilatation and stent placement) and duct brushings	Difficult in postbiliary-enteric anastomosis patients Limited ability to opacify ducts upstream from stricture Risk of post-ERCP pancreatitis/cholangitis
PTC		Evaluation of ducts upstream from level of obstruction Identification of isolated ducts in iatrogenic bile duct injuries Potential for therapeutic intervention (drainage catheter placement) and duct brushings	Risk of vascular injury and cholangitis

CBD, common bile duct; ERCP, endoscopic retrograde cholangiopancreatography; MRCP, magnetic resonance cholangiopancreatography; MRI, magnetic resonance imaging; PTC, percutaneous transhepatic cholangiography.

strictures, primary sclerosing cholangitis, and cholangiocarcinoma [53]. In the setting of suspected primary sclerosing cholangitis, MRCP performs well as an initial imaging test, which is often followed up with an ERCP [54]. There is a paucity of diagnostic accuracy studies comparing the performance of US, CT, and MRI in the evaluation of hilar cholangiocarcinoma [55] (Figure 5.15). Most studies have investigated the diagnostic performance of CT in staging cholangiocarcinoma, with an accuracy of 86% in determining ductal extent of tumor [55].

Endoscopic retrograde cholangiopancreatography and PTC both employ the common principle of injection of contrast directly into the biliary tree (Figure 5.16). Both of

these techniques are invasive and can yield highly detailed images of the bile ducts. ERCP is performed under sedation, with endoscopists cannulating the common bile duct or pancreatic duct and injecting contrast agent under force in a retrograde fashion. The advantage of this technique is the potential for intervention, such as balloon sweep of filling defect, balloon dilatation of strictures, and placement of decompressive stents upon identification of pathology. PTC involves percutaneous needle injection of contrast agent into the liver and not uncommonly involves multiple attempts to opacify an appropriate bile duct. This technique is useful in the evaluation of intrahepatic ductal dilatation, which may not be evaluated by ERCP owing to prior biliary

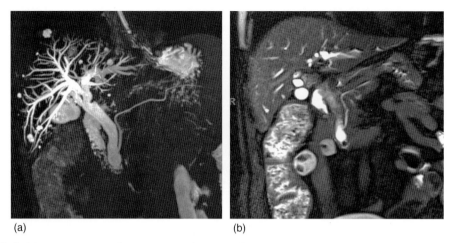

(a)   (b)

Figure 5.14 Thick slab MRCP image (a) demonstrates intrahepatic and extrahepatic biliary duct dilatation, the reason for which is not evident until examining the coronal T2 fat-saturated thin-slice image of the biliary tree (b). This reveals an obstructing stone in the distalmost common bile duct.

enteric surgery or high-grade stricture, or in the assessment of iatrogenic bile duct injury, especially when intervention such as placement of an internal/external biliary drain or U tube is a therapeutic necessity [56]. PTC and ERCP are typically performed after an initial assessment of the biliary tree with noninvasive cross-sectional imaging.

In the setting of suspected bile leak, usually from iatrogenic injury, several diagnostic imaging modalities are available. Patients are often first imaged by CT in the postoperative setting because of abdominal pain or liver function test abnormalities. This may reveal intraperitoneal or perihepatic fluid suspicious for biloma. The etiology of these fluid collections can be further evaluated by MRCP with Eovist hepatobiliary contrast agent [57] (Figure 5.17) or with a HIDA scan which will show extraluminal extravasation of excreted contrast or radiotracer, respectively. Hepatobiliary phase MRCP images may demonstrate the duct responsible for the biloma, but often ERCP and/or PTC are required for definitive identification and preoperative planning for repair.

5.2.3 Gallbladder
The gallbladder is affected by many benign entities as well as carcinoma and, rarely, metastatic disease. The most

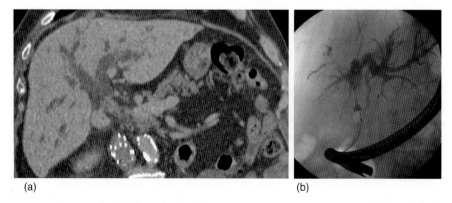

(a)   (b)

Figure 5.15 An 87-year-old man with multiple medical problems presented after his family noticed increased jaundice. CT examination with image in an oblique coronal reformatted plane (a) demonstrates enhancing intraductal mass within the common hepatic duct which causes intrahepatic biliary duct dilatation. This malignant stricture secondary to cholangiocarcinoma is confirmed on ERCP (b) with brushings. IVC filter is also noted.

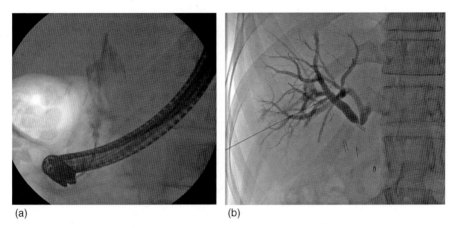

(a)   (b)

Figure 5.16 A 48-year-old woman with bile duct injury from laparoscopic cholecystectomy. Fluoroscopic spot image from ERCP demonstrates amorphous contrast extravasation upon cannulation and injection of the common bile duct (a) consistent with bile duct injury. Percutaneous transhepatic cholangiogram demonstrates opacification of the intrahepatic bile ducts on the right to the level of the confluence of the right and left hepatic ducts where surgical clips are present (b). Incidentally noted is variant biliary anatomy with right posterior sectional duct inserting on the left hepatic duct.

common symptomatic abnormality of the gallbladder is acute cholecystitis. The most appropriate imaging options for suspected acute cholecystitis are ultrasound or cholescintigraphy. Acute cholecystitis is typically manifest by gallbladder wall thickening, pericholecystic fluid, stones, and a positive sonographic Murphy's sign (tendernesss elicited by the ultrasound probe directly over the gallbladder). Two separate meta-analyses compared cholescintigraphy with ultrasound and found that ultrasound had a sensitivity of 81–88% and specificity of 80–83% and cholescintigraphy a sensitivity of 96–97% and specificity

of 90% [58,59]. Ultrasound is generally more easily accessible and avoids the need for radiation, making it a good choice for initial evaluation. Cholecscintigraphy may be used in the setting of equivocal ultrasound findings (see Figure 5.5).

In addition to acute cholecystitis, adenomyomatosis is a frequently encountered benign gallbladder process. This is often seen as an incidental imaging finding of focal wall thickening with characteristic cystic spaces on MRI or with classic comet tail artifact on ultrasound related to crystal formation within intramural mucosal diverticula

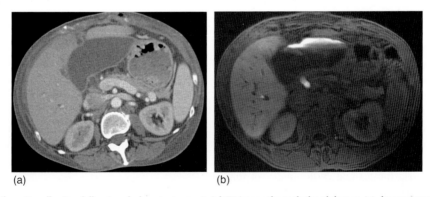

(a)   (b)

Figure 5.17 Perihepatic collection following cholecystectomy. Axial CT image through the abdomen (a) demonstrates large perihepatic fluid collection. Postcontrast axial MR image through the abdomen obtained 40 minutes after injection of Eovist intravenous contrast (b) demonstrates Eovist hepatobiliary contrast excretion through the bile duct layering in the nondependent portion of the perihepatic fluid collection, confirming that this fluid collection represents a biloma.

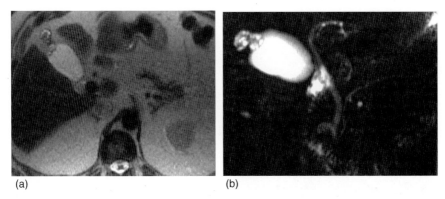

(a)   (b)

Figure 5.18 Adenomyomatosis. Axial T2-weighted MR image demonstrates luminal narrowing of the fundus of the gallbladder with thickened wall containing small T2 bright cystic spaces in the gallbladder wall which correspond to Rokitansky–Aschoff sinuses. These findings are consistent with fundal adenomyomatosis. The remainder of the gallbladder is normal. These same findings are redemonstrated on a thick slab MRCP image (b).

known as Rokitansky–Aschoff sinuses [60] (Figure 5.18). Adenomyomatosis is a benign process that has no malignant potential, and when the classic imaging features are present, no further work-up is required. The more focal mass-like presentation of adenomyomatosis may mimic malignancy and can be difficult to differentiate on preoperative imaging.

Gallbladder carcinoma has a poor prognosis and often presents with advanced disease. The most common imaging presentation is of a large intraluminal mass with invasion of the adjacent liver followed by the less common presentation of intraluminal polyp or diffuse/focal wall thickening [61]. No prospective studies have compared MR, CT, and PET/CT for preoperative staging. CT provides accurate information regarding liver involvement, nodal enlargement, and presence of distant metastases [62]. MR/MRCP may provide supplemental information regarding involvement of the bile duct in cancers that involve the gallbladder neck [63].

5.2.4 Pancreas
5.2.4.1 Cystic pancreatic lesions
Focal pancreatic lesions are best assessed by CT or MRI, and both modalities have similar diagnostic accuracy [64–66]. Although there are classic radiological appearances of solid tumors and cystic tumors of the pancreas, there may also be overlap in the imaging appearance of some cystic entities [65], and ultimately the lesions may require aspiration and analysis of fluid contents under endoscopic ultrasound [67,68].

Classically, a rim-enhancing peripancreatic cystic lesion containing nonenhancing debris, in the setting of prior pancreatitis, will represent a pseudocyst [69] (Figure 5.19a,b). This is in contradistinction to intrapancreatic cystic lesions, which in the setting of prior pancreatitis may represent walled-off necrosis. In the absence of prior pancreatitis, cystic lesions should raise concern for neoplasm. While there is considerable overlap in the imaging appearance of cystic lesions, there are some features that help to differentiate them [70]. A multilobulated, "sponge-like" lesion will represent a serous cystic neoplasm (Figure 5.19c,d). Intraductal papillary mucinous neoplasms (IPMN) will demonstrate communication with the pancreatic duct and may appear tubular or like a "cluster of grapes." A cystic lesion with a thick wall and no or only a few septations, usually in the body or tail of the pancreas, will represent a mucinous cystic neoplasm (Figure 5.19e). These features provide a general framework but there are exceptions such as the following: Some serous neoplasms may be oligocystic and mimic mucinous neoplasms. Neuroendocrine tumors can present with primarily cystic appearance. The communication with the pancreatic duct in the setting of IPMN may not be discernible on imaging. When there is doubt as to the diagnosis, endoscopic US with cytology and fluid sampling may be indicated.

5.2.4.2 Solid pancreatic lesions
Pancreatic adenocarcinomas account for the vast majority of pancreatic malignancies. These tumors are often infiltrative hypoenhancing masses which can occur in any

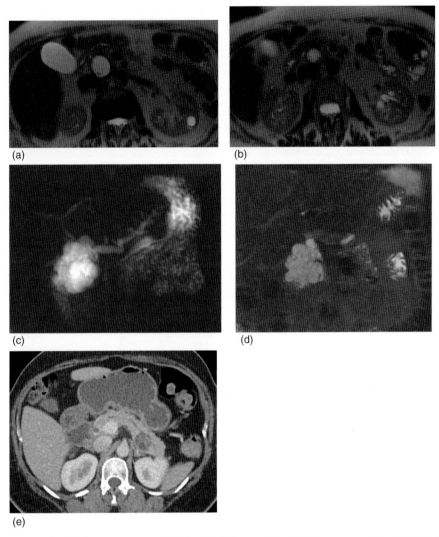

(a)

(b)

(c)

(d)

(e)

Figure 5.19 Classic examples of select cystic pancreatic lesions including pseudocyst (a,b), serous cystadenoma (c,d) and mucinous cystic neoplasm (e). Axial T2-weighted images through a T2 hyperintense cystic lesion in the pancreatic head (a,b) demonstrate T2 hypointense debris within the dependent portion of the lesion which did not demonstrate contrast enhancement, consistent with pseudocyst. Thick slab MRCP (c) and thin section T2 fat sat coronal (d) images demonstrate a large lobulated lesion in the pancreatic head which contains innumerable thin septations consistent with a serous cystadenoma, confirmed on EUS with fluid sampling. Axial CT image through the pancreatic tail (e) demonstrates a cystic lesion with several thick septations, confirmed as mucinous cystic neoplasm on aspiration and distal pancreatectomy.

portion of the pancreas and are equally well evaluated for potential surgical resection by CT and MRI [71]. These tumors classically produce pancreatic duct and/or common bile duct obstruction (Figure 5.20) and are locally advanced at presentation in about three quarters of patients [72]. Other solid lesions in the pancreas include neuroendocrine tumors which are usually distinguished from pancreatic adenocarcinoma by their hyperenhancement on arterial phase imaging. Other solid lesions to consider in the pancreas include solid pseudopapillary tumor, metastases, and lymphoma, in addition to mimics of tumor such as focal pancreatitis.

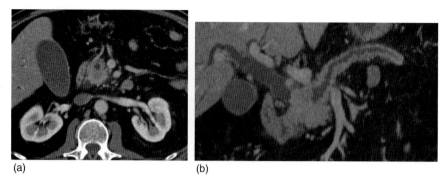

(a)   (b)

Figure 5.20 A 58-year-old man with right upper quadrant pain and elevated liver function tests. Axial arterial phase CT image through the pancreatic head demonstrates pancreatic and common bile duct dilatation secondary to ill-defined hypoenhancing mass in the pancreatic head. These findings are consistent with pancreatic adenocarcinoma with "double duct sign," better depicted on a curved multiplanar reformatted image (b). The patient underwent a successful Whipple procedure.

KEY POINTS

- Various imaging modalities are available for the assessment of HPB diseases, and modalities are often complementary. Discussion with the radiologist can help with determination of modality and customizing an examination, if necessary.

- CT contrast can be nephrotoxic and should generally not be administered to patients with acute renal failure; patients with end-stage renal disease on hemodialysis may receive contrast which can then be dialyzed.

- MR contrast agents are not nephrotoxic and generally can be administered to patients with eGFR greater than 30 mL/min. However, contrast administration policies vary by institution.

- While ultrasound is an acceptable modality for focal liver lesion screening in patients with chronic liver disease, the characterization of focal liver lesions is best performed with contrast-enhanced liver CT or MRI.

- Detailed anatomical information regarding HPB diseases is best achieved with CT or MRI, but nuclear scintigraphy examinations can provide valuable complementary physiological information.

References

1 Middleton WD, Kurtz AB, Hertzberg BS. Ultrasound. In: Thrall JH (ed.) Ultrasound: The Requisites. St Louis: Mosby; 2004.

2 Buckley O, Ward E, Ryan A, Colin W, Snow A, Torreggiani WC. European obesity and the radiology department. What can we do to help? Eur Radiol 2009; 19(2):298–309.

3 Konno K, Ishida H, Sato M, et al. Liver tumors in fatty liver: difficulty in ultrasonographic interpretation. Abdom Imag 2001; 26(5):487–491.

4 Di Martino M, de Filippis G, de Santis A, et al. Hepatocellular carcinoma in cirrhotic patients: prospective comparison of US, CT and MR imaging. Eur Radio 2013; 23(4):887–896.

5 Marcal LP, Patnana M, Bhosale P, Bedi DG. Intraoperative abdominal ultrasound in oncologic imaging. World J Radiol 2013; 5(3):51–60.

6 Kruskal JB, Kane RA. Intraoperative US of the liver: techniques and clinical applications. Radiographics 2006; 26(4):1067–1084.

7 D'Onofrio M, Vecchiato F, Faccioli N, Falconi M, Pozzi Mucelli R. Ultrasonography of the pancreas. 7. Intraoperative imaging. Abdom Imag 2007; 32(2):200–206.

8 Kamel IR, Liapi E, Fishman EK. Liver and biliary system: evaluation by multidetector CT. Radiol Clin North Am 2005; 43(6):977–997, vii.

9 ACR Manual on Contrast Media Version 9. 2013. Available at: www.acr.org/quality-safety/resources/contrast-manual (accessed 3 January 2016)

10 Cohan RH, Davenport MS, Dillman JR, et al. ACR Manual on Contrast Media Version 9. 2013. Available at: http://geiselmed.dartmouth.edu/radiology/pdf/ACR_manual.pdf (accessed 3 January 2016)

11 Johnson PT, Fishman EK. Routine use of precontrast and delayed acquisitions in abdominal CT: time for change. Abdom Imag 2013; 38(2):215–223.

12 Rengo M, Bellini D, de Cecco CN, et al. The optimal contrast media policy in CT of the liver. Part II: Clinical protocols. Acta Radiol 2011; 52(5):473–480.

13 Foley WD, Kerimoglu U. Abdominal MDCT: liver, pancreas, and biliary tract. Semin Ultrasound CT MR 2004; 25(2):122–144.

14 Maher MM, Kalra MK, Sahani DV, et al. Techniques, clinical applications and limitations of 3D reconstruction in CT of the abdomen. Korean J Radiol 2004; 5(1):55–67.

15 Oto A, Tamm EP, Szklaruk J. Multidetector row CT of the liver. Radiol Clin North Am 2005; 43(5):827–848, vii.

16 Van Leeuwen MS, Noordzij J, Feldberg MA, Hennipman AH, Doornewaard H. Focal liver lesions: characterization with triphasic spiral CT. Radiology 1996; 201(2):327–336.

17 Choi BI, Chung MJ, Han JK, Han MC, Yoon YB. Detection of pancreatic adenocarcinoma: relative value of arterial and late phases of spiral CT. Abdom Imag 1997; 22(2):199–203.

18 Takeshita K, Furui S, Takada K. Multidetector row helical CT of the pancreas: value of three-dimensional images, two-dimensional reformations, and contrast-enhanced multiphasic imaging. J Hepato-Biliary-Pancreatic Surg 2002; 9(5):576–582.

19 Kim HJ, Lee DH, Lim JW, Ko YT. Multidetector computed tomography in the preoperative workup of hilar cholangiocarcinoma. Acta Radiol 2009; 50(8):845–853.

20 Makarawo TP, Negussie E, Malde S, et al. Water as a contrast medium: a re-evaluation using the multidetector-row computed tomography. Am Surg 2013; 7 9(7):728–733.

21 Hammerstingl RM, Vogl TJ. Abdominal MDCT: protocols and contrast considerations. Eur Radiol 2005; 15(suppl 5):E78–90.

22 Bitar R, Leung G, Perng R, et al. MR pulse sequences: what every radiologist wants to know but is afraid to ask. Radiographics 2006; 26(2):513–537.

23 Wang PI, Chong ST, Kielar AZ, et al. Imaging of pregnant and lactating patients: part 1, evidence-based review and recommendations. Am J Roentgenol 2012; 198(4):778–784.

24 Kaewlai R, Abujudeh H. Nephrogenic systemic fibrosis. Am J Roentgenol 2012; 199(1):W17–23.

25 Shellock FG. Available from: http://mrisafety.com (accessed 17 December 2015).

26 Schillaci O, Filippi L, Danieli R, Simonetti G. Single-photon emission computed tomography/computed tomography in abdominal diseases. Semin Nucl Med 2007; 37(1):48–61.

27 Ziessman HA. Nuclear medicine hepatobiliary imaging. Clin Gastroenterol Hepatol 2010; 8(2):111–116.

28 De Gaetano AM, Rufini V, Castaldi P, et al. Clinical applications of (18)F-FDG PET in the management of hepatobiliary and pancreatic tumors. Abdom Imag 2012; 37(6):983–1003.

29 Kawamoto S, Johnson PT, Hall H, Cameron JL, Hruban RH, Fishman EK. Intrapancreatic accessory spleen: CT appearance and differential diagnosis. Abdom Imag 2012; 37(5):812–827.

30 Gunes I, Yilmazlar T, Sarikaya I, Akbunar T, Irgil C. Scintigraphic detection of splenosis: superiority of tomographic selective spleen scintigraphy. Clin Radiol 1994; 49(2):115–117.

31 Spencer LA, Spizarny DL, Williams TR. Imaging features of intrapancreatic accessory spleen. Br J Radiol 2010; 83(992):668–673.

32 Van Essen M, Sundin A, Krenning EP, Kwekkeboom DJ. Neuroendocrine tumours: the role of imaging for diagnosis and therapy. Nat Rev Endocrinol 2013.

33 Reubi JC, Waser B, Schaer JC, Laissue JA. Somatostatin receptor sst1-sst5 expression in normal and neoplastic human tissues using receptor autoradiography with subtype-selective ligands. Eur J Nucl Med 2001; 28(7):836–846.

34 Fowler KJ, Brown JJ, Narra VR. Magnetic resonance imaging of focal liver lesions: approach to imaging diagnosis. Hepatology 2011; 54(6):2227–2237.

35 Semelka RC, Martin DR, Balci C, Lance T. Focal liver lesions: comparison of dual-phase CT and multisequence multiplanar MR imaging including dynamic gadolinium enhancement. J Magn Reson Imag 2001; 13(3):397–401.

36 Lebedis C, Luna A, Soto JA. Use of magnetic resonance imaging contrast agents in the liver and biliary tract. Magn Reson Imag Clin North Am 2012; 20(4):715–737.

37 Zech CJ, Bartolozzi C, Bioulac-Sage P, et al. Consensus report of the Fifth International Forum for Liver MRI. Am J Roentgenol 2013; 201(1):97–107.

38 Grazioli L, Morana G, Federle MP, et al. Focal nodular hyperplasia: morphologic and functional information from MR imaging with gadobenate dimeglumine. Radiology 2001; 221(3):731–739.

39 Grazioli L, Bondioni MP, Haradome H, et al. Hepatocellular adenoma and focal nodular hyperplasia: value of gadoxetic acid-enhanced MR imaging in differential diagnosis. Radiology 2012; 262(2):520–529.

40 Grazioli L, Olivetti L, Mazza G, Bondioni MP. MR imaging of hepatocellular adenomas and differential diagnosis dilemma. Int J Hepatol 2013; 374170. http://dx.doi.org/10.1155/2013/374170

41 Fowler KJ, Karimova EJ, Arauz AR, et al. Validation of organ procurement and transplant network (OPTN)/united network for organ sharing (UNOS) criteria for imaging diagnosis of hepatocellular carcinoma. Transplantation 2013; 95(12):1506–1511.

42 Chung YE, Kim MJ, Park YN, et al. Varying appearances of cholangiocarcinoma: radiologic-pathologic correlation. Radiographics 2009; 29(3):683–700.

43 Kanematsu M, Kondo H, Goshima S, et al. Imaging liver metastases: review and update. Eur J Radiol 2006; 58(2):217–228.

44 Soyer P, Poccard M, Boudiaf M, et al. Detection of hypovascular hepatic metastases at triple-phase helical CT: sensitivity of phases and comparison with surgical and histopathologic findings. Radiology 2004; 231(2):413–420.

45 Motosugi U, Ichikawa T, Morisaka H, et al. Detection of pancreatic carcinoma and liver metastases with gadoxetic acid-enhanced MR imaging: comparison with contrast-enhanced multi-detector row CT. Radiology 2011; 260(2):446–453.

46 Kamaya A, Maturen KE, Tye GA, Liu YI, Parti NN, Desser TS. Hypervascular liver lesions. Semin Ultrasound CT MR 2009; 30(5):387–407.

47 Schwenzer NF, Springer F, Schraml C, Stefan N, Machann J, Schick F. Non-invasive assessment and quantification of liver steatosis by ultrasound, computed tomography and magnetic resonance. J Hepatol 2009; 51(3):433–445.

48 Reeder SB, Cruite I, Hamilton G, Sirlin CB. Quantitative assessment of liver fat with magnetic resonance imaging and spectroscopy. J Magn Reson Imag 2011; 34(4):729–749.

49 Ma X, Holalkere NS, Kambadakone RA, Mino-Kenudson M, Hahn PF, Sahani DV. Imaging-based quantification of hepatic fat: methods and clinical applications. Radiographics 2009; 29(5):1253–1277.

50 Merkle EM, Nelson RC. Dual gradient-echo in-phase and opposed-phase hepatic MR imaging: a useful tool for evaluating more than fatty infiltration or fatty sparing. Radiographics 2006; 26(5):1409–1418.

51 Varghese JC, Liddell RP, Farrell MA, Murray FE, Osborne DH, Lee MJ. Diagnostic accuracy of magnetic resonance cholangiopancreatography and ultrasound compared with direct cholangiography in the detection of choledocholithiasis. Clin Radiol 2000; 55(1):25–35.

52 Maurea S, Caleo O, Mollica C, et al. Comparative diagnostic evaluation with MR cholangiopancreatography, ultrasonography and CT in patients with pancreatobiliary disease. Radiol Med 2009; 114(3):390–402.

53 Bilgin M, Shaikh F, Semelka RC, Bilgin SS, Balci NC, Erdogan A. Magnetic resonance imaging of gallbladder and biliary system. Top Magn Reson Imag 2009; 20(1):31–42.

54 Weber C, Kuhlencordt R, Grotelueschen R, et al. Magnetic resonance cholangiopancreatography in the diagnosis of primary sclerosing cholangitis. Endoscopy 2008; 40(9):739–745.

55 Ruys AT, van Beem BE, Engelbrecht MR, Bipat S, Stoker J, van Gulik TM. Radiological staging in patients with hilar cholangiocarcinoma: a systematic review and meta-analysis. Br J Radiol 2012; 85(1017):1255–1262.

56 Thompson CM, Saad NE, Quazi RR, Darcy MD, Picus DD, Menias CO. Management of iatrogenic bile duct injuries: role of the interventional radiologist. Radiographics 2013; 33(1):117–134.

57 Marin D, Bova V, Agnello F, Youngblood R, Midiri M, Brancatelli G. Gadoxetate disodium-enhanced magnetic resonance cholangiography for the noninvasive detection of an active bile duct leak after laparoscopic cholecystectomy. J Comput Assist Tomogr 2010; 34(2):213–216.

58 Shea JA, Berlin JA, Escarce JJ, et al. Revised estimates of diagnostic test sensitivity and specificity in suspected biliary tract disease. Arch Intern Med 1994; 154(22):2573–2581.

59 Kiewiet JJ, Leeuwenburgh MM, Bipat S, Bossuyt PM, Stoker J, Boermeester MA. A systematic review and meta-analysis of diagnostic performance of imaging in acute cholecystitis. Radiology 2012; 264(3):708–720.

60 Stunell H, Buckley O, Geoghegan T, O'Brien J, Ward E, Torreggiani W. Imaging of adenomyomatosis of the gall bladder. J Med Imag Radiat Oncol 2008; 52(2):109–117.

61 Furlan A, Ferris JV, Hosseinzadeh K, Borhani AA. Gallbladder carcinoma update: multimodality imaging evaluation, staging, and treatment options. Am J Roentgenol 2008; 191 (5):1440–1447.

62 Kalra N, Suri S, Gupta R, et al. MDCT in the staging of gallbladder carcinoma. Am J Roentgenol 2006; 186(3):758–762.

63 Kim JH, Kim TK, Eun HW, et al. Preoperative evaluation of gallbladder carcinoma: efficacy of combined use of MR imaging, MR cholangiography, and contrast-enhanced dual-phase three-dimensional MR angiography. J Magn Reson Imag 2002; 16(6):676–684.

64 Lee HJ, Kim MJ, Choi JY, Hong HS, Kim KA. Relative accuracy of CT and MRI in the differentiation of benign from malignant pancreatic cystic lesions. Clin Radiol 2011; 66(4):315–321.

65 Sahani DV, Kambadakone A, Macari M, Takahashi N, Chari S, Fernandez-del Castillo C. Diagnosis and management of cystic pancreatic lesions. Am J Roentgenol 2013; 200(2):343–354.

66 Ichikawa T, Peterson MS, Federle MP, et al. Islet cell tumor of the pancreas: biphasic CT versus MR imaging in tumor detection. Radiology 2000; 216(1):163–171.

67 Rafique A, Freeman S, Carroll N. A clinical algorithm for the assessment of pancreatic lesions: utilization of 16- and 64-section multidetector CT and endoscopic ultrasound. Clin Radiol 2007; 62(12):1142–1153.

68 Khashab MA, Kim K, Lennon AM, et al. Should we do EUS/FNA on patients with pancreatic cysts? The incremental diagnostic yield of EUS over CT/MRI for prediction of cystic neoplasms. Pancreas 2013; 42(4):717–721.

69 Macari M, Finn ME, Bennett GL, et al. Differentiating pancreatic cystic neoplasms from pancreatic pseudocysts at MR imaging: value of perceived internal debris. Radiology 2009; 251(1):77–84.

70 Grieser C, Heine G, Stelter L, et al. Morphological analysis and differentiation of benign cystic neoplasms of the pancreas using computed tomography and magnetic resonance imaging. Rofo 2013; 185(3):219–227.

71 Park HS, Lee JM, Choi HK, Hong SH, Han JK, Choi BI. Preoperative evaluation of pancreatic cancer: comparison of gadolinium-enhanced dynamic MRI with MR cholangiopancreatography versus MDCT. J Magn Reson Imag 2009; 30(3):586–595.

72 Low G, Panu A, Millo N, Leen E. Multimodality imaging of neoplastic and nonneoplastic solid lesions of the pancreas. Radiographics 2011; 31(4):993–1015.

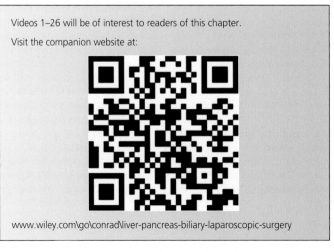

Videos 1–26 will be of interest to readers of this chapter.

Visit the companion website at:

www.wiley.com\go\conrad\liver-pancreas-biliary-laparoscopic-surgery

CHAPTER 6

Role of staging laparoscopy in hepatopancreatobiliary malignancies

Anil K. Agarwal, Raja Kalayarasan, and Amit Javed

Department of Gastrointestinal Surgery and Liver Transplant, Govind Ballabh Pant Hospital and Maulana Azad Medical College, Delhi University, New Delhi, India

EDITOR COMMENT

In this comprehensive chapter on staging laparoscopy for HPB diseases, the authors report the technique and respective evidence for performing staging laparoscopy, extended staging laparoscopy, and regional lymph node sampling to avoid non-therapeutic laparotomies. The chapter summarizes the available data for pancreatic cancer, intra- and extrahepatic biliary cancer, hepatocellular carcinoma, gallbladder cancer, and metastatic colorectal cancer. The value of including palliative biliary and enteric bypass in pancreatic cancer patients with positive staging laparoscopy is reviewed. Further, the technique and value of peritoneal lavage are shown and the optimal timing (prior to planned resection or as a separate procedure) is explored. The authors expand on how the yield of staging laparoscopy could be increased through optimal indications, performing regional lymph node sampling, and staging laparoscopic ultrasound.

Keywords: carcinomatosis, extended staging laparoscopy, minimally invasive lymph node staging, minimally invasive palliation, occult metastases, peritoneal lavage, staging laparoscopic ultrasound, staging laparoscopy, staging of hepatopancreatobiliary disease, timing of staging laparoscopy

The objective of preoperative evaluation for any malignancy, including pancreatic and hepatobiliary malignancy, is to identify patients who would benefit from surgical exploration and exclude those with metastatic or locally advanced unresectable disease. Despite significant advancements in imaging technology for preoperative assessment of accurate stage of pancreatic and hepatobiliary tumors, some patients with metastatic disease are not diagnosed preoperatively and are detected for the first time after surgical exploration, resulting in a nontherapeutic laparotomy. Staging laparoscopy (SL) is a minimally invasive tool that has conventionally been used to detect these radiologically occult metastatic diseases in various gastrointestinal malignancies to avoid unnecessary laparotomies [1,2]. Avoidance of a nontherapeutic laparotomy results in decreased morbidity related to the incision and the procedure, faster recovery, shorter hospital stay, and reduced time to initiation of chemotherapy/radiotherapy [1,2].

The concept of SL was introduced in the era when all definitive procedures were being performed by an open approach. Staging laparoscopy enabled direct visualization of the peritoneal cavity to detect small peritoneal and surface liver metastases which precluded a curative surgical resection. Over the years, there has been a significant change in the role of staging laparoscopy. On one hand, there have been significant improvements in cross-sectional imaging (computed tomography [CT] and magnetic resonance imaging [MRI]), widespread use of newer modalities like positron emission tomography (PET) scans, endoscopic ultrasound (EUS), and increasing role of tumor markers. This has led to increased

Laparoscopic Liver, Pancreas, and Biliary Surgery, First Edition.
Edited by Claudius Conrad and Brice Gayet.
© 2017 John Wiley & Sons, Ltd. Published 2017 by John Wiley & Sons, Ltd.

preoperative detection of metastatic disease with a resultant decrease in the overall yield of staging laparoscopy [3,4]. On the other hand, the procedure of SL itself has evolved and it is not just limited to the detection of radiologically occult metastases (like peritoneal and surface liver deposits). It is now often performed in conjunction with laparoscopic ultrasound (LUS) and has become a valuable tool in determining not just metastatic disease but also locoregional resectability of the tumor [5]. Additional dissection can be performed to better assess inaccessible areas, determine locoregional extent, and sample distant lymph nodes. In addition, it has gained a new role in the era of portal vein embolization and neoadjuvant treatment protocols for downstaging hepatopancreatobiliary tumors.

Widespread adoption of laparoscopy for tumor ablation (like radiofrequency ablation) and curative surgical resection has redefined the role of staging laparoscopy [6,7]. As more and more complex surgical resections for cancers are performed laparoscopically, SL has become an integral initial part of the procedure itself and its role is thus not limited to the avoidance of a nontherapeutic laparotomy. While newer techniques like PET scans have the potential to decrease the yield of SL, it may be associated with false-positive and -negative rates which would need further confirmation [8]. This chapter aims to highlight the current status of SL in the management of pancreatic and hepatobiliary malignancies.

6.1 Indications for staging laparoscopy

The principal indication for SL has been detection of radiologically occult metastatic disease [9]. This is done with the primary aim of preventing a nontherapeutic laparotomy. Occult intra-abdominal metastatic disease could be in the form of liver metastases (surface/deep intraparenchymal), peritoneal carcinomatosis or distant metastatic lymph nodes. While the presence of peritoneal and distant lymph nodal metastases may contraindicate a surgical resection, detection of additional tumors in the liver (primary and secondary) may alter the magnitude of proposed resection or change the management plan altogether.

Another important aim of SL is assessment of locoregional extent of disease [3,4]. This is important because of a change in philosophy as more and more centers perform increasingly radical operations to achieve complete resection. Locoregional resectability can be ascertained by direct visualization or a limited laparoscopic dissection. The accuracy is further improved by combining laparoscopic ultrasound [10]. Laparoscopic ultrasound Doppler probes not only help to assess involvement of locoregional vessels (e.g. portal vein/hepatic veins in hepatobiliary malignancies; superior mesenteric/portal vein and superior mesenteric artery in pancreatic malignancies) but also to qualify the extent of involvement (limited/circumferential/tumor thrombus, etc.).

Recently, SL has also been used to exclude metastatic disease in patients with borderline resectable/locally advanced tumors before planning neoadjuvant therapy or an invasive interventional procedure such as portal vein embolization [11]. This approach may be used to plan neoadjuvant therapy for downstaging such tumors. If axial imaging is indeterminate, a second-look SL can then be performed after completion of such treatment to assess locoregional tumor response or disease progression. Patients especially with colorectal cancer liver metastases who receive neoadjuvant chemotherapy may develop chemotherapy-associated steatohepatitis [9]. A SL with a liver biopsy may be useful in these cases in addition to evaluation of the extent of tumor. A SL with a liver biopsy may also be performed to evaluate the extent of fibrosis/cirrhosis in patients with hepatocellular carcinoma (HCC) [12]. In tumors necessitating extended liver resections (hilar cholangiocarcinoma/gallbladder cancer [GBC]), SL has also been proposed to exclude metastatic disease prior to performing portal vein embolization [3]. A repeat SL may then be performed after four to six weeks (at the time of surgery), which helps to rule out disease progression (new lesions that may contraindicate the planned resection) and assess the adequacy of the hypertrophy of the future liver remnant. In very selected cases, laparoscopic portal vein ligation can be performed during SL, which combines the benefits of SL and portal vein embolization in a single procedure but has the downsides of facing a dissected porta during the actual resection and some concerns as to the same degree of liver hypertrophy resulting from portal vein embolization and ligation [13].

Staging laparoscopy may also have a role in differentiating benign from malignant lesions. In certain thick-walled gallbladders (on cross-sectional imaging), the differential diagnosis includes cancer and other malignant masqueraders such as chronic cholecystitis or xanthogranulomatous cholecystitis [14]. A SL in such patients may provide additional clues that may help in making a diagnosis. If the probability of the lesion being benign in such a scenario is higher, the gallbladder with a wedge of adjacent liver may be resected laparoscopically and sent for frozen section. In the current era of significant advancements in complex laparoscopic surgery, a SL in such situations is useful and often an inseparable part of the surgical plan.

6.2 Technique of staging laparoscopy

In the simplest form, a SL is performed by inserting a laparoscope (usually 30°) through an abdominal port and systematically assessing the abdominal cavity [15]. This can visualize peritoneal metastases and surface liver metastases. We have defined these lesions as detectable lesions (DLs), which can be seen by simple SL without any additional dissection or gadgets [16]. If there are concerns for metastatic disease, DLs are biopsied and frozen section histopathological examination is performed. To biopsy a suspected metastasis and to visualize hidden areas such as the undersurface of the liver, SL is usually performed using two ports [16]. Additional ports are inserted as required for lysing adhesions, performing more complex biopsies or when an extended SL is performed.

The first trocar may be inserted by open or closed technique as per surgeon preference. While most surgeons insert the first trocar in the periumbilical region, the site of the second trocar is usually chosen within the line of the planned incision, should the disease be found to be resectable. The second port needs to be 10 mm if laparoscopic ultrasound is to be performed. Any significant ascites is aspirated and sampled for cytology examination. To allow for a systematic examination of all four quadrants of the peritoneal cavity, obstructing adhesions are divided [17]. Placement of additional ports facilitates complete systematic examination of the peritoneal cavity. After inspection of the peritoneum, the anterior and posterior surfaces of the right and left lobes of the liver are examined. The hepatoduodenal ligament, the foramen of Winslow, and hilum of the liver are examined for lymphadenopathy.

The patient is then placed in 10–15° Trendelenburg position. The omentum is retracted into the left upper quadrant after inspection of its surface for any evidence of omental deposits. The ligament of Treitz and the inferior

surface of the transverse mesocolon are then inspected for evidence of metastatic deposits and for lymphadenopathy. In standard SL, no additional dissection is performed except for minimal adhesiolysis to facilitate complete examination of the peritoneal cavity. The term "undetectable lesions" refers to those lesions which are not detected by a simple SL alone and require additional dissection to assess resectability and sample distant lymph nodes or need the help of gadgetry like an intraoperative ultrasound. Extended staging laparoscopy is performed to assess resectability in situations where a "simple staging laparoscopy" (SSL) does not reveal any metastatic lesions.

6.3 Extended staging laparoscopy

Extended SL is defined as an SL procedure which entails more than a simple visualization of the peritoneal cavity. It includes additional dissection to visualize inaccessible areas, assess locoregional resectability, distant (celiac/interaortocaval) lymph nodal sampling, addition of laparoscopic ultrasound, and/or peritoneal lavage cytology. For examination of the lesser sac, the gastrohepatic omentum is divided and the caudate lobe and inferior vena cava are examined [17]. Division of the gastrohepatic omentum also facilitates the examination of the anterior aspect of the head of the pancreas.

6.3.1 Lymph node biopsy
While biopsy of the nodes in the hepatoduodenal ligament can be performed, it is not routinely recommended as evidence of disease in this region does not contraindicate a curative resection for primary pancreatic and hepatobiliary malignancies. Hence, it should be selectively performed (e.g. in patients with colorectal liver metastases) where it can alter the management decision. However, it may be advisable to assess the distant celiac and aortocaval lymph nodes. Division of the gastrohepatic omentum and superior traction on the stomach facilitate identification of the left gastric artery. The left gastric artery can then be followed to its origin to allow inspection of the celiac axis and biopsy of any enlarged celiac nodes [17]. For aortocaval lymph node biopsy, a duodenal kocherization is performed to adequately expose the aortocaval space. Any enlarged lymph nodes in the aortocaval region below the level of the left renal vein are excised and sent for frozen section examination. Positive aortocaval/celiac lymph nodes on frozen section analysis are considered

as metastatic disease in the majority of the pancreatic and hepatobiliary malignancies, and the planned surgical resection is abandoned [18].

6.3.2 Peritoneal lavage cytology

Some authors have advocated peritoneal cytology to further increase the yield in hepatic, biliary, and pancreatic cancers [19,20]. In this procedure, approximately 150–200 mL of normal saline is instilled and aspirated in each of the following areas of the peritoneal cavity sequentially: the right upper quadrant, the left upper quadrant, and the pelvis. Specimens are then centrifuged and stained using the Papanicolaou technique. Positive peritoneal cytology is defined as peritoneal cytology that is highly suspicious or positive for adenocarcinoma [19]. To avoid false-positive results, cytological washings are taken prior to any biopsy. The principal drawback of including peritoneal lavage cytology routinely as a part of single stage SL is that the results are not immediately available and usually take at least 24 hours [19]. This precludes SL and operative exploration at the same sitting. Also, the increase in the yield above a standard SL alone is unclear and therefore may not justify routine use.

6.3.3 Laparoscopic ultrasound

Laparoscopic ultrasound consists of placement of a 6–10 MHz linear or curvilinear array transducer through a 10 mm port and systematic examination of the anterior, lateral, and inferior surfaces of the liver for evidence of intraparenchymal liver metastases [21]. The hepatoduodenal ligament, peripancreatic, aortocaval, and celiac axis lymph nodes are then evaluated. Laparoscopic ultrasound is also used to assess the locoregional extent of the tumor with respect to critical vascular structures. In the case of HCC, intrahepatic cholangiocarcinoma (IHC), and colorectal liver metastases, LUS is used to determine the proximity of the tumor to major hepatic veins. In a recent study, Viganò *et al.* reported that LUS is a reliable tool for staging liver tumors with a performance similar to that of open intraoperative ultrasound in detecting new nodules [5]. For hilar cholangiocarcinoma, an LUS probe is placed in a transverse direction over the hepatoduodenal ligament to determine portal vein invasion and hepatic artery involvement. For pancreatic cancers, it is used to determine the relationship of the tumor with the portal vein, superior mesenteric veins–splenic vein confluence, superior mesenteric artery, and celiac axis. It is also used to locate small pancreatic tumors and detect

additional lesions within the pancreas as in the case of islet cell tumors [21]. Laparoscopic ultrasound Doppler flow pattern also helps in the assessment of vascular involvement. Proper assessment of the hepatoduodenal ligament and porta hepatis can be performed by filling the right upper quadrant with saline or releasing most of the pneumoperitoneum.

6.4 Yield of staging laparoscopy

Yield of staging laparoscopy refers to the probablity of avoiding nontherapeutic laparotomy. The yield of SL is calculated by dividing the number of patients detected to have unresectable disease at SL by all patients undergoing staging laparoscopy [16]. The accuracy of SL for unresectable disease is calculated by dividing the number of patients detected to have unresectable disease at SL by all those with unresectable disease [16]. This definition is limited by varying assessments of unresectable disease. For example, some centers will define nonlocoregional metastatic lymph nodes as unsuitable for resection, and there are various definitions of locally unresectable disease. These differences in definition should be taken into consideration before making definitive conclusions regarding the yield and utility of staging laparoscopy.

Over the years, there has been a decline in the reported overall yield of SL [3,4] (Table 6.1). This is attributed to the advancements in cross-sectional imaging (CT scan and MRI) and the emergence of newer techniques like PET and EUS which have the potential to detect both metastatic disease and locally advanced disease [22,23]. Simultaneously, there have been advancements in

Table 6.1 Evolution in the yield of staging laparoscopy in pancreatic and hepatobiliary malignancies with advancements in imaging technology.

Malignancy type	Yield of staging laparoscopy	
	Studies published up to 2005	Studies published after 2005
Pancreatic cancer	25–40%	2–34%
Hepatocellular carcinoma	16–39%	7–40%
Hilar cholangiocarcinoma	25–53%	14–45%
Gallbladder cancer	38–83%	23–62%

surgical techniques and better understanding of tumor biology. More advanced resections, including vascular resection and reconstructions, are now being performed for tumors which were earlier considered inoperable, which has further contributed to a lower yield of staging laparoscopy [24]. However, as SL has evolved from simple SL to extended SL, its usefulness has changed. In addition to detecting metastatic disease, the scope of SL has extended to assessing locoregional extent of disease, detecting additional liver lesions, sampling distant lymph nodes, assessing the quality and quantity of future liver remnant, and performing additional procedures such as portal vein embolization and palliative procedures such as gastrointestinal bypass and celiac plexus block. Hence, the overall yield of SL will be affected by the extent of preoperative work-up, the extent of SL (simple or extended) performed, the aggressiveness of the center for resecting locoregionally advanced disease, and the surgical expertise to perform palliative/therapeutic procedures laparoscopically.

6.5 Timing of staging laparoscopy: single versus two stage

A SL can be performed as a single-stage or two-stage procedure [3,25]. In the single-stage procedure, SL is performed as an initial step before a planned curative surgical resection. If there is any evidence of suspicious metastatic lesion on the initial SL, it is biopsied, a frozen section analysis is performed, and the procedure terminated or a palliative bypass/procedure performed, if metastases are confirmed. Patients without evidence of metastases on SL can undergo a surgical exploration during the same sitting. A two-stage SL is performed as a part of staging work-up; a curative resection is not performed in the same setting even if there is no evidence of dissemination. This may frequently be performed prior to commencing neoadjuvant chemo-, radio- or combination therapy. The advantages of a single-stage procedure include a single operation and anesthesia for the patient and thereby a reduction of the overall cost, while the two-stage SL allows for an accurate assessment of disease extent before multimodality therapy.

In our practice, we perform two-stage SL in patients with a high risk for metastatic disease (suspicious metastatic lesions on preoperative imaging), where there is a need for an aggressive surgical procedure, and in patients positive for hepatitis (hepatitis B or C) or retrovirus (HIV). We prefer a two-stage procedure in patients planned for portal vein embolization and those deemed to be high risk for surgery because of associated comorbidities which might require extensive perioperative monitoring by the anesthesiologist.

6.6 Complications of staging laparoscopy

Complications associated with SL are uncommon, occurring in only 2–3% of cases [21]. These include wound infection, hemorrhage, port site herniation, and visceral perforation. One of the initial fears about SL was tumor implantation at the port site. This stemmed from isolated reports of port site recurrence after SL. However, this fear was put to rest by concrete evidence derived from landmark publications. Shoup *et al.* analyzed the incidence of port site recurrence in 1650 SL procedures carried out for upper gastrointestinal malignancies, including pancreatic and hepatobiliary tumors, and reported that port site recurrence occurred only in 0.8% (n = 13) of patients [26]. Of these 13 patients, eight had documented metastatic disease at the time of SL. These findings suggest that port site recurrence is a marker of more advanced disease and is not due to the SL itself. This finding was supported by Velanovich who reported that the incidence of port site recurrence (3%) following SL was equivalent to that of abdominal scar site recurrence in patients who had an exploratory laparotomy alone (3.9%) for pancreatic cancer [27].

6.7 Role of staging laparoscopy in pancreatic and hepatobiliary malignancies

6.7.1 Pancreatic cancer
Pancreatic adenocarcinoma is an aggressive tumor with a high incidence of metastatic disease. It has been estimated that at presentation, only 10–20% of patients with pancreatic adenocarcinoma are candidates for resection [17]. Hence SL has been advocated to detect radiologically occult disease. In 1978, Cuschieri *et al.* first described the use of SL in 23 patients with pancreatic malignancy and reported that 11 (47.8%) patients had metastatic disease on SL [28]. In their subsequent updated report of 73 patients in 1988, SL detected metastatic disease in

Table 6.2 Recent series (2005–2014) evaluating the role of staging laparoscopy (SL) in patients with pancreatic adenocarcinoma.

Author [ref]	Year of publication	Study period	Type of tumor	No of patients (n)	Yield of SL, n (%)
Karachristos et al. [30]	2005	1996–2003	Potentially resectable	63	12 (19)
Liu et al. [31]	2005	2000–2004	Locally advanced	74	25 (34)
Ahmed et al. [32]	2006	2001–2005	Potentially resectable	37	9 (24)
White et al. [33]	2008	1995–2005	Potentially resectable locally advanced	45	8 (18)
				55	13 (24)
Contreras et al. [34]	2009	2002–2006	Potentially resectable locally advanced	25	7 (28)
				33	11 (33)
Mayo et al. [35]	2009	1996–2003	Potentially resectable	86	24 (28)
Schnelldorfer et al. [36]	2014	2003–2012	Potentially resectable	136	3 (2)

57% (42/73) of patients deemed resectable on pre-operative imaging [29]. Since then, there have been significant improvements in imaging technology, and the yield of SL in the subsequent reports has shown a progressive decline (Table 6.2). The current yield of SL in patients with potentially resectable tumors who undergo preoperative high-quality multidetector CT is only 3–14% [33,34,36]. This has prompted a few authors to advocate against the routine use of SL in patients with pancreatic cancer.

The drawback in most of these studies, however, is the inclusion of periampullary tumors with pancreatic head carcinoma. Since periampullary tumors have a lower incidence of distant metastases in comparison with pancreatic adenocarcinoma, their inclusion has a confounding effect on the overall yield of SL. When results of SL for pancreatic cancer alone are analyzed, the yield in patients with potentially resectable tumors is 11–28% [31,33]. The yield is even higher in patients with locally advanced pancreatic adenocarcinoma (24–34%) and patients with tumors located in the body and tail of pancreas (25–36%) [31–37]. In locally advanced pancreatic adenocarcinoma planned for neoadjuvant therapy, SL may aid in avoiding the morbidity of neoadjuvant therapy. Further, in our opinion, findings from neoadjuvant trials for locally advanced pancreatic adenocarcinoma that do not incorporate pretherapy SL must be interpreted with caution.

While high-resolution CT can improve the preoperative detection of metastatic disease, a significant number of surface liver metastases and peritoneal deposits are too small (<3 mm) for detection, even with high-resolution helical CT scans. This is evident in the study by White et al. in which, even after the use of high-resolution imaging, 11% of patients with potentially resectable tumor on imaging had metastatic disease on SL [33]. A similar result was reported recently by Schnelldorfer et al., although SL failed to identify metastatic disease in 9% of patients [36].

Since elevated CA 19-9 value is associated with metastatic disease in patients with pancreatic cancer, it was suggested that this marker could be used for selecting patients for SL. Karachristos et al. reported that none of the patients with CA 19-9 levels below 100 U/mL had metastatic disease on SL [30]. However, in the study by Contreras et al., 12% of patients with potentially resectable pancreatic adenocarcinoma and CA 19-9 levels below 100 U/mL had occult liver metastases at laparoscopy [34].

Hence, from the current evidence, it is reasonable to conclude that all patients with locally advanced pancreatic adenocarcinoma and patients with tumor in the region of body and tail should undergo routine SL. In our opinion, in patients with potentially resectable head tumors, it is preferable to add routine SL before proceeding with curative resection considering the favorable risk/benefit ratio. The recent Cochrane review on the role of SL following CT scan also recommended routine SL before surgical resection in patients with pancreatic cancer [38].

The need to perform palliative biliary and/or gastric bypass has been cited as one of the principal reasons for not performing routine SL in many institutions [39,40]. Palliative surgical bypass was the only available treatment option for patients with unresectable disease in earlier decades. However, with the advances in endoscopic and percutaneous biliary stenting, there has been a drastic decrease in the need for surgical biliary bypass [41]. Prophylactic gastric bypass is no longer indicated in pancreatic cancer patients with metastatic disease since the expected survival is less than six months [42]. Nevertheless, a surgical bypass may be more durable than stenting and associated with less need for reintervention in patients who are expected to have a significant life expectancy. It may be performed laparoscopically as part of the SL [43].

Addition of peritoneal lavage fluid cytology to SL may have an important role in pancreatic cancer. A 7–30% incidence of positive peritoneal cytology has been reported in different series [44,45]. The tumor cells in peritoneal washings are considered as precursors of macroscopic dissemination, and several studies have reported that patients with positive peritoneal cytology have advanced-stage disease, early metastases, and a poor prognosis. In the current American Joint Committee on Cancer (AJCC) staging and National Comprehensive Cancer Network (NCCN) pancreatic adenocarcinoma guidelines, pancreatic cancer patients with positive peritoneal cytology are considered to have stage IV metastatic disease and only palliative treatment is recommended for these patients [46,47]. Recently, Yamada *et al.* reported that the survival period of patients with positive peritoneal cytology (n = 51) who underwent resection was significantly shorter than that of resected patients (n = 339) with negative peritoneal cytology (14.3 versus 18.0 months, P = 0.009). However, it was significantly better than the unresected cytology-positive patients (14.3 versus 6.8 months, P < 0.001) [48]. Others have also reported similar survival benefit with resection in patients with positive peritoneal lavage cytology without obvious peritoneal metastases [49]. Since surgical resection remains the only curative treatment option, and with the recent advent of better chemotherapeutic agents which can potentially eliminate micrometastases, further studies are required to determine the role of routine peritoneal lavage as a part of SL in patients with pancreatic cancer.

Lymph nodal involvement is one of the important factors which predicts prognosis in patients with pancreatic ductal adenocarcinoma. Lymph node metastases initially occur in the peripancreatic nodes and finally spread to the para-aortic lymph nodes through the nodes along the superior mesenteric artery [50,51]. Yoshida *et al.* reported that pancreatic cancer patients with para-aortic lymph node metastases have a poor prognosis following resection and recommended against resection in patients with para-aortic lymph node metastases on sampling biopsy and frozen section histopathological examination [50]. Murakami *et al.* reported a similarly poor outcome in patients with para-aortic lymph node metastases [51]. However, despite the importance of these lymph node stations, only a few centers perform routine sampling as part of SL or at the beginning of a curative resection. Considering the importance of prognostication, routine sampling of para-aortic lymph node station as part of SL may be considered in the future.

To summarize, all patients with locally advanced pancreatic adenocarcinoma and patients with tumor in the region of body and tail may benefit from routine SL. A routine SL should be strongly considered in patients with potentially resectable pancreatic cancer especially if they have elevated CA 19-9 levels or other high-risk factors for occult metastatic disease. Addition of laparosocpic para-aortic lymph node sampling as part of SL may be considered to improve the yield in pancreatic cancer, but this needs further study. Our current practice is to perform SL in all cases of pancreatic cancer, usually as a single-stage procedure, and as two stages in cases where the imaging suggests locally advanced disease, a very high CA 19-9 level or other high risks (significant cardiopulmonary disease, chronic liver disease). We do not perform para-aortic lymphadenectomy, laparoscopic ultrasound or peritoneal cytology as part of SL for pancreatic cancer.

6.7.2 Periampullary carcinomas

Periampullary carcinomas (PACA) include patients with ampullary, duodenal (second part of duodenum), and lower end cholangiocarcinoma. As already mentioned, the incidence of distant metastases is less in these tumors in comparison with pancreatic adenocarcinoma. Hence, it is a matter of debate whether SL should be performed routinely in these patients. White *et al.* reported that the yield of SL was less than 5% in patients with PACA and routine use of SL for these tumors is not warranted [33]. Similar low yield was reported in other studies where patients with PACA were analyzed together with pancreatic adenocarcinoma [52,53]. Involvement of para-aortic lymph nodes is considered as metastatic disease in PACA according to the current AJCC staging classification [46]. However, Yoshida *et al.* reported that PACA patients with para-aortic lymph node metastases had better survival than pancreatic adenocarcinoma patients with these involved nodes [50]. Murakami *et al.* reported a five-year survival rate of 24% in PACA patients with para-aortic lymph node metastases and concluded that surgical resection should not be contraindicated in these patients [51].

To summarize, the low yield of SL in patients with PACA does not support its routine use. However, considering the benefit to the patient in terms of morbidity and early postoperative recovery, it is reasonable to consider SL in high-risk PACA patients. There is no strong evidence to support extended SL in the form of laparoscopic para-aortic lymph node biopsy or peritoneal lavage cytology in patients with periampullary cancer.

6.7.3 Primary liver tumors: hepatocellular carcinoma

A significant proportion of patients with HCC present at an advanced stage and are not candidates for surgical resection [54]. In contrast to other tumors where distant metastases are the most common cause for unresectable disease, the principal oncological reason for unresectability is the presence of multifocal intrahepatic disease and, less commonly, extrahepatic spread. The extent of cirrhosis and liver function determines resectability in a significant proportion of patients [54]. The potential role of SL in HCC includes assessment of severity of cirrhosis and size of the liver remnant in addition to tumor assessment. In addition, SL may aid in planning a staged or a major liver resection and portal vein ligation may be performed simultaneously. However, the role of SL is less extensively studied in HCC in spite of the fact that the morbidity associated with nontherapeutic laparotomy is more in the cirrhotic patients with HCC [55–60].

The first report on the role of SL came from the Hong Kong group in which 91 patients deemed resectable on preoperative evaluation underwent SL [55]. Preoperative radiological studies included ultrasound, CT abdomen, and hepatic angiogram. Laparoscopic ultrasound was performed as part of SL in all patients. Fifteen patients

had evidence of unresectable disease on SL secondary to inadequate liver remnant/severe cirrhosis (n = 6), peritoneal metastases (n = 1), bilobar intrahepatic metastasis (n = 11), main portal vein tumor thrombus (n = 2), or inferior vena cava tumor thrombus (n = 1). Of the remaining 76 patients who underwent laparotomy, nine had unresectable disease secondary to inadequate liver remnant/severe cirrhosis (n = 1), bilobar intrahepatic metastasis (n = 2), main portal vein tumor thrombus (n = 3), inferior vena cava tumor thrombus (n = 1), or invasion of adjacent organs (n = 3). Overall, SL avoided nontherapeutic laparotomy and its related morbidity in 63% (15/24) of patients with unresectable disease. In this study, SL with laparoscopic ultrasound was highly accurate in assessing the future liver remnant and the presence of intrahepatic metastases. However, SL was less accurate than laparotomy and intraoperative ultrasound in determining the presence of tumor thrombi in major vascular structures and the extent of invasion of adjacent organs. These limitations of SL were most obvious in patients with large tumors (>10 cm) as bulky tumors interfered with assessment of extrahepatic adjacent organ involvement and adequate scanning with laparoscopic ultrasound [55].

In a small series from the Netherlands, SL combined with laparoscopic ultrasound spared nontherapeutic laparotomy in 13 (39%) patients and identified 81% (13/16) of unresectable patients [56]. In another study from the Memorial Sloan-Kettering Cancer Center (MSKCC), Weitz et al. reported that SL combined with laparoscopic ultrasound changed management in 22% (13/60) of patients deemed resectable on preoperative evaluation [57]. Staging laparoscopy identified unresectable disease in 13 of 18 patients, resulting in an accuracy of approximately 72%.

The routine use of SL in HCC was questioned in a recent report by Hoekstra et al. since the yield of SL was only 7% in their study (Table 6.3) [12]. The proposed reason for

Table 6.3 Recent series (2005–2014) evaluating the role of staging laparoscopy (SL) in patients with hepatocellular carcinoma.

Author [ref]	Year of publication	Study period	No of patients (n)	Yield of SL – change in management strategy after SL, n (%)	Accuracy of SL – ability to predict unresectable disease, n (%)
Klegar et al. [58]	2005	2001–2003	20	7 (35)	7 (100)
Lai et al. [59]	2008	2001–2007	119	44 (40)	44 (96)
Hoekstra [12]	2013	1999–2011	56	4 (7)	4 (27)

the low yield was the improvement in imaging technology. In addition, remnant liver volume can be predicted accurately using volumetric analysis. Improvement in the noninvasive assessment of fibrosis and cirrhosis using transient elastography also contributed to the low yield of SL in the present era. In the study by Hoekstra *et al.*, the median (range) time interval between SL and definitive operative exploration was 39 (7–83) days which could have contributed to the very low accuracy of 27% compared with other series [12]. Reddy *et al.* assessed the role of SL with laparoscopic ultrasound in 16 patients with HCC being evaluated for transplantation and reported that SL did not improve staging or alter the management [60]. However, in this study, two patients who were deemed nontransplantable were secondary to peritoneal metastases (n = 1) and lesser curve lymphadenopathy (n = 1). The result of this study can be extrapolated to living donor liver transplantation (LDLT) in which, before starting the donor operation, a SL of the recipient can be performed to rule out metastatic disease. Additionally, in contrast to pancreatic adenocarcinoma, the role of peritoneal lavage cytology in HCC patients remains unclear.

To summarize, from the current evidence, it appears that in low-risk HCC patients without significant cirrhosis, major vascular invasion or bilobar tumors, the yield of SL is low and routine use may not be recommended. However, with the increasing use of the laparoscopic treatment approach for HCC, in the form of laparoscopic-assisted radiofrequency ablation and laparoscopic resection, the role of advanced staging may increase.

6.7.4 Primary liver tumors: intrahepatic cholangiocarcinoma

Intrahepatic cholangiocarcinoma (IHC) is increasing in incidence worldwide, especially in western countries. While surgical resection remains the main curative treatment option, approximately 20–50% of patients have unresectable disease at the time of laparotomy [61]. The causes for unresectable disease include peritoneal metastases, intrahepatic metastases, lymph node metastases, and locally advanced disease. In view of the rarity of this tumor, only limited data are available regarding the role of SL in this malignancy. Goere *et al.* analyzed the role of SL in a small subgroup of 11 patients with IHC and reported that nontherapeutic laparotomy was avoided in 36% (4/11) of patients [62]. In another study, Weber *et al.* reported a yield of 27% (6/22) in a small subset of 22 patients [63]. Causes for unresectability in these

patients included peritoneal metastases (n = 4) and distant intrahepatic metastases (n = 2). Of the remaining 16 patients, five were found to be unresectable at laparotomy owing to distant lymph node metastases, resulting in an accuracy of approximately 54.5% [63]. Hence, to improve the yield of SL in selected cases of borderline resectable intrahepatic cholangiocarcinoma, laparoscopic assessment of lymph nodes should be performed.

To summarize, although the results of the relatively small series support routine use of SL in patients with intrahepatic cholangiocarcinoma, more evidence is required before making a conclusive recommendation for routine SL in these patients. Extended SL with the addition of laparoscopic lymph node biopsy and laparoscopic ultrasound can improve the yield. Addition of routine peritoneal lavage cytology as a part of SL is not recommended in patients with intrahepatic cholangiocarcinoma.

6.7.5 Metastatic liver tumors: colorectal liver metastases

Colorectal cancer (CRC) is the third most common malignant neoplasm, and the incidence is increasing in many countries. Approximately 50–60% of patients with colorectal cancer develop liver metastases, either synchronous or metachronous, during the course of their disease [64]. Surgical resection of colorectal liver metastases is the realistic curative option. However, only 10–25% of patients with colorectal liver metastases are candidates for a curative resection [64]. Hence, accurate preoperative staging is imperative, and SL has been widely used in these patients to decrease nontherapeutic laparotomy. However, in the era of modern imaging, the role of SL in this group of patients needs to be defined.

In one of the earlier studies, Rahusen *et al.* evaluated the role of SL in 50 patients with colorectal liver metastases [65]. The reported yield of SL in that study was 36% (18/50), and the addition of laparoscopic US improved the yield by detecting additional hepatic metastases and vascular involvement. The high yield in that study was probably due to inferior imaging quality as one of the more recent studies showed a yield of only 6% (3/54) [66]. This decline in the yield of SL was predominantly due to improvement in the imaging technology. One of the landmark studies which helped to choose patients for SL was published from the MSKCC by Grobmyer *et al.* [67]. Of the 264 patients evaluated with SL, 26 (10%) had unresectable disease and were spared a nontherapeutic laparotomy. Based on the

Table 6.4 Recent series (2005–2014) evaluating the role of staging laparoscopy (SL) in patients with colorectal liver metastasis.

Author [ref]	Year of publication	Study period	No of patients (n)	CRC risk score	Yield of SL – change in management strategy after SL, n (%)
Thaler et al. [68]	2005	1996–2004	138	–	34 (25)
Pilkington et al. [69]	2007	2000–2003	77	–	16 (21)
Mann et al. [70]	2007	2000–2004	200	0–1 (n = 31)	0 (0)
				2 or more (n = 169)	39 (23.1)
Li Destri et al. [71]	2008	1997–2003	43	0–2 (n = 25)	3 (12)
				2 or more (n = 18)	7 (38.9)
Shah et al. [72]	2010	2001–2005	71	0–3 (n = 48)	3 (7)
				3 or more (n = 23)	6 (24)

CRC, colorectal cancer.

extensive analysis of the patients who had unresectable disease on SL, a clinical risk score (CRS) was formulated with score ranging from 0 to 5 based on the presence of the following characteristics: node-positive primary tumor, prehepatectomy CEA greater than 200 ng/mL, more than one liver tumor, liver tumor size greater than 5 cm, and a disease-free interval of less than one year. Only 4% of patients with CRS of 0 and 1 had unresectable disease on SL; however, 21% of patients with a score of 2 or 3 and 24% of patients with scores of 4–5 had unresectable disease [67]. The predictive value of CRS to determine the need for SL has been validated in other studies (Table 6.4) [68–72]. In a recent meta-analysis, Hariharan et al. questioned the role of routine SL in the present era and recommended its selective use in patients with high incidence of peritoneal disease [73]. The result of this meta-analysis was supported by Dunne et al. who reported a very low incidence of unresectable disease (4.4%) among 295 patients who underwent open hepatectomy [4].

To summarize, the yield of SL has decreased with advances in imaging technology in patients with colorectal liver metastases. Hence, selective use of SL in high-risk patients with CRS 2 or more is recommended to improve the yield of SL and minimize unnecessary examinations. However, this approach is likely to change as more and more colorectal liver metastases are being managed by laparoscopic liver resection and therefore laparoscopy as it is becomes the first step. An extended SL with the addition of laparoscopic US without peritoneal lavage cytology is the recommended technique in patients with colorectal liver metastases.

6.7.6 Biliary tract tumor: hilar cholangiocarcinoma

Only 50–60% of patients with hilar cholangiocarcinoma or Klatskin's tumor considered for surgery after preoperative evaluation undergo potentially curative resection [74]. To avoid nontherapeutic laparotomy, SL has been evaluated in these patients. Locoregional advanced disease rather than distant metastases is the most common cause for unresectable disease. Hence, it is imperative to select appropriate candidates for staging laparoscopy.

Weber et al. from the MSKCC analyzed the role of SL in 56 patients with hilar cholangiocarcinoma and reported a yield of 25%. However, the yield of SL improved to 38% if only patients with stage T2 and T3 tumor were included [75]. Hence, selective use of SL for patients with locally advanced hilar cholangiocarcinoma was advocated by the authors. In a large series from the University of Edinburgh, SL had an overall yield of 25% which increased to 48% with the addition of laparoscopic ultrasonography [76]. Based on these results, the authors recommended the routine use of SL with the addition of laparoscopic ultrasound in hilar cholangiocarcinoma. However, laparoscopic ultrasound is not recommended universally for locoregional staging as it cannot accurately differentiate malignant infiltration from tissue inflammation especially in cases of preoperative biliary drainage. In a recent series published by Ruys et al., the overall yield of SL was only 14% (Table 6.5) [77]. The authors attributed this low yield to improvements in imaging technology.

While SL may not be very accurate in determining locally advanced disease, nodal metastases could be

Table 6.5 Recent series (2005–2014) evaluating the role of staging laparoscopy (SL) in patients with hilar cholangiocarcinoma.

Author [ref]	Year of publication	Study period	No of patients (n)	Yield of SL – change in management strategy after SL, n (%)	Accuracy of SL – ability to predict unresectable disease, n (%)
Connor et al. [76]	2005	2002–2004	84	35(42)	35 (53)
Goere et al. [62]	2006	2002–2004	20	5 (25)	5 (45)
Ruys et al. [77]	2012	2000–2010	175	24 (14)	24 (32)
Barlow et al. [78]	2013	1998–2011	100	45 (45)	45 (71)

potentially identified by performing extended SL. In a recent study, Barlow et al. refuted the findings of Ruys et al. and reported that SL should be performed in all patients with hilar cholangiocarcinoma [78]. In this study, SL with LUS had a yield of 45% with 71% accuracy. In contrast to previous reports, preoperative T stage, neutrophil lymphocyte ratio, and CA 19-9 levels were not found to predict metastatic disease in patients with hilar cholangiocarcinoma. However, the high yield reported in this series could be due to the less aggressive surgical approach (portal vein involvement considered as a contraindication) and the long study period (1998–2011).

Martin et al. studied the role of peritoneal lavage cytology in 26 patients with hilar cholangiocarcinoma and reported positive cytology in two patients [20]. However, both these patients had obvious peritoneal metastases. Nine other patients in this study, including four with actual peritoneal metastases, had negative peritoneal lavage. Based on these results, the authors concluded that peritoneal lavage cytology was not predictive of occult metastatic disease in hilar cholangiocarcinoma.

To summarize, staging laparoscopy is helpful in high-risk patients (T2/T3 or Bismuth type 3/4 and patients with suspicion of metastases). Several authors have suggested that SL is useful in all stages of hilar cholangiocarcinoma, which is also our approach. Extended SL including lymph node biopsy and laparoscopic ultrasound has not been recommended to be performed routinely. Peritoneal cytology is not recommended as a part of SL in patients with hilar cholangiocarcinoma.

6.7.7 Biliary tract tumor: gallbladder cancer

Gallbladder cancer (GBC) is the most common malignancy of the biliary tract [79]. A considerable proportion of patients have advanced disease at the time of presentation and, despite improvements in imaging studies, a significant proportion

undergo nontherapeutic laparotomy owing to radiologically occult metastatic disease. Since GBC is an aggressive tumor with a high incidence of metastatic disease, SL plays a significant role in the management of these patients.

The yield of SL in GBC reported in earlier series ranges from 38% to 62% [15,62,75]. However, is it indeed possible that the yield of SL is really high in GBC? To answer this question, the results of these series need to be critically analyzed. In the series reported by Goere et al. (35 patients with biliary cancer), the yield of SL was 62%; however, this result was based on only eight GBC patients [62]. Similarly, in the series from the MSKCC by Weber et al., the reported yield of SL (48%) for GBC was based on an analysis of only 44 patients [75]. Thus, the high yield reported in a few series could be due to relatively lower numbers of patients included in the analysis. In the series reported by Weber et al., the overall resectability rate was only 18.2% and any involved node outside the hepatoduodenal ligament was considered as an unresectable tumor [75]. In another study, Agrawal et al. reported a 38% yield with SL based on an analysis of 91 GBC patients; however, the overall resectability rate was only 35.2% [15]. In this series, in addition to distant metastases, patients with locally advanced disease (n = 6) on SL were also considered unresectable, which could have contributed to a higher yield of SL. In a recent report from our center of 409 patients, an overall resectability rate of 58.4% was found with the yield of SL being 23.2% (Table 6.6) [16].

A few opponents of SL suggest that with the advent of PET and improved imaging technology, SL is no longer indicated in GBC patients [80]. Although PET is a valuable investigation tool for detection of occult metastatic disease, its sensitivity in detecting peritoneal carcinomatosis is low. Moreover, a yield of 23% suggests that, even in the present era, SL may be routinely indicated in GBC patients [81].

However, when the GBC is incidentally discovered on histopathology following routine cholecystectomy,

Table 6.6 Recent series (2005–2014) evaluating the role of staging laparoscopy (SL) in patients with gallbladder cancer.

Author [ref]	Year of publication	Study period	No of patients (n)	Yield of SL – change in management strategy after SL, n (%)	Accuracy of SL – ability to predict unresectable disease, n (%)
Agrawal et al. [15]	2005	1989–2001	91	34 (37)	34 (68)
Goere et al. [62]	2006	2002–2004	8	5 (62)	5 (83
Butte et al. [82]*	2011	1998–2009	46	2 (4)	2 (20)
Agarwal et al. [16]	2012	2006–2011	409	95 (23)	95 (56)

*Only incidental gallbladder cancer patients included in the study.

routine SL has been reported to have low yield. In the series reported by Butte et al., the overall yield of SL in incidental GBC patients was 4.3% (2/46) [82]. The possible reasons for the low yield in this group are that the majority of patients had relatively early disease with perhaps a lower incidence of distant metastases, and some of the lesions may have been missed because of intra-abdominal adhesions from the previous cholecystectomy. The use of additional ports during SL to perform adhesiolysis and targeting high-risk incidental GBC patients like those with poorly differenti-ated, advanced-stage tumors, bile spillage during the index cholecystectomy or late presentation after the original pro-cedure might improve the yield of SL in these patients. Additionally, distant lymph node metastases was the main factor in up to 60% of patients deemed operable after SL but found to be unresectable at the time of attempted resection [16,18]. Hence, extending SL to include aorto-caval lymph node biopsy may improve the yield and accuracy of SL. A study assessing the role of extended SL to perform 16b lymph node biopsy is currently under way in our department.

To summarize, routine SL may be helpful in primary GBC patients as it avoids nontherapeutic laparotomy in as many as 23% of patients. In incidental GBC, use of SL is recom-mended in high-risk patients. Extended SL with lymph node biopsy (e.g. station 16) may improve the overall yield of SL in GBC patients. Future studies should focus on the role of peritoneal lavage cytology in these patients.

6.8 Summary and future of staging laparoscopy in pancreatic and hepatobiliary malignancies

Staging laparoscopy is a useful tool to stage pancreatic and hepatobiliary malignancy. It avoids nontherapeutic laparotomy, guides treatment by accurate assessment of tumor stage, avoids major interventions (portal vein embolization and neoadjuvant therapy) in patients with metastatic disease, and facilitates palliative proce-dures via a minimally invasive approach. The overall yield of SL has decreased in the past two decades owing to improvements in imaging and a more aggressive approach to locoregionally advanced disease. However, considering that SL is a brief, innocuous procedure, it is cost-effective to perform SL and obviate morbidity related to unnecessary laparotomy.

Technical modifications of SL have been described recently which include single-incision extended SL, transgastric natural orifice peritoneoscopy, fluorescence laparoscopy, and contrast-enhanced intraoperative lapa-roscopic ultrasound [10,83–85]. However, experience with these novel techniques is limited. The additional cost of SL has been proposed as a reason against its routine use. However, if a single-stage SL can be performed, the additional procedure-related cost may be offset by shorter hospital stay and saving thanks to avoidance of more extensive surgical procedure in patients detected to have metastatic disease on staging laparoscopy.

The goals for future development would be to decrease the need for SL and to increase the accuracy of detecting unresectable (metastatic and locoregional advanced) dis-ease by SL. With advancements in preoperative imaging and diagnostic techniques, one would hope that disease may be more accurately staged so that all potentially unre-sectable disease can be detected. Until this can be achieved, the main goal of SL is to accurately diagnose all cases of unresectable pancreatic and hepatobiliary tumors and thereby avoid 100% nontherapeutic laparotomy. However, even with an aggressive SL protocol in place, a major challenge remaining is accurately detecting unresectable locoregional advanced disease.

KEY POINTS

- To avoid nontherapeutic laparotomies, staging laparoscopy, extended staging laparoscopy and regional lymph node sampling are important tools in the armamentarium of hepatopancreatobiliary surgeons.

- Staging laparoscopy has a critical role in the management of pancreatic cancer, intra- and extrahepatic biliary cancer, hepatocellular carcinoma, gallbladder cancer, and metastatic colorectal cancer.

- Palliative biliary and enteric bypass in pancreatic cancer patients with positive staging laparoscopy can be a minimally invasive option for selected patients who are poor candidates for an endoscopic approach.

- Good technique of laparoscopic peritoneal lavage is important for accurate staging.

- Regional lymph node sampling and staging laparoscopic ultrasound may increase the yield of a staging laparoscopy.

References

1 Chang L, Stefanidis D, Richardson WS, *et al.* The role of staging laparoscopy for intraabdominal cancers: an evidence-based review. Surg Endosc 2009; 23:231–241.

2 Nieveen van Dijkum EJ, de Wit LT, Gouma DJ. Staging laparoscopy and laparoscopic ultrasonography in more than 400 patients with upper gastrointestinal carcinoma. J Am Coll Surg 1999; 189:459–465.

3 Rotellar F, Pardo F. Laparoscopic staging in hilar cholangio-carcinoma: is it still justified? World J Gastrointest Oncol 2013; 5:127–131.

4 Dunne DF, Gaughran J, Jones RP, *et al.* Routine staging laparoscopy has no place in the management of colorectal liver metastases. Eur J Surg Oncol 2013; 39:721–725.

5 Viganò L, Ferrero A, Amisano M, *et al.* Comparison of laparoscopic and open intraoperative ultrasonography for staging liver tumours. Br J Surg 2013; 100:535–542.

6 Aliyev S, Agcaoglu O, Aksoy E, *et al.* Efficacy of laparoscopic radiofrequency ablation for the treatment of patients with small solitary colorectal liver metastasis. Surgery 2013; 154:556–562.

7 Tan-Tam C, Chung SW. Mini review on laparoscopic hepatobiliary and pancreatic surgery. World J Gastrointest Endosc 2014; 6:60–67.

8 Garcea G, Ong SL, Maddern GJ. The current role of PET-CT in the characterization of hepatobiliary malignancies. HPB (Oxford) 2009; 11:4–17.

9 Kim HJ, d'Angelica M, Hiotis SP, *et al.* Laparoscopic staging for liver, biliary, pancreas, and gastric cancer. Curr Probl Surg 2007; 44:228–269.

10 Itabashi T, Sasaki A, Otsuka K, *et al.* Potential value of sonazoid-enhanced intraoperative laparoscopic ultrasonography for liver assessment during laparoscopy-assisted colectomy. Surg Today 2014; 44:696–701.

11 Katz MH, Crane CH, Varadhachary G. Management of borderline resectable pancreatic cancer. Semin Radiat Oncol 2014; 24:105–112.

12 Hoekstra LT, Bieze M, Busch OR, *et al.* Staging laparoscopy in patients with hepatocellular carcinoma: is it useful? Surg Endosc 2013; 27:826–831.

13 Ayiomamitis GD, Low JK, Alkari B, *et al.* Role of laparoscopic right portal vein ligation in planning staged or major liver resection. J Laparoendosc Adv Surg Tech A 2009; 19:409–413.

14 Agarwal AK, Kalayarasan R, Javed A, Sakhuja P. Mass-forming xanthogranulomatous cholecystitis masquerading as gallbladder cancer. J Gastrointest Surg 2013; 17:1257–1264.

15 Agrawal S, Sonawane RN, Behari A, *et al.* Laparoscopic staging in gallbladder cancer. Dig Surg 2005; 22:440–445.

16 Agarwal AK, Kalayarasan R, Javed A, *et al.* The role of staging laparoscopy in primary gall bladder cancer – an analysis of 409 patients: a prospective study to evaluate the role of staging laparoscopy in the management of gallbladder cancer. Ann Surg 2013; 258:318–323.

17 Conlon KC, Minnard EA. The value of laparoscopic staging in upper gastrointestinal malignancy. Oncologist 1997; 2:10–17.

18 Agarwal AK, Kalayarasan R, Javed A, *et al.* Role of routine 16b1 lymph node biopsy in the management of gallbladder cancer: an analysis. HPB (Oxford) 2014; 16:229–234.

19 Warshaw AL. Implications of peritoneal cytology for staging of early pancreatic cancer. Am J Surg 1991; 161:26–29.

20 Martin RC 2nd, Fong Y, DeMatteo RP, *et al.* Peritoneal washings are not predictive of occult peritoneal disease in patients with hilar cholangiocarcinoma. J Am Coll Surg 2001; 193:620–625.

21 Callery MP, Strasberg SM, Doherty GM, *et al.* Staging laparoscopy with laparoscopic ultrasonography: optimizing resectability in hepatobiliary and pancreatic malignancy. J Am Coll Surg 1997; 185:33–39.

22 De Angelis C, Manfrè SF, Pellicano R. Endoscopic ultrasonography for diagnosis and staging of pancreatic adenocarcinoma: key messages for clinicians. Minerva Med 2014; 105:121–128.

23 Serrano OK, Chaudhry MA, Leach SD. The role of PET scanning in pancreatic cancer. Adv Surg 2010; 44:313–325.

24 Igami T, Nishio H, Ebata T, *et al.* Surgical treatment of hilar cholangiocarcinoma in the "new era": the Nagoya University experience. J Hepatobiliary Pancreat Sci 2010; 17:449–454.

25 Tilleman EH, de Castro SM, Busch OR, *et al*. Diagnostic laparoscopy and laparoscopic ultrasound for staging of patients with malignant proximal bile duct obstruction. J Gastrointest Surg 2002; 6:426–430.

26 Shoup M, Brennan MF, Karpeh MS, *et al*. Port site metastasis after diagnostic laparoscopy for upper gastrointestinal tract malignancies: an uncommon entity. Ann Surg Oncol 2002; 9:632–636.

27 Velanovich V. The effects of staging laparoscopy on trocar site and peritoneal recurrence of pancreatic cancer. Surg Endosc 2004; 18:310–313.

28 Cuschieri A, Hall AW, Clark J. Value of laparoscopy in the diagnosis and management of pancreatic carcinoma. Gut 1978; 19:672–677.

29 Cuschieri A. Laparoscopy for pancreatic cancer: does it benefit the patient? Eur J Surg Oncol 1988; 14:41–44.

30 Karachristos A, Scarmeas N, Hoffman JP. CA 19-9 levels predict results of staging laparoscopy in pancreatic cancer. J Gastrointest Surg 2005; 9:1286–1292.

31 Liu RC, Traverso LW. Diagnostic laparoscopy improves staging of pancreatic cancer deemed locally unresectable by computed tomography. Surg Endosc 2005; 19:638–642.

32 Ahmed SI, Bochkarev V, Oleynikov D, *et al*. Patients with pancreatic adenocarcinoma benefit from staging laparoscopy. J Laparoendosc Adv Surg Tech A 2006; 16:458–463.

33 White R, Winston C, Gonen M, *et al*. Current utility of staging laparoscopy for pancreatic and peripancreatic neoplasms. J Am Coll Surg 2008; 206:445–450.

34 Contreras CM, Stanelle EJ, Mansour J, *et al*. Staging laparoscopy enhances the detection of occult metastases in patients with pancreatic adenocarcinoma. J Surg Oncol 2009; 100: 663–669.

35 Mayo SC, Austin DF, Sheppard BC, *et al*. Evolving preoperative evaluation of patients with pancreatic cancer: does laparoscopy have a role in the current era? J Am Coll Surg 2009; 208:87–95.

36 Schnelldorfer T, Gagnon AI, Birkett RT, *et al*. Staging laparoscopy in pancreatic cancer: a potential role for advanced laparoscopic techniques. J Am Coll Surg 2014; 218: 1201–1206.

37 Jimenez RE, Warshaw AL, Rattner DW, *et al*. Impact of laparoscopic staging in the treatment of pancreatic cancer. Arch Surg 2000; 135:409–414.

38 Allen VB, Gurusamy KS, Takwoingi Y, *et al*. Diagnostic accuracy of laparoscopy following computed tomography (CT) scanning for assessing the resectability with curative intent in pancreatic and periampullary cancer. Cochrane Database Syst Rev 2013; 11:CD009323.

39 Nieveen van Dijkum EJ, Romijn MG, Terwee C, *et al*. Laparoscopic staging and subsequent palliation in patients with peripancreatic carcinoma. Ann Surg 2003; 237:66–73.

40 Friess H, Kleeff J, Silva JC, *et al*. The role of diagnostic laparoscopy in pancreatic and periampullary malignancies. J Am Coll Surg 1998; 186:675–682.

41 Ferreira LE, Baron TH. Endoscopic stenting for palliation of malignant biliary obstruction. Expert Rev Med Devices 2010; 7:681–691.

42 Jeurnink SM, Steyerberg EW, van Hooft JE, *et al*. Dutch SUSTENT Study Group. Surgical gastrojejunostomy or endoscopic stent placement for the palliation of malignant gastric outlet obstruction (SUSTENT study): a multicenter randomized trial. Gastrointest Endosc 2010; 71:490–499.

43 Navarra G, Musolino C, Venneri A, *et al*. Palliative antecolic isoperistaltic gastrojejunostomy: a randomized controlled trial comparing open and laparoscopic approaches. Surg Endosc 2006; 20:1831–1834.

44 Merchant NB, Conlon KC, Saigo P, *et al*. Positive peritoneal cytology predicts unresectability of pancreatic adenocarcinoma. J Am Coll Surg 1999; 188:421–426.

45 Yachida S, Fukushima N, Sakamoto M, *et al*. Implications of peritoneal washing cytology in patients with potentially resectable pancreatic cancer. Br J Surg 2002; 89:573–578.

46 Sobin LH, Gospodarowicz MK, Wittekind C. (eds). International Union Against Cancer. *TNM Classification of Malignant Tumors*. New York: Wiley-Blackwell, 2009.

47 National Comprehensive Cancer Network. NCCN Clinical Practice Guidelines in Oncology. Pancreatic Adenocarcinoma. Version 1.2013. Available at: www.nccn.org/ professionals/physician_gls/f_guidelines.asp#site NCCN.org (accessed 17 December 2015).

48 Yamada S, Fujii T, Kanda M, *et al*. Value of peritoneal cytology in potentially resectable pancreatic cancer. Br J Surg 2013; 100:1791–1796.

49 Yoshioka R, Saiura A, Koga R, *et al*. The implications of positive peritoneal lavage cytology in potentially resectable pancreatic cancer. World J Surg 2012; 36:2187–2191.

50 Yoshida T, Matsumoto T, Sasaki A, *et al*. Outcome of paraaortic node-positive pancreatic head and bile duct adenocarcinoma. Am J Surg 2004; 187:736–740.

51 Murakami Y, Uemura K, Sudo T, *et al*. Is para-aortic lymph node metastasis a contraindication for radical resection in biliary carcinoma? World J Surg 2011; 35:1085–1093.

52 Garcea G, Cairns V, Berry DP, *et al*. Improving the diagnostic yield from staging laparoscopy for periampullary malignancies: the value of preoperative inflammatory markers and radiological tumor size. Pancreas 2012; 41:233–237.

53 Brooks AD, Mallis MJ, Brennan MF, *et al*. The value of laparoscopy in the management of ampullary, duodenal, and distal bile duct tumors. J Gastrointest Surg 2002; 6:139–145.

54 Ribero D, Abdalla EK, Thomas MB, *et al*. Liver resection in the treatment of hepatocellular carcinoma. Expert Rev Anticancer Ther 2006; 6:567–579.

55 Lo CM. Determining resectability for hepatocellular carcinoma: the role of laparoscopy and laparoscopic ultrasonography. J Hepatobiliary Pancreat Surg 2000; 7:260–264.

56 De Castro SMM, Tilleman EHBM, Busch ORC, *et al*. Diagnostic laparoscopy for primary and secondary liver malignancies:

impact of improved imaging and changed criteria for resection. Ann Surg Oncol 2004; 11:522–529.

57 Weitz J, d'Angelica M, Jarnagin W, *et al.* Selective use of diagnostic laparoscopy prior to planned hepatectomy for patients with hepatocellular carcinoma. Surgery 2004; 135:273–281.

58 Klegar EK. Diagnostic laparoscopy in the evaluation of the viral hepatitis patient with potentially resectable hepatocellular carcinoma. HPB Surg 2005; 7:204–207.

59 Lai EC, Tang CN, Ha JP, *et al.* The evolving influence of laparoscopy and laparoscopic ultrasonography on patients with hepatocellular carcinoma. Am J Surg 2008; 196: 736–740.

60 Reddy MS, Smith L, Jaques BC, *et al.* Do laparoscopy and intraoperative ultrasound have a role in the assessment of patients with end-stage liver disease and hepatocellular carcinoma for liver transplantation? Transplant Proc 2007; 39:1474–1476.

61 Bridgewater J, Galle PR, Khan SA, *et al.* Guidelines for the diagnosis and management of intrahepatic cholangiocarcinoma. J Hepatol 2014; 60:1268–1289.

62 Goere D, Wagholikar GD, Pessaux P, *et al.* Utility of staging laparoscopy in subsets of biliary cancers: laparoscopy is a powerful diagnostic tool in patients with intrahepatic and gallbladder carcinoma. Surg Endosc Other Intervent Tech 2006; 20:721–725.

63 Weber SM, Jarnagin WR, Klimstra D, *et al.* Intrahepatic cholangiocarcinoma: resectability, recurrence pattern, and outcomes. J Am Coll Surg 2001; 193:384–391.

64 Weitz J, Koch M, Debus J, *et al.* Colorectal cancer. Lancet. 2005; 365:153–165.

65 Rahusen FD, Cuesta MA, Borgstein PJ, *et al.* Selection of patients for resection of colorectal metastases to the liver using diagnostic laparoscopy and laparoscopic ultrasonography. Ann Surg 1999; 230:31–37.

66 Koea J, Rodgers M, Thompson P, *et al.* Laparoscopy in the management of colorectal cancer metastatic to the liver. ANZ J Surg 2004; 74:1056–1059.

67 Grobmyer SR, Fong YM, d'Angelica M, *et al.* Diagnostic laparoscopy prior to planned hepatic resection for colorectal metastases. Arch Surg 2004; 139:1326–1330.

68 Thaler K, Kanneganti S, Khajanchee Y, *et al.* The evolving role of staging laparoscopy in the treatment of colorectal hepatic metastasis. Arch Surg 2005; 140(8): 727–734.

69 Pilkington SA, Rees M, Peppercorn D, *et al.* Laparoscopic staging in selected patients with colorectal liver metastases as a prelude to liver resection. HPB(Oxford) 2007; 9:58–63.

70 Mann CD, Neal CP, Metcalfe MS, *et al.* Clinical Risk Score predicts yield of staging laparoscopy in patients with colorectal liver metastases. Br J Surg 2007; 94:855–859.

71 Li Destri G, di Benedetto F, Torrisi B, *et al.* Metachronous liver metastases and resectability: Fong's score and laparoscopic evaluation. HPB (Oxford) 2008; 10:13–17.

72 Shah AJ, Phull J, Finch-Jones MD. Clinical risk score can be used to select patients for staging laparoscopy and laparoscopic ultrasound for colorectal liver metastases. World J Surg 2010; 34:2141–2145.

73 Hariharan D, Constantinides V, Kocher HM, *et al.* The role of laparoscopy and laparoscopic ultrasound in the preoperative staging of patients with resectable colorectal liver metastases: a meta-analysis. Am J Surg 2012; 204:84–92.

74 Matsuo K, Rocha FG, Ito K, *et al.* The Blumgart preoperative staging system for hilar cholangiocarcinoma: analysis of resectability and outcomes in 380 patients. J Am Coll Surg 2012; 215:343–355.

75 Weber SM, DeMatteo RP, Fong YM, *et al.* Staging laparoscopy in patients with extrahepatic biliary carcinoma – analysis of 100 patients. Ann Surg 2002; 235:392–399.

76 Connor S, Barron E, Wigmore SJ, *et al.* The utility of laparoscopic assessment in the preoperative staging of suspected hilar cholangiocarcinoma. J Gastrointest Surg 2005; 9:476–480.

77 Ruys AT, Busch OR, Gouma DJ, *et al.* Staging laparoscopy for hilar cholangiocarcinoma: is it still worthwhile? Indian J Surg Oncol 2012; 3:147–153.

78 Barlow AD, Garcea G, Berry DP, *et al.* Staging laparoscopy for hilar cholangiocarcinoma in 100 patients. Langenbecks Arch Surg 2013; 398:983–988.

79 Nishio H, Ebata T, Yokoyama Y, *et al.* Gallbladder cancer involving the extrahepatic bile duct is worthy of resection. Ann Surg 2011; 253:953–960.

80 Cai X, Yu T, Yu H. Staging laparoscopy is not the best option to identify unresectable gallbladder cancer with 100% of accuracy. Ann Surg 2015; 262:e57.

81 Agarwal AK, Kalayarasan R, Javed A. Reply to letter: "Staging laparoscopy is the best option to avoid a nontherapeutic laparotomy for gallbladder cancer deemed operable on preoperative workup." Ann Surg 2015; 262:e57–58.

82 Butte JM, Gönen M, Allen PJ, *et al.* The role of laparoscopic staging in patients with incidental gallbladder cancer. HPB (Oxford) 2011; 13:463–472.

83 Maemura K, Shinchi H, Mataki Y, *et al.* Advanced staging laparoscopy using single-incision approach for unresectable pancreatic cancer. Surg Laparosc Endosc Percutan Tech 2011; 21:e301–305.

84 Nau P, Anderson J, Yuh B, *et al.* Diagnostic transgastric endoscopic peritoneoscopy: extension of the initial human trial for staging of pancreatic head masses. Surg Endosc 2010; 24:1440–1446.

85 Tran Cao HS, Kaushal S, Lee C, *et al.* Fluorescence laparoscopy imaging of pancreatic tumor progression in an orthotopic mouse model. Surg Endosc 2011; 25:48–54.

CHAPTER 7

Interventional radiology in the management of hepatopancreatobiliary malignancy and surgical complications

Steven Y. Huang and Michael J. Wallace

Department of Interventional Radiology, Division of Diagnostic Imaging, University of Texas MD Anderson Cancer Center, Houston, USA

EDITOR COMMENT

The best friend of the HPB surgeon is the interventional radiologist. Advanced laparoscopic HPB surgery can be done safely only in an environment where skillful interventional radiology exists. Therefore excellent communication between HPB surgeon and interventional radiologist is critical for accurate diagnostic and challenging therapeutic interventions. This chapter reviews the important role that interventional radiology plays in the management of HPB patients from diagnosis to management of surgical complications. In addition, options for unresectable patients (i.e. chemoembolization, radioembolization, and thermal ablation) are presented.

Keywords: biopsy, drainage, interventional radiology, locoregional therapy, palliation

---

7.1 Diagnosis

Percutaneous biopsy is one of the most commonly performed procedures in radiology departments [1]. Traditionally, the role of image-guided biopsy was to differentiate benign from malignant disease, to stage known malignancy, and to culture an organism in the case of infection. The recent explosion of molecular techniques (i.e. immunohistochemistry staining, polymerase chain reaction, fluorescence in situ hybridization, and gene sequencing) has expanded these baseline indications to include molecular profiling and genomic analysis of oncological specimens to guide treatment. Percutaneous techniques are particularly well suited for the liver, while lesions originating from the biliary system and pancreas should be evaluated on a case-by-case basis.

The liver is the most common solid organ biopsied in the abdomen and pelvis. The liver tolerates needle transgression well, with percutaneous techniques yielding an accuracy of approximately 96% for focal liver lesions [2].

Major complications are rare and include hemorrhage, abscess, and needle track seeding. The risk of hemorrhage can be minimized by choosing a biopsy path which transgresses at least 1 cm of normal liver parenchyma. Plugging the biopsy track with gelatin particles and coils has been described to decrease the risk of hemorrhage following biopsy [3,4].

Percutaneous biopsy of the pancreas and biliary system has largely been supplanted by endoscopic techniques utilizing brush cytology, forceps biopsy, and endoscopic ultrasound-guided fine needle aspiration (EUS-guided FNA). When endoscopy has failed or is contraindicated, needle biopsy of the pancreas can be used to effectively delineate focal pancreatitis, malignancy, and metastasis. Sensitivity of computed tomography (CT)-guided pancreatic biopsy for pancreatic neoplasm ranges from 45% to 90% [5,6] (Figure 7.1). A concern with pancreatic biopsies is the potential for peritoneal tumor seeding [7]. This concern, however, is difficult to substantiate, given that many of these patients are inoperable

---

Laparoscopic Liver, Pancreas, and Biliary Surgery, First Edition.
Edited by Claudius Conrad and Brice Gayet.
© 2017 John Wiley & Sons, Ltd. Published 2017 by John Wiley & Sons, Ltd.

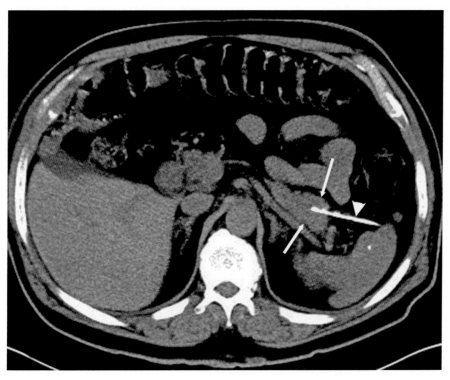

Figure 7.1 Axial CT image during CT-guided biopsy of a pancreatic tail mass (*arrows*). Biopsy needle passes anterior to the spleen (*arrowhead*).

and suffer from limited survival, making tissue confirmation and long-term imaging follow-up difficult. Needle biopsy of the biliary system can be accomplished when the obstructing lesion, such as cholangiocarcinoma, is visible with US, CT, or is located adjacent to an endoscopically placed stent. For biliary strictures, brush biopsy can be performed, though diagnostic yield is limited. In a study of 65 patients over a five-year period, Rabinovitz *et al.* found that biliary brushing from a percutaneous approach was useful to exclude malignancy, especially after multiple attempts with a probability of 6% of having bile duct carcinoma following three sequential negative cytological brushings [8].

In addition to percutaneous tissue acquisition, interventional radiologists are occasionally asked to evaluate patients with persistent hypoglycemia due to endogenous insulin production. When insulinoma, often associated with multiple endocrine neoplasia type 1, or nesidioblastosis, a form of acquired hyperinsulinism, are potential

diagnoses, preoperative localization is crucial to guide surgical resection. In spite of recent advances in imaging, localizing pancreatic lesions <2 cm in diameter and differentiating them from other lesions is challenging. Therefore, calcium arterial stimulation with hepatic venous sampling (ASVS) was developed by Doppman *et al.* in 1989 to localize insulin-secreting tumor cells to regions of the pancreas based on arterial supply [9] (Figure 7.2). The physiological rationale of the test is that a high concentration of extracellular calcium triggers release of insulin from insulinoma cells, while there is no increase in insulin secretion from normal pancreatic β-cells. ASVS has the highest accuracy for localization of insulinomas (84–88%), in comparison with magnetic resonance imaging (43%), arteriography (36%), CT (17%), and transabdominal US (17%) [10,11]. ASVS is especially important in the era of laparoscopic surgery, where accurate localization of lesions may help surgeons determine which procedures are amenable to laparoscopy versus laparotomy.

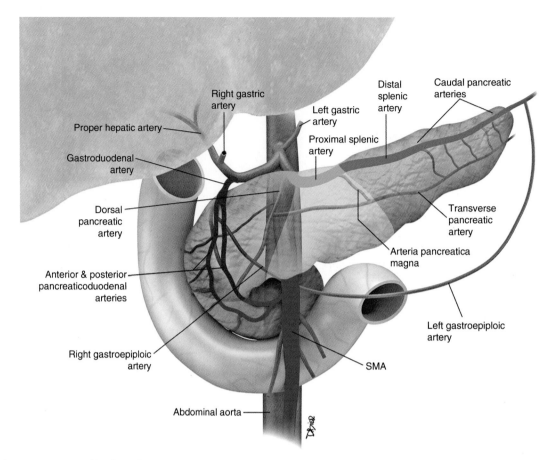

Figure 7.2 Pancreatic blood supply.

7.2 Interventional radiology management of postoperative complications

7.2.1 Catheter drainage of postoperative fluid collections

Following laparoscopic liver resection, intra-abdominal abscess, intra-abdominal fluid collection not otherwise specified, and liver abscess are relatively infrequent occurrences with a combined frequency of approximately 0.5% [12]. Percutaneous drainage can be safely performed with CT, US, or a combination of US with fluoroscopy. In a prospective multicenter trial of 96 patients with 137 intra-abdominal abscesses, percutaneous catheter drainage was effective as a single treatment in 70% of patients and increased to 82% with a second attempt [13]. In subgroup analysis, the success varied by the organ of origin: appendix, 95% (18/19); liver or biliary tract, 85% (17/20); colon and rectum, 78% (21/27); pancreas, 58% (7/12); other, 100% (18/18) (analysis of variance; P = 0.04). Importantly, negative predictors of successful outcome included the presence of yeast (odds ratio [OR] = 0.63; 95% confidence interval [95% CI] 0.51–0.78; P < 0.001) and pancreatic origin (OR = 0.78; 95% CI 0.63–0.96; P = 0.002).

The mainstays of the treatment of pyogenic liver abscesses are catheter-directed drainage and antibiotics [14]. However, in the setting of hepatobiliary-pancreatic malignancy, percutaneous drainage is successful in only 66% of cases [15]. Independent predictors of failure include presence of yeast, biliary communication, and multiloculation [15,16]. Lai *et al.* found that patients who fail management with percutaneous drainage have a significantly higher mortality than patients successfully treated (60% versus 17%, P = 0.007) [16].

Subphrenic abscesses are typically encountered in the postoperative patient following surgery involving the liver, pancreas, stomach or spleen. The pleura is attached to the eighth rib anteriorly, 10th rib laterally, and 12th rib posteriorly. Ideally, the drainage approach of a subphrenic abscess follows an extrapleural approach to avoid contamination of the pleural space by infected abdominal contents. This angled approach can be obtained most easily with ultrasonography, allowing direct, real-time visualization using an off-axis approach [17] (Figure 7.3).

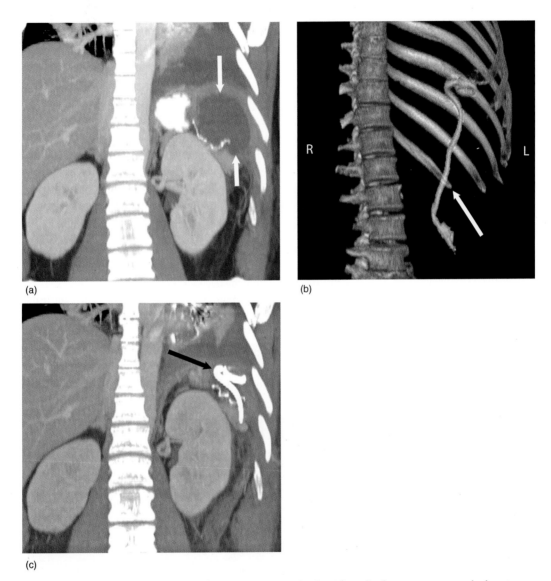

(a)

(b)

(c)

Figure 7.3 A 48-year-old man with pancreatic tail cancer at postoperative day 5 from distal pancreatectomy and splenectomy presents with fever and left upper upper quadrant pain. (a) Thick-slab coronal reformatted CT image of the upper abdomen demonstrates a fluid collection (*arrows*). (b) Given the location of the collection immediately underneath the diaphragm, there is the potential risk of causing an ipsilateral empyema with placement of a drainage catheter through the pleural space. Volume-rendered CT image demonstrates the steep trajectory of the drainage catheter (*arrow*) entering the abdomen below the 12th rib to avoid the pleural space. (c) Thick-slab coronal reformatted CT image of the upper abdomen 10 days following drainage catheter placement (*black arrow*) demonstrates near-complete interval resolution of the subphrenic fluid collection. The patient's fever and left upper quadrant quickly subsided after catheter placement. Source: Reproduced with permission of Sanjay Gupta MD.

However, shadowing from adjacent bones and air-filled loops of bowel may obscure visualization. CT is limited to the axial plane, but the ability to angle the gantry up to 30° allows some limited flexibility in needle placement. An alternative to angling the gantry is the triangulation method [18]. While every attempt to avoid the pleural space should be made, most patients with a subphrenic abscess will be successfully drained following either extrapleural or transpleural catheter drainage. In a study of 62 patients with subphrenic abscesses treated percutaneously, catheter-directed drainage was successful in 85% of cases [17]. Six (10%) patients in this study were drained through an intercostal approach, with one patient developing an empyema. Concern about transgression of the pleural space to drain an infected subphrenic collection may be mitigated by the fact that the pleural space adjacent to an inflammatory reaction arising from the adjacent abscess can be obliterated. In a small study of 28 drainage procedures for left subphrenic abscess following splenectomy, 20 drainages were transpleural and eight were extrapleural [19]; no patient developed empyema. At the authors' institution, every attempt is made to follow an extrapleural approach. When a transpleural route is used, the authors prefer to place an ipsilateral pleural drainage catheter.

Following pancreatic surgery, fluid collections from anastomotic leaks of gastrointestinal, biliary or pancreatic origin develop in 29–34% of patients [20–24]. The presence of a fluid collection does not warrant immediate intervention, as many postoperative pancreatic leaks are simple and resolve spontaneously [25]. In the setting of inadequate drainage by surgical drains, signs of suprainfection (e.g. rim enhancement, air) or patient decompensation (e.g. pain, leukocytosis, fever, tachycardia), interventional radiologists may be asked to place a drainage catheter (Figure 7.4). Depending on fluid viscosity, catheters as large as 30 Fr may be needed, with inadequate catheter size representing a known independent predictor of drainage failure [20]. Cronin *et al.* examined catheter-directed management of peripancreatic fluid collections in a single-center retrospective review of 51 patients who underwent 57 image-guided procedures following distal pancreatectomy [20]. The primary clinical success rate, defined as resolution of the peripancreatic collection with percutaneous drainage only, was 60%. Owing to the complex nature of peripancreatic collections and the relatively high rate of pancreatic fistulas following surgery, 20 of 57 cases (35%) required secondary catheter manipulation, ERCP or stenting to resolve the collection and seal the leak. The success of catheter-directed drainage increased to 95% following secondary intervention, obviating the need for re-exploration.

The importance of identifying a pancreatic fistula cannot be overstated as fistulas are difficult to treat and may lead to recurrent collections if the catheter is prematurely removed. Fluid location following pancreatic surgery is important as location adjacent to the pancreas has been

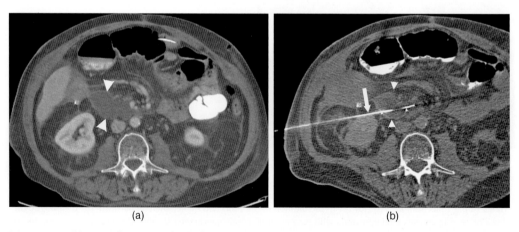

(a)　　　　　　　　　　　　　　　　(b)

Figure 7.4 A 62-year-old man with pancreatic head adenocarcinoma, who is nine days post pancreaticoduodenectomy, presents with fever and elevated white blood cell count. (a) Axial image from a CT scan with contrast demonstrates a rim-enhancing collection in the surgical resection bed (*arrowheads*). (b) Axial image from a CT scan following CT-guided placement of a 12 Fr drainage catheter; 30 mL of purulent fluid was aspirated. Follow-up CT scan (not shown) performed two weeks later demonstrated resolution of the collection.

shown to correlate with pancreatic duct leaks [24,26]. In the study by Cronin *et al.*, the authors noted that amylase was present in 88% of the collections drained (mean 11 557 IU/L, range 33–68 915 IU/L); however, the number of patients with a pancreatic fistula, as defined by the International Study Group [27] as output on or after postoperative day 3 with amylase content >3 times serum amylase, was unclear. The high reintervention rate of patients in their study (35%) suggests that many of the collections represented pancreatic fistulas. Cabay *et al.* reported on 20 patients with external pancreatic fistulas treated by percutaneous drainage [28]. Treatment was successful in 16 of 20 patients with high-output fistula (>200 mL/day), but only two of four patients with low-output fistula. Thus, while pancreatic fistulas are difficult entities to treat, conservative management with percutaneous catheter-directed drainage appears to be a reasonable alternative following medical management.

7.2.2 Biliary duct injury with and without biloma

Iatrogenic injury to the biliary system is relatively rare, occurring most often following laparoscopic cholecystectomy with an incidence of 0.6% [29–31]. Optimal management is provided by a multidisciplinary team incorporating hepatobiliary surgeons, endoscopists, and interventional radiologists. Initial management of bile duct injury is focused on draining any collections, biliary diversion, and completely characterizing the injury. Image-guided catheter drainage of collections with communication to the biliary tree is more likely to be successful than collections with a communication to the pancreatic duct. In a retrospective review of 57 patients, the success rates of catheter drainage for abdominal collections containing biliary and pancreatic ductal communication were 93% (39/42) and 67% (10/15), respectively (P = 0.01) [32]. Delayed drainage of bilomas is associated with abscess formation, cholangitis, and sepsis [33].

When biliary injury is suspected, endoscopic or percutaneous biliary drainage is often requested. The goal of biliary drainage is to eliminate the transpapillary pressure gradient to prevent extravasation at the site of the leak. Endoscopic therapy is largely successful with postcholecystectomy biliary leak, preventing any additional surgery. When there is complete ductal ligation, injury to an intrahepatic duct or ligation of an aberrant right hepatic bile duct, percutaneous transhepatic cholangiography with biliary drain placement is often needed for diagnosis and decompression [34–38] (Figure 7.5). Percutaneous drainage of nondilated biliary systems is technically challenging, with a success rate of 65–75% [39]. Some patients may require more than one session to place a drainage catheter, and in some cases, the area of extravasation may not be crossed.

Biliary drainage will not be effective when the injury does not communicate with the common bile duct and small bowel. In these cases, some authors advocate the use of repeated ethanol injection to sclerose the biliary epithelium [40,41]. Others have described the use of glue (n-butyl-cyanoacrylate) to obliterate the isolated duct(s) and seal the fistula [42–44]. Though the data on utilizing glue arise from small retrospective case series, the early clinical success warrants further attention.

7.2.3 Arterial injury

Intra-abdominal bleeding following laparoscopic liver resection is a relatively rare occurrence with a frequency of 10 out of 2804 (0.4%) patients [12]. Postpancreatectomy hemorrhage occurs in less than 10% of patients but accounts for 11–38% of mortality [45]; it is also correlated with bile leaks, pancreatic fistula, abscess, and sepsis [46–48]. Hemorrhagic scenarios include gastroduodenal artery stump leak, common and proper hepatic artery erosion, celiac axis erosion, splenic artery erosion, inferior pancreaticoduodenal artery aneurysm, and arc of Buehler aneurysm and pseudoaneurysm [49]. Depending on the location, embolization can be performed with coils, absorbable gelatin powder, n-butyl-cyanoacrylate, thrombin or flow-diverting stent grafts. Arterial embolization of postpancreatectomy hemorrhage is successful in 77–88% of cases (Figure 7.6) [50,51].

7.2.4 Portal venous hypertension
7.2.4.1 Prehepatic portal hypertension from portal vein obstruction
Prehepatic portal hypertension can result from hypercoagulable states (portal vein thrombosis), alterations in the portal vein wall from adjacent inflammation or surgery, and in association with malignancy (e.g. hepatocellular carcinoma [HCC], pancreatic cancer, bile duct cancer) [52,53]. Based on results from small retrospective studies, transhepatic portography with stent placement appears to be an effective procedure to relieve portal hypertension in patients with prehepatic portal vein

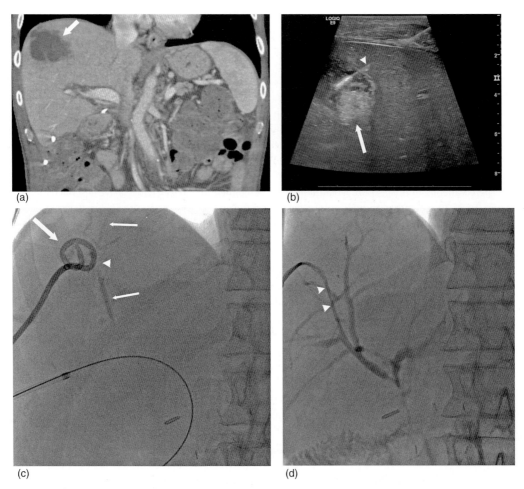

Figure 7.5 A 62-year-old man with pancreatic cancer status post pancreaticoduodenectomy. Postoperative course was complicated by an intrahepatic biloma. (a) Coronal reformation from a CT scan obtained two months following pancreaticoduodenectomy demonstrates a low-density intrahepatic fluid collection (*arrow*). (b) Intrahepatic fluid collection (*arrow*) was aspirated through a 22 gauge Chiba needle yielding bile with ultrasound guidance. A 12 Fr drain was subsequently placed. (c) One month following drainage, contrast injection through the intrahepatic biloma drainage catheter (*thick arrow*) demonstrated multiple segment VIII biliary radicles (*thin arrows*). A segment of the biliary tree was conspicuously absent (*arrowhead*) and likely represented the region of injury. (d) The biloma drainage catheter was successfully converted into an internal/external biliary drain, which crossed the segment of biliary injury. Six weeks later, the previously injured intrahepatic duct is normal (*arrowheads*) and communicates with the remainder of the biliary tree. The intrahepatic biloma was also resolved (not shown).

obstruction (Figure 7.7) [53,54]. In a study of 14 patients, Novellas *et al.* found that symptoms of portal venous hypertension were relieved in 10 patients (71%) following stent placement [54], with occlusion rates ranging from 21% to 40% [53,54]. The reason for occlusion appears to be a combination of tumor in-growth and thrombosis [55].

7.2.4.2 Portal hypertension and malignancy

The transjugular intrahepatic portosystemic shunt (TIPS) is a mainstay in the treatment of complications of portal hypertension. It has been proven that early use of TIPS could control acute variceal hemorrhage with significant reductions in treatment failure and mortality [56]. We reported our preliminary experience

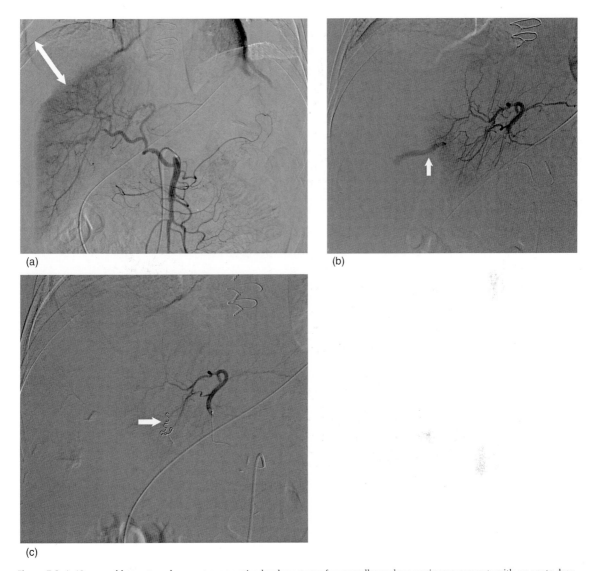

(a)

(b)

(c)

Figure 7.6 A 68-year-old man two days post pancreaticoduodenectomy for ampullary adenocarcinoma presents with an acute drop in hematocrit. (a) Superior mesenteric arteriography demonstrates a replaced right hepatic artery. There is a large subcapsular hepatic hematoma, as evidenced by the space between the diaphragm and enhancing liver margin (*double arrow*). (b) Left hepatic arteriogram demonstrates frank extravasation of contrast from a branch of a segment IVb hepatic artery. (c) The injured hepatic segment IVb branch was successfully coil embolized (*arrow*) and the patient's hemodynamic status immediately improved. Source: Reproduced with permission of Sanjay Gupta MD.

with TIPS in oncology patients and found that TIPS could be performed safely without increasing procedure-related complications [57]. We encountered no overt tumor seeding, despite shunt formation through tumor in nine patients. In our series, all TIPS were created with bare metal stents. With the use of polytetrafluoroethylene-covered stent grafts designed specifically for TIPS procedures [58], the theoretical risk of tumor seeding from TIPS which traverse tumor is likely reduced further.

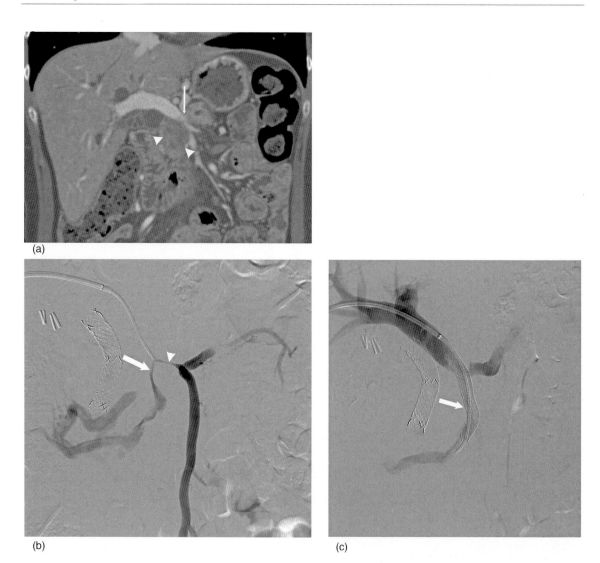

Figure 7.7 A 52-year-old woman with pancreatic cancer presents with ascites requiring serial large-volume paracentesis. Cytology from the fluid failed to demonstrate malignant cells. (a) Coronal reformation from a CT scan demonstrates a mass in the pancreatic head (*arrowheads*) and narrowing of the portal vein (*arrow*). (b) Transhepatic portography through a 5 Fr Kumpe catheter (Cook Medical Inc., Bloomington, IN) advanced to the portal vein stenosis demonstrates high-grade, short-segment narrowing of the superior mesenteric vein (*arrow*) and inferior mesenteric vein (*arrowhead*). There is an incidental biliary stent. (c) Venogram following placement of an 8 mm balloon-expandable stent (*arrow*) across the segment of SMV stenosis demonstrates brisk flow into the portal vein. The patient's ascites subsequently resolved.

7.3 Image-guided locoregional therapy of hepatobiliary-pancreatic malignancy

Therapy for liver cancer includes surgical resection, hepatic transplantation (in cases of HCC), systemic chemotherapy, external beam radiation, ablation, and transarterial embolization. Only 10–20% of patients with HCC and metastatic colorectal carcinoma (CRC) are amenable to surgical resection [59,60]. Ablative and transarterial techniques have been developed as minimally invasive options to treat patients who would otherwise be unsuitable for liver surgery.

7.3.1 Outcomes of image-guided therapy of hepatocellular carcinoma

Ablative techniques for the liver can be grouped into chemical (i.e. ethanol and acetic acid injection), thermal (i.e. radiofrequency, microwave, cryoablation), and non-thermal (i.e. cell membrane perforation with electroporation). Laser and US ablation will not be discussed in this chapter given the paucity of long-term survival data. Ablation can be used for local control and to downstage patients who are outside Milan or UCSF criteria, so that they can receive liver transplants [61,62].

Chemical ablation can be performed with ethanol or acetic acid. Ethanol was one of the earliest ablation agents and induces coagulative necrosis by a combination of cytoplasmic dehydration, denaturation of cellular proteins, and small vessel thrombosis [63]. Acetic acid dissolves lipids, extracts collagen [64], and has been shown to cause hepatocyte necrosis at concentrations of up to 50% [65]. In a meta-analysis evaluating the clinical outcomes of radiofrequency ablation (RFA), percutaneous ethanol injection (PEI), and percutaneous acetic acid injection (PAI) for HCC involving 1035 patients, RFA was superior to PEI for survival (OR 0.52; 95% CI 0.35–0.78; P = 0.001), complete tumor necrosis, and local recurrence. Of note, RFA was not superior to PEI for tumors ≤2 cm in size. PEI and PAI did not differ significantly for survival (OR 0.55; 95% CI 0.23–1.33; P = 0.18) and local recurrence, although PAI required fewer sessions [66]. Risk factors for local recurrence include tumor size >3 cm [67], lesion multiplicity, and elevated α-fetoprotein level [68].

Radiofrequency ablation passes an electric current through an electrode to destroy nearby tissue. The success of local control is largely dependent on tumor size (<3 cm is associated with complete necrosis in 90% of cases) and presence of adjacent vessels, the so-called heat sink effect (vessels >3 mm in size contiguous to hepatic tumors are an independent predictor of incomplete tumor destruction) [69,70]. Randomized studies comparing RFA to surgical resection for small HCC have found conflicting results with respect to overall survival (OS). Chen *et al.* randomized 180 patients to RFA or surgery and found no significant difference in four-year survival rates, which measured 67.9% and 64.0%, respectively [71]. This result, however, should be interpreted with caution as the study was not powered a priori to detect noninferiority. Huang *et al.* randomized 230 HCC patients who met Milan criteria to RFA or surgery [72]. Difference in OS at five years was statistically significant and measured 54.8% and 75.7%

for the RFA and surgery groups, respectively. For RFA as salvage therapy for recurrent HCC after hepatectomy, the technique is effective and safe [73]. Cumulative survival rates at one, two, three, four, and five years were 93.9%, 83.7%, 65.7%, 56.6%, and 51.6%, respectively, with a major complication rate of 1%.

Local tumor progression following RFA of HCC is a negative prognostic factor [74]. To prolong patient survival, minimizing local tumor progression is paramount. The combination of transarterial chemoembolization (TACE) followed by RFA may reduce local tumor progression by several mechanisms. The elimination of blood flow by TACE reduces heat loss and improves thermal ablation of micrometastases around the visible tumor. This is important because it has been shown that recurrent tumors often occur in the surgical remnant near the resection margin [75]. In addition, TACE is effective in treating these nodules immediately adjacent to the dominant tumor. The combination of TACE and RFA (TACE-RFA) reduces local tumor progression and improves OS and disease-free survival (DFS) in patients with small and medium HCCs [76–78]. In a recent study by Takuma *et al.* comparing the outcome of TACE-RFA with surgical resection in patients with HCC within the Milan criteria, after adjustment with propensity score matching, the respective one-, three-, and five-year OS rates were 99%, 88%, and 70% for the TACE-RFA group and 95%, 87%, and 75% for the surgical resection group; OS was comparable between the two groups (P = 0.393) [79]. One-, three-, and five-year DFS rates were 85%, 35%, and 17% in the TACE-RFA group and 79%, 53%, and 32% for the surgical resection group. DFS was superior in the surgical resection group (P < 0.048). Of note, when the patients were censored for HCC <2 cm in diameter, OS and DFS rates did not differ significantly between TACE-RFA and surgical resection groups (P = 0.348 and P = 0.614, respectively).

Microwave ablation (MWA) offers many potential advantages over RFA. MWA achieves larger ablation zones in a shorter amount of time [80] and does not require grounding pads, reducing the risk of skin thermal injury (Figure 7.8). Also, MWA appears to be less susceptible to the effects of heat sink [81]. Lu *et al.* demonstrated that complete ablation following MWA appears similar to RFA, 95% versus 93%, respectively [82]. In a recent retrospective study by Zhang *et al.* comparing RFA and MWA, one-, three-, and five-year OS rates were 91.0%, 64.1%, and 41.3% for the RFA group and 92.2%, 51.7%, and 38.5% for the MWA group (log-rank test, P = 0.780) [83].

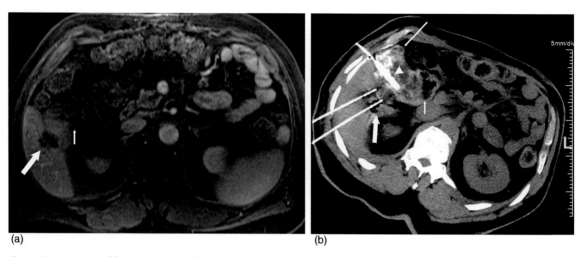

(a)   (b)

Figure 7.8 Microwave ablation of a 3 cm HCC. (a) T1-weighted contrast-enhanced axial image through the lower margin of the liver demonstrates a 2.8 cm hepatic nodule (*thick arrow*) with arterial enhancement (not shown) and early washout. Note the close proximity of a loop of colon (*thin arrow*). (b) Microwave ablation with two NeuWave (NeuWave Medical, Madison WI) microwave PR15 probes spaced 2 cm apart. Gas adjacent to the probes (*thick arrow*) is typical during ablation. A mixture of 5% dextrose solution mixed with ionic contrast (*long, thin arrow*) and a 10 mm balloon (*arrowhead*) was used to displace the colon (*short, thin arrow*) a safe distance away from the zone of ablation.

Transarterial chemoembolization involves the injection of a chemotherapeutic agent mixed with embolic particles selectively into feeding arteries to obtain selectively higher intratumoral concentrations of drug as well as blood vessel occlusion causing infarction and necrosis [84]. In a review of 14 randomized trials (n = 545 patients) for unresectable HCC, arterial embolization improved two-year survival compared with control (P = 0.017) [85]. However, OS at three years for those with intermediate HCC remained low (<30%). Post-TACE complications can also be severe [86]. Drug-eluting beads (DEBs) were developed in the hope of improving response rates and survival, while reducing post-TACE complications. DEBs are nonresorbable hydrogel beads capable of being loaded with anthracycline derivatives, such as doxorubicin [87]. In a recent phase II trial comparing DEBs loaded with doxorubicin with conventional TACE, the DEB group showed higher rates of complete response, objective response, and disease control compared with the conventional TACE group, though the hypothesis of superiority was not met (P = 0.11) [88]. DEBs, however, were associated with improved tolerability, reduction of serious liver toxicities (P < 0.001), and lower rates of doxorubicin-related side-effects (P = 0.0001).

Hepatocellular carcinoma has traditionally been regarded as a radio-resistant tumor because of the inability to deliver lethal doses of external radiation. Radioembolization is performed with microspheres labeled with the β-emitting isotope yttrium-90 (Y90). These are radiolabelled particles which are injected through the hepatic artery, where they become trapped at the precapillary level and emit internal radiation. In a large cohort study of 291 patients with HCC, Salem *et al.* reported response rates of 57% based on EASL criteria [89]. Importantly, survival times differed between patients with Child–Pugh A and Child–Pugh B disease (A, 17.2 months; B, 7.7 months; P = 0.002), highlighting the importance of patient selection. There has been recent interest in combining Y90 with systemic sorafenib in order to capitalize on the antiangiogenic effects of the latter. In a prospective study, Vouche *et al.* reported on the combination therapy as a bridge to transplantation in HCC relative to a comparison group composed of patients treated with Y90 only. While the study was limited by small patient size, the adjunct of sorafenib to Y90 for HCC did not augment pathological or radiological response [90].

7.3.2 Outcomes of image-guided therapy of hepatic metastases

A detailed review of the safety and efficacy of locoregional therapies for hepatic metastatic disease is beyond the scope of this chapter. In brief, liver ablation is largely

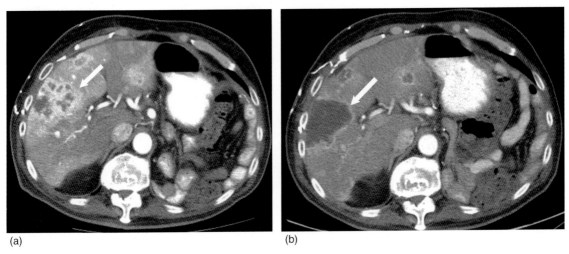

(a)   (b)

Figure 7.9 A 48-year-old man presents with metastatic neuroendocrine carcinoma to the liver. (a) Axial contrast-enhanced CT image before Y90 radioembolization demonstrates bilobar hyperenhancing masses with the largest mass in the right hepatic lobe (*arrow*). (b) Three months following bilobar radioembolization, there is marked decrease in arterial enhancement consistent with an excellent partial response by modified Response Evaluation Criteria for Solid Tumors (mRECIST) criteria.

performed using thermal-based techniques, particularly RFA and MWA, for purposes of local control [91–95]. In addition to local control, an additional niche for percutaneous thermal ablation may be cytoreduction of liver metastases, which preliminary data indicate may yield a survival benefit [96]. The data for PEI for liver metastases are sparse. Intra-arterial chemoembolization and radioembolization (Figure 7.9) have also been shown to prolong survival and improve quality of life for patients with a variety of liver metastases [16,97,98].

7.3.3 Outcomes of image-guided therapy of cholangiocarcinoma

Patients with unresectable cholangiocarcinoma have a dismal prognosis with reported median survival of 3.9 months [99]. A recent meta-analysis of 16 articles (n = 542 patients) reported that OS in patients with cholangiocarcinoma following chemotherapy-based transarterial therapy was 15.7 +/– 5.8 months [100]; 76.8% of patients exhibited a response or stable disease on follow-up imaging. Based on this analysis, transarterial therapy appeared to confer a survival benefit of 2–7 months compared with systemic therapies. Admittedly, the study was limited by insufficient data, lack of randomized controlled trials, and heterogeneous patient population. Several recent studies have evaluated the use of selective internal radiation therapy with Y90 for cholangiocarcinoma [101–104]. Early

data are promising with median survival ranging from 9.3 to 22.0 months. Mouli *et al.* reported that survival was decreased with multifocal, infiltrative, and bilobar tumor patterns [104].

One of the limitations of intra-arterial therapy for cholangiocarcinoma is tumor hypovascularity, limiting the amount of intra-arterial chemotherapeutic and embolic agent which can be delivered. For patients with small (<3 cm diameter) and intermediate (3–5 cm diameter) size tumors, thermal ablation may provide benefit [105]. Kim *et al.* reported on 13 patients with 17 primary intrahepatic cholangiocarcinomas who underwent RFA. Immediate technical success was achieved in 15/17 patients (88%); two failures occurred in tumors >5 cm in diameter. Median local progression-free survival and OS were 32.2 and 38.5 months, respectively. The one-, three-, and five-year survival rates were 85%, 51%, and 15%, respectively. While initial data appear promising, additional studies are needed to delineate the role of locoregional therapy for unresectable cholangiocarcinoma [105].

7.3.4 Outcomes of image-guided therapy of pancreatic cancer

Most intra-arterial and ablative therapies for metastatic pancreatic cancer are palliative. Kim *et al.* reported on the results of intra-arterial chemoembolization with cisplatin, ethiodol, and gel foam on 15 patients with liver-dominant pancreatic metastases [106]. Median survival was 7.5 months, with responders surviving 11.3 months versus 4.9 months for the rest of the group (P < 0.0001). Survival as long as 15 months has also been reported following the use of Y90 microspheres. Thermal ablation of liver metastases can also be performed. Park *et al.* demonstrated the utility of RFA for liver metastases in a study involving 34 patients with tumors less than 3 cm in diameter [107]. Median survival for the group was 15 months.

Locally advanced pancreatic cancer is defined as non-metastatic but unresectable disease because of vascular involvement [108]. Therapy with thermal ablation techniques suffers from unacceptably high complication rates [109,110]. Irreversible electroporation (IRE) is a nonthermal ablative technique in which a strong but short electric field is created to induce permanent nanopores in the cell membrane with resulting cell death from apoptosis [111,112]. The advantage of IRE is that tumors in direct contact with vessels may be treated without comprising the vessel or loss of ablation effect from heat sink. In one of the largest studies to date, 27 patients underwent IRE for locally advanced pancreatic cancer [113]. Nineteen patients had in situ IRE, while eight had IRE performed in conjunction with surgical resection. At 90-day follow-up, there was no evidence of local recurrence. Complications at 90 days occurred in nine patients (33%). While the complications were variable, they were most commonly associated with the open surgical procedure. Still early in its evaluation phase, further studies with larger number of patients are needed to validate the safety and efficacy of IRE for pancreatic cancer.

7.4 Palliation

7.4.1 Diversionary percutaneous biliary drainage for malignant occlusion

The prognosis for patients with obstructive jaundice secondary to malignant obstruction, most often from pancreatic carcinoma, cholangiocarcinoma, and metastatic disease, is poor, with a two-year mortality of 95% [114]. Curative surgery is often not feasible in these patients, with interventions being directed at palliation [115,116]. In these situations, biliary drainage relieves pruritus, cholangitis, and cholestasis, a risk factor for infectious complications [55,117,118]. ERCP with stent placement is the procedure of choice. However, endoscopic retrograde cholangiopancreatography may not be successful in certain clinical scenarios, such as common bile duct (CBD) obstructions above the cystic duct, failure to locate the papilla, tumor obstructing the gastric outlet or papilla, or altered postsurgical anatomy. For these cases, percutaneous transhepatic biliary drainage is often requested.

When a percutaneous drain is requested, it is important to prepare the patient emotionally for the burden of multiple potential external catheters along with the requisite fluid and electrolyte losses. Determination of the number of catheters placed is multifactorial. For obstructions involving the CBD, a single catheter can often effectively drain both lobes of the liver while more peripheral biliary obstructions may require multiple catheters. In patients who have otherwise normal underlying liver parenchyma, draining as little as 30% of the liver with a single catheter in one lobe may be adequate for symptom resolution.

Metallic biliary endoprostheses placed percutaneously are viable alternatives to external catheters for palliation. In a study of 34 patients with malignant biliary obstruction in which metallic stents were used to bridge the area of narrowing, relief of obstruction with alleviation of jaundice and pruritus occurred in 31 of 34 patients (91%) within 2–6 weeks after stent insertion [119]. Metallic stents can also be safely placed in a one-step approach, bypassing the need for a two-stage approach in which a percutaneous drainage catheter is placed followed by conversion to a metallic stent days to weeks later [119,120]. Stents are generally placed across the entire region of narrowing to limit tumor ingrowth from the end of the stent.

The main issue with metallic stents has long been the relatively high occlusion rate, ranging from 43% to 81% at six months (Figure 7.10) [121–123]. Covered stents were developed to improve stent patency by preventing tumor ingrowth through the stent interstices. One study involving 80 patients with malignant biliary obstruction treated with nitinol stents covered with polytetrafluoroethylene/fluorinated ethylene propylene (Viabil, WL Gore & Associates, Flagstaff, AZ) demonstrated encouraging results [124]. Immediate technical success was 100% and primary stent graft patency rates at three, six, and 12 months were 95.5%, 92.6%, and 85.78%, respectively. There were three cases of

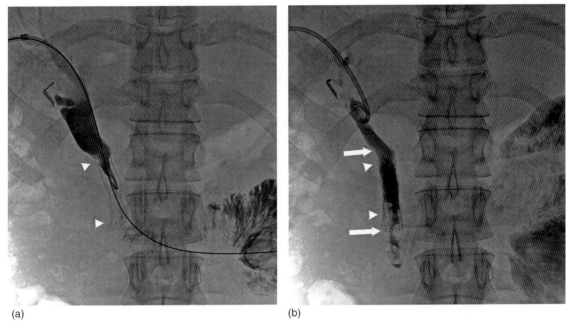

(a)   (b)

Figure 7.10 A 46-year-old man with metastatic carcinoid tumor, who received a bare metal stent to the inferior common bile duct for obstruction six months previously, presents with new-onset obstructive jaundice. (a) Percutaneous transhepatic cholangiogram demonstrates complete obstruction in the stent (*arrowheads*). (b) Despite balloon cholangioplasty, flow could not be restored. A new 8 mm × 6 cm bare metal stent (*arrows*) was deployed across the old one (*arrowheads*) with excellent result.

acute cholecystitis, which developed when the cystic duct was covered. In a meta-analysis by Saleem *et al.*, outcomes of bare metal stents were compared with covered stents [125]. The authors found that while the use of covered stents was associated with longer primary stent patency (weighted mean difference, 60.6 days, P = 0.001), rates of stent migration, tumor overgrowth at the stent margins, and sludge formation were significantly higher for covered stents.

Hyperbilirubinemia can also limit the use of certain chemotherapeutic agents, which are excreted via the biliary system. In a retrospective study of 647 patients, Thornton *et al.* found that 168 (26%) cases were being performed for this indication. The success of decreasing total bilirubin to a level of 1 mg/dL or lower was associated with predrainage bilirubin level (P = 0.004), predrainage INR (P = 0.002), and successful drainage of >75% of the liver (P = 0.001) [126]. It is interesting to note that no maximum predrainage value of total bilirubin was found in which drainage universally failed, as three of 17 patients in this study with predrainage bilirubin values of >20 mg/dL achieved a final bilirubin level of <1 mg/dL.

7.4.2 Enteral nutrition feeding options

Patients with pancreatitis, gastroesophageal reflux disease, and gastroparesis often require postpyloric feeding. Interventional radiologists can place gastrojejunal feeding tubes, which provide one port for gastric decompression or medication administration and a second port for jejunal feeds. In the setting of altered gastric anatomy (e.g. Bilroth II), partial or total gastrectomy, or intrathoracic stomach (e.g. large sliding-type hiatal hernia or history of Ivor–Lewis esophagectomy), percutaneous transgastric jejunal feeding tube placement is not possible. In these circumstances, jejunostomy tubes can be placed using fluoroscopic and/or sonographic techniques by interventional radiologists. Unlike obtaining gastric access for gastrojejunostomy tubes, direct jejunal access is considered highly challenging because of jejunal mobility. Both fluoroscopic and sonographic techniques have been described following the infusion of air or saline, respectively (Figure 7.11) [127,128]. Technical success rates of primary percutaneous jejunostomy range from 87% to 98% [127–129]. Major complications are extremely rare. Minor complications are tube related, including tube occlusion, malposition, pericatheter leakage, and cellulitis.

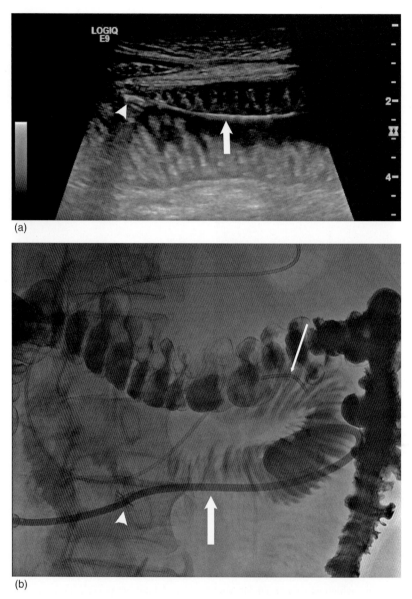

Figure 7.11 Primary percutaneous jejunostomy tube. (a) After instillation of saline via a nasojejunal tube, ultrasound demonstrates a loop of distended small bowel in anterior abdomen. T-tacks (*arrowhead*) secure the loop of bowel to the anterior abdomen and a wire (*arrow*) maintains access to place the feeding tube using a Seldinger technique. (b) Oblique abdominal radiograph following percutaneous jejunostomy tube placement demonstrates the feeding tube (*thick arrow*) located in a loop of small bowel and T-tacks (*arrowhead*). The nasojejunal tube (*thin arrow*) is used to instill saline for bowel distension.

7.4.3 Ascites management

Treatment of malignant ascites is directed towards the underlying cancer. The pathophysiology of ascites from peritoneal carcinomatosis is believed to be from fluid efflux from tumor implants and inability to appropriately resorb fluid across the peritoneum [130]. Conservative measures, such as dietary salt restriction and diuretics (i.e. spironolactone and/or furosemide), are reasonable interventions for patients with an element of portal hypertension. More often than not, the management of malignant ascites consists of large-volume paracentesis of up to 6 L at once [131]. Interventions such as peritoneal venous shunting as well as nontunneled and tunneled peritoneal drainage catheters are helpful adjuncts to address patient symptoms, such as abdominal distension, bloating, pain, dyspnea, and nausea.

7.5 Conclusion

In conclusion, interventional radiologists play an important role in the management of patients with hepatobiliary-pancreatic malignancy, providing options for diagnosis and management of surgical complications. While the bulk of the literature for locoregional therapy (i.e. chemical and thermal ablation, arterial embolization) is devoted to HCC, expansion of these techniques to other tumors is an area of active investigation.

KEY POINTS

- Optimal communication and the availability of advanced interventional radiology capabilities are the basis for an environment in which advanced minimally invasive HPB procedures can be performed safely.

- Interventional radiology has the ability to provide critical diagnostic information prior to surgery.

- There is an increasing role for interventional radiology in liver direct therapy to treat malignant disease. Effective and durable palliation can be accomplished by interventional radiology but it requires the input of the HPB surgeon to determine goals, extent, and type of palliation.

References

1 Kwan SW, Bhargavan M, Kerlan RK Jr, Sunshine JH. Effect of advanced imaging technology on how biopsies are done and who does them. Radiology 2010; 256:751–758.

2 Reading CC, Charboneau JW, James EM, Hurt MR. Sonographically guided percutaneous biopsy of small (3 cm or less) masses. Am J Roentgenol 1988; 151:189–192.

3 Riley SA, Ellis WR, Irving HC, Lintott DJ, Axon AT, Losowsky MS. Percutaneous liver biopsy with plugging of needle track: a safe method for use in patients with impaired coagulation. Lancet 1984; 2:436.

4 Allison DJ, Adam A. Percutaneous liver biopsy and track embolization with steel coils. Radiology 1988; 169:261–263.

5 Rodriguez J, Kasberg C, Nipper M, Schoolar J, Riggs MW, Dyck WP. CT-guided needle biopsy of the pancreas: a retrospective analysis of diagnostic accuracy. Am J Gastroenterol 1992; 87:1610–1613.

6 Amin Z, Theis B, Russell RC, House C, Novelli M, Lees WR. Diagnosing pancreatic cancer: the role of percutaneous biopsy and CT. Clin Radiol 2006; 61:996–1002.

7 Smith FP, Macdonald JS, Schein PS, Ornitz RD. Cutaneous seeding of pancreatic cancer by skinny-needle aspiration biopsy. Arch Intern Med 1980; 140:855.

8 Rabinovitz M, Zajko AB, Hassanein T, et al. Diagnostic value of brush cytology in the diagnosis of bile duct carcinoma: a study in 65 patients with bile duct strictures. Hepatology 1990; 12:747–752.

9 Doppman JL, Miller DL, Chang R, Shawker TH, Gorden P, Norton JA. Insulinomas: localization with selective intraarterial injection of calcium. Radiology 1991; 178:237–241.

10 Guettier JM, Kam A, Chang R, et al. Localization of insulinomas to regions of the pancreas by intraarterial calcium stimulation: the NIH experience. J Clin Endocrinol Metab 2009; 94:1074–1080.

11 Brown CK, Bartlett DL, Doppman JL, et al. Intraarterial calcium stimulation and intraoperative ultrasonography in the localization and resection of insulinomas. Surgery 1997; 122:1189–1193; discussion 1193–1194.

12 Nguyen KT, Gamblin TC, Geller DA. World review of laparoscopic liver resection – 2,804 patients. Ann Surg 2009; 250:831–841.

13 Cinat ME, Wilson SE, Din AM. Determinants for successful percutaneous image-guided drainage of intra-abdominal abscess. Arch Surg 2002; 137:845–849.

14 Huang CJ, Pitt HA, Lipsett PA, et al. Pyogenic hepatic abscess. Changing trends over 42 years. Ann Surg 1996; 223:600–607; discussion 607–609.

15 Mezhir JJ, Fong Y, Jacks LM, et al. Current management of pyogenic liver abscess: surgery is now second-line treatment. J Am Coll Surg 2010; 210:975–983.

16 Lai KC, Cheng KS, Jeng LB, et al. Factors associated with treatment failure of percutaneous catheter drainage for pyogenic liver abscess in patients with hepatobiliary–pancreatic cancer. Am J Surg 2013; 205:52–57.

17 Mueller PR, Simeone JF, Butch RJ, et al. Percutaneous drainage of subphrenic abscess: a review of 62 patients. Am J Roentgenol 1986; 147:1237–1240.

18 Van Sonnenberg E, Wittenberg J, Ferrucci JT Jr, Mueller PR, Simeone JF. Triangulation method for percutaneous needle guidance: the angled approach to upper abdominal masses. Am J Roentgenol 1981; 137:757–761.

19 McNicholas MM, Mueller PR, Lee MJ, *et al*. Percutaneous drainage of subphrenic fluid collections that occur after splenectomy: efficacy and safety of transpleural versus extrapleural approach. Am J Roentgenol 1995; 165:355–359.

20 Cronin CG, Gervais DA, Castillo CF, Mueller PR, Arellano RS. Interventional radiology in the management of abdominal collections after distal pancreatectomy: a retrospective review. Am J Roentgenol 2011; 197:241–246.

21 Ferrone CR, Warshaw AL, Rattner DW, *et al*. Pancreatic fistula rates after 462 distal pancreatectomies: staplers do not decrease fistula rates. J Gastrointest Surg 2008; 12: 1691–1697; discussion 1697–1698.

22 Knaebel HP, Diener MK, Wente MN, Buchler MW, Seiler CM. Systematic review and meta-analysis of technique for closure of the pancreatic remnant after distal pancreatectomy. Br J Surg 2005; 92:539–546.

23 Kleeff J, Diener MK, ZGraggen K, *et al*. Distal pancreatectomy: risk factors for surgical failure in 302 consecutive cases. Ann Surg 2007; 245:573–582.

24 Zink SI, Soloff EV, White RR, *et al*. Pancreaticoduodenectomy: frequency and outcome of post-operative imaging-guided percutaneous drainage. Abdom Imaging 2009; 34:767–771.

25 Brown DB, Narayanan G. Interventional radiology and the pancreatic cancer patient. Cancer J 2012; 18:591–601.

26 Hashimoto M, Koga M, Ishiyama K, *et al*. CT features of pancreatic fistula after pancreaticoduodenectomy. Am J Roentgenol 2007; 188:W323–327.

27 Bassi C, Dervenis C, Butturini G, *et al*. Postoperative pancreatic fistula: an international study group (ISGPF) definition. Surgery 2005; 138:8–13.

28 Cabay JE, Boverie JH, Dondelinger RF. Percutaneous catheter drainage of external fistulas of the pancreatic ducts. Eur Radiol 1998; 8:445–448.

29 Southern Surgeons Club. A prospective analysis of 1518 laparoscopic cholecystectomies. N Engl J Med 1991; 324: 1073–1078.

30 Deziel DJ, Millikan KW, Economou SG, Doolas A, Ko ST, Airan MC. Complications of laparoscopic cholecystectomy: a national survey of 4,292 hospitals and an analysis of 77,604 cases. Am J Surg 1993; 165:9–14.

31 McMahon AJ, Fullarton G, Baxter JN, O'Dwyer PJ. Bile duct injury and bile leakage in laparoscopic cholecystectomy. Br J Surg 1995; 82:307–313.

32 Singh AK, Gervais DA, Alhilali LM, Hahn PF, Mueller PR. Imaging-guided catheter drainage of abdominal collections with fistulous pancreaticobiliary communication. Am J Roentgenol 2006; 187:1591–1596.

33 Lee CM, Stewart L, Way LW. Postcholecystectomy abdominal bile collections. Arch Surg 2000; 135:538–542; discussion 42–44.

34 Perini RF, Uflacker R, Cunningham JT, Selby JB, Adams D. Isolated right segmental hepatic duct injury following

35 Pomerantz BJ. Biliary tract interventions. Tech Vasc Interv Radiol 2009; 12:162–170.

36 Chapman WC, Abecassis M, Jarnagin W, Mulvihill S, Strasberg SM. Bile duct injuries 12 years after the introduction of laparoscopic cholecystectomy. J Gastrointest Surg 2003; 7: 412–416.

37 Covey AM, Brown KT. Percutaneous transhepatic biliary drainage. Tech Vasc Interv Radiol 2008; 11:14–20.

38 Saad N, Darcy M. Iatrogenic bile duct injury during laparoscopic cholecystectomy. Tech Vasc Interv Radiol 2008; 11: 102–110.

39 Saad WE, Wallace MJ, Wojak JC, Kundu S, Cardella JF. Quality improvement guidelines for percutaneous transhepatic cholangiography, biliary drainage, and percutaneous cholecystostomy. J Vasc Interv Radiol 2010; 21:789–795.

40 Yamashita Y, Hamatsu T, Rikimaru T, *et al*. Bile leakage after hepatic resection. Ann Surg 2001; 233:45–50.

41 Kyokane T, Nagino M, Sano T, Nimura Y. Ethanol ablation for segmental bile duct leakage after hepatobiliary resection. Surgery 2002; 131:111–113.

42 Tanaka S, Hirohashi K, Tanaka H, *et al*. Incidence and management of bile leakage after hepatic resection for malignant hepatic tumors. J Am Coll Surg 2002; 195: 484–489.

43 Vu DN, Strub WM, Nguyen PM. Biliary duct ablation with N-butyl cyanoacrylate. J Vasc Interv Radiol 2006; 17:63–69.

44 Seewald S, Groth S, Sriram PV, *et al*. Endoscopic treatment of biliary leakage with n-butyl-2 cyanoacrylate. Gastrointest Endosc 2002; 56:916–919.

45 Jagad RB, Koshariya M, Kawamoto J, Chude GS, Neeraj RV, Lygidakis NJ. Postoperative hemorrhage after major pancreatobiliary surgery: an update. Hepatogastroenterology 2008; 55:729–737.

46 Tien YW, Lee PH, Yang CY, Ho MC, Chiu YF. Risk factors of massive bleeding related to pancreatic leak after pancreaticoduodenectomy. J Am Coll Surg 2005; 201:554–559.

47 Koukoutsis I, Bellagamba R, Morris-Stiff G, *et al*. Haemorrhage following pancreaticoduodenectomy: risk factors and the importance of sentinel bleed. Dig Surg 2006; 23:224–228.

48 Choi SH, Moon HJ, Heo JS, Joh JW, Kim YI. Delayed hemorrhage after pancreaticoduodenectomy. J Am Coll Surg 2004; 199:186–191.

49 Puppala S, Patel J, McPherson S, Nicholson A, Kessel D. Hemorrhagic complications after Whipple surgery: imaging and radiologic intervention. Am J Roentgenol 2011; 196: 192–197.

50 Sohn TA, Yeo CJ, Cameron JL, *et al*. Pancreaticoduodenectomy: role of interventional radiologists in managing patients and complications. J Gastrointest Surg 2003; 7:209–219.

51 Hur S, Yoon CJ, Kang SG, *et al*. Transcatheter arterial embolization of gastroduodenal artery stump pseudoaneurysms after pancreaticoduodenectomy: safety and efficacy of two embolization techniques. J Vasc Interv Radiol 2011; 22:294–301.

52 Sarin SK, Agarwal SR. Extrahepatic portal vein obstruction. Semin Liver Dis 2002; 22:43–58.

53 Yamakado K, Nakatsuka A, Tanaka N, Fujii A, Terada N, Takeda K. Malignant portal venous obstructions treated by stent placement: significant factors affecting patency. J Vasc Interv Radiol 2001; 12:1407–415.

54 Novellas S, Denys A, Bize P, et al. Palliative portal vein stent placement in malignant and symptomatic extrinsic portal vein stenosis or occlusion. Cardiovasc Intervent Radiol 2009; 32:462–470.

55 Tomioka M, Iinuma H, Okinaga K. Impaired Kupffer cell function and effect of immunotherapy in obstructive jaundice. J Surg Res 2000; 92:276–282.

56 Garcia-Pagan JC, Caca K, Bureau C, et al. Early use of TIPS in patients with cirrhosis and variceal bleeding. N Engl J Med 2010; 362:2370–2379.

57 Wallace MJ, Madoff DC, Ahrar K, Warneke CL. Transjugular intrahepatic portosystemic shunts: experience in the oncology setting. Cancer 2004; 101:337–345.

58 Otal P, Smayra T, Bureau C, et al. Preliminary results of a new expanded-polytetrafluoroethylene-covered stent-graft for transjugular intrahepatic portosystemic shunt procedures. Am J Roentgenol 2002; 178:141–147.

59 Scheele J, Stang R, Altendorf-Hofmann A, Paul M. Resection of colorectal liver metastases. World J Surg 1995; 19:59–71.

60 Mor E, Tur-Kaspa R, Sheiner P, Schwartz M. Treatment of hepatocellular carcinoma associated with cirrhosis in the era of liver transplantation. Ann Intern Med 1998; 129:643–653.

61 Gordon-Weeks AN, Snaith A, Petrinic T, Friend PJ, Burls A, Silva MA. Systematic review of outcome of downstaging hepatocellular cancer before liver transplantation in patients outside the Milan criteria. Br J Surg 2011; 98:1201–1208.

62 Livraghi T, Goldberg SN, Lazzaroni S, Meloni F, Solbiati L, Gazelle GS. Small hepatocellular carcinoma: treatment with radio-frequency ablation versus ethanol injection. Radiology 1999; 210:655–661.

63 Shiina S, Tagawa K, Unuma T, et al. Percutaneous ethanol injection therapy for hepatocellular carcinoma. A histopathologic study. Cancer 1991; 68:1524–1530.

64 Timpl R, Wiedemann H, van Delden V, Furthmayr H, Kuhn K. A network model for the organization of type IV collagen molecules in basement membranes. Eur J Biochem/FEBS 1981; 120:203–211.

65 Ohnishi K, Ohyama N, Ito S, Fujiwara K. Small hepatocellular carcinoma: treatment with US-guided intratumoral injection of acetic acid. Radiology 1994; 193:747–752.

66 Germani G, Pleguezuelo M, Gurusamy K, Meyer T, Isgro G, Burroughs AK. Clinical outcomes of radiofrequency ablation, percutaneous alcohol and acetic acid injection for hepatocelullar carcinoma: a meta-analysis. J Hepatol 2010; 52:380–388.

67 Ishii H, Okada S, Nose H, et al. Local recurrence of hepatocellular carcinoma after percutaneous ethanol injection. Cancer 1996; 77:1792–1796.

68 Koda M, Murawaki Y, Mitsuda A, et al. Predictive factors for intrahepatic recurrence after percutaneous ethanol injection therapy for small hepatocellular carcinoma. Cancer 2000; 88:529–537.

69 Livraghi T, Goldberg SN, Lazzaroni S, et al. Hepatocellular carcinoma: radio-frequency ablation of medium and large lesions. Radiology 2000; 214:761–768.

70 Lu DS, Raman SS, Limanond P, et al. Influence of large peritumoral vessels on outcome of radiofrequency ablation of liver tumors. J Vasc Interv Radiol 2003; 14:1267–1274.

71 Chen MS, Li JQ, Zheng Y, et al. A prospective randomized trial comparing percutaneous local ablative therapy and partial hepatectomy for small hepatocellular carcinoma. Ann Surg 2006; 243:321–328.

72 Huang J, Yan L, Cheng Z, et al. A randomized trial comparing radiofrequency ablation and surgical resection for HCC conforming to the Milan criteria. Ann Surg 2010; 252:903–912.

73 Choi D, Lim HK, Rhim H, et al. Percutaneous radiofrequency ablation for recurrent hepatocellular carcinoma after hepatectomy: long-term results and prognostic factors. Ann Surg Oncol 2007; 14:2319–2329.

74 Lam VW, Ng KK, Chok KS, et al. Incomplete ablation after radiofrequency ablation of hepatocellular carcinoma: analysis of risk factors and prognostic factors. Ann Surg Oncol 2008; 15:782–790.

75 Yoshida Y, Kanematsu T, Matsumata T, Takenaka K, Sugimachi K. Surgical margin and recurrence after resection of hepatocellular carcinoma in patients with cirrhosis. Further evaluation of limited hepatic resection. Ann Surg 1989; 209:297–301.

76 Yamakado K, Nakatsuka A, Ohmori S, et al. Radiofrequency ablation combined with chemoembolization in hepatocellular carcinoma: treatment response based on tumor size and morphology. J Vasc Interv Radiol 2002; 13:1225–1232.

77 Peng ZW, Zhang YJ, Chen MS, et al. Radiofrequency ablation with or without transcatheter arterial chemoembolization in the treatment of hepatocellular carcinoma: a prospective randomized trial. J Clin Oncol 2013; 31:426–432.

78 Takaki H, Yamakado K, Nakatsuka A, et al. Radiofrequency ablation combined with chemoembolization for the treatment of hepatocellular carcinomas 5 cm or smaller: risk factors for local tumor progression. J Vasc Interv Radiol 2007; 18:856–861.

79 Takuma Y, Takabatake H, Morimoto Y, et al. Comparison of combined transcatheter arterial chemoembolization and radiofrequency ablation with surgical resection by using propensity score matching in patients with hepatocellular carcinoma within Milan criteria. Radiology 2013; 269: 927–937.

80 Lubner MG, Brace CL, Hinshaw JL, Lee FT Jr. Microwave tumor ablation: mechanism of action, clinical results, and devices. J Vasc Interv Radiol 2010; 21:S192–203.

81 Yu NC, Raman SS, Kim YJ, Lassman C, Chang X, Lu DS. Microwave liver ablation: influence of hepatic vein size on heat-sink effect in a porcine model. J Vasc Interv Radiol 2008; 19:1087–1092.

82 Lu MD, Xu HX, Xie XY, et al. Percutaneous microwave and radiofrequency ablation for hepatocellular carcinoma: a

retrospective comparative study. J Gastroenterol 2005; 40:1054–1060.

83 Zhang L, Wang N, Shen Q, Cheng W, Qian GJ. Therapeutic efficacy of percutaneous radiofrequency ablation versus microwave ablation for hepatocellular carcinoma. PLoS One 2013; 8:e76119.

84 Raoul JL, Heresbach D, Bretagne JF, et al. Chemoemboliza-tion of hepatocellular carcinomas. A study of the biodistri-bution and pharmacokinetics of doxorubicin. Cancer 1992; 70:585–590.

85 Llovet JM, Bruix J. Systematic review of randomized trials for unresectable hepatocellular carcinoma: Chemoemboli-zation improves survival. Hepatology 2003; 37:429–442.

86 Marelli L, Stigliano R, Triantos C, et al. Transarterial therapy for hepatocellular carcinoma: which technique is more effective? A systematic review of cohort and randomized studies. Cardiovasc Intervent Radiol 2007; 30:6–25.

87 Lewis AL, Gonzalez MV, Lloyd AW, et al. DC bead: in vitro characterization of a drug-delivery device for transarterial che-moembolization. J Vasc Interv Radiol 2006; 17:335–342.

88 Lammer J, Malagari K, Vogl T, et al. Prospective randomized study of doxorubicin-eluting-bead embolization in the treat-ment of hepatocellular carcinoma: results of the PRECISION V study. Cardiovasc Intervent Radiol 2010; 33:41–52.

89 Salem R, Lewandowski RJ, Mulcahy MF, et al. Radioembo-lization for hepatocellular carcinoma using Yttrium-90 microspheres: a comprehensive report of long-term out-comes. Gastroenterology 2010; 138:52–64.

90 Vouche M, Kulik L, Atassi R, et al. Radiological-pathological analysis of WHO, RECIST, EASL, mRECIST and DWI: imag-ing analysis from a prospective randomized trial of Y90 +/− sorafenib. Hepatology 2013; 58:1655–1666.

91 Abdalla EK, Vauthey JN, Ellis LM, et al. Recurrence and outcomes following hepatic resection, radiofrequency ablation, and combined resection/ablation for colorectal liver metasta-ses. Ann Surg 2004; 239:818–825; discussion 825–827.

92 Martin RC, Scoggins CR, McMasters KM. Safety and efficacy of microwave ablation of hepatic tumors: a prospective review of a 5-year experience. Ann Surg Oncol 2010; 17:171–178.

93 Stang A, Fischbach R, Teichmann W, Bokemeyer C, Brau-mann D. A systematic review on the clinical benefit and role of radiofrequency ablation as treatment of colorectal liver metastases. Eur J Cancer 2009; 45:1748–1756.

94 Meloni MF, Andreano A, Laeseke PF, Livraghi T, Sironi S, Lee FT Jr. Breast cancer liver metastases: US-guided per-cutaneous radiofrequency ablation – intermediate and long-term survival rates. Radiology 2009; 253:861–869.

95 Livraghi T, Goldberg SN, Solbiati L, Meloni F, Ierace T, Gazelle GS. Percutaneous radio-frequency ablation of liver metastases from breast cancer: initial experience in 24 patients. Radiology 2001; 220:145–149.

96 Lawes D, Chopada A, Gillams A, Lees W, Taylor I. Radio-frequency ablation (RFA) as a cytoreductive strategy for hepatic metastasis from breast cancer. Ann Roy Coll Surg Engl 2006; 88:639–642.

97 Ho AS, Picus J, Darcy MD, et al. Long-term outcome after chemoembolization and embolization of hepatic metastatic lesions from neuroendocrine tumors. Am J Roentgenol 2007; 188:1201–1207.

98 Stuart JE, Tan B, Myerson RJ, et al. Salvage radioembolization of liver-dominant metastases with a resin-based microsphere: initial outcomes. J Vasc Interv Radiol 2008; 19:1427–1433.

99 Park J, Kim MH, Kim KP, et al. Natural history and prognostic factors of advanced cholangiocarcinoma without surgery, chemotherapy, or radiotherapy: a large-scale observational study. Gut Liver 2009; 3:298–305.

100 Ray CE Jr, Edwards A, Smith MT, et al. Metaanalysis of survival, complications, and imaging response following chemotherapy-based transarterial therapy in patients with unresectable intrahepatic cholangiocarcinoma. J Vasc Interv Radiol 2013; 24:1218–1226.

101 Hoffmann RT, Paprottka PM, Schon A, et al. Transarterial hepatic yttrium-90 radioembolization in patients with unresectable intrahepatic cholangiocarcinoma: factors associated with pro-longed survival. Cardiovasc Intervent Radiol 2012; 35:105–116.

102 Saxena A, Bester L, Chua TC, Chu FC, Morris DL. Yttrium-90 radiotherapy for unresectable intrahepatic cholangiocar-cinoma: a preliminary assessment of this novel treatment option. Ann Surg Oncol 2010; 17:484–491.

103 Ibrahim SM, Mulcahy MF, Lewandowski RJ, et al. Treatment of unresectable cholangiocarcinoma using yttrium-90 micro-spheres: results from a pilot study. Cancer 2008; 113:2119–2128.

104 Mouli S, Memon K, Baker T, et al. Yttrium-90 radioemboliza-tion for intrahepatic cholangiocarcinoma: safety, response, and survival analysis. J Vasc Interv Radiol 2013; 24:1227–1234.

105 Kim JH, Won HJ, Shin YM, Kim KA, Kim PN. Radiofrequency ablation for the treatment of primary intrahepatic cholangio-carcinoma. Am J Roentgenol 2011; 196:W205–209.

106 Kim JH, Choi EK, Yoon HK, Ko GY, Sung KB, Gwon DI. Transcatheter arterial chemoembolization for hepatic recur-rence after curative resection of pancreatic adenocarcinoma. Gut Liver 2010; 4:384–388.

107 Park JB, Kim YH, Kim J, et al. Radiofrequency ablation of liver metastasis in patients with locally controlled pancreatic duc-tal adenocarcinoma. J Vasc Interv Radiol 2012; 23:635–641.

108 Callery MP, Chang KJ, Fishman EK, Talamonti MS, William Traverso L, Linehan DC. Pretreatment assessment of resectable and borderline resectable pancreatic cancer: expert consensus statement. Ann Surg Oncol 2009; 16:1727–1733.

109 Girelli R, Frigerio I, Salvia R, Barbi E, Tinazzi Martini P, Bassi C. Feasibility and safety of radiofrequency ablation for locally advanced pancreatic cancer. Br J Surg 2010; 97:220–225.

110 Wu Y, Tang Z, Fang H, et al. High operative risk of cool-tip radiofrequency ablation for unresectable pancreatic head cancer. J Surg Oncol 2006; 94:392–395.

111 Maor E, Ivorra A, Leor J, Rubinsky B. The effect of irreversible electroporation on blood vessels. Technol Can-cer Res Treat 2007; 6:307–312.

112 Jose A, Sobrevals L, Ivorra A, Fillat C. Irreversible electro-poration shows efficacy against pancreatic carcinoma

without systemic toxicity in mouse models. Cancer Lett 2012; 317:16–23.

113 Martin RC 2nd, McFarland K, Ellis S, Velanovich V. Irreversible electroporation therapy in the management of locally advanced pancreatic adenocarcinoma. J Am Coll Surg 2012; 215:361–369.

114 Bjornsson E, Gustafsson J, Borkman J, Kilander A. Fate of patients with obstructive jaundice. J Hosp Med 2008; 3:117–123.

115 De Groen PC, Gores GJ, LaRusso NF, Gunderson LL, Nagorney DM. Biliary tract cancers. N Engl J Med 1999; 341:1368–1378.

116 Yip D, Karapetis C, Strickland A, Steer CB, Goldstein D. Chemotherapy and radiotherapy for inoperable advanced pancreatic cancer. Cochrane Database Syst Rev 2006; 3:CD002093.

117 Covey AM, Brown KT. Palliative percutaneous drainage in malignant biliary obstruction. Part 1: indications and pre-procedure evaluation. J Support Oncol 2006; 4:269–273.

118 Katz S, Yang R, Rodefeld MJ, Folkening WJ, Grosfeld JL. Impaired hepatic bacterial clearance is reversed by surgical relief of obstructive jaundice. J Pediatr Surg 1991; 26:401–405; discussion 405–406.

119 Lee MJ, Dawson SL, Mueller PR, Krebs TL, Saini S, Hahn PF. Palliation of malignant bile duct obstruction with metallic biliary endoprostheses: technique, results, and complications. J Vasc Interv Radiol 1992; 3:665–671.

120 Lammer J, Hausegger KA, Fluckiger F, et al. Common bile duct obstruction due to malignancy: treatment with plastic versus metal stents. Radiology 1996; 201:167–172.

121 Tesdal IK, Adamus R, Poeckler C, Koepke J, Jaschke W, Georgi M. Therapy for biliary stenoses and occlusions with use of three different metallic stents: single-center experience. J Vasc Interv Radiol 1997; 8:869–879.

122 Gordon RL, Ring EJ, LaBerge JM, Doherty MM. Malignant biliary obstruction: treatment with expandable metallic stents – follow-up of 50 consecutive patients. Radiology 1992; 182:697–701.

123 Lee BH, Choe DH, Lee JH, Kim KH, Chin SY. Metallic stents in malignant biliary obstruction: prospective long-term clinical results. Am J Roentgenol 1997; 168:741–745.

124 Fanelli F, Orgera G, Bezzi M, Rossi P, Allegritti M, Passariello R. Management of malignant biliary obstruction: technical and clinical results using an expanded polytetrafluoroethylene fluorinated ethylene propylene (ePTFE/FEP)-covered metallic stent after 6-year experience. Eur Radiol 2008; 18:911–919.

125 Saleem A, Leggett CL, Murad MH, Baron TH. Meta-analysis of randomized trials comparing the patency of covered and uncovered self-expandable metal stents for palliation of distal malignant bile duct obstruction. Gastrointest Endosc 2011; 74:321–327 e1–3.

126 Thornton RH, Ulrich R, Hsu M, Moskowitz C, Reidy-Lagunes D, Covey AM, et al. Outcomes of patients undergoing percutaneous biliary drainage to reduce bilirubin for administration of chemotherapy. J Vasc Interv Radiol. 2012 Jan; 23(1):89–95.

127 Cope C, Davis AG, Baum RA, Haskal ZJ, Soulen MC, Shlansky-Goldberg RD. Direct percutaneous jejunostomy: techniques and applications – ten years experience. Radiology 1998; 209:747–754.

128 Van Overhagen H, Ludviksson MA, Lameris JS, et al. US and fluoroscopic-guided percutaneous jejunostomy: experience in 49 patients. J Vasc Interv Radiol 2000; 11: 101–106.

129 Kim CY, Engstrom BI, Horvath JJ, Lungren MP, Suhocki PV, Smith TP. Comparison of primary jejunostomy tubes versus gastrojejunostomy tubes for percutaneous enteral nutrition. J Vasc Interv Radiol 2013; 24:1845–1852.

130 Lee CW, Bociek G, Faught W. A survey of practice in management of malignant ascites. J Pain Symptom Manage 1998; 16:96–101.

131 Covey AM. Management of malignant pleural effusions and ascites. J Support Oncol 2005; 3:169–173, 176.

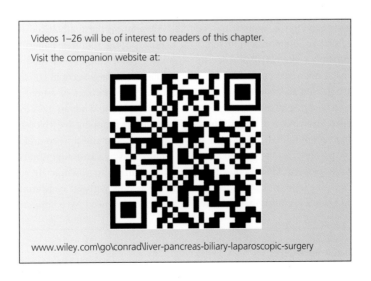

Videos 1–26 will be of interest to readers of this chapter.

Visit the companion website at:

www.wiley.com\go\conrad\liver-pancreas-biliary-laparoscopic-surgery

CHAPTER 8

Robotic hepatopancreatic surgery

Hop S. Tran Cao,[1] Claudius Conrad,[2] and Matthew H.G. Katz[2]

[1]Department of Surgery, Baylor College of Medicine, Houston, TX, USA
[2]Department of Surgical Oncology, University of Texas MD Anderson Cancer Center, Houston, USA

EDITOR COMMENT

The authors detail the available literature on robotic hepatic and pancreatic surgery. The robotic approach is contrasted with laparoscopic and open hepatopancreatobiliary surgery. Issues pertaining to learning curves and the dearth of oncological outcome data are detailed. Finally, the authors demonstrate their approach to a robotic distal pancreatectomy that can be very useful for pancreatic surgeons who wish to expand their operative armamentarium to robotic surgery. The authors sound a cautionary note that robotic and laparoscopic hepatopancreatic surgery are merely techniques and excellence in oncological outcomes and morbidity rates should not suffer when these techniques are used.

Keywords: robotic-assisted hepatopancreatobiliary surgery, robotic distal pancreatectomy, robotic liver surgery, robotic pancreas surgery, robotic pancreaticoduodenectomy

---

8.1 Introduction

If there were ever a final frontier in minimally invasive surgery, one would be hard pressed to point to anything other than hepatopancreatic (HP) surgery. Indeed, although the first reports of laparoscopic liver and pancreatic surgery date back to the early 1990s [1–3], laparoscopic HP surgery has been slow in gaining broad acceptance until recent years and remains limited, for the most part, to the hands of expert surgeons with considerable laparoscopic experience practicing in high-volume centers. The slower adoption and dissemination of this technique into broad general HP practice, in comparison to other organs, is not unexpected. Liver and pancreatic resections are regarded as some of the most intricate and technically challenging abdominal operations undertaken. A detailed knowledge of the complex liver anatomy, with its high preponderance of vascular supply and biliary system variability, and advanced laparoscopic skills are required to perform laparoscopic liver surgery, especially when tackling lesions situated deep in the liver parenchyma or in a posterior location. Similarly,

operating on the pancreas represents an inherently difficult task: the pancreatic gland is notoriously intolerant of even minor trauma, while its retroperitoneal location and intimate relationship with major vascular structures contribute to a technically demanding dissection, particularly when dealing with malignant lesions where tumor margins are of paramount importance. Furthermore, in the case of pancreatic head lesions, tumor resection results in the need to perform three anastomoses to restore biliary, pancreatic, and enteric continuity.

Translating these advanced operations to the laparoscopic setting requires expertise in hepatic/pancreatic surgery and mastery of laparoscopic skills. Although challenging, laparoscopic HP surgery has been demonstrated in a number of studies to be feasible and safe, offering potential advantages over the open approach of reduced intraoperative blood loss, decreased postoperative pain and time to oral intake, a shorter hospital length of stay, and superior complication rates [4–7]. Importantly, laparoscopic HP surgery appears to deliver these results without compromising oncological principles, as evidenced by comparable short-term outcomes

---

Laparoscopic Liver, Pancreas, and Biliary Surgery, First Edition.
Edited by Claudius Conrad and Brice Gayet.
© 2017 John Wiley & Sons, Ltd. Published 2017 by John Wiley & Sons, Ltd.

with regard to margin status and lymph node yield [8,9], and in the case of liver resection, similar disease-free and overall survival rates for patients with hepatocellular carcinoma (HCC) and colorectal metastases (CRM) relative to open surgery [10,11].

Achieving these types of results, however, requires overcoming the inherent shortcomings of laparoscopy, which include the limitation of laparoscopic equipment to four degrees of freedom, the fulcrum effect exerted by the ports on the rigid instruments, the amplification of physiological tremors, the two-dimensional visual field, and the awkward ergonomics. These challenges combine to create a steep learning curve, especially when performing tasks that demand a great degree of dexterity, such as delicate vascular dissection or precision suturing, both of which are routinely required in HP surgery. The advent of three-dimensional and flexible laparoscopic cameras, along with improvements in laparoscopic instruments and energy devices and a greater focus during operative set-up on optimizing eye–target axis, have helped to overcome some of these challenges.

Nevertheless, in an effort to address these limitations, surgeons have increasingly turned to the use of computer-assisted robotic platforms, with some having abandoned the laparoscopic approach to HP surgery in favor of the robot [12]. Robotic-assisted surgery incorporates a number of technological tools that render its application intuitive and, in our opinion, reduce the slope of the learning curve. First, EndoWrist articulated instruments recapitulate the seven degrees of freedom of the human hand, permitting more fluid movement and improved dexterity. Next, motion scaling and tremor filtration enhance the precision of surgical motions and add a novel element of ambidexterity to otherwise unidextrous individuals [13]. A three-dimensional view, combined with powerful magnification capabilities, allows for accurate depth perception and a truer optical representation of the surgical field, while placing control of the camera in the hands (or feet, to be exact) of the operating surgeon translates to improved surgical flow. Emerging data suggest that it is the three-dimensional visual field, which can now be provided by some laparoscopic cameras, rather than the addition of wrist articulation, that is the dominant factor in decreasing the learning curve slope for robotic HP surgery. Finally, the ergonomics of robotic surgery, where the operating surgeon is seated comfortably at the console, decrease fatigue and weariness associated with these challenging and often tedious operations.

Still, robotic-assisted surgery does come with its own set of drawbacks, including a lack of haptic feedback, which some authors have suggested is partly compensated for by enhanced visual feedback [14]; the high initial cost of the robot along with significant maintenance costs; and the bulkiness of the robotic cart and arms that obligates judicious port placement and makes it difficult to tilt or otherwise adjust the patient's position once the robot has been docked. Finally, emergency undocking of the robot in the event of hemorrhage may present a significant time delay during conversion to open surgery.

The aforementioned limitations notwithstanding, robotic-assisted HP surgery has generated considerable enthusiasm and interest, with a rapidly expanding literature reporting on its feasibility, safety, and outcomes. In this chapter, we review the available literature on both liver and pancreatic robotic-assisted surgery, focusing on perioperative and oncological outcomes, when available. We will then describe our technique for robotic-assisted distal pancreatectomy, the HP procedure we believe will be most likely to permeate general practice in the near future.

8.2 Robotic-assisted liver surgery

In 2008, a consensus statement was released by a consortium of 45 world experts in hepatobiliary surgery regarding the state and role of laparoscopic liver surgery [15]. While the laparoscopic approach was deemed safe and effective in dealing with all types of liver resection, only limited resections were performed minimally invasively at that time.

Therefore the 2008 guidelines were reflective of actual practice prior to the consensus conference. A review of 2804 worldwide laparoscopic liver resections determined that segmentectomies, wedge resections, and anatomical left lateral sectionectomies made up the vast majority of reported cases, while major hepatectomies – anatomical resection of three or more segments – accounted for only 17% of the cases (9% right, 7% left, and 1% extended hepatectomies) [16]. By facilitating more precise, finer movements and greater ease of vessel control, the robotic platform has been proposed as a better tool for minimally invasive liver surgery. First reported in 2003 [17,18], robotic-assisted liver resection has since generated a number of case series and comparative analyses that have demonstrated its feasibility and safety. The largest of these series [19–25] are outlined and summarized in Table 8.1 and Table 8.2.

Table 8.1 Intra- and perioperative outcomes of selected major series of robotic-assisted liver surgery.

First author	Country	Year	No. of cases – major/total	Conversion rate (%)	Operative time (min)	EBL (mL)	Transfusion rate (%)	Morbidity rate (%)	30-day mortality rate (%)	Hospital LOS (d)
Giulianotti [19]	USA/Italy	2011	27/70	5.7	270	262	21.4	21.4	0	7
Tsung [20]	USA	2013	21/57	7.0	253	200	3.8	19.3	0	4
Lai [21]	China	2013	10/42	7.2*	229	413	7.1	7.1	0	6.2
Troisi [22]	Belgium/Italy	2013	0/40	20.0	271	330	NR	12.5	0	6.1
Choi [23]	Korea	2012	20/30	6.7	507	343	13.3	43.3	0	11.7
Ji [24]	China	2011	9/13	0	338	280	0	7.8	0	6.7
Berber [25]	USA	2010	0/9	11.1	259	136	NR	11.1	0	NR

EBL, estimated blood loss; LOS, length of stay; NR, not reported.
*Includes 2.4% conversion rate to hand-assisted approach.

8.2.1 Feasibility and operative outcomes

As experience with the robotic platform has increased, so has the number of major hepatectomies reported in the literature. In a recent systematic review of robotic liver resection, Abood and Tsung found that major hepatectomies made up 86 of 236 cases reviewed (36.4%) [26].

Despite lagging the laparoscopic liver experience by nearly a decade, this rate is already more than double that reported by Nguyen *et al.* in their review of worldwide laparoscopic hepatectomies [16]. The seemingly greater comfort level with which surgeons tackle liver surgery robotically may be due to the precise instrument

Table 8.2 Oncological parameters and outcomes of selected major series of robotic-assisted liver surgery.

First author	No. of cases – malignant/total	Mean (largest) tumor size (cm) (range or SD)	R0 rate (%)	Mean margin size (mm) (range or SD)	Median FU (months)	Survival data
Giulianotti [19]	42/70	4.7 (1.1–11.0)	100	18 (1–70)	NR	NR
	HCC: 13	4.7 (1.1–9.7)	100	13 (1–20)		
	CRM: 16	4.7 (1.2–11.0)	100	25 (5–70)		
Tsung [20]	40/57	3.2 (2.05–5.0)	95	NR	NR	NR
	(7 HCC; 21 CRM)					
Lai [21]	42/42 (all HCC)	3.4 (1.9)	93	NR	14	2-yr DFS: 74%
						2-yr OS: 94%
Troisi [22]	28/40	1.97 (1.4)	92.5	NR	NR	NR
	(3 HCC; 24 CRM)					
Choi [23]	21/30	–	–	–	–	–
	HCC: 13	3.1 (0.8–5.0)	100	21 (1–35)	11	No recurrence; no death
	CRM: 4	–	–	–	12*	1 recurrence*; no death
Ji [24]	8/13	NR	100	#	NR	NR
Berber [25]	9/9	3.2 (1.3)	100	11 (8)	14	2 recurrences
	(3 HCC; 4 CRM)					

CRM, colorectal metastases; FU, follow-up; HCC, hepatocellular carcinoma; NR, not reported; DFS, disease-free survival; OS, overall survival; SD, standard deviation.
*Refers to outcomes of liver metastases group (4 CRM, 1 small bowel metastasis).
Margin >10 mm for 3 patients, 5–10 mm for 3 patients, <5 mm for 2 patients.

handling permitted by the stable robotic platform, which in turn improves hilar and hepatocaval dissection, as proposed by Giulianotti *et al.* [19]. Similarly, Lai *et al.* report that wrist articulation and three-dimensional vision afforded by the robot facilitate anatomical hepatectomies by allowing precise portal dissection and possibly early control of the hepatic veins prior to parenchymal transection [21].

A second marker of feasibility when evaluating minimally invasive technologies is the rate at which the operation needs to be converted to hand-assisted or open surgery, an event shown to be associated with worse outcomes. In series that compare the two modalities, robotic-assisted liver surgery was found to have a lower conversion rate than laparoscopic hepatectomy. Tsung *et al.* achieved a 93% rate of purely minimally invasive hepatectomy with the robot, compared with only 49% with laparoscopy [20]. Similarly, Ji *et al.* reported a 0% conversion rate in their robotic series of 13 hepatectomies, including nine major resections, compared with a 10% rate with laparoscopy [24]. Troisi *et al.* were the only group to report a higher conversion rate with the robot (20%) than with laparoscopy (7.6%) [22]. A study limitation was that the bi-institutional series compared the robotic experience from one institution with the laparoscopic experience from another. Conversion rates among the remaining major published series of robotic liver resection range from 5.7% to 11.1% (see Table 8.1), which compares favorably with the 5–15% range reported in the literature for laparoscopic liver resection.

Operative times (OT) and estimated blood loss (EBL) have been among the most heavily reported operative outcomes in minimally invasive series dealing with novel applications of technology. In the case of robotic-assisted liver surgery, results have been variable, with OT ranging between 229 minutes and 507 minutes, and EBL between 136 mL and 413 mL (see Table 8.1). This degree of heterogeneity is a function of both case distribution between major and minor hepatectomies and operator robotic experience. It also highlights the learning curve associated with new technologies and reflects individual surgeons' inherent comfort level and adaptability.

As expected, OT diminished as the number of cases performed increased. Choi *et al.* experienced a sharp downturn in their OT after the seventh case in their series of 30 robotic hepatectomies [23]. Likewise, when Tsung *et al.* compared their early (first 13 cases) and late (last 44 cases) robotic experience, they found a drop in OT

from an average of 381 minutes to 232 minutes and further identified a threefold decrease in EBL over the same time frame [20]. Overall, most series reported longer OT with the robot than with laparoscopy [20–24] but equivalent or even lower EBL. The ability to first achieve extraparenchymal vascular control and then identify vessels during parenchymal transection afforded by the robot has been cited as a reason for diminished blood loss. In fact, Giulianotti [19] and Ji [24] both made the point that the Pringle maneuver, which is used during laparoscopic hepatectomy, was not necessary in their robotic series. The difference in EBL has been even more pronounced in favor of robotic hepatectomy when compared with open surgery [20,24].

The safety profile of robotic-assisted liver resection has also been reassuring, even while acknowledging publication bias. No mortality has been reported in any of the major series, and the morbidity rate ranges from 7.1% to 43.3% (see Table 8.1). In their recent review of the robotic liver surgery literature, which includes most of the series reported here, Abood and Tsung reported a cumulative complication rate of 14.6% that is comparable to the laparoscopic liver resection literature [26]. Also comparable between the two approaches was the median length of stay (LOS). Tsung *et al.*, in their case-matched comparison of 57 robotic and 114 laparoscopic hepatectomies that bore similar major/minor resection extents, found that both groups had a median LOS of four days [20]. Yet, in the same series, the authors reported shorter median LOS for major hepatectomy with the robotic approach (five days) than with the open approach (eight days). Remaining series report median LOS ranging between 5.1 and 11.7 days (see Table 8.1). The Giulianotti series is interesting in that it represents the author's experience with robotic hepatectomy with two separate populations in two different countries (Italy and USA) [19]. While the cumulative median LOS for the entire series was seven days, median LOS was seven days for the Italian cohort compared to only five days for the American cohort. The difference was not due to any reported differences in surgical outcomes; it seems instead to reflect the cultural bias inherent to the two healthcare systems.

8.2.2 Oncological outcomes

Because robotic-assisted hepatic surgery is in its nascency, few long-term oncological data are currently available. Instead, pathological results have been cited as the most significant surrogate markers of oncological adequacy (see Table 8.2). First, it is important to point out that malignant tumors account for the vast majority of all reported cases in these series, with hepatocellular carcinoma and colorectal liver metastases as the leading indications. While most robotic series have adhered to the Louisville consensus guidelines for laparoscopic hepatectomy in limiting tumor size to 5 cm and location to peripheral segments, Giulianotti *et al.* argue that these criteria were adopted in part because of the limitations of laparoscopic instruments. Instead, in their robotic series, the authors did not observe any size limitations, performing surgery for tumors greater than 8 cm in 21.4% of all their cases, with the largest tumors measuring 11 cm [19]. Despite this, Giulianotti, along with every other major robotic hepatectomy series, achieved high R0 resection rates (see Table 8.2).

Early survival results from robotic hepatectomy series for malignancies have been encouraging. In their series of 42 robotic resections for HCC, including 10 major hepatectomies, after a median follow-up time of 14 months, Lai *et al.* reported two-year rates of disease-free survival (DFS) and overall survival (OS) of 74% and 94%, respectively [21]. Choi *et al.* have found no recurrence or death among 13 robotic hepatectomies performed for HCC after a median follow-up (FU) time of 11 months [23]. Based on their review of the currently available literature, which is limited to data from four series [19,23–25], Abood and Tsung reported the overall recurrence rate following robotic liver resection to be 15%, with no reported port site recurrences [26].

Although long-term survival data are still incomplete for robotic-assisted hepatic resection, results from the laparoscopic experience – with comparable DFS and OS rates to open surgery – should provide some degree of optimism. It is conceivable that the robotic approach, thanks to its greater freedom of movement, routine 3D vision, and lower conversion rate, may in fact improve upon outcomes so far achieved with laparoscopy.

8.2.3 Summary

The robotic approach to liver surgery has so far been shown to be both feasible and safe. When compared with the laparoscopic approach, it is associated with a lower conversion rate, equivalent or lower EBL, but longer OT. Short-term oncological outcomes appear acceptable, but long-term outcomes are sorely needed. It is important to emphasize that the results reported in these series, which were obtained from highly selected patients and achieved by experts in robotic surgery, are unlikely to translate easily into general practice today.

8.3 Robotic-assisted pancreatic surgery

Pancreatic resection has long represented a major challenge to minimally invasive surgery, especially in the case of pancreaticoduodenectomy, where the dissection is tedious, tumor margins are critical, and the complex reconstruction demands meticulous technical skills. This point is made even more significant when major venous involvement is present, mandating vascular resection and reconstruction. Although some experts have been able to accomplish this challenging task laparoscopically [27], many surgeons are not comfortable with a minimally invasive approach to pancreatectomy, especially for right-sided lesions.

Despite first having been reported nearly two decades ago, laparoscopic pancreatic resection has been slow to gain widespread adoption, and enthusiasm for laparoscopic pancreaticoduodenectomy in particular has been tepid. Criticism for the laparoscopic approach to pancreatic surgery has focused on the significantly longer operative time for little demonstrated benefit. Additional issues include the steep learning curve and the lack of long-term oncological data. In a review of 285 published laparoscopic pancreaticoduodenectomies, Gumbs *et al.* reported morbidity (48%) and mortality (2%) rates that were comparable to those from open series, with an improvement in EBL but at the cost of longer OT and LOS (weighted average of 12 days) [28]. The data for laparoscopic distal pancreatectomy (LDP), on the other hand, have been more favorable. In a meta-analysis examining perioperative outcomes of LDP, Venkat *et al.* found lower blood loss, shorter LOS, and a lower risk of overall complications and infections, with similar rates of pancreatic fistula, mortality, and margin positivity, compared with the open approach [7]. These results have engendered excitement about laparoscopic distal pancreatectomy, which has seen a rapid rise in its application in the treatment of pancreatic body and tail lesions in the last few years [29]. Still, some have postulated that dissection of the splenic vessels and separation of the pancreatic tail from the splenic hilum are two particularly challenging aspects of distal pancreatectomy that may be ameliorated with the use of the computer-assisted robotic technique.

Table 8.3 Intra- and perioperative outcomes of selected major series of robotic-assisted pancreatic surgery.

First author	Country	Year	No. of cases	Conversion rate (%)	Operative time (min)	EBL (mL)	Morbidity rate (%)	Fistula rate* All/B+ (%)	30-day mortality rate (%)	Hospital LOS (d)
Robotic-assisted pancreaticoduodenectomy										
Zureikat [35]	USA	2013	132	8	527	300**	63	17/8	1.5	10
Giulianotti [36]	USA/Italy	2010	60	18.3	421	394	NR	31.3/NR	1.5	28.7/12.5ᵃ
Chalikonda [37]	USA	2012	30	10	476	485	30	6.7/6.7	3	9.8
Lai [38]	China	2012	20	5	491	247	50	35/35	0	13.7
Zhou [39]	China	2011	8	20	718	153	25	25/12.5	0	16.4
Robotic-assisted central pancreatectomy										
Zureikat [35]	USA	2013	13	15	394	200**	100	92/77	0	8
Kang [40]	Korea	2011	5	0	432	287	20	20/20	0	14.6
Giulianotti [41]	Italy	2010	3	0	320	233	33.3	33.3/33.3	0	9–27
Robotic-assisted distal pancreatectomy										
Zureikat [35]	USA	2013	83	2	256	160**	72	43/17	0	6
Giulianotti [36]	Italy/USA	2010	46	6.5	NR	NR	NR	19.6/NR	2.2	NR
Hwang [42]	Korea	2013	22	0	399	361	NR	NR/9.1	0	7
Waters [43]	USA	2010	17	12 ᵇ	298	279	18	0/0	0	3.8

EBL, estimated blood loss; LOS, length of stay; NR, not reported.

*B+ refers to clinically relevant fistulas per ISGPF criteria (B and C); **estimated from graph; ᵃ results from author's experience in Italy and USA, respectively; ᵇ includes 1 conversion from robotic to laparoscopic (6%).

In 2003, Melvin *et al.* were the first to describe a robotic distal pancreatectomy in the treatment of a neuroendocrine tumor [30]. In the same year, Giulianotti *et al.* reported on the author's personal robotic experience, a series that included eight robotic pancreaticoduodenectomies and five distal pancreatectomies [17]. Since then, several series have been published on the robotic pancreatic experience, along with nearly as many comprehensive reviews and meta-analyses [31–34]. The largest series [35–43] are presented in Table 8.3 and Table 8.4.

Table 8.4 Oncological parameters and outcomes of selected major series of robotic-assisted pancreatic surgery.

First author	Malignant cases (% of total)	Mean tumor size (cm) (range or SD)	R0 rate (%)	Median/mean LN (range or SD)	Median FU (months)	Survival data
Robotic-assisted pancreaticoduodenectomy						
Zureikat [26]	106 (80)	NR	87.7	19 (4–61)	NR	NR
Giulianotti [27]	45 (75)	2.1 (0.6–5.2)/3.6 (1.5–6.6)*	100/79*	21 (5–37)/14 (12–45)*	Incomplete	Incomplete
Chalikonda [28]	14 (46)	2.9 (0.6–6.5)	100	13.2 (1–37)	NR	NR
Lai [29]	15 (75)	2.1 (0.7)	73.3	10 (6)	NR	NR
Zhou [30]	8 (100)	NR	100	NR	NR	NR
Robotic-assisted distal pancreatectomy						
Zureikat [26]	60 (72.3)	NR	97	14 (NR)	NR	NR
Giulianotti [27]	18 (39.1)	NR	NR	NR	NR	NR
Hwang [33]	0 (0)	3.2 (1.5)	NR	NR	NR	NR
Waters [34]	0 (0)	2 (1)	100	5	NR	NR

FU, follow-up; LN, lymph node; NR, not reported; SD, standard deviation.

*Results from author's experience in Italy and USA, respectively.

8.3.1 Robotic-assisted pancreaticoduodenectomy (RAPD)

Zureikat *et al.* have published the largest series of robotic pancreatic resections to date, a series of 250 cases that include 132 pancreaticoduodenectomies, 13 central pancreatectomies, and 83 distal pancreatectomies [35]. Results for the entire series feature adequate safety metrics, including a 0.8% 30-day mortality rate, a 20% rate of Clavien–Dindo 3 and 4 complications, and a 16% rate of clinically significant pancreatic fistula (International Study Group Pancreatic Fistula [ISGPF] grades B and C). Not surprisingly, the morbidity profile of the RAPD subset was slightly worse than that of other pancreatectomies. In fact, all Clavien–Dindo grades 4 and 5 (deaths) complications came from the pancreaticoduodenectomy group, but the 3.8% 90-day mortality rate still compared favorably with documented rates, ranging between 3% and 5%. Impressively, the rates of overall and clinically significant pancreatic fistulas among the RAPD subset were only 17% and 7.6%, respectively (see Table 8.3).

As their experience grew, the authors detected a significant drop in their rate of Clavien–Dindo grades 3–5 complications (30.7% in their first 88 cases compared with 13.6% in their last 44 cases) and a trend toward improvements in clinically significant fistula rates as well. While the median OT for the entire PD cohort was 527 minutes, this too improved with experience, dropping to 360 minutes in their last 50 cases. These times are comparable to those published in series of laparoscopic PD [9] and approach those of open series. Their conversion rate has also experienced a dramatic drop over time, from six conversions in the authors' first 20 cases to only five conversions in their last 112 cases. Based on the results of their robotic pancreatic resection experience, Zureikat *et al.* are now using the robotic platform as their preferred minimally invasive technique for pancreatic surgery.

Another large series was published by Giulianotti *et al.*, who reported on the author's personal experience of 134 robotic-assisted pancreatic operations [36]. As was the case with his robotic-assisted liver series [19], Giulianotti's pancreatic experience featured a prolific number of cases that spanned two countries (Italy and USA). Among the 134 cases were 60 RAPD; interestingly, rather than perform a pancreaticoenteric anastomosis, the authors chose to sclerose the pancreatic remnant in over two-thirds of the cases by injecting biological glue into the pancreatic duct, a maneuver that was reserved for older,

frailer patients or those with smaller ducts or friable pancreatic parenchyma. For the remaining one third of the cases, a standard pancreaticojejunostomy was performed. The rate of pancreatic fistula in the sclerosis cohort was 36.5%, compared with a 21% rate among the anastomosis cohort. Importantly, no information on exocrine insufficiency was given.

More recently, the authors have transitioned to a transgastric dunking pancreaticogastrostomy as a means of reducing pancreatic anastomotic leak [44]. Among the reported results, LOS was markedly different based on the setting – 28.7 days in Italy versus 12.5 days in the USA, a variation the authors attribute to the differences in health systems. In a later analysis of their American subset of RAPD that overlapped heavily with this larger series, the authors compared 44 RAPD with 39 open pancreaticoduodenectomies performed over the same time frame. They reported superior results with the robotic technique, including shorter OT (444 versus 559 minutes), reduced EBL (387 versus 827 mL), and a higher number of lymph nodes harvested (16.8 versus 11), with no difference in complications, perioperative mortality or LOS [45]. However, it should be pointed out that both the OT and EBL reported for the open cohort in this study were inordinately high, and the lymph node yield relatively low, compared with most published series of open pancreaticoduodenectomy.

The next three large series of RAPD all sought to compare the robotic and open techniques [37–39]. All three reported longer OT, less EBL, and significantly reduced LOS with the robotic approach. Conversion rates in these series ranged from 5% to 20%, while fistula rates varied from 6.7% to 35% (see Table 8.3). In each case, the authors concluded that the robotic approach to pancreaticoduodenectomy was safe and feasible in appropriately selected patients.

8.3.2 Robotic-assisted distal pancreatectomy (RADP)

The two largest series of RADP were also the two studies with the largest number of RAPD detailed above [35,36]. Zureikat *et al.* reported outcomes of 83 RADP performed as part of their series of 250 robotic-assisted pancreatic resections [35]. The authors demonstrated great feasibility metrics, including a low conversion rate with fair OT. Their safety profile was acceptable, with no mortality, a 13% rate of clinically significant complications, and a 17% rate of clinically relevant pancreatic fistula. Mean hospital LOS was six days. In an earlier report in which the same group compared their early RADP experience of 30 cases with a historical cohort of 94 consecutive laparoscopic distal pancreatectomies [46], they found equivalent results in most outcome parameters but detected a significantly lower rate of conversion (0% versus 16%) and a shorter operative time with the robotic technique. Importantly, they also achieved significantly reduced positive margin status (0% versus 36%) and improved lymph node harvest (19 versus nine) in the RADP group. The authors concluded that in their hands, the robotic platform constituted a superior minimally invasive approach to distal pancreatectomy to the laparoscopic technique.

Two additional studies on RADP are worth highlighting in our review (see Table 8.3). First, Hwang *et al.* described their experience with RADP for benign and premalignant tumors with a particular focus on the rate of spleen preservation [42]. In their series of 22 cases, the success rate for spleen preservation was an impressive 95.5%, including four cases in which the Warshaw technique for splenic preservation was utilized. This rate was superior to that achieved by the same group with the laparoscopic technique (64%) [47]. In this earlier report, the authors also compared the cost incurred by the patient with the two techniques and found a twofold increase in the cost associated with the robot [47]. Waters *et al.*, for their part, conducted a retrospective analysis comparing 32 open DP, 28 LDP, and 17 RADP; the primary focus of their series was cost-effectiveness [43]. Review of the short-term outcomes revealed a longer OT with the robotic compared with the laparoscopic and open approaches (298 minutes versus 245 minutes and 222 minutes, respectively), while EBL, morbidity, and mortality did not differ. The rate of splenic preservation was highest in the robotic cohort (65% versus 29% in the laparoscopic group) and lowest in the open cohort (12%), although it is important to point out that malignancies accounted for a greater proportion of the open cases (47%) than for the minimally invasive cases (29%). Hospital costs were found to be comparable among the three groups, thanks to a significant reduction in hospital LOS for the robotic group (four days) over the laparoscopic group (six days) and the open group (eight days) [43].

One caveat to consider when addressing the issues of both LOS and hospital costs is that, as reported, these parameters often reflect only results from the original hospitalization associated with the operation. Baker *et al.* analyzed the rate of readmission following distal

pancreatectomy performed at their institution over a two-year period. The authors reported a significantly higher rate of readmission with the laparoscopic approach when compared with the open approach (25% versus 8%, P < 0.05), which negated the benefit of reduced LOS on the original hospitalization detected in the laparoscopic cohort [48]. This study might have been underpowered to demonstrate a statistically significant difference, as cumulative LOS was 7.2 ± 0.3 days for LDP (n = 20) and 9.3 ± 0.1 days for open DP (n = 50), P = 0.20. Still, it highlights the importance of collecting and reporting on the readmission rates and their associated outcomes for robotic HP surgery.

8.3.3 Robotic-assisted central pancreatectomy (RACP)

Current data on RACP are limited, with the three largest series combining for only 21 cases. As can be expected when such a small number of studies and patients is available, outcomes are highly variable, with conversion rates ranging from 0% to 15%, morbidity rates from 20% to 100%, fistula rates from 20% to 92%, and hospital LOS from eight to 27 days (see Table 8.3).

8.3.4 Oncological outcomes

A concern regarding the application of minimally invasive techniques to cancer surgery is that oncological principles will be violated in order to achieve the operation either laparoscopically or robotically; in other words, that surgeons will adjust treatment of the disease to fit the technique rather than adjusting the technique to treat the disease. Such fears are justified and need to be addressed. Currently, as is the case with other minimally invasive approaches to cancer, long-term oncological data for robotic-assisted pancreatectomy are still accruing, with no clear results yet available. Surrogate markers of appropriateness of oncological operation do exist, and they include rate of positive margins and lymph node yield. In the case of pancreatic cancer, both of these parameters have been linked to prognosis and are well identified as immediate markers of technical adequacy. In the RAPD experience, negative margins (R0 rates) in cancer cases were achieved in between 73.3% and 100% of the cases (see Table 8.4), with the 73.3% R0 rate in the Lai *et al.* series comparing favorably with the 64.1% R0 rate achieved in their open cohort [38]. Likewise, lymph node yield was adequate, ranging from 10 to 21 mean or median lymph nodes; again, although Lai *et al.* achieved the lowest lymph node yield with 10, this was comparable to results from their open cohort, indicating no difference in the oncological completeness of their operative techniques [38].

Among these major series, only one offered any long-term, albeit incomplete, survival data. Giulianotti *et al.* performed RAPD for 27 cases of pancreatic head ductal adenocarcinoma; eight of these patients were lost to long-term follow-up, two died in the postoperative period, five more died from recurrent disease between seven and 20 months after surgery, three were alive with recurrences at one year, and nine were disease free at a mean follow-up of 16.8 months [36]. An additional parameter to take into account with regard to oncological therapy is the rate of multimodal therapy completion, a concept proved to be of paramount importance [49]. In an earlier report that over-lapped heavily with the Zureikat series [35], Zeh *et al.* were able to report that, of 15 patients who underwent RAPD and met criteria for adjuvant chemotherapy following surgery, 11 (73.3%) were able to progress to receive adjuvant therapy at a mean of 11.5 weeks after surgery [50].

Among the distal pancreatectomy studies, even less information on oncological outcomes is available presently. Based on the two studies that reported on immediate oncological outcomes [35,43], R0 resection rates were excellent (97–100%). Lymph node yield was adequate in one series but low in the Waters series, especially when compared with the authors' laparoscopic and open cohorts (five versus 11 versus 14 lymph nodes, P = 0.06). That being said, no clear conclusions at this time can be drawn from the currently available data. The dearth of long-term survival outcome is especially pronounced for the RADP experience (see Table 8.4).

8.3.5 Summary
The robotic approach to pancreatectomy has garnered significant attention in recent years, and is becoming more widespread, especially for distal pancreatectomy. In general, robotic-assisted pancreatic surgery can be accomplished safely, with acceptable short-term oncological outcomes. Advantages may include reduced EBL and possibly shorter LOS, at the cost of longer OT. Long-term oncological outcomes are essential and constitute, in our opinion, the ultimate metric of applicability for this technology. It bears repeating that, as was the case with robotic-assisted liver surgery, results from published robotic pancreatectomy series are not generalizable.

The learning curve is steep, especially for PD, and attempts to overcome it should be conducted in such a way as to never compromise the basic tenets of safe surgery or violate oncological principles.

8.4 Laparoscopic-assisted robotic distal pancreatectomy

8.4.1 Indications and contraindications
Distal pancreatectomy is performed for benign to malignant lesions located in the body and tail of the pancreas, to the left of the superior mesenteric vessels. While pancreatic ductal adenocarcinoma (PDAC) of the pancreatic tail is often diagnosed at advanced stages, when curative surgery is no longer feasible, distal pancreatectomy with negative margins may be achieved if the tumor is caught early and is localized to the gland, in the absence of metastatic disease. Locally advanced tumors that involve the splenic vein and/or a distal segment of the splenic artery away from the celiac trunk do not contraindicate surgical resectability.

Premalignant and benign pathologies of the pancreas that are amenable to surgical resection include mucinous tumors (mucinous cystic neoplasms [MCN] and intraductal papillary mucinous neoplasms [IPMN]), solid pseudopapillary tumors of the pancreas (SPPT), and functional pancreatic islet cell (neuroendocrine) tumors that cannot be enucleated. We reserve enucleation for those neuroendocrine tumors that are small (<1–2 cm) and superficial, located a safe distance away from the pancreatic duct. It is important to note that enucleation is not an appropriate surgical option for mucinous neoplasms from an oncological perspective, as these lesions carry a risk of malignancy and must be resected with clear margins.

Finally, cases of chronic pancreatitis limited to the body and tail of the pancreas may be encountered, especially in the presence of a main duct stricture. Distal pancreatectomy can offer these patients a chance at significant quality of life improvement. Not uncommonly, however, inflammation from the pancreatitis will have caused splenic vein thrombosis, with resultant splenomegaly and sinistral hypertension. In such cases, a pancreatectomy with en bloc splenectomy is the preferred operation.

When discussing distal pancreatectomy, the subject of splenic preservation deserves a special mention. The primary benefit of avoiding a splenectomy, of course, is preservation of intact immunity against encapsulated organisms and avoiding overwhelming postsplenectomy sepsis. This is of particular importance for younger patients, such as those with SPPT. Moreover, splenic preservation has also been reported to be associated with a decreased incidence of postpancreatectomy diabetes mellitus. In our practice, splenic preservation is attempted whenever possible when performing distal pancreatectomy for benign and premalignant tumors. Malignant tumors, on the other hand, are still resected with en bloc splenectomy.

Contraindications to robotic-assisted distal pancreatectomy include the same contraindications to open distal pancreatectomy (e.g. metastatic disease, locally unresectable tumors) in addition to pneumoperitoneum intolerance, elevated intracranial pressure, and presence of significant adhesive disease that would prohibit a safe operation.

8.4.2 Preoperative planning

In planning a distal pancreatectomy for PDAC, a thorough staging work-up must be undertaken. A high-quality computed tomography (CT) scan of the abdomen and pelvis with intravenous contrast is obtained to assess the extent of tumor invasion and look for metastatic disease. Although thin-cut CT scans are accurate in determining local tumor extent, their sensitivity in detecting small peritoneal or liver surface implants remains suboptimal, with failure rates up to 30%. Since pancreatic body and tail tumors do not produce early symptoms, they bear a high probability of having metastasized by the time of diagnosis.

Conversely, cross-sectional imaging is of tremendous value in distinguishing benign from malignant pancreatic cystic neoplasms, a distinction that is critical in guiding management. Serous cystadenomas (SCA) are benign and do not warrant surgical resection, unless they cause symptoms, whereas MCNs and main duct IPMNs may harbor invasive components and should be completely resected with clear margins in many cases. On imaging, SCAs may appear either as a nonenhancing mass containing multiple small cysts separated by internal septations, possibly with a central starburst calcification (polycystic microcystic variant), or as a macrocyst with a distinctive lobulated contour that is most commonly found in the pancreatic head

(oligocystic variant). MCNs, on the other hand, appear as a thick-walled, usually septated macrocyst with smooth sharp boundaries, with no surrounding inflamed pancreatic tissue. They are most often located in the pancreatic body or tail, and may contain papillary excrescences or mural nodules and possibly calcifications within the cyst walls. Finally, IPMNs appear as lobulated, poorly demarcated, polycystic masses associated with dilatation of the main pancreatic duct or its side branches; findings suggestive of malignant main duct disease include mural nodules, main pancreatic duct dilatation (>10 mm), and presence of intraluminal calcifications [51].

Preoperative imaging must be carefully reviewed to identify potential anatomical variations, especially with regard to vascular aberrancies, and in the case of a spleen-preserving distal pancreatectomy, to define the degree of pancreatic tail extension into the splenic hilum.

Basic blood tests, including liver function tests and coagulation parameters, are checked. If splenectomy is anticipated, appropriate vaccinations are provided two weeks prior to surgery.

8.4.3 Surgery

While several robotic-assisted distal pancreatectomy approaches have been described in the literature, our preferred technique is the hybrid method, whereby the operation is begun laparoscopically to gain access to the lesser sac and expose the pancreas, and the robot – the da Vinci Surgical System (Intuitive Surgical, Sunnyvale, CA) – is then docked to complete the dissection and resection.

8.4.3.1 Positioning

The patient is placed in the supine position on the operating table, with a bump or wedge behind the left side so as to tilt him/her towards the right. The bed is then tilted in slight (30°) reverse Trendelenburg position, and the patient's arms are tucked. Care must be taken to properly pad the patient's head and all pressure points along the extremities and to preserve safe access to the patient's head and neck for anesthesia monitoring and airway protection. A Foley catheter and an orogastric tube are inserted, and the abdomen is prepped and draped widely. The patient is provided with appropriate prophylactic antibiotics as well as pharmacological and mechanical thromboprophylaxis.

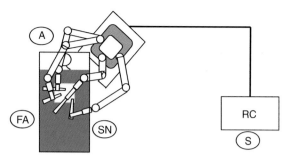

Figure 8.1 Operating room set-up after robot docking. The robotic cart is brought in from above the patient's left shoulder. The anesthesia team (A) remains above the patient's right shoulder. The first assistant (FA) is situated to the patient's right side, while the scrub nurse (SN) stands on the left side of the patient and is responsible for instrument exchanges. The surgeon (S) is seated at the robotic console (RC).

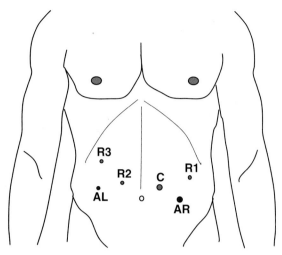

Figure 8.2 Port placement for robotic assisted distal pancreatectomy. Robotic ports are represented in blue; laparoscopic ports are represented in red. The 12 mm robotic camera trocar (C) is placed in the left paraumbilical area. The robotic working arms 1 and 2 are placed through 8 mm ports R1 and R2, respectively. The third robotic arm (8 mm) is placed in the right upper quadrant (R3) and is used primarily for retraction. The assistant's right-hand instrument is placed through a 12 mm port (AR). The assistant's left-hand 8 mm port (AL) may be optional.

When the robotic portion of the operation is reached, the bulky robot cart will be brought in from above the patient's left shoulder; it is imperative to properly situate all operating personnel accordingly. The anesthesia team will remain above the patient's right shoulder and ensure adequate access to the patient's head and airway. The first assistant, who must be skilled in laparoscopy, will be situated to the patient's right side while the scrub nurse will stand to the patient's left side (Figure 8.1).

8.4.3.2 Incision/exposure

The operation is commenced with establishment of pneumoperitoneum. A 12 mm trocar is placed to the left of the midline, 2–3 cm above the level of the umbilicus, using the Hassan technique, and the abdominal cavity is insufflated to 14 mmHg. This will also serve as the camera port. A 30° laparoscope is introduced to visually inspect peritoneal surfaces before proceeding with additional port placement under direct visualization. In total, six ports are placed – four for the robotic arms (including the camera port) and two for the assistant, as illustrated in Figure 8.2.

8.4.3.3 Surgical technique

The laparoscopic-assisted robotic distal pancreatectomy can be broken down into five main steps:
1 entry into lesser sac and exposure of the pancreas
2 pancreatic mobilization and dissection
3 vascular control and pancreatic transection

4 posterior dissection and separation of the pancreas from splenic vessels and retroperitoneum in a medial to lateral direction
5 specimen removal and closure.

Exposure of pancreas

After pneumoperitoneum has been established and upon completion of peritoneal surface inspection to rule out metastatic disease, additional ports are placed to carry out this step laparoscopically.

- The small bowel is mobilized to the patient's right and the transverse colon is retracted cephalad to expose the mesentery of the left colon. The left colon is then medialized in a caudad to cephalad manner toward the splenic flexure.
- Next, the transverse colon is deflected inferiorly by mobilizing the splenic flexure from its lateral and retroperitoneal attachments. The greater omentum is dissected away from the transverse colon along the avascular plane. Conversely, it can also be divided below and along the course of the gastroepiploic arcade, ligating the minimum number of short gastric vessels

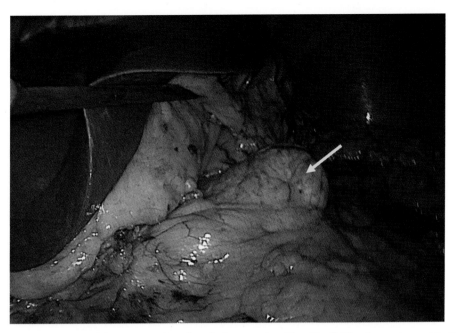

Figure 8.3 Laparoscopic exposure of the pancreas. Entry into the lesser sac is achieved by dividing the greater omentum below the gastroepiploic arcade. The transverse colon is retracted caudally, and the stomach lifted to expose the anterior surface of the pancreas. A tumor can be seen protruding from the body of the pancreas (*arrow*).

necessary to provide good exposure to the pancreatic tail if the spleen is to be preserved.

- The colon is then retracted inferiorly and the omentum lifted up to enter the lesser sac, exposing the anterior surface of the pancreas and the transverse mesocolon (Figure 8.3).
- Separation of the posterior wall of the stomach from the pancreas can be accomplished bluntly with relative ease but may at times require sharp dissection in the setting of prior inflammation. Medially, near the pylorus, we routinely look for and divide a communicating vein between the right gastroepiploic vein and the middle colic vein so as to avoid tearing it during upward retraction of the stomach.
- To aid in retraction of the stomach, we tack it to the anterior abdominal wall with a suture which will then be removed upon completion of the pancreatic resection.
- Laparoscopic ultrasound can be performed, if necessary, along the anterior surface of the pancreas to confirm tumor location. Some of the inferior pancreatic dissection can be performed at this time as well (Figure 8.4).

At this stage of the operation, the remaining trocars are placed and the robot is docked. The robotic cart is brought in over the patient's left shoulder and oriented obliquely, aiming toward the patient's right foot.

Pancreatic mobilization and dissection

With the pancreas now fully exposed anteriorly, the transverse mesocolon is stretched caudally to outline the pancreatic inferior border. Dissection is begun at the pancreatic neck.

- Using the monopolar cautery hook, the peritoneal layer overlying the inferior pancreatic border is incised and the areolar tissue layer is entered and gently dissected to elevate the pancreas. This dissection is carried out towards the tail of the pancreas, exposing the splenic vein along its course (Figure 8.5).
- Medially, the superior mesenteric vein (SMV) is identified and, with the pancreas retracted upwards by the third robotic arm, gentle blunt dissection is carried out along the anterior surface of the SMV as it transitions into the portal vein (PV) upon joining the splenic vein, thereby creating the retropancreatic tunnel and identifying the pancreatic neck (Figure 8.6).

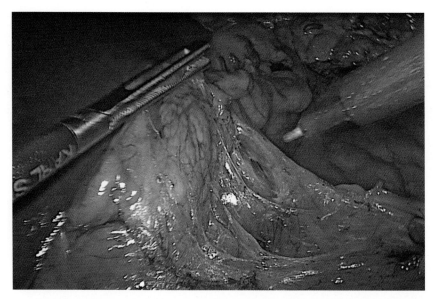

Figure 8.4 Dissection of the inferior border of the pancreas. The laparoscopic equipment can be used to commence dissection of the inferior pancreatic border along a relatively avascular plane. Care must be taken to avoid dissecting into the transverse mesocolon.

- Retraction of the pancreas can be more gently achieved by lifting it with the flat surface of the instrument's closed jaws while providing additional traction with the elbow of the instrument rather than by grasping the gland between the jaws of the instrument.
- Surgical tape is then used to encircle the pancreatic neck to assist in retraction (Figure 8.7).

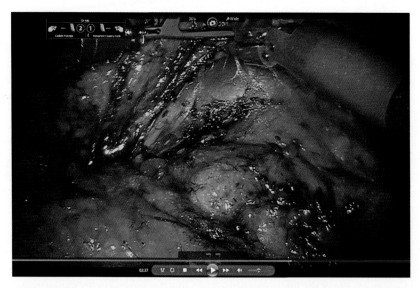

Figure 8.5 Exposure of the splenic vein along the inferior border of the pancreas. Following docking of the robot, the plane below the inferior pancreatic border is further developed so as to expose the splenic vein. This dissection is carried laterally toward the tail of the pancreas.

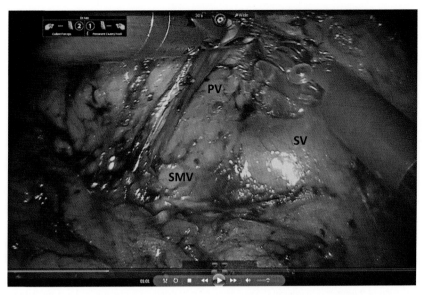

Figure 8.6 Development of the retropancreatic tunnel at the level of the pancreatic neck. Medial dissection exposes the junction of the splenic vein (SV) and superior mesenteric vein (SMV) as they merge to form the portal vein (PV). This represents the area of pancreatic transection for this pancreatic body tumor.

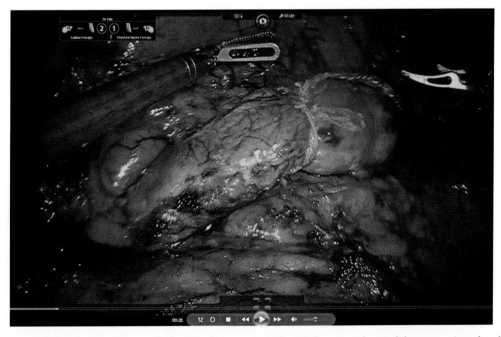

Figure 8.7 Encircling of the pancreatic neck with surgical tape. A piece of surgical tape is tied around the pancreatic neck to facilitate retraction of the pancreas for further dissection and pancreatic transection.

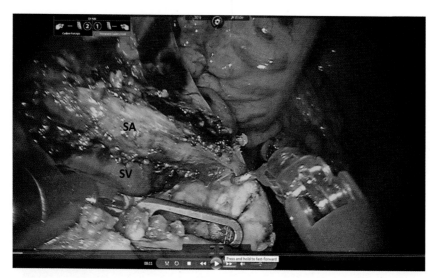

Figure 8.8 Skeletonization of the splenic artery during dissection along the superior border of the pancreas. The splenic artery (SA) is identified during dissection of the superior border of the pancreas, near its origin. It is skeletonized in a medial to lateral fashion. The splenic vein (SV) can be seen inferiorly.

We next turn our attention to the superior border of the pancreas to obtain vascular control.

Vascular control and pancreatic transection

Beginning at the level of the pancreatic neck, with the pancreas retracted caudally, the arterial dissection is addressed. Vascular dissection can be accomplished with great precision thanks to the fine controlled movements afforded by the robotic platform.

- The common hepatic artery is identified and skeletonized back to the celiac axis, sweeping the lymphatic tissue toward the specimen.
- The splenic artery is identified next and dissected distally towards the pancreatic tail (Figure 8.8). If the artery runs behind the pancreas rather than above it, we prefer to delay this distal dissection until after having initiated our retropancreatic dissection.

In our experience, dividing the pancreatic neck early helps with the rest of the pancreatic mobilization. This step is completed prior to the retropancreatic dissection.

- The neck of the pancreas is divided with an EndoGIA stapler loaded with a vascular staple load fitted with a Seamguard attachment, introduced through the assistant's 12 mm port (Figure 8.9). The stapler should be applied slowly to minimize trauma. We typically take 2–3 minutes to fire the stapler completely. We do not oversew the staple line (Figure 8.10).

- If the neck of the pancreas is particularly thick, the pancreas is divided instead with a combination of cautery and suture ligation. The pancreatic stump is closed with a running 3-0 prolene suture, and the pancreatic duct is oversewn with a vertical mattress, nonabsorbable suture. While some authors have advocated using fibrin glue to reinforce the suture line, its efficacy in reducing pancreatic leak or fistulization remains questionable.

If en bloc splenectomy is planned, we prefer to control the splenic vessels as the next step after pancreatic neck transection.

- The splenic artery is skeletonized, locking clips are applied, and the artery is sharply divided. The arterial stump is then suture-ligated, which can be accomplished with relative ease using the robot.
- Similarly, the splenic vein is dissected free starting from the splenomesenteric junction, and divided with a vascular stapler.

Retropancreatic dissection and vascular separation

The distal pancreatic stump can now be grasped with the third robotic arm and retracted laterally to expose the posterior pancreatic surface.

- The pancreas is gently dissected off the retroperitoneum and off the splenic artery and vein in a medial to lateral direction. There are invariably several tributaries behind the pancreas draining directly into the

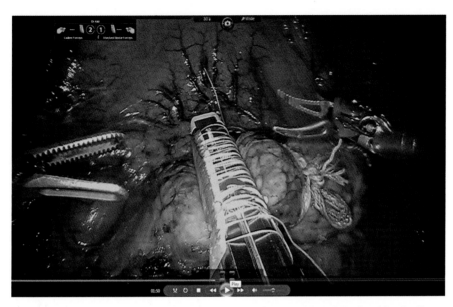

Figure 8.9 Division of the pancreatic neck. An endoGIA stapler loaded with a vascular staple load and fitted with a Seamguard attachment is introduced by the assistant through the 12 mm trocar. After closing the stapler, we typically wait 15 seconds before firing the staple load.

splenic vein (Figure 8.11). These must be meticulously dissected and controlled; they can usually be divided with ultrasonic shears (Figure 8.12).

• With adequate traction, the plane of dissection should be kept anterior to Gerota's fascia, avoiding

potential injury to the left adrenal gland and left renal vein.

• The pancreatic tail is next dissected off the splenic hilum; large branches in this area may necessitate suture ligation. In some patients, the pancreatic tail

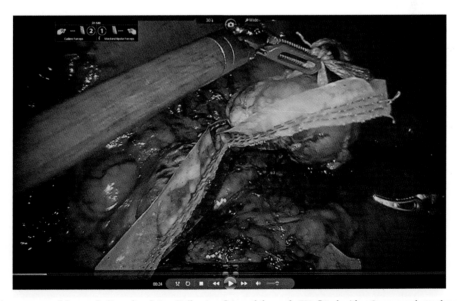

Figure 8.10 Appearance of the staple line after firing. Following firing of the endoGIA fitted with a Seamguard attachment, the staple line on the pancreatic remnant does not need to be oversewn.

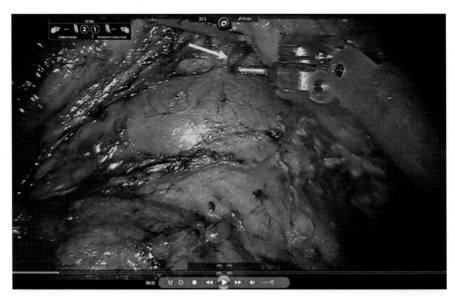

Figure 8.11 Identification of a tributary draining into the splenic vein (*arrow*). During the retropancreatic dissection, tributaries from the posterior surface of the pancreas must be carefully dissected and controlled as they drain directly into the splenic vein.

does not extend into the splenic hilum; the specimen will be freed upon separation of the pancreatic tail for the splenic vessels instead (Figure 8.13).

- When the goal is en bloc distal pancreatectomy with splenectomy, hilar dissection is avoided. Lateral and retroperitoneal attachments of the spleen are dissected with shears instead, and short gastric vessels are completely ligated.

Completion of these steps will have completely freed up the specimen, which is then placed in an endoscopic bag for extraction.

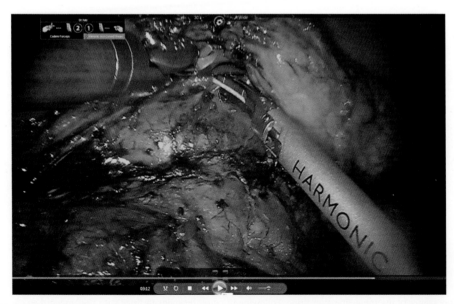

Figure 8.12 Ligation of splenic vein tributaries during retropancreatic dissection. Ultrasonic shears are used to ligate splenic vein tributaries.

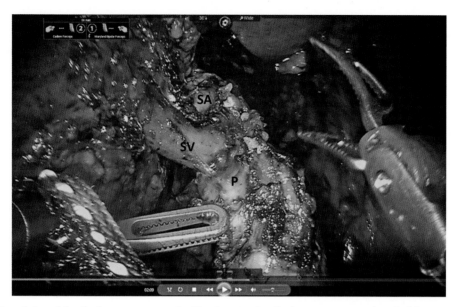

Figure 8.13 Completion of the distal pancreatectomy. In this spleen-sparing distal pancreatectomy, the tail of the pancreas ends short of the splenic hilum, such that the lateral attachments between the splenic artery (SA) and splenic vein (SV) and the tail of the pancreas (P) represent the last step of our dissection. The specimen is then retrieved in an endobag and extracted through an extension of the assistant's right-hand port.

Specimen extraction and abdominal closure

To allow for removal of the specimen, a small incision is made, either in the lower abdomen through a Pfannenstiel incision or locally in the left upper quadrant, extending from one of the ports.

- Following specimen removal, the extraction site is closed, and the abdominal cavity reinsufflated. Hemostasis is verified, paying special attention to the pancreatic bed.
- A 19 Fr silastic drain is placed near the pancreatic stump under direct visualization, exiting laterally through the left robotic arm port site.
- The robot is undocked, and the 12 mm port sites are closed under laparoscopic visualization using an endoscopic suture passer device.

The abdomen is desufflated, the remaining ports are removed, and each wound is closed with subcuticular absorbable sutures. The patient is extubated and taken to the recovery room.

8.4.4 Postoperative management/ complications

The patient is admitted to the regular ward postoperatively, and analgesia is provided with IV narcotics. A clear liquid diet is started on postoperative day 1 and advanced as tolerated. As with all patients undergoing abdominal surgery, pulmonary exercises with incentive spirometry are instituted.

Laboratory checks include close monitoring of blood sugar levels, as a permanent or transient diabetic state may develop. We do not routinely check serial serum amylase levels.

The drain output is closely monitored, and if minimal, the drain is removed prior to discharge. Conversely, if the output is high or rising, a drain amylase is sent along with a serum amylase level to diagnose a pancreatic fistula. If present, the drain is left in place until its output diminishes to minimal levels, a process that may take several weeks. In our experience, rates of clinically significant pancreatic fistulas (grades B and C) are low when proper surgical techniques are employed.

8.5 Conclusion

Hepatic and pancreatic resections are among the most advanced, technically challenging abdominal operations encountered. While enthusiasm for minimally invasive surgery has been widespread, the field of HP surgery has been relatively slow to adopt the laparoscopic technique because of inherent limitations of this technology. The computer-assisted robot, by offering a stable platform that allows for precise maneuvering, seven degrees of freedom, a 3D visual field, and improved ergonomics, may present some advantages over laparoscopy for HP surgery. So far, robotic-assisted HP surgery has yielded encouraging results. Perioperative outcomes, including morbidity and mortality, have been mostly similar between the two groups, while the robotic approach is generally associated with shorter hospital LOS, especially when compared with the open HP experience. The main drawbacks of robotic-assisted HP are the longer OT, the lack of haptic feedback, and the higher cost of the equipment, although this may be offset by the financial savings associated with a shorter hospital LOS. Short-term surrogate markers of oncological adequacy have been encouraging, with excellent rates of negative margins and

adequate lymph node yield. Long-term oncological outcomes are eagerly awaited.

Enthusiasm for robotic-assisted HP surgery must be tempered by both this dearth of long-term oncological outcomes and the realization that the currently available data are derived from highly selected patients, operated on by highly skilled surgeons, in highly specialized centers. It is likely that the robotic approach to HP surgery will be assimilated into the treatment of liver and pancreatic pathologies before any randomized controlled trial will demonstrate its noninferiority, much less its superiority, to the open and laparoscopic approaches. It is therefore important to be reminded that the robot is but a tool in the surgeon's armamentarium, albeit an advanced one, and, like the laparoscope before it, should always serve as a means to an end and never become an end in itself.

KEY POINTS

- Among the minimally invasive approaches to hepatopancreatobiliary surgery, there are important differences between a laparoscopic and a robotic approach.

- The advantages of a robotic approach are improved ergonomics, three-dimensional vision, and greater degrees of freedom of the instruments.

- The disadvantages are the need for an additional experienced hepatopancreatobiliary surgeon at the table to manage acute complications, inferior three-dimensional vision compared with the view provided by newer laparoscopic three-dimensional cameras, limited options in advanced energy devices that facilitate liver surgery.

- In particular, reconstruction is facilitated with a robotic approach.

- A robotic approach may help surgeons to transition from an open to a minimally invasive technique.

- Key concepts of advanced minimally invasive surgery regarding acute complication management must be comprehended before performing robotic hepatopancreatobiliary surgery.

- Further innovation at the instrument-surgeon interface will elevate robotic surgery from "tele-manipulation" (the surgeon is remote from the operative field) to true automatically enhanced surgery.

- Proctoring, supervision, case selection, and noncompromised oncological outcomes are important concepts when gaining robotic experience.

References

1 Gagner M, Rheault M, Dubuc J. Laparoscopic partial hepatectomy for liver tumours (abstract). Surg Endosc 1992; 6:99.

2 Gagner M, Pomp A. Laparoscopic pylorus-preserving pancreatoduodenectomy. Surg Endosc 1994; 8:408–410.

3 Cushieri A. Laparoscopic surgery of the pancreas. J Roy Coll Surg Edinb 1994; 39:178–184.

4 Reddy SK, Tsung A, Geller DA. Laparoscopic liver resection. World J Surg 2011; 35:1478–1486.

5 Vanounou T, Steel JL, Nguyen KT, et al. Comparing the clinical and economic impact of laparoscopic versus resection. Ann Surg Oncol 2010; 17:998–1009.

6 Kooby DA, Gillespie T, Bentrem D, et al. Left-sided pancreatectomy: a multicenter comparison of laparoscopic and open approaches. Ann Surg 2008; 248:438–446.

7 Venkat R, Edil BH, Schulick RD, *et al.* Laparoscopic distal pancreatectomy is associated with significantly less overall morbidity compared to the open technique: a systematic review and meta–analysis. Ann Surg 2012; 255:1048–1059.

8 Simillis C, Constantinides VA, Tekkis PP, *et al.* Laparoscopic versus open hepatic resections for benign and malignant neoplasms – a meta-analysis. Surgery 2007; 141:203–211.

9 Kendrick ML, Cusati D. Total laparoscopic pancreaticoduodenectomy: feasibility and outcome in an early experience. Arch Surg 2010; 145:19–23.

10 Sarpel U, Hefti MM, Wisnievsky JP, *et al.* Outcome for patients treated with laparoscopic versus open resection of hepatocellular carcinoma: case-matched analysis. Ann Surg Oncol 2009; 16:1572–1577.

11 Castaing D, Vibert E, Ricca L, *et al.* Oncologic results of laparoscopic versus open hepatectomy for colorectal liver metastases in two specialized centers. Ann Surg 2009; 250: 849–855.

12 Daouadi M, Zureikat AH, Zenati MS, *et al.* Robot-assisted minimally invasive distal pancreatectomy is superior to the laparoscopic technique. Ann Surg 2013; 257:128–132.

13 Prasad SM, Prasad SM, Maniar HS, *et al.* Surgical robotics: impact of motion scaling on task performance. J Am Coll Surg 2004; 199:863–868.

14 Giulianotti PC, Sbrana F, Bianco FM, *et al.* Robot-assisted laparoscopic pancreatic surgery: single-surgeon experience. Surg Endosc 2010; 24:1646–1657.

15 Buell JF, Cherqui D, Geller DA, *et al.* The international position on laparoscopic liver surgery: The Louisville Statement, 2008. Ann Surg 2009; 250:825–830.

16 Nguyen KT, Gamblin TC, Geller DA. World review of laparoscopic liver resection –2,804 patients. Ann Surg 2009; 250:831–841.

17 Giulianotti PC, Coratti A, Angelini M, *et al.* Robotics in general surgery: personal experience in a large community hospital. Arch Surg 2003; 138:777–784.

18 Vibert E, Denet C, Gayet B. Major digestive surgery using a remote-controlled robot: the next revolution. Arch Surg 2003; 138:1002–1006.

19 Giulianotti PC, Coratti A, Sbrana F, *et al.* Robotic liver surgery: results for 70 resections. Surgery 2011; 149:29–39.

20 Tsung A, Geller DA, Sukato DC, *et al.* Robotic versus laparoscopic hepatectomy: a matched comparison. Ann Surg 2014; 249:549–555.

21 Lai EC, Yang GP, Tang CN. Robot-assisted laparoscopic liver resection for hepatocellular carcinoma: short-term outcome. Am J Surg 2013; 205:697–702.

22 Troisi RI, Patriti A, Montalti R, *et al.* Robot assistance in liver surgery: a real advantage over a fully laparoscopic approach? Results of a comparative bi-institutional analysis. Int J Med Robot 2013; 9:160–166.

23 Choi GH, Choi SH, Kim SH, *et al.* Robotic liver resection: technique and results of 30 consecutive procedures. Surg Endosc 2012; 26:2247–2258.

24 Ji WB, Wang HG, Zhao ZM, *et al.* Robotic-assisted laparoscopic anatomic hepatectomy in China: initial experience. Ann Surg 2011; 253:342–348.

25 Berber E, Akyildiz HY, Aucejo F, *et al.* Robotic versus laparoscopic resection of liver tumours. HPB (Oxford) 2010; 12: 583–586.

26 Abood GJ, Tsung A. Robot-assisted surgery: improved tool for major liver resections? J Hepatobiliary Pancreat Sci 2013; 20:151–156.

27 Kendrick ML, Sclabas GM. Major venous resection during total laparoscopic pancreaticoduodenectomy. HPB (Oxford) 2011; 13:454–458.

28 Gumbs AA, Rodriguez Rivera AM, Milone L, *et al.* Laparoscopic pancreatoduodenectomy: a review of 285 published cases. Ann Surg Oncol 2011; 18:1335–1341.

29 Tran Cao HS, Lopez N, Chang DC, *et al.* Improved perioperative outcomes with minimally invasive distal pancreatectomy: results from a population-based analysis. JAMA Surg 2014; 149:237–243.

30 Melvin WS, Needleman BJ, Krause KR, *et al.* Robotic resection of pancreatic neuroendocrine tumor. J Laparoendosc Adv Surg Tech A 2003; 13:33–36.

31 Winer J, Can MF, Bartlett DL, *et al.* The current state of robotic-assisted pancreatic surgery. Nat Rev Gastroenterol Hepatol 2012; 9:468–476.

32 Milone L, Daskalaki D, Wang X, *et al.* State of the art in robotic pancreatic surgery. World J Surg 2013; 37:2761–2770.

33 Strijker M, van Santvoort HC, Besselink MG, *et al.* Robot-assisted pancreatic surgery: a systematic review of the literature. HPB (Oxford) 2013; 15:1–10.

34 Zhang J, Wu WM, You L, *et al.* Robotic versus open pancreatectomy: a systematic review and meta-analysis. Ann Surg Oncol 2013; 20:1774–1780.

35 Zureikat AH, Moser AJ, Boone BA, *et al.* 250 robotic pancreatic resections: safety and feasibility. Ann Surg 2013; 258: 554–559.

36 Giulianotti PC, Sbrana F, Bianco FM, *et al.* Robot-assisted laparoscopic pancreatic surgery: single-surgeon experience. Surg Endosc 2010; 24:1646–1657.

37 Chalikonda S, Aguilar-Saavedra JR, Walsh RM. Laparoscopic robotic-assisted pancreaticoduodenectomy: a case-matched comparison with open resection. Surg Endosc 2012; 26: 2397–2402.

38 Lai EC, Yang GP, Tang CN. Robot-assisted laparoscopic pancreaticoduodenectomy versus open pancreaticoduodenectomy – a comparative study. Int J Surg 2012; 10: 475–479.

39 Zhou NX, Chen JZ, Liu Q, *et al.* Outcomes of pancreatoduodenectomy with robotic surgery versus open surgery. Int J Med Robot 2011; 7:131–137.

40 Kang CM, Kim DH, Lee WJ, *et al.* Initial experiences using robot-assisted central pancreatectomy with pancreaticogastrostomy: a potential way to advanced laparoscopic pancreatectomy. Surg Endosc 2011; 25:1101–1106.

41 Giulianotti PC, Sbrana F, Blanco FM, *et al*. Robot-assisted laparoscopic middle pancreatectomy. J Laparoendosc Adv Surg Tech A 2010; 20:135–139.

42 Hwang HK, Kang CM, Chung YE, *et al*. Robot-assisted spleen-preserving distal pancreatectomy: a single surgeon's experiences and proposal of clinical application. Surg Endosc 2013; 27:774–781.

43 Waters JA, Canal DF, Wiebke EA, *et al*. Robotic distal pancreatectomy: cost effective? Surgery 2010; 148: 814–823.

44 Fernandes E, Giulianotti PC. Robotic-assisted pancreatic surgery. J Hepatobiliary Pancreat Sci 2013; 20:583–589.

45 Buchs NC, Addeo P, Bianco FM, *et al*. Robotic versus open pancreaticoduodenectomy: a comparative study at a single institution. World J Surg 2011; 35:2739–2746.

46 Daouadi M, Zureikat AH, Zenati MS, *et al*. Robot-assisted minimally invasive distal pancreatectomy is superior to the laparoscopic technique. Ann Surg 2013; 257:128–132.

47 Kang CM, Kim DH, Lee WJ, *et al*. Conventional laparoscopic and robot-assisted spleen-preserving pancreatectomy: does da Vinci have clinical advantages? Surg Endosc 2011; 25:2004–2009.

48 Baker MS, Bentrem DJ, Ujiki MB, *et al*. Adding days spent in readmission to the initial postoperative length of stay limits the perceived benefit of laparoscopic distal pancreatectomy when compared with open distal pancreatectomy. Am J Surg 2011; 201:295–299.

49 Tzeng CW, Tran Cao HS, Lee JE, *et al*. Treatment sequencing for resectable pancreatic cancer: influence of early metastases and surgical complications on multimodality therapy completion and survival. J Gastrointest Surg 2014; 18:16–25.

50 Zeh HJ, Zureikat AH, Secrest A, *et al*. Outcomes after robot-assisted pancreaticoduodenectomy for periampullary lesions. Ann Surg Oncol 2012; 19:864–870.

51 Tran Cao HS, Kellogg B, Lowy AM, *et al*. Cystic neoplasms of the pancreas. Surg Oncol Clin N Am 2010; 19:267–295.

CHAPTER 9

Enhanced recovery after hepatopancreatobiliary surgery

David Fuks,[1] Thomas A. Aloia,[2] and Brice Gayet[1]

[1]Department of Digestive Diseases, Institut Mutualiste Montsouris, Paris, France
[2]Department of Surgical Oncology, University of Texas MD Anderson Cancer Center, Houston, USA

EDITOR COMMENT

In this chapter, the authors provide an overview of the available evidence regarding enhanced recovery after hepatopancreatobiliary surgery. They remind us that optimal recovery for the major procedures we perform in liver and pancreas surgery begins prior to surgery. Meticulous patient selection and optimization of medical comorbidities are key contributors to the goals of any fast-track program, shortening length of stay while lowering perioperative morbidity. During surgery, the surgeon must strive for a transfusion rate of zero, while communicating clearly with the anesthesia team regarding fluid, pain, and analgesic management. While the results of published literature on enhanced and fast-track recovery programs can be difficult to interpret because of variations in protocol adherence, uncontrolled confounders, and nonweighted composite outcome measures, a programmatic approach to optimizing recovery is important. In addition to programmatic policies of early enteral nutrition, early mobilization, and restrictive transfusion policies, excellent communication among the patient, family, nursing, anesthesia, and surgery staff is critical for ensuring optimal recovery with faster discharge. As advanced laparoscopic hepatopancreatobiliary surgeons, we must remind ourselves that low complication rate is the most important component in earlier discharge.

Keywords: enhanced recovery after hepatic surgery, enhanced recovery after hepatopancreatobiliary surgery, enhanced recovery after pancreas surgery, fast-track surgery, length of stay

---

9.1 Introduction

Major abdominal surgical procedures such as hepatic or pancreatic resections cause a considerable surgical stress reaction and derangements in metabolic and cardiopulmonary function [1,2]. In past decades, advances in diagnostic and surgical techniques and improved anesthetic/intensive care management have led to better outcomes after both liver and pancreatic resections. Mortality for the most common liver and pancreatic resection has been reported to be consistently below 5% in specialized centers [3,4]. However, morbidity, especially for pancreatic surgery, remains high at a rate of 40–60% [3,4]. Complications, such as anastomotic leak, hemorrhage, biliary and pancreatic fistula, delayed gastric emptying

(DGE), and intra-abdominal abscess, are the main reasons for delayed recovery and frequently require additional percutaneous or surgical interventions.

In the past decade, fast-track surgery protocols have been used for various types of surgery, to attenuate the stress response to surgical trauma and improve recovery, thereby decreasing postoperative complications and postoperative length of stay (LOS) [5]. The intention is to prevent complications associated with an exaggerated inflammatory reaction to surgery, such as poor healing, infections, and organ dysfunction [6]. Fast-track surgery incorporating intensive optimization of early patient mobility, intestinal function, and analgesia [7] contributes to expediting recovery and minimizing morbidity [8].

Laparoscopic Liver, Pancreas, and Biliary Surgery, First Edition.
Edited by Claudius Conrad and Brice Gayet.
© 2017 John Wiley & Sons, Ltd. Published 2017 by John Wiley & Sons, Ltd.

Table 9.1 Elements included in the fast-track programme applicable to both liver and pancreatic surgery.

Evidence-based factors	Probably useful factors
No oral bowel preparation	Preoperative counseling
Preoperative feeding: carbohydrate loading up to 2 h before surgery	Provision of intravenous analgesia
No preanaesthetic medication	Stimulation of bowel movement with laxatives
Antithrombotic prophylaxis	Early and scheduled mobilization
Single-dose antibiotics	Audit
Epidural analgesia	
Prevention of postoperative nausea and vomiting	
Avoidance of hypothermia	
No routine drainage of peritoneal cavity*	
Preoperative biliary drainage if total bilirubinemia >250 μmol/L**	
No postoperative nasogastric intubation	
Optimized fluid balance	
Removal of urinary catheter on day 1	
Normal food at will after surgery from day 1	

* Specific to liver surgery.
** Specific to pancreas surgery.

Fast-track surgery protocols have gained ground quickly because of the associated cost efficiency derived from the reduction in LOS, an important issue in today's context of rapidly increasing healthcare costs and the consequent need for optimization. Studies showing fast-track surgery protocols that reduce LOS and morbidity rates and improved patient satisfaction have been published for vascular [9], orthopedic [10], gynecological [11], breast [12], bariatric [13], and prostate surgery [14], as well as other forms of abdominal (including major) surgery [15]. However, although fast-track surgery protocols have also been implemented in hepatopancreatobiliary (HPB) surgery, their widespread acceptance remains limited. A summary of fast-track protocols applicable to both liver and pancreas surgery is detailed in Table 9.1.

9.2 Fast-track liver surgery

Liver resection is associated with specific postoperative changes which need to be recognized when optimizing outcomes of patients following liver surgery. The surgical outcomes of liver resection are largely dependent on the complexity of the procedure and the host liver function. To maximize the potential benefit of fast-track liver surgery programs, future research needs to aim at establishing perioperative care plans specific to liver surgery. We have identified a total of 257 relevant articles on fast-track

liver surgery. These include studies investigating outcomes of open hepatic surgery, including two randomized controlled trials (RCTs) [16,17], two prospective cohort studies [18,19], one retrospective cohort study [20], and two case-control studies [21,22].

The two case–control trials compared outcomes of fast-track surgery protocols with those of conventional care after laparoscopic surgery [23,24]. As expected, fast-track surgery programs in those two studies reduced LOS, a result seen in all studies on fast-track surgery in open liver resection. However, fast-track programs have the ability to reduce not only LOS but also complication rates. Similar to the colorectal literature [5], in hepatic surgery, fast-track programs reduced complication rates: a meta-analysis of two published RCTs [16,17] shows a reduction in overall complication rates. This reduction was not reproduced in non-RCT studies, though this may be due to selection bias or to the methodology of those particular protocols. In the randomized series reported by Ni *et al.* [17], the selected population was particularly young and fit, and it is possible that better general health in the study populations leads to no difference between fast-track and conventional care with respect to complication rate [16,17].

Compliance with fast-track protocols is an additional factor that has been examined in several studies. Compliance with a fast-track program incorporating 19 components was exceptionally high in the series published by Jones *et al.* [16]. While only three trials commented on adherence to the protocol, higher rates of compliance are associated with reduced LOS. Further, low compliance is associated with higher readmission rates [16,18,22]. Compliance with fast-track programs is clearly an area which has potential to increase the efficacy of fast-track liver surgery protocols.

Although the rates of general complications were reduced in the two RCTs, no difference in liver-specific surgical complications was observed. Liver resection offers a unique set of postoperative circumstances as a result of liver regeneration, the anatomical complexity of biliary drainage and intraoperative vascular inflow control, and the transient impairment of liver function following resection [25]. It is therefore not surprising that a fast-track surgery approach does not reduce liver-specific complications. However, while fast-track surgery protocols focus on general pre- and postoperative considerations, the liver surgeon must not forget to optimize intraoperative care for best possible outcome. For example, minimizing blood loss is one area that may reduce liver-specific surgical complications [26–28].

Overload of salt and free water, as well as hypovolemia in the perioperative period, all increase postoperative complication rates [29], suggesting that near-zero fluid balance should be achieved around the time of surgery. Determining the correct amount required is complicated by the use of epidural anesthesia as it causes vasodilatation and intravascular depletion with hypotension, often treated with fluid resuscitation. This may result in the administration of unnecessary and large volumes of fluid [30]. Importantly, elevated central venous pressure (CVP) has been shown to be associated with intraoperative blood loss during liver resection [31]. Six of the nine trials included a care component based on the reduction of intraoperative fluid, but only two [21,22] commented on titration of intravenous fluid according to CVP. Jones *et al.* used goal-directed fluid therapy guided by cardiac output monitoring to prevent fluid overload, although they only monitored this in the early postoperative period [16].

Since the successful report of the first laparoscopic liver wedge resection in 1991 [32], laparoscopic liver resection has progressively gained popularity. For minor liver resections, comparative studies of open and laparoscopic procedures have shown that laparoscopic liver resection resulted in decreased intraoperative bleeding, fewer complications, and shorter postoperative hospital stays [33–37]. Over the last few years, technological and instrumental improvements have resulted in several centers reporting better hemostasis during laparoscopic liver resection [38–41].

Fast-track surgery protocols in liver surgery should incorporate preoperative, intraoperative, and postoperative components to maximize their benefits. Interestingly, use of a thoracic epidural was not explored in any of the studies. Although a thoracic epidural is recommended in fast-track surgery in the context of colorectal surgery [42], its use has been questioned in liver surgery [43]. There is conflicting evidence regarding the impact of epidurals on recovery in liver surgery, and this continues to be an active area of investigation [44,45]. Further evaluation of analgesia in liver surgery within the context of a fast-track surgery program is required to establish optimal practice. Indeed, paracetamol (acetaminophen) is routinely utilized as the backbone of analgesic regimens [46,47], but in major hepatic resections it is often withheld for fear of inducing liver damage, which increases opiate requirements.

In summary, the level I evidence investigating fast-track surgery protocols following liver surgery is limited and only two RCTS have been conducted. Fast track liver surgery programs seem to reduce complication rates, although surgical morbidity remains high and is currently unaffected by fast-track surgery protocols following liver surgery. Postoperative LOS is reduced in the context of fast-track surgery in comparison with conventional care (Table 9.2). Future research should concentrate on perioperative care components specific to liver surgery, such as optimal analgesic regimens and intraoperative manipulations to reduce blood loss, rather than simply transferring fast-track concepts from colorectal to liver surgery.

9.3 Fast-track pancreas surgery

Most series focusing on fast-track surgery in pancreatic surgery concern pancreatoduodenectomy (PD). No RCTs have been conducted in pancreatic surgery. This is probably due to the fact that RCTs are difficult to organize for multimodal recovery programs under greatly varying conditions (according to the complexity of liver resection). Problems are likely to be encountered with blinding when various interventions and professionals are involved. The incidence of specific complications, such as DGE and pancreatic fistula, tended to be lower in the fast-track surgery group, but meta-analysis in patients undergoing PD did not show statistically significant differences [48,49]. The included studies were either retrospective or prospective case series, or comparative studies

Table 9.2 Postoperative outcomes after implementation of a clinical pathway in liver surgery.

Study	Length of stay Study vs control group	Morbidity % Study vs control group	Mortality % Study vs control group	Readmissions % Study vs control group
Lin et al. 2011 [21]	7 vs 11 days*	46 vs 43%	1.8 vs 1.6%	7 vs 3%
Hendry et al. 2010 [62]	3 vs 5 days*	17	2	5
Stoot et al. 2009 [24]	5 vs 7 days	15 vs 15%	0 vs 0%	0 vs 0%
Koea et al. 2009 [44]	4 vs 6 days	19	0	4
Van Dam et al. 2008 [22]	6 vs 8 days*	41 vs 31%	0 vs 2%	13 vs 10%
MacKay & O'Dwyer 2008 [63]	4 days (2–7)	17	0	0

* Significant difference.

based on historical controls. Indeed, there seemed to be little replication of methodology in the studies examined. Individual studies used different study protocols incorporating a variety of elements, and some protocols may have included elements that are more conservative than others. For example, postoperative feeding started from postoperative days 1–2 in some studies [50,51], whereas other studies began with liquid intake with a gradual increase from clear to full liquids and solid food from days 3–4 [52–57]. Unfortunately, it is still unclear which elements are important in perioperative care in pancreatic resections, and therefore we cannot draw definitive conclusions as to the precise benefit of fast-track programs in pancreas surgery.

Similar to liver fast-track programs, most studies on pancreatic fast-track surgery do not investigate compliance with the protocol. Therefore, it remains unclear what the actual measurable difference in perioperative care between study and control group is. Policies to improve postoperative protocol adherence, in particular, should be considered. For instance, reorganization of surgical wards and continuous education of nurses and staff [58] may provide helpful information on which portions of a fast-track program have improved outcomes. A study by Ahmed et al. showed that an overall protocol compliance of 77% compared with 88% compliance in patients participating in a clinical trial does not negatively affect outcome [59].

The consistency between criteria defining minor and major complications after pancreatic surgery in the included studies is also limited. Only one study reported complications according to a validated classification scheme (Clavien–Dindo classification) [60]. Therefore, comparing morbidity between different centers is difficult, as shown by the variations in leakage rates ranging from 2% to 62% (Table 9.3). A suggestion would be to use

Table 9.3 Postoperative outcomes after implementation of a clinical pathway in pancreatic surgery.

Study	Length of stay Study vs control group	Morbidity % Study vs control group	Mortality % Study vs control group	Readmissions % Study vs control group
Robertson et al. 2012 [56]	10 days (8–17)	46%	4%	4%
Di Sebastiano et al. 2011 [51]	10 days (6–69)	39%	2.7%	6%
Kennedy et al. 2009 [57]	7 vs 10 days *	16 vs 37%	1.1 vs 2.3%	7 vs 25% *
Balzano et al. 2008 [54]	13 vs 15 days *	47 vs 59% *	3.6 vs 2.8%	7 vs 6%
Berberat et al. 2007 [52]	10 days (4–115)	25%	2%	3%
Vanounou et al. 2007 [53]	8 vs 8 days	54 vs 62%	1.4 vs 1.6%	9 vs 6%
Kennedy et al. 2007 [55]	7 vs 13 days *	37 vs 44%	1.1 vs 2.3%	8 vs 7%
Porter et al. 2000 [64]	13 vs 16 days *	24 vs 20%	1 vs 3%	9 vs 10%

* Significant difference.

a composite endpoint [61], which would reduce the required sample sizes for studies and improve objectivity and comparability.

In a meta-analysis of fast-track programs for pancreas surgery, readmission rates were not significantly higher in the fast-track surgery group. One study reported a nonsignificant 1% higher mortality rate in the fast-track surgery group [54]. Also, in a meta-analysis of the four studies addressing PDs, mortality was not significantly different. Additionally, hospital costs were significantly lower in three of the four studies that reported a cost-effectiveness analysis. As for liver surgery, few data on functional recovery or predefined discharge criteria were available, and accordingly, no conclusion could be drawn.

In summary, although the available evidence is still limited, implementation of a fast-track surgery program in pancreatic resections, particularly PD, is feasible. Such programs may contribute to a shorter hospital stay and do not seem to compromise outcome measures, such as morbidity, mortality, and readmissions. Future studies should report on predefined discharge criteria and time to functional recovery to assess whether postoperative recovery is in fact accelerated.

KEY POINTS

- Recognition of specific postoperative changes is associated with optimal outcomes for patients following liver resection. Outcomes are largely dependent on complexity of the procedure and the host liver function.

- Fast-track programs have the ability to reduce LOS and complication rates. Future research in establishing perioperative care plans specific to liver surgery can help maximize the potential benefit of fast-track programs.

- Fast-track surgery protocols in liver surgery should incorporate preoperative, intraoperative, and postoperative components.

- Most studies on pancreatic fast-track surgery have not investigated compliance with protocol. Policies to improve postoperative protocol adherence should be considered.

- Although available evidence is limited, a fast-track surgery program in pancreatic resections, particularly PD, is feasible. It may contribute to shorter hospital stay without compromising morbidity, mortality, and readmissions.

- Future studies should report predefined discharge criteria and time to functional recovery to assess whether postoperative recovery is in fact accelerated.

References

1 Reissfelder C, Rahbari NN, Koch M, et al. Postoperative course and clinical significance of biochemical blood tests following hepatic resection. Br J Surg 2011; 98:836–844.

2 Lassen K, Coolsen MME, Slim K, et al. Guidelines for perioperative care for pancreaticoduodenectomy: Enhanced Recovery After Surgery (ERAS®) Society Recommendations. World J Surg 2013; 37:240–258.

3 Virani S, Michaelson J, Hutter M, et al. Morbidity and mortality after liver resections: results of the patient safety in surgery study. J Am Coll Surg 2007; 204:1248–1292.

4 Sewnath ME, Karsten TM, Prins MH, et al. A metaanalysis on the efficacy of preoperative biliary drainage for tumors causing obstructive jaundice. Ann Surg 2002; 236:17–27.

5 Varadhan KK, Neal KR, Dejong CH, et al. The enhanced recovery after surgery (ERAS) pathway for patients undergoing major elective open colorectal surgery: a meta-analysis of randomized controlled trials. Clin Nutr 2010; 29:434–440.

6 Holte K, Kehlet H. Epidural anaesthesia and analgesia – effects on surgical stress response and implications for postoperative nutrition. Clin Nutr 2002; 21:199–206.

7 Grade M, Quintel M, Ghadimi M. Standard perioperative management in gastrointestinal surgery. Langenbecks Arch Surg 2011; 396:591–606.

8 Kehlet H. Multimodal approach to control postoperative pathophysiology and rehabilitation. Br J Anaesth 1997; 78:606–617.

9 Brustia P, Renghi A, Gramaglia L, et al. Mininvasive abdominal aortic surgery. Early recovery and reduced hospitalization after multidisciplinary approach. J Cardiovasc Surg (Torino) 2003; 44:629–635.

10 Scott N, McDonald D, Campbell J, et al. The use of enhanced recovery after surgery (ERAS) principles in Scottish orthopaedic units – an implementation and follow-up at 1 year, 2010–2011: a report from the Muculoskeletal Audit, Scotland. Arch Orthop Trauma Surg 2013; 133:117–124.

11 Lv D, Wang X, Shi G. Perioperative enhanced recovery programmes for gynaecological cancer patients. Cochrane Database Syst Rev 2010; 6:CD008239.

12 Arsalani-Zadaeh R, El Fadl D, Yassin N, MacFie J. Evidence-based review of enhancing postoperative recovery after breast surgery. Br J Surg 2011; 98:181–196.

13 McCarty TM, Arnold DT, Lamont JP, Fisher TL, Kuhn JA. Optimizing outcomes in bariatric surgery: outpatient laparoscopic gastric bypass. Ann Surg 2005; 242:494–498; discussion 498–501.

14 Kirsh EJ, Worwag EM, Sinner M, Chodak GW. Using outcome data and patient satisfaction surveys to develop policies regarding minimum length of hospitalization after radical prostatectomy. Urology 2000; 56:101–106; discussion 106–107.

15 Cerfolio RJ, Bryant AS, Bass CS, Alexander JR, Bartolucci AA. Fast tracking after Ivor Lewis esophagogastrectomy. Chest 2004; 126:1187–1194.

16 Jones C, Kelliher L, Dickinson M, et al. Randomized clinical trial on enhanced recovery versus standard care following open liver resection. Br J Surg 2013; 100:1015–1024.

17 Ni C, Yang Y, Chang Y, et al. Fast-track surgery improves postoperative recovery in patients undergoing partial hepatectomy for primary liver cancer: a prospective randomized controlled trial. Eur J Surg Oncol 2013; 39:542–547.

18 MacKay G, O'Dwyer P. Early discharge following liver resection for colorectal metastases. Scott Med J 2008; 53:22–24.

19 Schultz N, Larsen P, Klarskov B, et al. Evaluation of a fast-track programme for patients undergoing liver resection. Br J Surg 2013; 100:138–143.

20 Connor S, Cross A, Sakowska M, Linscott D, Woods J. Effects of introducing an enhanced recovery after surgery programme for patients undergoing open hepatic resection. HPB 2013; 15:294–301.

21 Lin D, Li X, Ye Q, Lin F, Li L, Zhang Q. Implementation of a fast-track clinical pathway decreases postoperative length of stay and hospital charges for liver resection. Cell Biochem Biophys 2011; 61:413–419.

22 Van Dam R, Hendry P, Coolsen M, et al. on behalf of the Enhanced Recovery After Surgery (ERAS) Group. Initial experience with a multimodal enhanced recovery programme in patients undergoing liver resection. Br J Surg 2008; 95:969–975.

23 Sànchez-Pérez B, Aranda-Narvaez J, Suarez-Munoz M, et al. Fast-track programme in laparoscopic liver surgery: theory of fact. World J Gastrointest Surg 2012; 4:246–250.

24 Stoot J, van Dam R, Busch O, et al. on behalf of the Enhanced Recovery After Surgery (ERAS) Group. The effect of multimodal fast-track programme on outcomes in laparoscopic liver surgery: a multicentre pilot study. HPB (Oxford) 2009; 11:140–144.

25 Hughes MJ, McNally S, Wigmore SJ. Enhanced recovery following liver surgery: a systematic review and meta-analysis. HPB (Oxford) 2014; 16(8):699–706.

26 Hammond J, Guha I, Beckingham I, Lobo D. Prediction, prevention and management of postresection liver failure. Br J Surg 2011; 98:1188–1200.

27 Zimmitti G, Roses R, Andreou A, et al. Greater complexity of liver surgery is not associated with an increased incidence of liver-related complications except for bile leak: an experience with 2628 consecutive resections. J Gastrointest Surg 2013; 17:57–64.

28 Poon R, Fan S, Lo C, et al. Improving perioperative outcome expands the role of hepatectomy in management of benign and malignant hepatobiliary diseases. Analysis of 1222 consecutive patients from a prospective database. Ann Surg 2004; 240:698–710.

29 Brandstrup B, Tønnesen H, Beier-Holgersen R, et al. Effects of intravenous fluid restriction on postoperative complications: comparison of two perioperative fluid regimens: a randomized assessor-blinded multicenter trial. Ann Surg 2003; 238 (5):641–648.

30 Holte K, Foss NB, Svensén C, Lund C, Madsen JL, Kehlet H. Epidural anesthesia, hypotension, and changes in intravascular volume. Anesthesiology 2004; 100(2):281–286.

31 McNally S, Revie E, Massie L, et al. Factors in perioperative care that determine blood loss in liver surgery. HPB (Oxford) 2012; 14:236–241.

32 Reich H, McGlynn F, DeCaprio J, Budin R. Laparoscopic excision of benign liver lesions. Obstet Gynecol 1991; 78:956–958.

33 Ito K, Ito H, Are C, et al. Laparoscopic versus open liver resection: a matched-pair case control study. J Gastrointest Surg 2009; 13:2276–2283.

34 Belli G, Limongelli P, Fantini C, et al. Laparoscopic and open treatment of hepatocellular carcinoma in patients with cirrhosis. Br J Surg 2009; 96:1041–1048.

35 Topal B, Fieuws S, Aerts R, et al. Laparoscopic versus open liver resection of hepatic neoplasms: comparative analysis of short-term results. Surg Endosc 2008; 22:2208–2213.

36 Tranchart H, Di Giuro G, Lainas P, et al. Laparoscopic resection for hepatocellular carcinoma: a matched-pair comparative study. Surg Endosc 2010; 24:1170–1176.

37 Buell JF, Cherqui D, Geller DA, et al. The international position on laparoscopic liver surgery: he Louisville Statement, 2008. Ann Surg 2009; 250:825–830.

38 Gayet B, Cavaliere D, Vibert E, et al. Totally laparoscopic right hepatectomy. Am J Surg 2007; 194:685–689.

39 Dagher I, O'Rourke N, Geller DA, et al. Laparoscopic major hepatectomy: an evolution in standard of care. Ann Surg 2009; 250:856–860.

40 Martin RC, Scoggins CR, McMasters KM. Laparoscopic hepatic lobectomy: advantages of a minimally invasive approach. J Am Coll Surg 2010; 210:627–634.

41 Nitta H, Sasaki A, Fujita T, et al. Laparoscopy-assisted major liver resections employing a hanging technique: the original procedure. Ann Surg 2010; 251:450–453.

42 Lassen K, Soop M, Nygren J, et al. for the Enhanced Recovery After Surgery (ERAS) Group. Consensus review of optimal perioperative care in colorectal surgery. Arch Surg 2009; 144:961–969.

43 Tzimas P, Prout J, Papadopolous G, Mallett S. Epidural anaesthesia and analgesia for liver resection. Anaesthesia 2013; 68:628–635.

44 Koea J, Young Y, Gunn K. Fast track liver resection: the effect of a comprehensive care package and analgesia with single dose intrathecal morphine with gabapentin or continuous epidural analgesia. HPB Surg 2009; 2009:271986

45 Revie E, McKeown D, Wilson J, Garden O, Wigmore S. Randomized clinical trial of local infiltration plus patient-controlled opiate analgesia vs epidural analgesia following liver resection surgery. HPB (Oxford) 2012; 14:611–618.

46 Galinski M, Delhotal-Landes B, Lockey D, et al. Reduction of paracetamol metabolism after hepatic resection. Pharmacology 2006; 77:161–165.

47 Hoffmann H, Kettelhack C. Fast-track surgery – conditions and challenges in postsurgical treatment: a review of elements of translational research in enhanced recovery after surgery. Eur Surg Res 2012; 49:24–34.

48 Coolsen MM, van Dam RM, van der Wilt AA, Slim K, Lassen K, Dejong CH. Systematic review and meta-analysis of enhanced recovery after pancreatic surgery with particular emphasis on pancreaticoduodenectomies. World J Surg 2013; 37(8):1909–1918.

49 Lassen K, Coolsen MM, Slim K, et al. Enhanced Recovery After Surgery (ERAS) Society for Perioperative Care; European Society for Clinical Nutrition and Metabolism (ESPEN); International Association for Surgical Metabolism and Nutrition (IASMEN). Guidelines for perioperative care for pancreaticoduodenectomy: Enhanced Recovery After Surgery (ERAS®) Society recommendations. World J Surg 2013; 37(2):240–258.

50 Maessen J, Dejong C, Kessels A, von Myenfeldt M. Length of stay: an inappropriate readout of the success of enhanced recovery programmes. World J Surg 2008; 32:971–997.

51 Di Sebastiano P, Festa L, de Bonis A, et al. A modified fast-track program for pancreatic surgery: a prospective single-center experience. Langenbecks Arch Surg 2011; 396(3):345–351.

52 Berberat PO, Ingold H, Gulbinas A, et al. Fast track – different implications in pancreatic surgery. J Gastrointest Surg 2007; 11(7):880–887.

53 Vanounou T, Pratt W, Fischer J, et al. Deviation-based cost modeling: a novel model to evaluate the clinical and economic impact of clinical pathways. J Am Coll Surg 2007; 204(4):570–579.

54 Balzano G, Zerbi A, Braga M, et al. Fast-track recovery programme after pancreatico-duodenectomy reduces delayed gastric emptying. Br J Surg 2008; 95(11):1387–1393.

55 Kennedy EP, Rosato E, Sauter P, et al. Initiation of a critical pathway for pancreaticoduodenectomy at an academic institution – the first step in multidisciplinary team building. J Am Coll Surg 2007; 204(5):917–923; discussion 923–924.

56 Robertson N, Gallacher P, Peel N, et al. Implementation of an enhanced recovery programme following pancreaticoduodenectomy. HPB (Oxford) 2012; 14(10):700–708.

57 Kennedy EP, Grenda T, Sauter P, et al. Implementation of a critical pathway for distal pancreatectomy at an academic institution. J Gastrointest Surg 2009; 13(5):938–944.

58 Maessen J, Dejong C, Hausel J, et al. A protocol is not enough to implement an enhanced recovery programme for colorectal resection. Br J Surg 2007; 94(2):224–231.

59 Ahmed J, Khan S, Gatt M, et al. Compliance with enhanced recovery programmes in elective colorectal surgery. Br J Surg 2010; 97:754–758.

60 Dindo D, Demartines N, Clavien PA. Classification of surgical complications: a new proposal with evaluation in a cohort of 6336 patients and results of a survey. Ann Surg 2004; 240:205–213.

61 Van den Broek MA, van Dam RM, van Breukelen GJ, et al. Development of a composite endpoint for randomized controlled trials in liver surgery. Br J Surg 2011; 98(8):1138–1145.

62 Hendry PO, van Dam RM, Bukkems SF, et al. Randomized clinical trial of laxatives and oral nutritional supplements within an enhanced recovery after surgery protocol following liver resection. Br J Surg 2010; 97(8):1198–1206.

63 MacKay G, O'Dwyer PJ. Early discharge following liver resection for colorectal metastases. Scott Med J 2008; 53(2):22–24.

64 Porter GA, Pisters PW, Mansyur C, et al. Cost and utilization impact of a clinical pathway for patients undergoing pancreaticoduodenectomy. Ann Surg Oncol 2000; 7(7):484–489.

CHAPTER 10

Relevant hepatobiliary anatomy

Tadatoshi Takayama,[1] Masatoshi Makuuchi,[2] and Kimitaka Kogure[3]

[1]*Department of Digestive Surgery, Nihon University School of Medicine, Tokyo, Japan*
[2]*Department of Hepato-Biliary-Pancreatic Surgery, Japanese Red Cross Medical Center, Tokyo, Japan*
[3]*Institute for Molecular and Cellular Regulation, Gunma University, Maebashi, Japan*

EDITOR COMMENT

This chapter, by world-renowned and pioneering liver surgeons, allows the reader to obtain an important in-depth understanding of liver anatomy. This level of understanding of liver anatomy is the basis for performing advanced laparoscopic liver surgery as shown in the video atlas portion. The chapter details anatomical classifications by Couinaud, Healey, and Schroy and the results of the Brisbane consensus conference on anatomical classification. The authors further detail the anatomy of each liver segment, including a thorough historical and in-depth account of the special anatomy of segment I. This chapter summarizes essential surgical landmarks that should be used in anatomical liver resection. Beautiful anatomical sketches and intraoperative pictures will allow in-depth comprehension of liver anatomy as we know it today.

Keywords: anatomical liver resection, bile duct anatomy, Brisbane classification, Couinaud classification, Healey classification, hepatic artery anatomy, hepatic vein anatomy, liver segmental resection, caudate lobe (segment I), portal vein anatomy

10.1 Introduction

Since the 1950s, our developing understanding of the surgical anatomy of the liver has enabled safe resection of hepatic malignancy [1]. A major breakthrough was the segmental anatomy proposed by Couinaud (1954), who divided the liver into eight segments based on the map of the portal vein [2]. The modern era of liver resection blossomed from this anatomical revolution, shifting from an inability to reference vasculature during surgery to major resection following anatomical planes. The credit for the first anatomical right hepatectomy with preliminary hilar ligation belongs to Lortat-Jacob (1952) in France [1]. In 1985, Makuuchi developed a systematic approach to segmentectomy through the implementation of intraoperative ultra-sound devices. This allowed any of Couinaud's segments to be removed anatomically [3,4]. The technical revolution of intraoperative ultrasound has allowed liver resection to become a potential cure for malignancies; it is now performed at high-volume centers worldwide, with low morbidity and mortality [5–7]. It is also the basis for a more recent development, laparoscopic liver resection, which in skillful hands is an alternative to open surgery in selected cases [8,9].

In this chapter, we outline the relevant hepatobiliary anatomy that forms the basis for advanced laparoscopic liver resections, which requires precise knowledge of hepatic division, vascular structures, and surgical landmarks. A clear understanding of these aspects of liver anatomy enables advanced laparoscopic and open liver resections to be performed safely.

Laparoscopic Liver, Pancreas, and Biliary Surgery, First Edition.
Edited by Claudius Conrad and Brice Gayet.

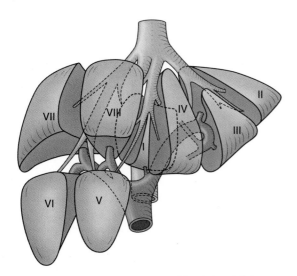

Figure 10.1 Hepatic division. Couinaud divided the left hemi-liver into left paramedian and lateral sectors, while Healey and Schroy divided the left lobe into medial and lateral segments. Source: Takayama [11]. Reproduced with permission of Wiley.

10.2 Basic liver anatomy

10.2.1 Hepatic division

In the 1950s, Couinaud [2] and Healey and Schroy [10] independently advocated two nomenclature systems for hepatic division based on the results of corrosion cast analyses (Figure 10.1). Both systems are widely accepted throughout the world, each dividing the liver into three levels. Couinaud's levels are (1) hemi-liver, (2) sector, and (3) segment, while Healey defined the levels as (1) lobe, (2) segment, and (3) area. The caudate lobe as defined by Healey corresponds to Couinaud's segment I, and Healey subdivided segment IV into the medial superior and inferior areas [11].

Although there are some inconsistencies between the two systems, surgeons have used either or both in their clinical practice. However, Couinaud's nomenclature, based on the intrahepatic portal and hepatic venous system, is more widely accepted in liver surgery today.

In Couinaud's nomenclature, the liver is divided into right and left hemi-liver along the middle hepatic vein (MHV) (corresponding to the Rex–Cantlie line). Each hemi-liver is subdivided into two sectors by the right hepatic vein (RHV) and left hepatic vein (LHV) (right/left lateral and paramedian sectors), respectively. Each sector (excluding the left lateral sector) is further subdivided into two segments, so that the overall number of

segments for the total liver is an eight-segment subdivision, including the caudate lobe (segments I–VIII), according to the third-order branches of the intrahepatic portal pedicles. The liver segments are denoted in a clockwise fashion by Roman numerals, starting from the caudate lobe as segment I. Interestingly, this clockwise designation is numbered similarly to the administrative districts (arrondisements) of Paris.

In Healey's nomenclature, Couinaud's hemi-livers correspond to lobes, sectors become segments, and segments become areas. The conceptual difference between the two nomenclature systems lies in the left side of the liver. Couinaud divided the left portal vein into an umbilical portion and a segment II branch. Consequently, the left hemi-liver was divided into the left paramedian sector (Couinaud's segments III and IV) and the lateral sector (segment II). Healey divided the left hepatic artery and bile duct into lateral and medial branches, causing the left lobe to be divided into the lateral segment (segments II and III) and the medial segment (segment IV). The fact that the term "segment" is used in both concepts, but indicates different parts of the liver, has created confusion [11].

From an embryological perspective, Couinaud's division is more accurate than Healey's [12]. In human embryos (Figure 10.2), the right and left hemi-livers emerge simultaneously, and the umbilical vein connects equally to the right and left portal veins. In the fifth week of gestation, the umbilical vein feeding the right liver obliterates while the vein feeding the left liver remains. This leads to an increase in the left liver volume. On closure of the umbilical vein after birth, the left liver gradually shrinks, triggering growth of the right liver. This process of development indicates that the right and left livers fundamentally share the same formation pathway and anatomy.

In Couinaud's definition, the right and left lateral sectors share the same anatomical features of receiving the first major branch from the right and left portal veins, of having a main hepatic vein at their medial sides, and of having a main portal pedicle at the center of the territory. Therefore, treating segment IV as an independent sector, as suggested by those who prefer the Healey nomenclature, primarily American surgeons, could be considered to be anatomically inaccurate. As we are striving for greater accuracy, it is believed by many that the use of the Healey nomenclature to describe anatomical landmarks of the liver should be abandoned.

From a surgical viewpoint, a left paramedian sectoriectomy (e.g. segment III and IV) [13] can be performed

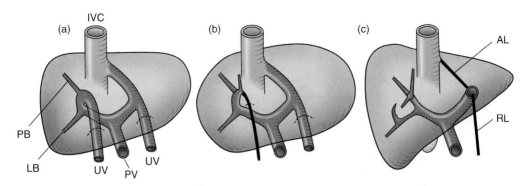

Figure 10.2 Liver development. (a) the umbilical veins (UV) enter both the right and left portal veins (PV); (b) the right UV obliterates, and the left UV remains; (c) the left UV closes and becomes the round ligament (RL) together with Arantius' ligament (AL). IVC, inferior vena cava; LB, lateral branch; PB, paramedian branch. Source: Makuuchi [12]. Reproduced with permission of Lippincott, Williams & Wilkins.

similarly to a right paramedian sectoriectomy (e.g. resection of segments V and VIII) [14], with the LHV or RHV running on the resected surface. In practice, however, surgeons' preference and a greater relevance for the encountered clinical scenarios mean that lateral (e.g. segment II and III) or medial segmentectomy (segmentectomy IV) is routinely performed in clinical practice today. Recently, the Hjortsjo's division of the right paramedian sector into the ventral and dorsal segments, which is clinically highly relevant, has been proposed [15,16].

In 2000, a committee of the International Hepato-Pancreatico-Biliary Association proposed the first universal terminology for liver anatomy and resection (the Brisbane 2000 Nomenclature) [17]. This classification system aimed to simplify the descriptions of different types of resections according to anatomically relevant structures. In this system, the anatomical terms for parts of the liver (hemi-liver, section, and segment) correspond to the terms used to describe hepatic resection (hemi-hepatectomy, sectionectomy, and segmentectomy), using Couinaud's segmental reference as the preferential anatomical source reference (segments I–VIII). The watersheds for the first-order, second-order, and third-order divisions are referred to as the midplane, the right and left intersectional planes, and the intersegmental planes, respectively. As a result, the Brisbane system is based on the anatomy described by Couinaud but changes the terminology (from sector to section), except for division of the left liver, and defines en bloc resection of segments II and III as a lateral sectionectomy [18]. Recently, Strasberg [19] evaluated the global dissemination of the terminology 10 years after its introduction and found that use of the Brisbane terms "hemihepatectomy"

and "sectionectomy" has increased dramatically in comparison with the discarded term "lobectomy," especially in America and Asia.

10.2.2 Portal vein

Of the vessels related to the liver, the portal venous system is the most easily identifiable on imaging and is therefore a good surgical landmark. The first-order branches of the portal vein include the right and left main branches; the second-order branches include the right anterior and posterior sectoral branches, left umbilical branch, and caudate (segment I) branch; and the third-order branches include the segmental (segments II–VIII) branches (Figure 10.3) [20]. Third-order branches are named after the major feeding area in the segmental domain (i.e. P8v is the Portal pedicle of segment VIII for the ventral portion) [3,11].

Portal mapping facilitates the surgeon's understanding of the segmental anatomy in each patient; all portal venous branches and hepatic veins can be traced by ultrasound mapping of the portal venous branches. In addition to mapping intrahepatic vessels, a precise understanding of the relationship between target tumor and related intrahepatic vessels is of critical surgical importance, especially when anatomical segmentectomies are performed [21].

10.2.3 Hepatic vein

The hepatic venous system consists of the three main hepatic veins (RHV, MHV, and LHV), which run along the right, main, and left portal fissures, respectively (Figure 10.4). In addition, the umbilical fissure vein runs along the umbilical fissure between the LHV and MHV, and the anterior fissure vein runs along the anterior fissure between the MHV and RHV. The drainage of these veins has several possible variations, in which the umbilical

(a) Anterior view

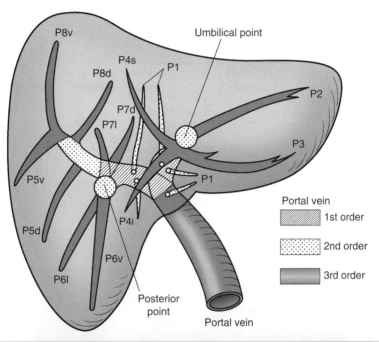

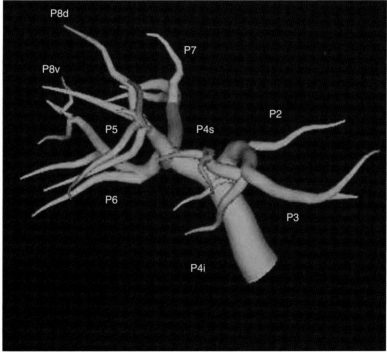

Figure 10.3 Portal venous system. (a) anterior view; (b) lateral view of the liver. P represents the portal venous branch, numbers refer to the eight segments of the liver, and lower-case letters refer to the segmental branches named after their major feeding portions in the segment (v, ventral portion; d, dorsal portion; l, lateral portion; s, superior portion; i, inferior portion). Source: Takayama [11]. Reproduced with permission of Wiley.

(b) Lateral view

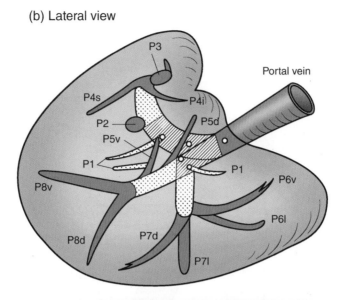

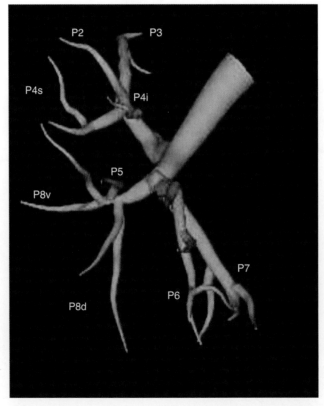

Figure 10.3 (*Continued*)

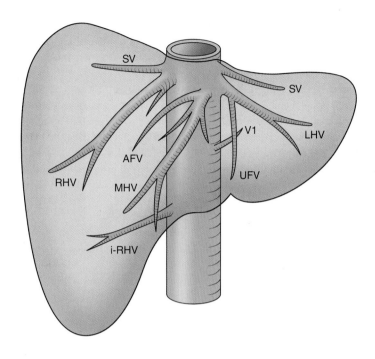

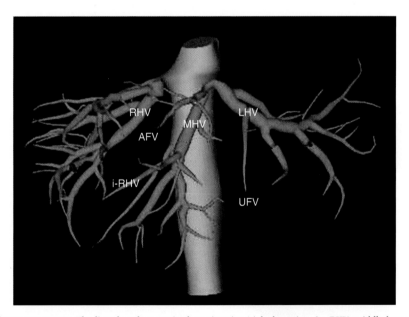

Figure 10.4 Hepatic venous system. The liver has three major hepatic veins (right hepatic vein, RHV; middle hepatic vein, MHV; left hepatic vein, LHV) and two fissure veins (umbilical fissure vein, UFV; anterior fissure vein, AFV). i-RHV, inferior RHV; SV, superficial vein; V1, venous branch of segment I.

fissure vein joins the LHV (90%), the MHV (7%) or the bifurcation of both veins (3%). Likewise, the junctures of the anterior fissure vein may include a juncture at the MHV (91%), RHV or inferior vena cava (IVC) (9%). There are accessory veins, such as the inferior RHV draining segment VI and the short hepatic vein draining segment I [22].

The hepatic veins are a crucial element that must be understood in order to perform anatomical liver resection and partial liver transplantation. The major hepatic veins represent a good landmark in resection and are, when damaged or resected, a source of congestion and subsequent atrophy of the graft.

10.3 Anatomy for hemihepatectomy

10.3.1 Hilar vessels and hepatic vein
The hepatic hilus consists of the hilar plate above the hepatic confluence, portal vein, hepatic artery, and bile duct (Figure 10.5). The umbilical portion of the left portal vein is located at the left distal end of the hilus, and the gallbladder covers the right distal end of the hilus with serosa [23].

The portal vein runs along the right back side of the proper hepatic artery and the back side of the

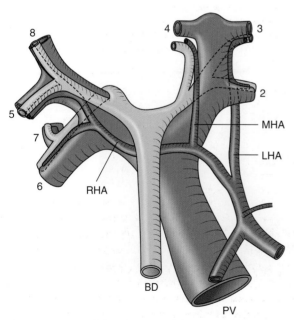

Figure 10.5 Hepatic hilus. The hepatic hilus is made of the hilar plate, including three vessels. Numbers refer to Couinaud's segments. BD, bile duct; LHA, left hepatic artery; MHA, middle hepatic artery; PV, portal vein; RHA, right hepatic artery.

hepatoduodenal ligament. The right portal vein usually bifurcates into anterior and posterior branches at Rouviere's sulcus. The left hepatic artery enters the liver through the left part of Rex's recessus, and the right hepatic artery bifurcates into an anterior branch which runs between the bile duct and the portal vein, and a posterior branch which runs caudally and enters the liver. The left bile duct is formed just above the left portal vein by the junction of the medial and lateral ducts. The right anterior bile duct lies on the right anterior portal vein and comes down to join with the right posterior bile duct [23].

10.3.1.1 Portal vein
At the hepatic hilus, the main portal trunk bifurcates into left and right portal veins. The left portal vein runs horizontally and then vertically with formation of the umbilical portion after giving off the portal vein branch to segment II (P2). A few branches run dorsally from the horizontal portion of the left portal vein to the caudate lobe. In contrast, the right portal vein has three ramification patterns (Figure 10.6):
- common type (86%), forming a long right portal vein
- posterior type (7%), in which the posterior branch arises directly from the main portal trunk
- trifurcation type (6%), in which the left, anterior, and posterior branches arise from the same point [24].

10.3.1.2 Hepatic artery
The ramification of the hepatic artery is classified into five patterns, including (i) common type (76%); (ii) replaced left hepatic artery (12%) arising from the left gastric artery; and (iii) replaced right hepatic artery (11%) originating from the superior mesenteric artery (Figure 10.7) [25]. In patients with the third pattern, surgeons need to be careful when the right (or posterior) hepatic artery runs behind the portal trunk, especially when performing a right hemihepatectomy. The frequency of a type (iv) pattern with double replaced left and right hepatic arteries arising from the left gastric and superior mesenteric arteries, and type (v), with replaced common hepatic artery developing as an independent branch of the superior mesenteric artery, is very low.

10.3.1.3 Bile duct
The bile duct in the right hemi-liver is classified into three types: (i) supraportal type (71%), in which the right posterior duct runs behind the portal vein and joins the anterior duct at the cranial side; (ii) supraportal type

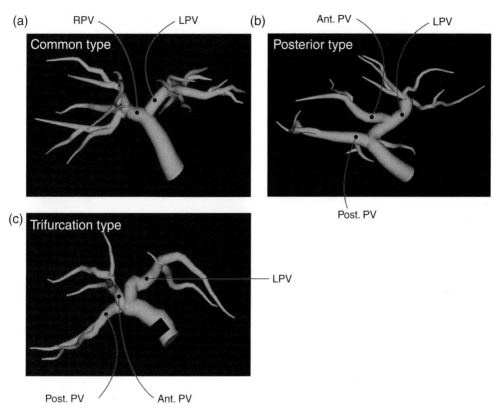

Figure 10.6 Portal vein anatomy. The portal vein (PV) has three ramification patterns: (a) common (86%), (b) posterior (7%), and (c) trifurcation (6%). Ant PV, anterior PV; LPV, left PV; Post PV, posterior PV; RPV, right PV.

joining left duct (17%), in which the right posterior duct directly enters the left hepatic duct; and (iii) infraportal type (12%), in which the right posterior duct runs caudal to the portal vein and joins the anterior duct at the caudal side (Figure 10.8) [26]. As for the bile duct in the left hemi-liver, there are three types: (i) B2/B3 common type (50%), in which B2 and B3 join to the left of the umbilical portion to form the common duct, which is joined by B4; (ii) B3/B4 common type (29%), in which B3 and B4 join to the right of the umbilical portion, which is joined by B2; and (iii) confluence type (13%), in which B2, B3, and B4 join at the same point [27]. The relationship between bile ducts and portal veins can be confusing, because the bile ducts and portal veins do not run parallel at the hepatic hilus. Therefore, three-dimensional (3D) computed tomography (CT) reconstruction images at the confluence of the posterior bile duct or left segmental

duct prior to surgery can be very helpful to the surgeon to avoid injury at the level of the hilus (Figure 10.9).

10.3.1.4 Hepatic vein

In hemihepatectomy, surgeons have to understand the precise anatomy of tributaries of the MHV because in true anatomical resection, the trunk needs to be exposed on the resected surface (Figure 10.10). The MHV has three distinct venous branches draining the anterior segment: V5v (for ventral segment V), V8v (for ventral segment VIII), and the anterior fissure vein. The MHV has two venous branches draining segment IV: V4a (for inferior segment IV) and V4b (for superior segment IV). V5v joins V4a and forms the main trunk of MHV, and V8v and V4b join MHV at the terminal portion. The anterior fissure vein usually joins the MHV but sometimes joins the RHV (6%) or IVC (2%). On the other hand, V4b joins the LHV

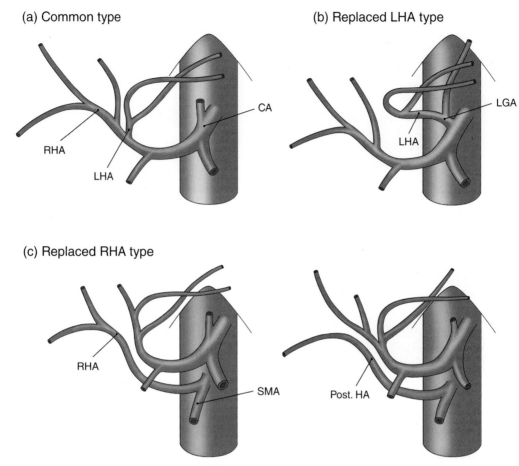

(a) Common type

(b) Replaced LHA type

CA

RHA

LHA

LGA

LHA

(c) Replaced RHA type

RHA

SMA

Post. HA

Figure 10.7 Hepatic artery anatomy. The hepatic artery has three branching patterns. (a) Common (76%). (b) Replaced left hepatic artery (LHA) (12%). (c) Replaced right hepatic artery (RHA) (11%). CA, celiac axis; LGA, left gastric artery; post HA, posterior HA; SMA, superior mesenteric artery.

(57%) or MHV (43%) [22]. Accessory hepatic veins such as the inferior RHV draining segment VI can be present (27%), requiring that surgeons exercise caution in mobilization of the right hemi-liver.

In hemihepatectomy by an anterior approach using a hanging maneuver [28], surgeons insert a pair of forceps into the potential space between the retrohepatic IVC and the liver. To identify a longitudinal avascular virtual plane, Hirai *et al.* [29] have defined three insertion courses: rightward, intermediate, and leftward. They recommend that in patients without an inferior RHV, the rightward course is the best approach, less frequently damaging the caudate vein. However, changing from a leftward to rightward approach to the retrohepatic space is required in patients with an inferior RHV.

10.3.2 Pericaval ligament
10.3.2.1 Inferior vena cava ligament
This ligament is a fibrous membrane around the IVC and attaches to the RHV and LHV at the cranial end. Division makes it possible to expose the insertions of the RHV and LHV to the IVC [30]. The attachment between the ligament and IVC is usually loose, and its mean length and width are 17 mm and 15 mm, respectively [31]. Therefore, when separating the IVC ligament, it is easier and safer to insert the forceps from the caudal to cranial side. The lymphatic vessels in the ligament are abundant and should be ligated and divided to prevent postoperative lymphorrhea, especially in patients who have cirrhosis or those undergoing liver transplantation.

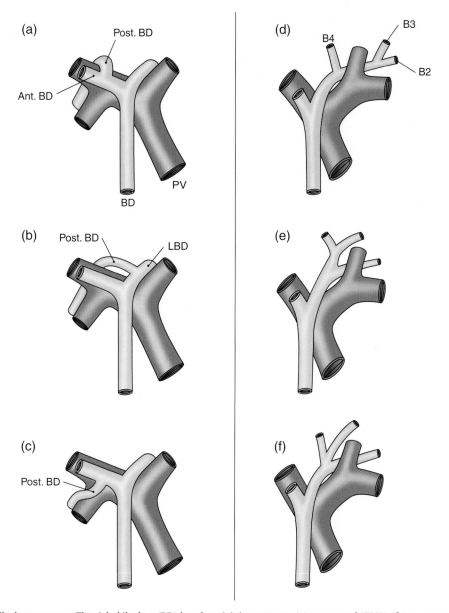

Figure 10.8 Bile duct anatomy. The right bile duct (BD) has three joining patterns: (a) supraportal (71%), (b) supraportal joining left duct (17%), and (c) infraportal (12%); and the left BD has three: (d) B2/B3 common (50%), (e) B3/B4 common (29%), and (f) confluence (13%).

10.3.2.2 Arantius' ligament

During the embryonic period, this ligament is a bypass between the umbilical portion of the left portal vein and the IVC and runs from the ventral side of the umbilical portion to the confluence of the LHV into the IVC (or directly connects to the IVC). The round ligament, umbilical portion, and Arantius' ligament line up on a straight line. Arantius' ligament is on the fossa between the left side of the caudate lobe and the left hemi-liver (fossa ductus venosi) and is attached to the surface of the liver.

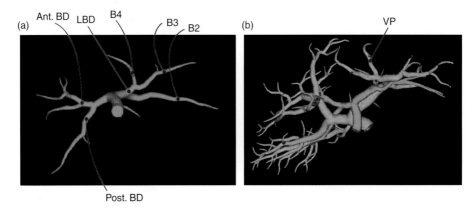

Figure 10.9 Three-dimensional image of the bile duct: (a) bile duct image and (b) bile duct with portal vein image. B3 and B4 form a common duct (B3/B4 common type), and then B2 joins (a) at the right side of the umbilical portion (UP) (b). The right anterior and posterior bile ducts join (a) at the ventro-cranial point of the right portal vein (supraportal type) (b).

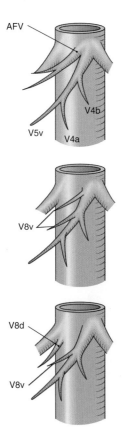

Figure 10.10 Hepatic vein anatomy. The middle hepatic vein has five distinct branches, including the vein for ventral segment V (V5v), the vein for ventral segment VIII (V8v), the anterior fissure vein (AFV), the vein for inferior segment IV (V4a), and the vein for superior segment IV (V4b). V8d, vein for dorsal segment VIII.

Arantius' ligament can be found as a band structure on the anterior surface of the caudate lobe, and its junctions must be divided to mobilize the caudate lobe.

10.3.3 Landmarks for surgeons

In hemihepatectomies, hepatic parenchymal transection [32] should be carried out along the demarcation line, which can be obtained by extrahepatic ligation of the hepatic artery and portal vein. To minimize hemorrhage and avoid transfusion [33] during transection it is important to confirm the branches of the MHV preoperatively, for which 3D imaging modalities such as CT-based simulation are useful [34].

10.3.3.1 Right hemihepatectomy

Anatomical resection requires complete exposure of the MHV, running along the midplane of the liver (Figure 10.11). At the initial stage of transection, the surgeon will seek and trace the tributary of the MHV (V5v) to reach the trunk of the MHV. Transection advances cranially with division of other tributaries (V8v, AFV) up to the caval insertion. At the hepatic hilum, the surgeon must be aware of the ramification pattern of the vessels to prevent injury to the anomalous hepatic artery and bile duct.

10.3.3.2 Left hemihepatectomy

Since the surgical landmark is again the MHV (Figure 10.12), the surgeon will trace the tributary of the MHV (V4a) to reach the trunk of the MHV. Transection advances cranially with division of other tributaries (V4b, occasionally the umbilical fissure vein) up to the caval

Middle hepatic vein

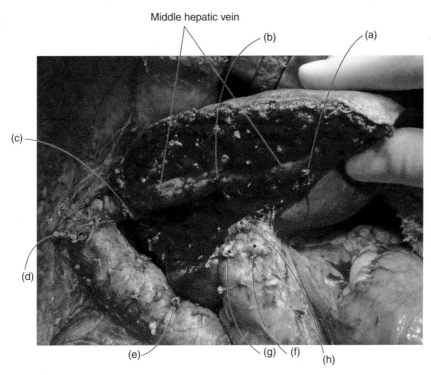

Figure 10.11 Right hemihepatectomy. On the cut surface, the middle hepatic vein is exposed completely. The cut stumps of (a) vein for ventral segment V (V5v); (b) vein for ventral segment VIII (V8v); (c) anterior fissure vein (AFV); (d) right hepatic vein (RHV); (e) inferior RHV; (f) right hepatic artery (g) right portal vein; (h) right bile duct.

Middle hepatic vein

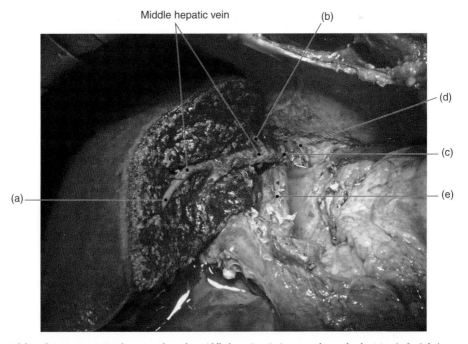

Figure 10.12 Left hemihepatectomy. On the cut surface, the middle hepatic vein is exposed completely. (a) vein for inferior segment IV (V4a); (b) anterior fissure vein (AFV); the cut stumps of (c) vein for superior segment IV (V4b); (d) left hepatic vein; (e) vein for segment I.

insertion. The MHV and LHV form a common trunk at the caval insertion.

10.4 Anatomy for hepatic segmentectomy

10.4.1 Hepatic segments

Couinaud's segment receives the portal pedicle (P) containing branches of the portal vein, hepatic artery, and bile duct and is defined by the hepatic veins or portal fissures (Figure 10.13).

- *Segment VIII* is located at the cranial and ventral territory between the MHV and RHV and has two branches, P8v and P8d (75%), or three branches, P8v, P8d, and P8l (20%). P8d is the first branch from the anterior portal

pedicle. A hepatic venous branch runs between P8v and P8d. P8d occasionally supplies the right side of segment I (Figure 10.14).

- *Segment VII* is located at the cranial side of the RHV and has usually one thick branch (P7d). In patients with several branches from the posterior portal trunk, the border between segment VII and segment VI is unclear. A superficial branch into the RHV is usually present.
- *Segment VI* is located at the caudal side of the RHV and has 1–3 branches of P6v. The presence of the inferior RHV is noted.
- *Segment V* is located at the caudal and dorsal territories between MHV and RHV and has two branches, P5v and P5d (60%), or three or more branches (40%). In the latter case, counterstaining of P8d is useful to totally identify segment V [35].

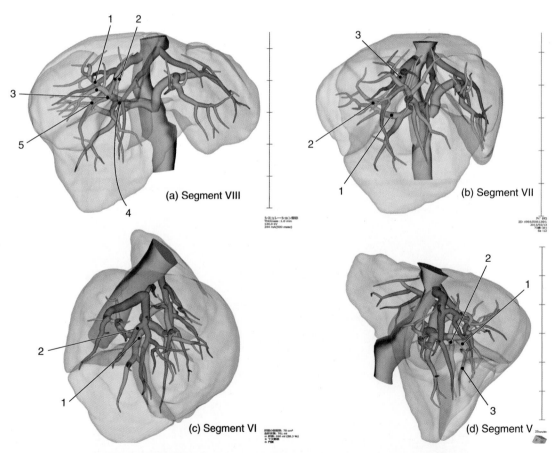

Figure 10.13 Segmental anatomy. Three-dimensional images showing the territory (green) of corresponding segment on virtual clipping of the portal pedicle (P) with the hepatic vein (V). (a) Segment VIII: 1, P8v, 2, P8d, 3, P8l, 4, V8v, 5, V8d; (b) Segment VII: 1, P7d, 2, 3, V7; (c) Segment VI: 1, P6v, 2, V6; (d) Segment V: 1, P5v, 2, P5d, 3, V5v; (e) Segment IV: 1, P4 s, 2, P4i, 3, V4a; (f) Segment III: 1, P3, 2, V3; (g) Segment II: 1, P2, 2, V2; (h) Segment I.

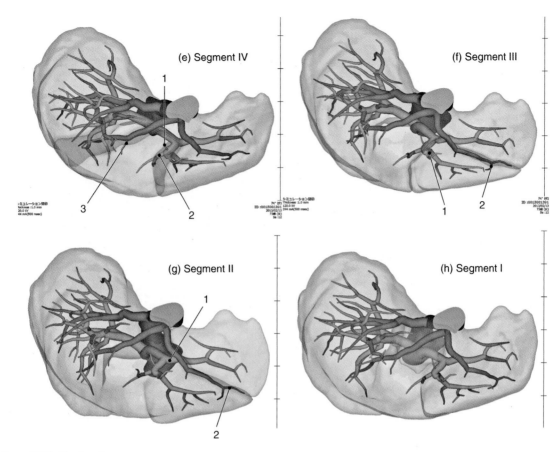

Figure 10.13 (*Continued*)

- *Segment IV* is located between the umbilical fissure and the MHV. P4 commonly arises from the right top of the umbilical portion and bifurcates superiorly (P4a) and inferiorly (P4b). The umbilical fissure vein runs in this segment when it drains into the MHV.
- *Segment III* is located at the left ventral side of the LHV. The right margin corresponds to the umbilical fissure. P3 branches at the left cranial top of the umbilical portion.
- *Segment II* is located at the left dorsal side of the LHV. P2 branches next to P1 (Spiegel's lobe) and is recognized at the most proximal side of the umbilical portion. A superficial branch into the RHV is usually present.

10.4.2 Intraoperative ultrasonography

The use of intraoperative ultrasonography (IUS) in routine practice includes the identification of intrahepatic vascular anatomy, the detection of tumors [36], and US-guided diagnostic and therapeutic procedures (see also Chapter 15) [21]. During hepatic resection, the transection line can be visualized through air artifacts on US as a glittering line. The relation between the transection and target vessels or tumors can be visualized by occasional identification of these air artifacts on US, thereby facilitating accurate resection of the liver. Ultrasound is of critical importance for advanced open and laparoscopic liver surgery, since the smallest surgical unit of the liver is Couinaud's segment. However, these segments cannot be accurately delineated in situ because of the lack of landmarks on the hepatic surface unless US is used.

In 1985, the concept of systematic segmentectomy (Makuuchi's procedure) was realized through the introduction of IUS to liver surgery, enabling segmental borders to be visualized by US-guided staining [3,21]. The main branch of the portal vein is visualized by ultrasound,

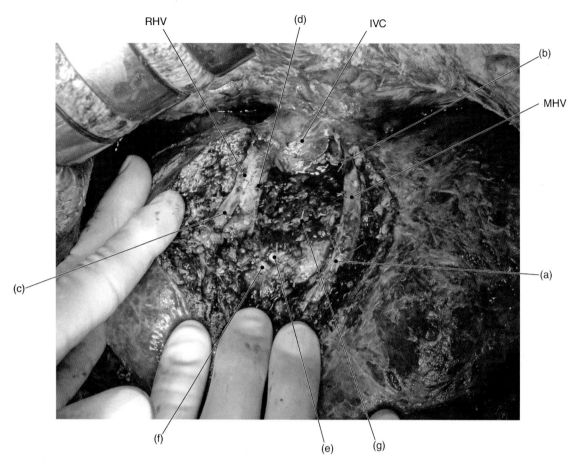

Figure 10.14 Segment VIII resection. The landmark vessels defining segment VIII are exposed, i.e. the middle hepatic vein (MHV), right hepatic vein (RHV), and inferior vena cava (IVC). The cut stumps of (a) vein for ventral segment VIII (V8v); (b) anterior fissure vein (AFV) (c) vein for segment VII (V7); (d) vein for dorsal segment VIII (V8d); (e) portal pedicle for segment VIII ventral area (P8v); (f) portal pedicle for segment VIII dorsal area (P8d); (g) portal pedicle for segment I.

and ultrasound-guided puncture of the relevant portal pedicle using a 23 gauge needle is performed. The tip of the needle is confirmed in the root of the portal vein using IUS, and blue dye (5 mL of indigo carmine) is injected. The liver transection can be performed along the borders of the stained area.

10.5 Anatomy for caudate lobe resection

Confusion has surrounded the anatomy of the caudate lobe because Couinaud's definition changed over the years [37]. Couinaud

- first defined the caudate lobe (classified as segment I) in the 1950s as only the left dorsal part of the liver (corresponding to Spiegel's lobe);
- redefined it in 1989 as the "dorsal liver," including a territory dorsal to the three hepatic veins, with division into two subsegments (segment I right and left);
- designated "segment I right" as segment IX in 1994;
- expanded segment IX to the periphery of the IVC and subdivided it into d and b in 1998; and
- finally renamed segments d and b as segments IXR and IXL respectively in 2000; and
- ultimately abandoned the concept of segment IX in 2002.

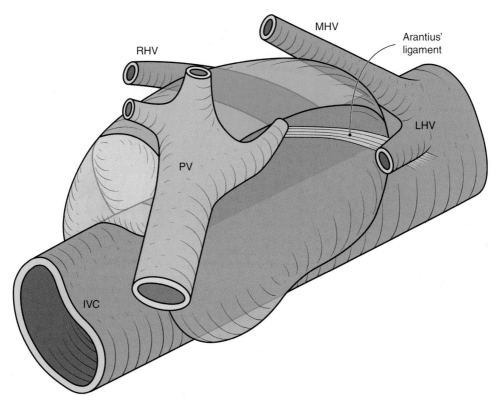

Figure 10.15 Caudate lobe division. Surgically, the caudate lobe is divided into Spiegel's portion (red area), the process portion (yellow area), and the caval portion (green area). IVC, inferior vena cava; LHV, left hepatic vein; MHV, middle hepatic vein; PV, portal vein; RHV, right hepatic vein.

Such rapid changes in nomenclature made it extremely difficult for the surgical community to maintain consistency in the definition of the caudate lobe.

For the purpose of clarity, we define the caudate lobe as an independent hepatic segment which is located at the centro-dorsal territory of the liver, at the left side of segment VII, and under part of segments II, III, IV, V, and VIII, like a fan (see Figure 10.13 h). In accordance with Kumon's classification [38], the caudate lobe is surgically classified into three portions with defined landmarks (Figure 10.15) [4,11,41]:

• Spiegel's portion (left protruding area from Arantius' ligament)
• process portion (protruding area caudal to the right portal pedicle)
• caval portion (paracaval area just below the RHV and MHV).

The caudate lobe feeds the portal vein branches fanning out in the posterior direction from the portal confluence and the left and right portal veins, respectively. The caudate lobe has 1–6 portal vein branches (Figure 10.16) [39]. The hepatic venous system consists of the caudate lobe proper hepatic vein, the caudate processus hepatic vein, and multiple accessory small hepatic veins [40]. These caudate lobe hepatic veins drain directly into the IVC and act effectively as a bypass of the hepatic veins in patients presenting with Budd–Chiari syndrome. The proper hepatic vein of the caudate lobe is a good landmark, indicating the border between Spiegel's portion and the caval portion. The external notch, usually observed at the caudal edge of the caudate lobe, is also a good landmark of this border (Figure 10.17).

Anatomical resection of the caudate lobe harboring a tumor is challenging because of its dorsal location and close attachment to the hepatic hilum, hepatic veins, and IVC. A tumor in Spiegel's portion or a process portion can be removed by a limited resection. In contrast, tumors located in the caval portion of the

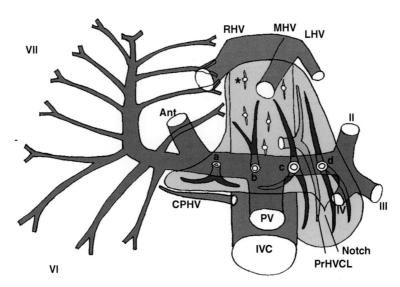

Figure 10.16 Caudate lobe vessels. **(a–d)**, portal vein branches to the caudate lobe; Ant, anterior PV; CPHV, caudate processus hepatic vein; LHV, left hepatic vein; MHV, middle hepatic vein; PrHVCL, proper hepatic vein of caudate lobe; PV, portal vein; RHV, right hepatic vein. Asterisk, accessory hepatic vein of caudate lobe. Numbers refer to Couinaud's segments.

liver (Couinaud's segment IX) can be resected in combination with an adjacent segment or hemi-liver in patients with adequate hepatic function. Such wider anatomical resection provides optimal exposure of the operative field and improves access to the tumor, facilitating resection [41]. Isolated total caudate lobe resection as described by Takayama ("high dorsal resection")

(Figure 10.18) is a procedure of choice in selected patients with moderate cirrhosis [4,42]. After the procedure, landmarks such as the IVC and the posterior surfaces of the RHV and MHV are exposed on the raw surface.

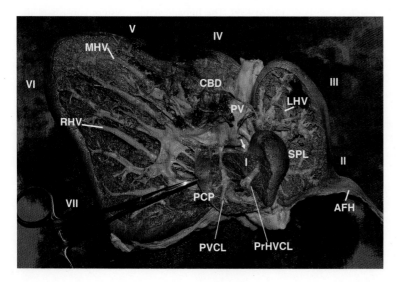

Figure 10.17 Proper hepatic vein. The caudate lobe is split according to the line indicated by the external notch (*arrow*). The proper hepatic vein of the caudate lobe (PrHVCL) is a landmark dividing the caudate lobe into portions. AFH, appendix fibrosa hepatis; CBD, common bile duct; LHV, left hepatic vein; MHV, middle hepatic vein; PCP, paracaval portion; PVCL, portal vein branch of the caudate lobe; RHV, right hepatic vein; SPL, Spiegel's lobe; Numbers refer to Couinaud's segments.

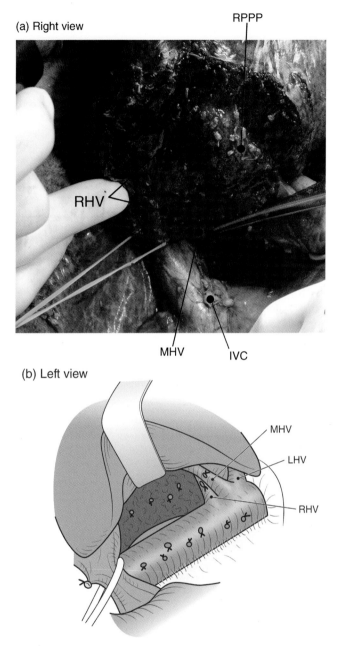

Figure 10.18 High dorsal resection. After isolated total caudate lobectomy (Takayama's procedure), the landmark vessels are exposed on the cut surface and include the right hepatic vein (RHV), middle hepatic vein (MHV), left hepatic vein (LHV), right posterior portal pedicle (RPPP) and inferior vena cava (IVC). Reproduced with permission from Modorikawa and Takayama [42].

10.6 Important points

To accomplish anatomical resection of the liver, it is important to acquire a thorough knowledge of the vascular anatomy and to recognize hepatic boundaries intraoperatively [43–46].

From a surgical point of view, there are notable landmarks that are visible from the hepatic surface, including

Table 10.1 Surgical landmarks in anatomical liver resection

Resection	Landmarks	How to identify the unknown border
Right hemi-liver	MHV, IVC	Rex–Cantlie's line by right P ligation
Left hemi-liver	MHV, IVC	Rex–Cantlie's line by left P ligation
Segment VIII	MHV, RHV, IVC	Caudal border by P8 staining
Segment VII	RHV, IVC	Caudal border by P7 staining
Segment VI	RHV	Cranial border by P6 staining
Segment V	MHV, RHV	Cranial border by P5 staining
Segment IV	UP, falciform ligament, MHV, IVC	Right border by P4 ligation
Segment III	UP, LHV	Upper border by P3 ligation
Segment II	LHV, IVC	Lower border by P2 ligation
Segment I	RHV, MHV, Arantius' ligament, IVC	Right border by P6 and P7 counterstaining

IVC, inferior vena cava; LHV, left hepatic vein; MHV, middle hepatic vein; P, portal pedicle; RHV, right hepatic vein; UP, umbilical portion of the left portal vein.

the umbilical portion of the left portal vein, Rouviere's sulcus, Arantius' ligament, the falciform ligament, and the IVC. Intrahepatic structures, such as the hepatic veins and portal pedicles, which comprise the borders of Couinaud's segments, are critical landmarks for anatomical resection. For example, total exposure of the cranial portions of the MHV and RHV as well as the cranial portion of the IVC on the transected plane guarantees that segment VIII can be accurately resected.

10.7 Conclusion

This chapter has summarized the essential surgical landmarks that can be used in anatomical liver resection (Table 10.1). The MHV is a remarkable landmark during parenchymal transection when resecting the right or left hemi-liver and segment VIII, V, IV, or I. The IVC is a target for transection when resecting the right or left hemi-liver and segment VIII, VII, IV, II, or I. Boundaries of the hemi-liver and segments IV, III, and II can be identified by extrahepatic ligation of the relevant portal pedicle(s), and the staining or counterstaining technique is the procedure of choice to define the territory of segments VIII, VII, VI, V, and I.

For successful liver surgery, a full understanding of the hemihepatic or segmental anatomy of the liver and biliary system is a clinical priority.

KEY POINTS

- Clear understanding of hepatobiliary anatomy, stemming from Couinaud's classification of the segmental liver anatomy, allows for safer liver resection and is the basis for advanced laparoscopic liver resection.

- The major hepatic veins represent important landmarks and are crucial elements to be understood in order to perform anatomical liver resection and partial liver transplantation.

- Because bile ducts and portal veins can be confusing, 3D CT reconstruction images at the confluence of the posterior bile duct or left segmental duct before surgery may be helpful in avoiding injury at the level of the hilus.

- Intraoperative ultrasonography is of critical importance in advanced open and laparoscopic liver surgery. Through identification of intrahepatic vascular anatomy and its relation between transection and target vessels, ultrasound accurately facilitates advanced liver resections.

References

1 Foster JH, Berman MM. Highlights in the history of liver tumors and their resection. In: Solid Liver Tumors. Major Problems in Clinical Surgery, vol. XXIII. Philadelphia: WB Saunders, 1977, pp. 9–27.

2 Couinaud C. Lobes et segments hepatiques. Note sur l'architecture anatomique et chirurgicale du foie. Presse Med 1954; 62:709–711.

3 Makuuchi M, Hasegawa H, Yamazaki S. Ultrasonically guided subsegmentectomy. Surg Gynecol Obstet 1985; 161:346–350.

4 Takayama T, Tanaka T, Higaki T, et al. High dorsal resection of the liver. J Am Coll Surg 1994; 179:72–75.

5 Takayama T, Makuuchi M, Hirohashi S, et al. Early hepatocellular carcinoma as an entity with a high rate of surgical cure. Hepatology 1998; 28:1241–1246.

6 Imamura H, Seyama Y, Kokudo N, et al. One thousand fifty-six hepatectomies without mortality in 8 years. Arch Surg 2003; 138:1198–1206.

7 Takayama T. Surgical treatment for hepatocellular carcinoma. Jpn J Clin Oncol 2011; 41:447–454.

8 Gayet B, Cavaliere D, Vibert E. Totally laparoscopic right hepatectomy. Am J Surg 2007; 194:685–689.

9 Ishizawa T, Gumbs AA, Kokudo N, Gayet B. Laparoscopic segmentectomy of the liver: from segment I to VIII. Ann Surg 2012; 256:959–964.

10 Healey JE, Schroy PC. Anatomy of the biliary ducts within the human liver: analysis of the prevailing pattern of branching and the major variations of biliary ducts. Arch Surg 1953; 66:599–616.

11 Takayama T, Makuuchi M. Liver resection of primary tumors: hepatocellular carcinoma, cholangiocarcinoma, and gallbladder cancer. In: Clavien PA (ed.) Malignant Liver Tumors: Current and Emerging Therapies, 3rd edn. Chichester: Wiley-Blackwell, 2010, pp. 177–191.

12 Makuuchi M. Could we or should we replace the conventional nomenclature of liver resections? Ann Surg 2013; 257:387–388.

13 Kawasaki S, Makuuchi M, Harada H, et al. A new alternative hepatectomy method for resection of segments 3 and 4 of the liver. Surg Gynecol Obstet 1992; 175:267–269.

14 Makuuchi M, Hashikura Y, Kawasaki S, et al. Personal experience of right anterior segmentectomy (segments V and VIII) for hepatic malignancies. Surgery 1993; 114:52–58.

15 Kogure K, Kuwano H, Fujimaki N, et al. Reproposal for Hjortsjo's segmental anatomy on the anterior segment in human liver. Arch Surg 2002; 137:1118–1124.

16 Cho A, Okazumi S, Makino H, et al. Anterior fissure of the right liver: the third door of the liver. J Hepatobiliary Pancreat Surg 2004; 11:390–396.

17 Strasberg SM. Nomenclature of hepatic anatomy and resections: a review of the Brisbane 2000 system. J Hepatobiliary Pancreat Surg 2005; 12:351–355.

18 Bismuth H. Revisiting liver anatomy and terminology of hepatectomies. Ann Surg 2013; 257:383–386.

19 Strasberg S, Phillips C. Use and dissemination of the Brisbane 2000 nomenclature of liver anatomy and resections. Ann Surg 2013; 257:377–382.

20 Takayasu K, Moriyama N, Muramatsu Y, et al. Intrahepatic portal vein branches studied by percutaneous transhepatic portography. Radiology 1985; 153:31–36.

21 Takayama T, Makuuchi M. Intraoperative ultrasonography and other techniques for segmental resections. Surg Oncol Clin North Am 1996; 5:261–269.

22 Ryu M, Cho A. Anatomy of the hepatic vein. In: New Liver Anatomy: Portal Segmentation and the Drainage Vein. New York: Springer, 2009, pp. 55–66.

23 Nimura Y, Hayakawa N, Kamiya J, et al. Hilar cholangiocarcinoma: surgical anatomy and curative resection. J Hepat Bil Pancreat Surg 1995; 2:239–248.

24 Varotti G, Gondolesi GE, Goldman J, et al. Anatomic variations in right liver living donors. J Am Coll Surg 2004; 198:577–582.

25 Hiatt JR, Gabbay J, Busuttil RW. Surgical anatomy of the hepatic arteries in 1000 cases. Ann Surg 1994; 220:50–52.

26 Ohkubo M, Nagino M, Kamiya J, et al. Surgical anatomy of the bile ducts at the hepatic hilum as applied to living donor liver transplantation. Ann Surg 2004; 239:82–86.

27 Kitami M, Takase K, Murakami G, et al. Types and frequencies of biliary tract variations associated with a major portal venous anomaly: analysis with multi-detector row CT cholangiography. Radiology 2006; 238:156–166.

28 Belghiti J, Guevara OA, Noun R, et al. Liver hanging maneuver: a safe approach to right hepatectomy without liver mobilization. J Am Coll Surg 2001; 193:109–111.

29 Hirai I, Murakami G, Kimura W, et al. How should we treat short hepatic veins and paracaval branches in anterior hepatectomy using the hanging maneuver without mobilization of the liver? An anatomical and experimental study. Clin Anat 2003; 16:224–232.

30 Makuuchi M, Yamamoto J, Takayama T, et al. Extrahepatic division of the right hepatic vein in hepatectomy. Hepatogastroenterology 1991; 38:176–179.

31 Hirai I, Kimura W, Murakami G, et al. Surgical anatomy of the inferior vena cava ligament. Hepatogastroenterology 2003; 50:983–987.

32 Takayama T, Makuuchi M, Kubota K, et al. Randomized comparison of ultrasonic vs clamp transection of the liver. Arch Surg 2001; 136:922–928.

33 Yamazaki S, Takayama T, Kimura Y, et al. Transfusion criteria for fresh frozen plasma in liver resection: a 3 + 3 cohort expansion study. Arch Surg 2011; 146:1293–1299.

34 Saito S, Yamanaka J, Miura K, et al. A novel 3D hepatectomy simulation based on liver circulation: application to liver resection and transplantation. Hepatology 2005; 41: 1297–1304.

35 Takayama T, Makuuchi M, Watanabe K, *et al*. A new method for mapping hepatic subsegment: counterstaining identification technique. Surgery 1991; 109:226–229.

36 Midorikawa Y, Takayama T, Shimada K, *et al*. Marginal survival benefit in the treatment of early hepatocellular carcinoma. J Hepatol 2013; 58:306–311.

37 Filipponi F, Romagnoli P, Mosca F, Couinaud C. The dorsal sector of human liver: embryological, anatomical and clinical relevance. Hepatogastroenterology 2000; 26:1726–1731.

38 Kumon M. Anatomy of the caudate lobe with special reference to portal vein and bile duct. Acta Hepatol Jpn 1985; 26:1193–1199.

39 Kogure K, Kuwano H, Fujimaki N, Makuuchi M. Relation among portal segmentation, proper hepatic vein, and external notch of the caudate lobe in the human liver. Ann Surg 2000; 231:223–228.

40 Kogure K, Kuwano H, Yorifuji H, Ishikawa H, Takata K, Makuuchi M. The caudate processus hepatic vein: a boundary hepatic vein between the caudate lobe and the right liver. Ann Surg 2008; 247:288–293.

41 Takayama T, Makuuchi M. Caudate lobe resection for liver tumors. Hepato-Gastroenterology 1998; 45:20–23.

42 Midorikawa Y, Takayama T. Caudate lobectomy (segmentectomy 1) *with video*. J Hepatobiliary Pancreat Sci 2012; 19: 48–53.

43 Sugawara Y, Makuuchi M, Takayama T, *et al*. Right lateral sector graft in adult living-related liver transplantation. Transplantation 2002; 73:111–114.

44 Makuuchi M, Hasegawa H, Yamazaki S, Takayasu K. Four new hepatectomy procedures for resection of the right hepatic vein and preservation of the inferior right hepatic vein. Surg Gynecol Obstet 1987; 164:68–72.

45 Baer HU, Dennison AR, Maddern GJ, Blumgart LH. Subtotal hepatectomy: a new procedure based on the inferior right hepatic vein. Br J Surg 1991; 78:1221–1222.

46 Takayama T, Nakatsuka T, Makuuchi M, *et al*. Re-reconstruction of a single remnant hepatic vein. Br J Surg 1996; 83:762–763.

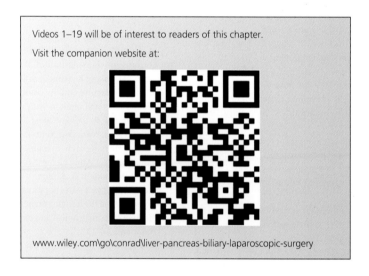

Videos 1–19 will be of interest to readers of this chapter.

Visit the companion website at:

www.wiley.com\go\conrad\liver-pancreas-biliary-laparoscopic-surgery

CHAPTER 11

Anesthesia for laparoscopic liver surgery

Jonathan A. Wilks and Vijaya N.R. Gottumukkala

Department of Anesthesiology and Perioperative Medicine, University of Texas MD Anderson Cancer Center, Houston, USA

EDITOR COMMENT

In this chapter by expert liver anesthesiologists, the authors describe key considerations for successful liver anesthesia to achieve optimal outcomes for patients undergoing laparoscopic liver resections. Each laparoscopic liver surgeon needs to be familiar with these concepts to achieve optimal patient outcomes. Concepts related to liver physiology of patients undergoing liver surgery as well as issues pertaining to anesthetic induction and anesthetic maintenance are described. Anesthetic as well as surgical strategies to reduce blood loss are detailed, the most important being low central venous pressure anesthesia. While this strategy has proven to be effective in reducing hepatic venous bleeding and in avoiding blood transfusions, it requires excellent communication and trust between surgery and anesthesia team. Advanced laparoscopic liver surgery can only be performed successfully if surgeon and anesthesiologist work closely together before, during, and after the liver resection.

Keywords: blood loss prevention strategies, complications, hepatic blood flow, liver anesthesia, low central venous pressure anesthesia, patient positioning, physiology of pneumoperitoneum

---

11.1 Introduction

Recent advances in surgical techniques and medical technology combined with a focus on patient-centered outcomes have led to greater adoption of minimally invasive techniques across the surgical practice. Mini-laparotomy, laparoscopy, and robotic-assisted surgery are increasingly being adopted in liver surgery. Robotic-assisted surgery has been gaining some popularity as it overcomes some of the limitations of laparoscopic surgery such as loss of three-dimensional vision, reduced surgeon hand–eye coordination, and instrument articulation. However, lack of haptic feedback, difficulties encountered in robot docking, cost issues, and the need for an additional experienced surgeon for emergency conversion remain limitations for widespread adoption.

In addition to the specific perioperative considerations for open liver surgery, critical issues for the anesthesiologist during laparoscopic and robotic procedures include factors related to the physiological consequences of pneumoperitoneum, patient positioning, restricted vascular access to the patient in an emergency, and venous gas embolism. In this chapter, key issues related to the anesthetic considerations for minimally invasive liver surgery are reviewed.

11.2 Liver pathophysiology

11.2.1 Hepatic blood flow

The liver receives nearly 25% of the total cardiac output. Portal venous inflow makes up three quarters of the total liver blood flow, and the remaining quarter is contributed by the hepatic arterial supply. The hepatic arterial buffer response (HABR) is an intrinsic mechanism that alters hepatic arterial resistance based on portal venous flow to maintain hepatic oxygen supply. In a fasted state for elective surgery, autoregulation is not present; portal venous flow is therefore directly related to systemic perfusion pressure [1].

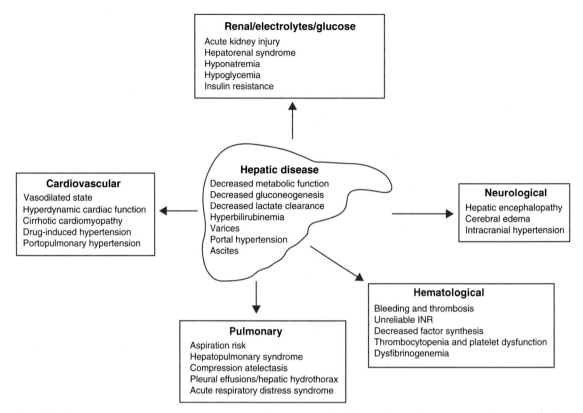

Figure 11.1 Organ response to hepatic dysfunction. Source: Kiamanesh *et al.* [2]. Reproduced with permission of Oxford University Press.

11.2.2 Disease state

Patients presenting for liver resections may have varying levels of hepatic dysfunction. More importantly, liver function changes immediately post resection because of decreased liver parenchymal volume as well as postoperative dysfunction of the remnant liver. Anesthetic goals for liver resection should therefore be to avoid exacerbation of pre-existing liver dysfunction and to preserve function of the future liver remnant. The sequelae of liver disease can impact every organ system and may have profound implications for anesthetic management as well as the postoperative course of the patient (Figure 11.1) [2]. Significant effects of portal hypertension include ascites and pleural effusions with impaired respiratory mechanics and aspiration risks; esophageal varices and risk of hemorrhage; and intra-abdominal venous collaterals with risk for significant intraoperative blood loss. Hemodynamic changes in patients with cirrhosis can mirror sepsis, and myocardial

changes could eventually lead to cardiomyopathy. The splanchnic vasodilatory patterns in advanced liver disease lead to the activation of the renin–angiotensin axis that results in renal hypoperfusion over time and a predisposition to acute kidney injury [2].

11.2.3 Changes in metabolism

Liver disease can profoundly impact the metabolism and clearance of medications, including those used in the course of an anesthetic (Box 11.1) [2]. Pharmacokinetic and pharmacodynamic changes, including drug interactions and impaired clearance of medications, can result in delayed emergence from anesthesia. The pharmacokinetic changes after liver resection are complex and influenced by reduced protein binding and increased free fraction of drug from decreased protein synthesis; decreased intrinsic hepatic clearance with hepatocyte injury; and decreased hepatic blood flow important for drugs with high extraction ratios [2,3].

Box 11.1 Pharmacological changes with liver dysfunction

Benzodiazepines	Increased sensitivity, may precipitate/exacerbate encephalopathy
Midazolam	Increased sensitivity, prolonged action
Diazepam	Increased sensitivity, prolonged action
Lorazepam	Increased sensitivity, minimal change
Opiates	Increased sensitivity, may precipitate/exacerbate encephalopathy
Morphine	Prolonged action
Hydromorphone	Prolonged action
Fentanyl	Unchanged in bolus administration
Sufentanil	Possible accumulation in continuous infusions
Remifentanil	Unchanged
Neuromuscular blockers	
Atracurium	No change
Cisatracurium	No change
Rocuronium	Increased dose requirement, decreased clearance, prolonged action
Vecuronium	Increased dose requirement, decreased clearance, prolonged action
Anesthetics	
Propofol	No change
Lidocaine	Decreased clearance, prolonged action
Dexmedetomidine	Decreased clearance, prolonged action
Ketamine	Decreased clearance, prolonged action
Volatiles	Minimal reduction in total hepatic blood flow

11.2.4 Coagulation

Intrinsic liver disease can result in a bleeding diathesis for several reasons: platelet sequestration and thrombocytopenia from hypersplenism in portal hypertension, coagulopathy from a defect in the synthetic function, and altered activity of the fibrinolytic system. Although lacking validation, thromboelastography may offer guidance in the objective evaluation and management of coagulation abnormalities [2].

11.2.5 Pathology

Patients with hepatocellular carcinoma from underlying hepatitis are more likely to have systemic manifestation of liver dysfunction because of the chronicity of their disease. Metastatic disease may occur in otherwise healthy livers but underlying parenchymal pathology (e.g. steatosis) may also adversely affect liver function. Intrahepatic carcinoid tumors may present anesthetic challenges depending on the secretory function of the tumor; octreotide administration may aid in their management [4,5]. Carcinoid crisis may manifest with diarrhea, bronchospasm, dysrhythmias, hypertension, hypotension, and right heart failure.

11.3 Physiology of pneumoperitoneum

11.3.1 Ventilatory effects

Pneumoperitoneum is known to increase peak inspiratory pressures by 35% and decrease pulmonary compliance as much as 27% [6]. Functional residual capacity decreases with laparoscopy; decreased lung volumes over time favor the development of atelectasis (Box 11.2) [7]. The absorption of carbon dioxide and resulting hypercarbia during pneumoperitoneum may require a 30% increase in minute ventilation to compensate for hypercarbia [8,9].

Box 11.2 Ventilatory effects of Trendelenburg positioning and pneumoperitoneum

- Increased peak airway pressures
- Decreased functional residual capacity
- Atelectasis
- Decreased lung compliance
- Hypercarbia
- Potential for endobronchial intubation

Table 11.1 Hemodynamic changes encountered in liver surgery.

	MAP	HR	CO	Pcwp	SVR	CVP
Pneumoperitoneum	↑	↑/↓ Prepare for vagal response	↓	↑	↑	↑
Trendelenburg	↑	↓	↑	↑	↑/↓	↑
Reverse Trendelenburg	↓	↑	↓	↓	↑/↓	↓
Pringle	↑	↑	↓	↓	↑	↓
Total vascular occlusion	↓	↑	↓	↓	↑	↓

CO, cardiac output; CVP, central venous pressure; HR, heart rate; MAP, mean arterial pressure; Pcwp, pulmonary capillary wedge pressure; SVR, systemic vascular resistance.

Lung protection ventilation strategies include limiting the inspired fraction of oxygen to maintain pulse plethysmographic value of greater than 94%, limiting tidal volume to decrease volume/barotrauma, utilizing positive end-expiratory pressure (PEEP) to avoid atelectasis, and application of lung recruitment maneuvers following desufflation [7]. Trendelenburg positioning has a distinct disadvantage, increasing respiratory resistance compared with supine or reverse Trendelenburg [10]. Care must be taken with Trendelenburg positioning as endotracheal tubes may get displaced, resulting in a mainstem endobronchial intubation as a result of the patient sliding down the OR table. Mainstem endobronchial intubation may cause significant intraoperative hypoxia as a result of atelectasis and an intrapulmonary shunt physiology. Permissive hypercapnia is increasingly being utilized/tolerated in contemporary anesthetic practice to favor oxygen delivery at the tissue and cellular level. However, given the increase in dead space ventilation with pneumoperitoneum, expired carbon dioxide levels may not be an accurate predictor of arterial carbon dioxide tension [11].

11.3.2 Hemodynamic changes

Invasive hemodynamic measurements in patients undergoing laparoscopic cholecystectomy revealed the predictable changes of (i) decreased central venous pressure (CVP), pulmonary capillary wedge pressure (Pcwp), and mean arterial pressure (MAP) with reverse Trendelenburg positioning; and (ii) increased CVP, Pcwp, MAP, and systemic vascular resistance (SVR) with intraperitoneal insufflation without significant changes in heart rate (Table 11.1) [12]. Abdominal insufflation of carbon dioxide causes a pressure-dependent increase in the intrathoracic and abdominal inferior vena cava (IVC) pressure gradient, resulting in a brief initial increase in cardiac filling followed by a decrease in filling with

insufflation pressures more than 10–15 mmHg [13]. Increased CVP or Pcwp during laparoscopy (pneumoperitoneum) may not necessarily indicate increased central blood volume; transmitted increased intrathoracic pressure may be possible [12,14,15].

Transesophageal echocardiography measurements and hemodynamic data taken before, during, and after insufflation for laparoscopic cholecystectomy reveal increased arterial pressure and afterload (left ventricular wall stress) and decreased cardiac output which all return to normal values prior to desufflation or postural changes, suggesting that factors other than increased intra-abdominal pressure may be contributory to these transient hemodynamic changes [16,17]. In addition to mechanical forces, plasma concentrations of vasopressin mirror the changes seen in systemic vascular resistance during insufflation and pneumoperitoneum [18].

Although heart rate does not predictably change during pneumoperitoneum, occasional vagal responses with insufflation can result in hemodynamically significant bradycardia requiring treatment. Absorbed carbon dioxide resulting in hypercarbia can cause sympathetic nervous system activation with increased heart rate, blood pressure, and myocardial contractility [19,20]. Furthermore, the respiratory acidosis and subsequent catecholamine release with carbon dioxide insufflation can result in cardiac dysrhythmias [21]. Intraperitoneal insufflation results in abdominal venous stasis and decreased lower extremity venous flow, creating a prothrombotic environment [9,22].

11.3.3 Central nervous system and ocular effects

The increased intra-abdominal pressure generated with pneumoperitoneum results in elevated intracranial pressure (ICP) [23]. Cerebral blood flow is increased with absorption of carbon dioxide (hypercapnia), further increasing ICP resulting from pneumoperitoneum [15]. ICP will similarly increase with Trendelenburg positioning. Cerebral oxygenation as measured by near-infrared spectroscopy in patients undergoing robotic-assisted prostatectomy was minimally decreased (less than 5%) with prolonged duration in steep Trendelenburg positioning [24]. Patients with ventriculoperitoneal shunts, however, require special considerations [19].

Increased MAP, hypercarbia, and elevated CVP (present with pneumoperitoneum) can all potentially elevate intraocular pressure (IOP). Concerns over exacerbating IOP have prompted multiple investigations in patients undergoing laparoscopic surgery. Pneumoperitoneum does not seem to have an adverse effect on IOP; Trendelenburg position, however, does cause a rise in IOP [25,26]. Furthermore, anesthetic choice may also influence these changes, with propofol having a protective effect on IOP changes secondary to positioning and pneumoperitoneum [26–28].

11.3.4 Effects on hepatic physiology

Portal blood flow decreases with pneumoperitoneum (pressures above 14 mmHg) with maintained hepatic arterial blood flow [29,30]. The degree to which decreases in portal blood flow cause acute hepatocyte injury in the setting of pneumoperitoneum is unknown. Reductions in portal blood flow with pneumoperitoneum have led some to urge caution with laparoscopy in patients with severe underlying liver disease [31]. Keeping intra-abdominal pressures lower than 16 mmHg, Meierhenrich and colleagues found unchanged hepatic blood flow as measured by hepatic vein blood flow index with transesophageal Doppler echocardiography during pneumoperitoneum [32].

11.4 Preoperative assessment

In addition to the regular preoperative assessment for any anesthetic (airway, relevant family history for anesthetic complications, and tolerance/complications with previous anesthetics), patients without significant medical comorbidities do not require extensive evaluation other than blood counts, serum chemistry, and a coagulation profile. Blood product availability may need to be arranged depending on the estimated need for intraoperative transfusion [33]. Additional evaluations are guided

by other medical comorbidities, nutritional state, and functional status of the patient.

11.4.1 Cardiac evaluation

Patients with limited cardiac reserve may not tolerate pneumoperitoneum with the accompanying marked increase in afterload (wall stress) and decrease in venous return [21]. Vascular control mechanisms utilized in hepatic resections can have equally profound implications for cardiac patients, necessitating thorough preoperative cardiac assessment. Intra-abdominal operations are intermediate risk for cardiac adverse events; preoperative cardiac evaluation is guided by a patient's comorbid conditions, risk factors, and functional status [34]. Although obesity may not necessarily justify exhaustive cardiac evaluation, transesophageal echocardiographic (TEE) evaluation of morbidly obese patients during pneumoperitoneum mirrors that of patients with poor cardiac reserve [35].

11.4.2 Pulmonary evaluation

Patients with pulmonary disease are more likely to benefit postoperatively from minimally invasive surgery by avoiding the profound respiratory morbidity associated with open upper abdominal surgery. However, the ventilation changes associated with pneumoperitoneum may present intraoperative challenges in patients with chronic obstructive pulmonary disease (COPD). Pulmonary function tests may guide the anesthesiologist in assessing the reversibility of an obstructive ventilatory defect in symptomatic patients. Decreased room air oxygen saturations may detect patients with hepatopulmonary syndrome: a ventilation/perfusion mismatch due to increased pulmonary blood flow from capillary dilation with unchanged ventilation and impaired hypoxic pulmonary vasoconstriction [33].

11.4.3 Hepatic evaluation

Liver anatomy and remnant liver volume are thoroughly evaluated preoperatively by appropriate imaging studies. When needed, preoperative portal vein embolization is performed to increase the size of the remnant liver volume and preserve function. Nevertheless, preoperative synthetic liver function is most often surveyed via albumin levels and coagulation studies. Often, determination of resectability may only be obtained intraoperatively. In these cases of possible inoperable anatomy, anesthetic plans should be tailored for potential short operative times.

11.5 Anesthetic management

11.5.1 Induction of anesthesia

Induction of anesthesia is guided by the overall condition of the patient. Rapid sequence induction may be required in patients who have a history of significant ascites or other risk factors for gastric regurgitation. Intravenous access (peripheral or central) sufficient for rapid, large-volume resuscitation is required. In the authors' clinical practice, invasive arterial blood pressure monitoring is routinely used during the procedure. Forced warm-air devices and fluid warmers should be used to guard against hypothermia and its potentiation of a coagulopathy. Benzodiazepines can precipitate hepatic encephalopathy, and the metabolism may be significantly altered, prolonging their effects – questioning the need for routine pre-operative anxiolysis with benzodiazepine agents.

11.5.2 Maintenance of anesthesia

General anesthesia is maintained with volatile anesthetics (isoflurane, sevoflurane, desflurane, nitrous oxide), intravenous anesthetics (propofol, dexmedetomidine, ketamine, opiates), or combinations of these. Muscle relaxation is accomplished with a nondepolarizing muscle blocker; changes in metabolism in hepatic disease necessitate careful monitoring of the degree of neuromuscular blockade (train-of-four) intraoperatively when dosing muscle relaxants. Cisatracurium is often preferred given its predictable Hoffman elimination (independent of hepatic function), as well as its lack of significant histamine release. Other short- and intermediate-acting muscle relaxants (atracurium, rocuronium, vecuronium) may also be used safely while bearing in mind their pharmacokinetic and pharmacodynamic profiles [36–40]. Comparing a total intravenous technique (propofol with sufentanil) with a volatile technique (isoflurane with fentanyl) in donor hepatectomies showed no significant advantages of one technique over the other [36]. Although no significant clinical difference was found, patients who were administered isoflurane anesthesia had higher postoperative international normalized ratio (INR) values and elevated liver enzymes compared with patients receiving propofol [41]. A recent randomized trial comparing desflurane with isoflurane in donor hepatectomies revealed higher postoperative INR and liver enzymes in patients anesthetized with isoflurane; the clinical significance of this observation in postoperative morbidity was not studied [42]. All volatile anesthetics

reduce total hepatic blood flow though current volatile agents (isoflurane, sevoflurane, desflurane) cause minimal reduction. Less is known about the effects of intravenous anesthetics; however, current evidence suggests minimal effects on hepatic blood flow assuming normal systemic arterial pressure and hemodynamic function [3].

11.5.3 Anesthetic techniques

Laparoscopic intra-abdominal surgery inevitably demands a general anesthetic because of the peritoneal stimulation from pneumoperitoneum (vagal stimulation) and the discomfort of increased abdominal pressure on the diaphragm. Regional anesthetic techniques are possible, and wound infiltration (local anesthesia) is frequently administered as an adjunct for postoperative analgesia [19,38].

Evaluation of perioperative factors with regard to their influence on recurrence-free survival (RFS) after oncological surgery is gaining interest [43]. The immunological effects of volatile anesthetic agents, opioids, IV anesthetic medications, sedatives, nonopiate analgesics, and other medications may have profound implications in the cancer microenvironment that remain poorly understood [44,45]. Research on the possible effects of regional anesthesia techniques (epidural analgesia) on RFS is ongoing [46]. Choosing the appropriate technique ultimately requires thoughtful consideration of the patient's underlying condition, comorbidities, and perioperative goals.

11.5.4 Patient positioning

Melendez *et al.* reported that a 15° Trendelenburg position not only aids renal perfusion and hemodynamic stability by an increase in venous return but also is ideal for hepatic resections [47]. Supine as well as reverse Trendelenburg positioning have also been reported for hepatic resections [48,49].

Trendelenburg positioning is thought to reduce the risk of air embolism [50]. Direct measurements of central venous pressures and hepatic venous pressures (IVC at the level of the hepatic veins) in supine, 20° head-down, and 20° head-up positions revealed significantly higher IVC and hepatic venous pressures in Trendelenburg without changing the gradient between the two (air is entrained with the development of a negative gradient) [51].

In an effort to maintain low CVP, Jones *et al.* propose head-up positioning to decrease CVP [48]. Indeed, prior to insufflation in laparoscopic cholecystectomies, reverse Trendelenburg positioning predictably decreases CVP, Pcwp, and MAP [12]. For surgical exposure, laparoscopic liver surgery and robotic-assisted hepatectomy are often performed in reverse Trendelenburg position [52].

11.5.5 Intraoperative monitoring

In addition to the standard American Society of Anesthesiologists (ASA) recommended monitoring of patients undergoing a general anesthetic for major procedures, patients undergoing laparoscopic/robotic liver resection have special considerations. Routine CVP monitoring in donor liver resections has been questioned [37,53]. As CVP in the presence of pneumoperitoneum does not reflect true ventricular filling pressure, routine central venous monitoring during laparoscopic liver resections is unlikely to benefit patient care. As opposed to static measures of hemodynamic function (CVP), dynamic measures such as stroke volume variation (SVV), pulse pressure variation (PPV), and stroke volume (SV) derived from the arterial pressure wave form (pulse contour analysis) have gained momentum in the intraoperative arena [54]. Low stroke volume variation (below 6%) was found to be associated with greater blood loss in donor hepatectomies, thought to be due to increased intravascular volume [40]. Should CVP be monitored, caution must be exercised in placing too much emphasis on an absolute number given vast differences in patient comorbidities and resulting physiology; trends are often of greater utility. Monitoring CVP in critical care patients has been shown to be of no value in predicting volume status or response to volume administration [55,56].

11.5.6 Hemodynamic changes

Intraoperative hemodynamic changes witnessed during hepatic resections vary considerably, depending on techniques used for vascular control (see Table 11.1). Hepatic pedicle clamping results in a predictable increase in MAP and SVR and a decrease in Pcwp and cardiac index; clamp release results in the return to normal values within three minutes [57]. Comparing hemodynamic variables related to hepatic pedicle clamping in laparoscopic resections with that in open resections revealed similar patterns and no significant differences between groups [58]. The hemodynamic changes associated with hepatic pedicle clamping in both open and laparoscopic resections are well tolerated [58–60]. Total vascular exclusion (clamping hepatic pedicle, suprahepatic IVC, and infrahepatic IVC) results in much more profound alterations in hemodynamics: decreases in MAP, Pcwp, and cardiac index with significant increases in heart rate and SVR [61]. Interruption of caval flow certainly influences anesthetic management, fluid management, and choices of intraoperative monitoring.

11.5.7 Fluid management

When choosing a fluid for intraoperative volume administration, the debate over crystalloids and colloids will likely continue until better monitoring of end-organ perfusion allows more precise measurement and comparison [62]. In critical care practice, no significant differences in mortality have been observed when albumin is compared with normal saline [63]. Hydroxyethyl starch solutions were once commonplace in critical care and perioperative settings; recent analyses (after exclusion of multiple retracted studies) reveal increased incidence of renal failure and mortality with their use [64,65].

Even though standard preoperative fasting requirements prior to elective surgery may create fluid deficits in patients at the time of anesthesia induction, continued volume sparing becomes important in minimizing blood loss during the parenchymal transection because low hydrostatic IVC pressures reduce hepatic venous bleeding. Nevertheless, the additive effects of intravenous fluid restriction prior to parenchymal transection, reverse Trendelenburg positioning, and pneumoperitoneum during laparoscopic liver resection decrease venous return significantly, which needs to be anticipated. Young and otherwise healthy patients may be able to tolerate this hypovolemic state without significant intervention; however, most patients will require goal-directed or intervention-assessed volume administration during the pre-resection period to sustain perfusion pressure [47].

11.6 Blood loss and preventive strategies

Although the estimated blood loss (EBL) for liver surgery has decreased in the recent past, hepatic resections will always carry a significant risk of hemorrhage. Improved surgical techniques, better understanding of the surgical procedures by anesthesiologists, improved communication between the surgical and anesthesia teams, and adopting active blood management strategies have resulted in reduced blood loss and consequent need for blood transfusions [66,67]. Nomograms have been published to predict the need for perioperative transfusion (based on the number of segments resected, other organ resections, preoperative anemia, and coagulation function) [68].

In a retrospective review of over 1300 liver resections at the Memorial Sloan Kettering Cancer Center, Kooby *et al.* found that even transfusion of only one or two units of allogeneic blood perioperatively (within 30 days of the operation) was related to significantly worse perioperative and long-term outcomes when compared with no transfusion. In addition, larger transfusion requirements were associated with even greater perioperative risk [69]. Similarly, Giuliante *et al.* found that blood transfusion was an independent risk factor for worse long-term and disease-free survival in their retrospective review of 251 liver resections [70]. With increasing risks related to transfusions, surgeon and anesthesiologist must work jointly to minimize the likelihood of transfusion and determine patient-specific transfusion thresholds.

11.6.1 Low CVP anesthesia
Increased retrohepatic IVC pressure (directly measured with a 2 mm umbilical catheter inserted intraoperatively into the IVC) has been reported to have a positive correlation with intraoperative blood loss [71]. Patients with CVP less than or equal to 5 cmH$_2$O had significantly less EBL and blood transfusions in early studies [48]. Jones *et al.* reported using nitroglycerine, diuretics, and reverse Trendelenburg positioning to maintain a low CVP [48]. A retrospective study comparing outcomes before and after the institution of hepatic pedicle clamping and low CVP anesthesia revealed these two maneuvers to be associated with lower morbidity, mortality, EBL, intensive care unit (ICU) stay, and length of hospital stay [50]. Smyrniotis *et al.* showed that the effect of low CVP in decreasing EBL was not present for all clamping methods; hepatic pedicle clamping alone resulted in lower EBL with low CVP whereas selective hepatic vascular exclusion was independent of CVP effects [72].

In early descriptions of total vascular exclusion, average CVP values were reported to be between 4 and 6 cmH$_2$O during the different phases of the operation. However, it should be noted that the range of CVPs encountered was wide (0–20 cmH$_2$O) [73]. Earlier methods of attaining low CVP during hepatic resections included thoracic epidural activation, nitroglycerine infusions (average of 50 µg/min and often higher), and dopamine infusions (3 µg/kg/min) [49].

Subsequent descriptions of fluid management relied on the anesthetic (volatile agent and opiate-related venodilation) combined with conservative fluid management (less than 75 mL/h until parenchymal resection was complete) to maintain low CVP (less than 5 mmHg); nitroglycerine infusions were only required in five of 496 resections to reduce CVP [47]. Fluid boluses were administered to keep urine output above 25 mL/h and systolic blood pressure above 90 mmHg before the resection was complete; a goal of euvolemia was only attempted following parenchymal resection [47]. Moug *et al.* describe fluid restriction and diuretic administration in addition to preoperative bowel preparation as one of the options for low CVP measures [74]. As CVP monitoring has decreased significantly in the authors' practice, creating an environment (low hydrostatic IVC pressures) which minimizes hepatic venous bleeding relies on a fasted state, volume-sparing anesthesia, reverse Trendelenburg positioning, and pneumoperitoneum. This technique requires a relationship of trust and good communication between surgeon and anesthesiologist to ensure minimal blood loss.

11.6.2 Pharmacological interventions
Very few studies evaluating the use of antifibrinolytics in hepatic resections have been performed despite a clear trend towards hyperfibrinolysis in patients undergoing liver resections [75]. Much of the data regarding these pharmacological interventions must be extrapolated from liver transplantation literature [66]. A double-blind, randomized, placebo-controlled trial of tranexamic acid in liver resections in 2006 revealed significantly less EBL, fewer transfusions, shorter operating times, and lower costs in patients receiving tranexamic acid [76]. Although aprotinin is no longer available in the United States, it was investigated in the only other double-blind, randomized, placebo-controlled trial in liver resections; EBL, transfusion rates, and transfusion amounts were significantly less in the aprotinin group [77]. A Cochrane review has concluded that none of these interventions seems to decrease perioperative morbidity or offer any long-term survival benefit [78].

11.6.3 Nonpharmacological interventions
The development of new instruments (ultrasonic and hydro-jet dissectors, argon coagulation, radiofrequency

ablation [RFA], and surgical staplers) for the surgeon's armamentarium has contributed significantly to decreasing the risk of hemorrhage in liver resections [66]. Acute normovolemic hemodilution has been advocated to reduce rates of intraoperative transfusion [79,80]. Efforts are being made to determine which patients would benefit most from hemodilution [81–83]. Increasing experience in liver resections has reduced the reported blood loss and, as a result, intraoperative blood salvage is seldom necessary. Furthermore, many surgeons and anesthesiologists are less likely to accept the theoretical (yet unproven) risk of bacterial and malignant contamination of the returned blood; some proponents have included immediate irradiation of the salvaged blood [84–87]. Reports of intraoperative blood salvage in liver surgery are confined to donor hepatectomies, which presumably eliminates the concern for spread of malignant cells [88]. Investigations in prostate and bladder cancer surgeries suggest no effect on recurrence when intraoperative blood salvage is used [89,90]. A Cochrane review evaluating cardiopulmonary interventions (low CVP anesthesia and acute normovolemic hemodilution) to decrease blood loss and blood transfusion requirements for liver resections concluded that none of the interventions seems to decrease perioperative morbidity or offer any long-term survival benefit [91].

11.6.4 Surgical techniques
11.6.4.1 Pringle maneuver
Obtaining vascular control of the portal vein and hepatic artery within the porta hepatis significantly reduces blood flow and is commonly used to reduce bleeding in parenchymal transection. As is now the standard in most institutions, intermittent hepatic pedicle clamping was found to result in less parenchymal damage than was the case with continuous pedicle clamping; total blood loss is similar in both techniques [92].

Chen *et al.* showed lower EBL with resections following the adoption of hepatic pedicle clamping [50]. A smaller retrospective comparison of resections with and without hepatic pedicle clamping concluded that hepatic pedicle clamping is associated with less EBL and fewer transfusions [93]. In contrast, others found similar blood loss and postoperative outcomes in both arms; parenchymal resection time was, however, shorter in the clamp group [94]. Giuliante *et al.* showed a lower rate of transfusions in resections with pedicle clamping (19.4%) than in those without (35.0%). Not surprisingly, they

confirmed that blood transfusion requirements increase with resections of increasing complexity and decrease with increasing surgical experience [70].

De Carlis *et al.* concluded that hepatic pedicle clamping offers a better prognosis in terms of a longer RFS compared with those without clamping in a recent case-matched retrospective review; the absence of clamping remained a significant predictor of worse prognosis in their Cox regression model [95]. Other trials have found no difference in oncological outcomes with hepatic pedicle clamping [96,97].

Hepatic pedicle clamping and selective vascular clamping are now also utilized in laparoscopic liver resections [52]. Depending on surgeon preference and experience, selective hepatic vascular exclusion (which may have lower EBL than hepatic pedicle clamping alone) may be employed [72].

11.6.4.2 Total vascular exclusion
Total vascular exclusion (TVE) requires control of all inflow and outflow vessels of the liver: porta hepatis with hepatic artery and portal vein, infrahepatic and suprahepatic IVC [98]. In order to tolerate the dramatic decrease in venous return, some degree of volume expansion is required prior to clamping. Early reports describe volume administration only up to a CVP of $12\,cmH_2O$ in order to avoid hepatic venous bleeding after clamp removal [73]. TVE carries additional operative time and morbidity without significant gains in reducing blood loss perioperatively [47,98–100].

11.7 Complications

11.7.1 Trocar related
Inadvertent vascular injury with Veress needle/trocar insertion or other mechanical trauma is a well-recognized complication of laparoscopic surgery that can result in significant hemorrhage [101]. Similarly, bowel injury from mechanical or thermal trauma can have profound influences not only on postoperative morbidity and recovery but also on the intraoperative course to treat the injury [101].

11.7.2 Pneumoperitoneum related
Pleural effusions, pneumothoraces with subsequent subcutaneous emphysema, pneumomediastinum, and air embolism are all recognized complications of

pneumoperitoneum that can have profound hemo-dynamic and respiratory effects intraoperatively [21].

11.7.3 Procedure related

Air embolism is a known intraoperative complication which can occur not only when a large vein is opened but also, as a result of the Venturi effect, with a slightly compressed IVC via small open hepatic veins [48,102]. Farges *et al.* found no increased risk of air embolism during laparoscopic resections than during open proce-dures [60]. Though not thoroughly studied, Melendez *et al.* concluded that TEE was not helpful in detecting clinically significant air emboli [47]. Minor air emboli can occur in as many as 60% of liver resections as detected by TEE [103]. Besides common surgical complications such as wound infections, urinary tract infection, pneumonia, venous thrombosis, and hemorrhage, complications spe-cific to liver resections include pleural effusions, ascites, subphrenic infections, biliary tract injury, and leak [104]. Posthepatectomy liver failure is an exceptionally serious complication with an incidence of 1.2–32% [105]. Risk factors for postoperative liver failure include chemo-therapy, blood transfusion requirements, remnant liver volume, extent of resection, and pre-existing liver dis-ease [106–108]. Research is ongoing to understand, treat, and prevent postresection liver failure, as liver transplan-tation is the only true cure for unresolved liver failure [109].

11.7.4 Positioning related

Nerve injuries may occur intraoperatively as a result of poor positioning (compression/stretch injury), low per-fusion states (ischemic injury), and not securing the patient adequately. Nerve injuries are the second most common cause (after death) of professional liability among anesthesiologists, accounting for 16% of claims in the ASA closed claims database [110]. Anesthesiolo-gists should be familiar with and follow the recommen-dations of the ASA practice advisory for the prevention of perioperative neuropathies (Box 11.3) [111]. It may be advisable to look for and document symptoms of nerve dysfunction preoperatively in high-risk patients (those with risk factors for perioperative neuropathies or those coming for high-risk surgery: long procedures or surgical positions at risk for injury). A description of the intra-operative positioning and measures taken to prevent injury should be documented in the anesthetic record

at the beginning of the procedure and thereafter on a regular basis.

11.8 Postoperative recovery

As recent as 1998, the standard protocol for some centers performing hepatic resections was to take the patient to the postanesthesia care unit (PACU) intubated [47]. Farges *et al.* reported a decreased narcotic requirement and reduced length of stay in their series of laparoscopic liver resections compared with open procedures [60]. A general trend towards reduced hospital stays has been noted, but institutional and geographic differences make large-scale analyses difficult [112].

While opioid use is generally safe for most patients, opioid analgesics are associated with adverse effects, the most serious effect being respiratory depression, which is generally preceded by sedation [113]. Other common adverse effects associated with opioid therapy include dizziness, nausea, vomiting, constipation, sedation, delir-ium, hallucinations, falls, hypotension, and aspiration pneumonia.

Oderda *et al.* have recently published results of their large retrospective study assessing the impact of opioid-related adverse events (ORADE) on patient outcomes following selected surgical procedures known to require postoperative pain control [114]. Among 319 898 surger-ies of interest, 12.2% of patients experienced an ORADE. The aim of a multimodal analgesia regimen is to avoid ORADE by incorporating nonopioid analgesics in the pain management strategies to minimize opioid use [115]. The ASA has recently advocated the use of multimodal pain management regimens when appropriate in the perio-perative period [116].

Enhanced recovery after surgery (ERAS) is an evi-dence-based perioperative clinical pathway developed to accelerate functional recovery of surgical patients. The goal of these programs is to reduce the incidence of postoperative symptoms and complications (through the use of multimodal opioid-sparing pain management strategies), accelerate functional recovery, increase patient satisfaction and safety after discharge with no increase in readmission rates or postdischarge complica-tions, and reduce the length of hospital stay. Multimodal regimens currently used in enhanced recovery in liver surgery (ERILS) include celecoxib, acetaminophen, gaba-pentinoids, and wound infiltration with local anesthetic agents at port or mini-incision sites [117,118].

Box 11.3 ASA advisory statements for patient positioning

Preoperative history and physical assessment

When judged appropriate, it is helpful to ascertain that patients can comfortably tolerate the anticipated operative position

Specific positioning strategies for the upper extremities

- Arm abduction in supine patients should be limited to 90°
- Supine patient with arm on an armboard
  - The upper extremity should be positioned to decrease pressure on the postcondylar groove of the humerus (ulnar groove)
  - Either supination or the neutral forearm position facilitates this action
- Supine patient with arms tucked at side
  - The forearm should be in a neutral position
  - Flexion of the elbow may increase the risk of ulnar neuropathy, but there is no consensus on an acceptable degree of flexion during the perioperative period
- Prolonged pressure on the radial nerve in the spiral groove of the humerus should be avoided
- Extension of the elbow beyond the range that is comfortable during the preoperative assessment may stretch the median nerve
- Periodic perioperative assessments may ensure maintenance of the desired position

Specific positioning strategies for the lower extremities

- Stretching of the hamstring muscle group
  - Positions that stretch the hamstring muscle group beyond the range that is comfortable during the preoperative assessment may stretch the sciatic nerve
- Limiting hip flexion
  - Because the sciatic nerve or its branches cross both the hip and the knee joints, extension and flexion of these joints, respectively, should be considered when determining the degree of hip flexion
- Neither extension nor flexion of the hip increases the risk of femoral neuropathy
- Prolonged pressure on the peroneal nerve at the fibular head should be avoided

Protective padding

- Padded armboards may decrease the risk of upper extremity neuropathy
- The use of chest rolls in the laterally positioned patient may decrease the risk of upper extremity neuropathy
- Padding at the elbow may decrease the risk of upper extremity neuropathy
- The use of specific padding to prevent pressure of a hard surface against the peroneal nerve at the fibular head may decrease the risk of peroneal neuropathy
- The inappropriate use of padding (e.g. padding too tight) may increase the risk of perioperative neuropathy

Equipment

- The use of properly functioning automated blood pressure cuffs on the arm (i.e. placed above the antecubital fossa) does not change the risk of upper extremity neuropathy
- The use of shoulder braces in a steep head-down position may increase the risk of perioperative neuropathies

Postoperative assessment

- A simple postoperative assessment of extremity nerve function may lead to early recognition of peripheral neuropathies

Documentation

- Documentation of specific perioperative positioning actions may be useful for continuous improvement processes and may result in improvements by (i) helping practitioners focus attention on relevant aspects of patient positioning, and (ii) providing information on positioning strategies that eventually leads to improvements in patient care

---

KEY POINTS

- Liver pathophysiology is dependent on underlying liver disease and tumor histology. Resulting changes in coagulation and metabolism have to be considered.

- A thorough preoperative patient assessment is important, taking specific aspects of laparoscopy and liver surgery into account.

- Establishment of pneumoperitoneum and patient positioning have critical effects on ventilation, hemodynamics, and end-organ perfusion, including the liver.

- Establishment and maintenance of anesthesia need to be accomplished with low IVC pressures to minimize hepatic venous bleeding.

- Complications specific to laparoscopic liver surgery such as gas embolism require prevention and management strategies.

- Successful advanced laparoscopic liver surgery can only be accomplished if surgeon and anesthesiologist establish a relationship of excellent communication and trust.

References

1 Mushlin PS, Gelman S. Hepatic physiology and pathophysiology. In: Miller RD (ed.) Miller's Anesthesia. Philadelphia: Churchill Livingstone/Elsevier, 2010.

2 Kiamanesh D, Rumley J, Moitra VK. Monitoring and managing hepatic disease in anaesthesia. Br J Anaesth 2013; 111(suppl 1):i50–i61.

3 Rothenberg DM, O'Connor CJ, Tuman KJ. Anesthesia and the hepatobiliary system. In: Miller RD (ed.) Miller's Anesthesia. Philadelphia: Churchill Livingstone/Elsevier, 2010.

4 Kinney MA, Warner M, Nagorney D, et al. Perianaesthetic risks and outcomes of abdominal surgery for metastatic carcinoid tumours. Br J Anaesth 2001; 87(3):447–452.

5 Massimino K, Harrskog O, Pommier S, et al. Octreotide LAR and bolus octreotide are insufficient for preventing intraoperative complications in carcinoid patients. J Surg Oncol 2013; 107(8):842–846.

6 Rauh R, Hemmerling T, Rist M, et al. Influence of pneumoperitoneum and patient positioning on respiratory system compliance. J Clin Anesth 2001; 13(5):361–365.

7 Valenza F, Chevallard G, Fossali T, et al. Management of mechanical ventilation during laparoscopic surgery. Best Pract Res Clin Anaesthesiol 2010; 24(2):227–241.

8 Tan PL, Lee TL, Tweed WA. Carbon dioxide absorption and gas exchange during pelvic laparoscopy. Can J Anaesth 1992; 39(7):677–681.

9 Neudecker J, Sauerland S, Neugebauer E, et al. The European Association for Endoscopic Surgery clinical practice guideline on the pneumoperitoneum for laparoscopic surgery. Surg Endosc 2002; 16(7):1121–1143.

10 Fahy BG, Barnas G, Nagel S, et al. Effects of Trendelenburg and reverse Trendelenburg postures on lung and chest wall mechanics. J Clin Anesth 1996; 8(3):236–244.

11 O'Croinin D, Ni Chonghaile M, Higgins B, et al. Bench-to-bedside review: permissive hypercapnia. Crit Care 2005; 9(1): 51–59.

12 Joris JL, Noirot D, Legrand M, et al. Hemodynamic changes during laparoscopic cholecystectomy. Anesth Analg 1993; 76(5):1067–1071.

13 Giebler RM, Behrends M, Steffens T, et al. Intraperitoneal and retroperitoneal carbon dioxide insufflation evoke different effects on caval vein pressure gradients in humans: evidence for the starling resistor concept of abdominal venous return. Anesthesiology 2000; 92(6):1568–1580.

14 Hein HA, Joshi G, Ramsay M, et al. Hemodynamic changes during laparoscopic cholecystectomy in patients with severe cardiac disease. J Clin Anesth 1997; 9(4):261–265.

15 O'Malley C, Cunningham AJ. Physiologic changes during laparoscopy. Anesthesiol Clin North Am 2001; 19(1):1–19.

16 Branche PE, Duperret S, Sagnard P, et al. Left ventricular loading modifications induced by pneumoperitoneum: a time course echocardiographic study. Anesth Analg 1998; 86(3):482–487.

17 Cunningham AJ, Turner J, Rosenbaum S, et al. Transoesophageal echocardiographic assessment of haemodynamic function during laparoscopic cholecystectomy. Br J Anaesth 1993; 70(6):621–625.

18 Joris JL, Chiche J, Canivet J, et al. Hemodynamic changes induced by laparoscopy and their endocrine correlates: effects of clonidine. J Am Coll Cardiol 1998; 32(5):1389–1396.

19 Gerges FJ, Kanazi GE, Jabbour-Khoury SI. Anesthesia for laparoscopy: a review. J Clin Anesth 2006; 18(1):67–78.

20 Nguyen NT, Wolfe BM. The physiologic effects of pneumoperitoneum in the morbidly obese. Ann Surg 2005; 241 (2):219–226.

21 Sharma KC, Kabinoff G, Ducheine Y, et al. Laparoscopic surgery and its potential for medical complications. Heart Lung 1997; 26(1):52–64; quiz 65–67.

22 Goodale RL, Beebe D, McNevin M, *et al.* Hemodynamic, respiratory, and metabolic effects of laparoscopic cholecystectomy. Am J Surg 1993; 166(5):533–537.

23 Bloomfield GL, Ridings P, Blocher C, *et al.* Effects of increased intra-abdominal pressure upon intracranial and cerebral perfusion pressure before and after volume expansion. J Trauma 1996; 40(6):936–941; discussion 941–943.

24 Closhen D, Treiber A, Berres M, *et al.* Robotic assisted prostatic surgery in the Trendelenburg position does not impair cerebral oxygenation measured using two different monitors: a clinical observational study. Eur J Anaesthesiol 2014; 31(2):104–109.

25 Hvidberg A, Kessing SV, Fernandes A. Effect of changes in PCO2 and body positions on intraocular pressure during general anaesthesia. Acta Ophthalmol (Copenh) 1981; 59 (4):465–475.

26 Lentschener C, Benhamou D, Neissen F, *et al.* Intra-ocular pressure changes during gynaecological laparoscopy. Anaesthesia 1996; 51(12):1106–1108.

27 Hwang JW, Oh A, Hwang D, *et al.* Does intraocular pressure increase during laparoscopic surgeries? It depends on anesthetic drugs and the surgical position. Surg Laparosc Endosc Percutan Tech 2013; 23(2):229–232.

28 Mowafi HA, Al-Ghamdi A, Rushood A. Intraocular pressure changes during laparoscopy in patients anesthetized with propofol total intravenous anesthesia versus isoflurane inhaled anesthesia. Anesth Analg 2003; 97(2):471–474.

29 Windberger UB, Auer R, Keplinger F, *et al.* The role of intra-abdominal pressure on splanchnic and pulmonary hemodynamic and metabolic changes during carbon dioxide pneumoperitoneum. Gastrointest Endosc 1999; 49(1):84–91.

30 Jakimowicz J, Stultiens G, Smulders F. Laparoscopic insufflation of the abdomen reduces portal venous flow. Surg Endosc 1998; 12(2):129–132.

31 Takagi S. Hepatic and portal vein blood flow during carbon dioxide pneumoperitoneum for laparoscopic hepatectomy. Surg Endosc 1998; 12(5):427–431.

32 Meierhenrich R, Gauss A, Vandenesch P, *et al.* The effects of intra-abdominally insufflated carbon dioxide on hepatic blood flow during laparoscopic surgery assessed by transesophageal echocardiography. Anesth Analg 2005; 100 (2):340–347.

33 Redai I, Emond J, Brentjens T. Anesthetic considerations during liver surgery. Surg Clin North Am 2004; 84 (2):401–411.

34 American College of Cardiology/American Heart Association Task Force on Practice. ACC/AHA 2007 guidelines on perioperative cardiovascular evaluation and care for noncardiac surgery: executive summary: a report of the American College of Cardiology/American Heart Association Task Force on Practice Guidelines (Writing Committee to Revise the 2002 Guidelines on Perioperative Cardiovascular Evaluation for Noncardiac Surgery). Anesth Analg 2008; 106 (3):685–712.

35 Popescu WM, Bell R, Duffy A, *et al.* A pilot study of patients with clinically severe obesity undergoing laparoscopic surgery: evidence for impaired cardiac performance. J Cardiothorac Vasc Anesth 2011; 25(6):943–949.

36 Rabie M, Negmi H, Hammad Y, *et al.* Living donor hepatectomy (LDH) – comparative study between two different anesthetic techniques. Middle East J Anesthesiol 2006; 18 (4):743–756.

37 Niemann CU, Feiner J, Behrends M, *et al.* Central venous pressure monitoring during living right donor hepatectomy. Liver Transpl 2007; 13(2):266–271.

38 Martucci G, Burgio G, Spada M, *et al.* Anesthetic management of totally robotic right lobe living-donor hepatectomy: new tools ask for perioperative care. Eur Rev Med Pharmacol Sci 2013; 17(14):1974–1977.

39 Siniscalchi A, Begliomini B, Matteo G, *et al.* Intraoperative effects of combined versus general anesthesia during major liver surgery. Minerva Anestesiol 2003; 69(12):885–895.

40 Kim YK, Shin W, Song J, *et al.* Does stroke volume variation predict intraoperative blood loss in living right donor hepatectomy? Transplant Proc 2011; 43(5):1407–1411.

41 Ozgul U, Ucar M, Erdogan M, *et al.* Effects of isoflurane and propofol on hepatic and renal functions and coagulation profile after right hepatectomy in living donors. Transplant Proc 2013; 45(3):966–970.

42 Toprak HI, Sahin T, Aslan S, *et al.* Effects of desflurane and isoflurane on hepatic and renal functions and coagulation profile during donor hepatectomy. Transplant Proc 2012; 44 (6):1635–1639.

43 Gottschalk A, Sharma S, Ford J, *et al.* Review article: the role of the perioperative period in recurrence after cancer surgery. Anesth Analg 2010; 110(6):1636–1643.

44 Kurosawa S. Anesthesia in patients with cancer disorders. Curr Opin Anaesthesiol 2012; 25(3):376–384.

45 Snyder GL, Greenberg S. Effect of anaesthetic technique and other perioperative factors on cancer recurrence. Br J Anaesth 2010; 105(2):106–115.

46 Biki B, Mascha E, Moriarty D, *et al.* Anesthetic technique for radical prostatectomy surgery affects cancer recurrence: a retrospective analysis. Anesthesiology 2008; 109(2): 180–187.

47 Melendez JA, Arslan V, Fischer M, *et al.* Perioperative outcomes of major hepatic resections under low central venous pressure anesthesia: blood loss, blood transfusion, and the risk of postoperative renal dysfunction. J Am Coll Surg 1998; 187(6):620–625.

48 Jones RM, Moulton CE, Hardy KJ. Central venous pressure and its effect on blood loss during liver resection. Br J Surg 1998; 85(8):1058–1060.

49 Rees M, Plant G, Wells J, *et al.* One hundred and fifty hepatic resections: evolution of technique towards bloodless surgery. Br J Surg 1996; 83(11):1526–1529.

50 Chen H, Merchant NB, Didolkar MS. Hepatic resection using intermittent vascular inflow occlusion and low central

venous pressure anesthesia improves morbidity and mortality. J Gastrointest Surg 2000; 4(2):162–167.

51 Moulton CA, Chui A, Mann D, et al. Does patient position during liver surgery influence the risk of venous air embolism? Am J Surg 2001; 181(4):366–367.

52 Yan CY, Cai XJ, Wang YF. Effect of selective inflow occlusion on hemodynamic conditions during laparoscopic left hemihepatectomy effect of selective inflow occlusion on hemodynamic conditions during laparoscopic left hemihepatectomy. Hepatogastroenterology 2012; 59 (114):501–504.

53 Kim YK, Chin J, Kang S, et al. Association between central venous pressure and blood loss during hepatic resection in 984 living donors. Acta Anaesthesiol Scand 2009; 53 (5):601–606.

54 Montenij LJ, de Waal EE, Buhre WF. Arterial waveform analysis in anesthesia and critical care. Curr Opin Anaesthesiol 2011; 24(6):651–656.

55 Marik PE, Baram M, Vahid B. Does central venous pressure predict fluid responsiveness? A systematic review of the literature and the tale of seven mares. Chest 2008; 134 (1):172–178.

56 Marik PE, Cavallazzi R. Does the central venous pressure predict fluid responsiveness? An updated meta-analysis and a plea for some common sense. Crit Care Med 2013; 41 (7):1774–1781.

57 Delva E, Camus Y, Paugam C, et al. Hemodynamic effects of portal triad clamping in humans. Anesth Analg 1987; 66 (9):864–868.

58 Decailliot F, Cherqui D, Leroux B, et al. Effects of portal triad clamping on haemodynamic conditions during laparoscopic liver resection. Br J Anaesth 2001; 87(3):493–496.

59 Decailliot F, Streich B, Heurtematte Y, et al. Hemodynamic effects of portal triad clamping with and without pneumoperitoneum: an echocardiographic study. Anesth Analg 2005; 100(3):617–622.

60 Farges O, Jagot P, Kirstetter P, et al. Prospective assessment of the safety and benefit of laparoscopic liver resections. J Hepatobiliary Pancreat Surg 2002; 9(2):242–248.

61 Eyraud D, Richard O, Borie D, et al. Hemodynamic and hormonal responses to the sudden interruption of caval flow: insights from a prospective study of hepatic vascular exclusion during major liver resections. Anesth Analg 2002; 95(5):1173–1178.

62 Perel P, Roberts I, Ker K. Colloids versus crystalloids for fluid resuscitation in critically ill patients. Cochrane Database Syst Rev 2013; 2:CD000567.

63 Finfer S, Bellomo R, Boyce N, et al. A comparison of albumin and saline for fluid resuscitation in the intensive care unit. N Engl J Med 2004; 350(22):2247–2256.

64 Antonelli M, Sandroni C. Hydroxyethyl starch for intravenous volume replacement: more harm than benefit. JAMA 2013; 309(7):723–724.

65 Zarychanski R, Abou-Setta A, Turgeon A, et al. Association of hydroxyethyl starch administration with mortality and acute kidney injury in critically ill patients requiring volume resuscitation: a systematic review and meta-analysis. JAMA 2013; 309(7):678–688.

66 Alkozai EM, Lisman T, Porte RJ. Bleeding in liver surgery: prevention and treatment. Clin Liver Dis 2009; 13 (1):145–154.

67 American Society of Anesthesiologists Task Force on Perioperative Blood Transfusion and Adjuvant Therapies. Practice guidelines for perioperative blood transfusion and adjuvant therapies: an updated report by the American Society of Anesthesiologists Task Force on Perioperative Blood Transfusion and Adjuvant Therapies. Anesthesiology 2006; 105(1):198–208.

68 Sima CS, Jarnagin W, Fong Y, et al. Predicting the risk of perioperative transfusion for patients undergoing elective hepatectomy. Ann Surg 2009; 250(6):914–921.

69 Kooby DA, Stockman J, Ben-Porat L, et al. Influence of transfusions on perioperative and long-term outcome in patients following hepatic resection for colorectal metastases. Ann Surg 2003; 237(6):860–869; discussion 869–870.

70 Giuliante F, Ardito F, Vellone M, et al. Role of the surgeon as a variable in long-term survival after liver resection for colorectal metastases. J Surg Oncol 2009; 100(7):538–545.

71 Johnson M, Mannar R, Wu AV. Correlation between blood loss and inferior vena caval pressure during liver resection. Br J Surg 1998; 85(2):188–190.

72 Smyrniotis V, Kostopanagiotou G, Theodoraki K, et al. The role of central venous pressure and type of vascular control in blood loss during major liver resections. Am J Surg 2004; 187(3):398–402.

73 Bismuth H, Castaing D, Garden OJ. Major hepatic resection under total vascular exclusion. Ann Surg 1989; 210 (1):13–19.

74 Moug SJ, Smith D, Leen E, et al. Selective continuous vascular occlusion and perioperative fluid restriction in partial hepatectomy. Outcomes in 101 consecutive patients. Eur J Surg Oncol 2007; 33(8):1036–1041.

75 Ortmann E, Besser MW, Klein AA. Antifibrinolytic agents in current anaesthetic practice. Br J Anaesth 2013; 111 (4):549–563.

76 Wu CC, Ho W, Cheng S, et al. Perioperative parenteral tranexamic acid in liver tumor resection: a prospective randomized trial toward a "blood transfusion"-free hepatectomy. Ann Surg 2006; 243(2):173–180.

77 Lentschener C, Benhamou D, Mercier F, et al. Aprotinin reduces blood loss in patients undergoing elective liver resection. Anesth Analg 1997; 84(4):875–881.

78 Gurusamy KS, Li J, Sharma D, et al. Pharmacological interventions to decrease blood loss and blood transfusion requirements for liver resection. Cochrane Database Syst Rev 2009; 4:CD008085.

79 Matot I, Scheinin O, Jurim O, *et al.* Effectiveness of acute normovolemic hemodilution to minimize allogeneic blood transfusion in major liver resections. Anesthesiology 2002. 97(4):794–800.

80 Putchakayala K, DiFronzo LA. Acute hemodilution is safe in patients with comorbid illness undergoing partial hepatectomy. Am Surg 2013; 79(10):1093–1097.

81 Frankel TL, Fischer M, Grant F, *et al.* Selecting patients for acute normovolemic hemodilution during hepatic resection: a prospective randomized evaluation of nomogram-based allocation. J Am Coll Surg 2013; 217(2):210–220.

82 Jarnagin WR, Gonen M, Maithel S, *et al.* A prospective randomized trial of acute normovolemic hemodilution compared to standard intraoperative management in patients undergoing major hepatic resection. Ann Surg 2008; 248 (3):360–369.

83 Maithel SK, Jarnagin WR. Adjuncts to liver surgery: is acute normovolemic hemodilution useful for major hepatic resections? Adv Surg 2009; 43:259–268.

84 Feltracco P, Michieletto E, Barbieri S, *et al.* Microbiologic contamination of intraoperative blood salvaged during liver transplantation. Transplant Proc 2007; 39 (6):1889–1891.

85 Valbonesi M, Bruni R, Lercari G, *et al.* Autoapheresis and intraoperative blood salvage in oncologic surgery. Transfus Sci 1999; 21(2):129–139.

86 Ashworth A, Klein AA. Cell salvage as part of a blood conservation strategy in anaesthesia. Br J Anaesth 2010; 105(4):401–416.

87 Hansen E, Bechmann V, Altmeppen J. Intraoperative blood salvage in cancer surgery: safe and effective? Transfus Apher Sci 2002; 27(2):153–157.

88 Lutz JT, Valentin-Gamazo C, Gorlinger K, *et al.* Blood-transfusion requirements and blood salvage in donors undergoing right hepatectomy for living related liver transplantation. Anesth Analg 2003; 96(2):351–355.

89 Nieder AM, Carmack A, Sved P, *et al.* Intraoperative cell salvage during radical prostatectomy is not associated with greater biochemical recurrence rate. Urology 2005; 65 (4):730–734.

90 Nieder AM, Manoharan M, Yang Y, *et al.* Intraoperative cell salvage during radical cystectomy does not affect long-term survival. Urology 2007; 69(5):881–884.

91 Gurusamy KS, Li J, Vaughan J, *et al.* Cardiopulmonary interventions to decrease blood loss and blood transfusion requirements for liver resection. Cochrane Database Syst Rev 2012; 5:CD007338.

92 Belghiti J, Noun R, Malafosse R, *et al.* Continuous versus intermittent portal triad clamping for liver resection: a controlled study. Ann Surg 1999; 229(3):369–375.

93 Arnoletti JP, Brodsky J. Reduction of transfusion requirements during major hepatic resection for metastatic disease. Surgery 1999; 125(2):166–171.

94 Capussotti L, Muratore A, Ferrero A, *et al.* Randomized clinical trial of liver resection with and without hepatic pedicle clamping. Br J Surg 2006; 93(6):685–689.

95 De Carlis L, di Sandro S, Giacomoni A, *et al.* Colorectal liver metastases: hepatic pedicle clamping during hepatectomy reduces the incidence of tumor recurrence in selected patients. Case-matched analysis. Eur J Surg Oncol 2013; 39(7):726–733.

96 Ferrero A, Russolillo N, Vigano L, *et al.* Does Pringle maneuver affect survival in patients with colorectal liver metastases? World J Surg 2010; 34(10):2418–2425.

97 Giuliante F, Ardito F, Pulitano C, *et al.* Does hepatic pedicle clamping affect disease-free survival following liver resection for colorectal metastases? Ann Surg 2010; 252 (6):1020–1026.

98 Abdalla EK, Noun R, Belghiti J. Hepatic vascular occlusion: which technique? Surg Clin North Am 2004; 84 (2):563–585.

99 Torzilli G, Makuuchi M, Midorikawa Y, *et al.* Liver resection without total vascular exclusion: hazardous or beneficial? An analysis of our experience. Ann Surg 2001; 233 (2):167–175.

100 Benoist S, Salabert A, Penna C, *et al.* Portal triad clamping (TC) or hepatic vascular exclusion (VE) for major liver resection after prolonged neoadjuvant chemotherapy? A case-matched study in 60 patients. Surgery 2006; 140 (3):396–403.

101 Deziel DJ, Millikan K, Economou S, *et al.* Complications of laparoscopic cholecystectomy: a national survey of 4,292 hospitals and an analysis of 77, 604 cases. Am J Surg 1993; 165(1):9–14.

102 Hatano Y, Murakawa M, Segawa H, *et al.* Venous air embolism during hepatic resection. Anesthesiology 1990; 73 (6):1282–1285.

103 Poznanska G, Grzelak P, Durczynski A, *et al.* Venous air embolism during major liver surgery: far more common than we think. Eur J Anaesthesiol 2014; 31(2):120–121.

104 Jin S, Fu Q, Wuyun G, *et al.* Management of post-hepatectomy complications. World J Gastroenterol 2013; 19(44):7983–7991.

105 Rahbari NN, Garden O, Padbury R, *et al.* Posthepatectomy liver failure: a definition and grading by the International Study Group of Liver Surgery (ISGLS). Surgery 2011; 149 (5):713–724.

106 Ribeiro HS, Costa W Jr, Diniz A, *et al.* Extended preoperative chemotherapy, extent of liver resection and blood transfusion are predictive factors of liver failure following resection of colorectal liver metastasis. Eur J Surg Oncol 2013; 39 (4):380–385.

107 Van den Broek MA, Olde Damink S, Dejong C, *et al.* Liver failure after partial hepatic resection: definition, pathophysiology, risk factors and treatment. Liver Int 2008; 28 (6):767–780.

108 Hammond JS, Guha I, Beckingham I, *et al.* Prediction, prevention and management of postresection liver failure. Br J Surg 2011; 98(9):1188–1200.

109 Golse N, Bucur P, Adam R, *et al.* New paradigms in post-hepatectomy liver failure. J Gastrointest Surg 2013; 17 (3):593–605.

110 Gottumukkala V. Positioning of patients for operation. In: Longnecker DE (ed.) *Anesthesiology*. New York: McGraw-Hill Medical, 2008.

111 American Society of Anesthesiologists Task Force on Prevention of Perioperative Peripheral Neuropathies. Practice advisory for the prevention of perioperative peripheral neuropathies: an updated report by the American Society of Anesthesiologists Task Force on prevention of perioperative peripheral neuropathies. Anesthesiology 2011; 114(4):741–754.

112 Reddy SK, Tsung A, Geller DA. Laparoscopic liver resection. World J Surg 2011; 35(7):1478–1486.

113 Vila H Jr, Smith R, Augustyniak M, *et al.* The efficacy and safety of pain management before and after implementation of hospital-wide pain management standards: is patient safety compromised by treatment based solely on numerical pain ratings? Anesth Analg 2005; 101(2):474–480.

114 Oderda GM, Gan T, Johnson B, *et al.* Effect of opioid-related adverse events on outcomes in selected surgical patients. J Pain Palliat Care Pharmacother 2013; 27(1):62–70.

115 Joshi GP. Multimodal analgesia techniques for ambulatory surgery. Int Anesthesiol Clin 2005; 43(3):197–204.

116 American Society of Anesthesiologists Task Force on Acute Pain Management. Practice guidelines for acute pain management in the perioperative setting: an updated report by the American Society of Anesthesiologists Task Force on Acute Pain Management. Anesthesiology 2012; 116(2): 248–273.

117 Schultz, NA, Larsen P, Klarskov B, *et al.* Evaluation of a fast-track programme for patients undergoing liver resection. Br J Surg 2013; 100(1):138–143.

118 Jones C, Kelliher M, Dickinson M, *et al.* Randomized clinical trial on enhanced recovery versus standard care following open liver resection. Br J Surg 2013; 100(8):1015–1024.

Videos 1–20 will be of interest to readers of this chapter.

Visit the companion website at:

www.wiley.com\go\conrad\liver-pancreas-biliary-laparoscopic-surgery

CHAPTER 12

Oncological management of primary liver cancer in the era of minimal access surgery

Jennifer Chan

Department of Medical Oncology, Dana-Farber Cancer Institute, Harvard Medical School, Boston, USA

EDITOR COMMENT

In this chapter, an expert view on the general oncological management of primary liver cancer is given. Primary liver cancers, which include hepatocellular carcinoma and biliary tract cancers, represent a major global health problem. For patients with early-stage disease, surgical resection represents an optimal curative treatment modality with a growing role for the minimally invasive approach; ablative therapy can also be considered for small hepatocellular carcinomas. The overall prognosis for primary liver cancers remains poor because of the presence of advanced-stage disease for most patients at the time of diagnosis, underlying liver dysfunction that limits treatment options and survival, and only modest benefits of systemic therapy. Despite these problems, advances in surgical, radiation, and hepatic artery-based techniques plus the development of molecularly targeted agents have led to improvements in patient outcome. The reader will learn how a dedicated multidisciplinary approach is critical for optimizing patient outcomes.

Keywords: chemotherapy, cholangiocarcinoma, hepatic artery embolization, hepatocellular carcinoma, laparoscopic resection of primary liver cancer, radiation, radiofrequency ablation, sorafenib

---

12.1 Introduction

As the second most common cause of cancer-related mortality worldwide, primary liver cancers, which include hepatocellular carcinoma and biliary tract cancers, represent a major global health problem [1]. Liver cancers are most prevalent in less developed regions of the world but also remain a challenge in developed nations. In the United States, the incidence and mortality rates are increasing for liver cancers, in contrast to stable or declining trends for most other cancers [2]. The prognosis for patients with primary liver cancers remains poor because of the presence of advanced, unresectable disease for most patients at the time of diagnosis, underlying liver disease that limits treatment options and survival, and only modest benefits of systemic therapy. Despite these problems, advances in surgical, radiation, and interventional radiology techniques plus the development of molecularly targeted agents have led to improvements in patient

outcome. A multidisciplinary approach is critical for optimizing outcome of patients with primary liver cancers.

12.2 Hepatocellular carcinoma

Several factors pose challenges to the management of patients with hepatocellular carcinoma (HCC). First, most patients present with advanced disease or vascular invasion that limits curative treatment options, including surgery, liver transplantation, or ablative therapy. Second, HCC arises in the setting of chronic liver disease and cirrhosis in over 80% of patients [3,4]. Underlying liver disease can adversely affect overall survival, limit surgical options, and influence tolerance to anticancer therapy by affecting drug metabolism and increasing risk of adverse events. Finally, HCC has a chemoresistant phenotype with a complex and heterogeneous biology that has posed challenges to the efficacy of systemic therapy.

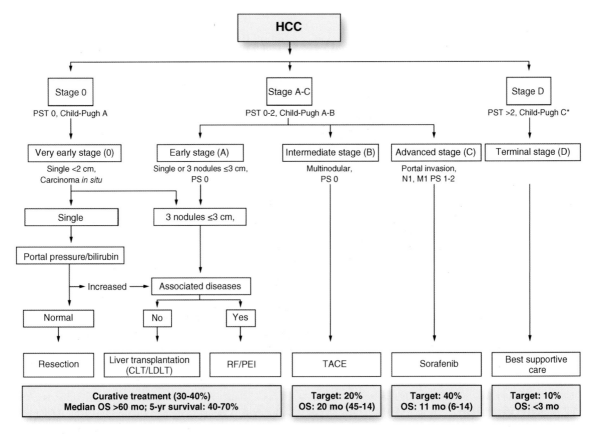

Figure 12.1 Staging, management recommendations, and prognosis of patients with HCC according to the Barcelona Clinic Liver Classification (BCLC). Source: Llovet [7]. Reproduced with permission of Elsevier.

Various staging schemes exist for stratifying patient outcome, each of which has its advantages and limitations. Whereas the TNM system of the American Joint Committee on Cancer (AJCC) incorporates pathological features of disease [5,6], others, such as the Barcelona Clinic Liver Cancer (BCLC) [7], Cancer of the Liver Italian Program (CLIP) [8], Okuda [9], Japan Integrated Staging Score [10], and Chinese University Prognostic Index (CUPI) [11] systems, take into account measures of underlying liver function in addition to an assessment of extent of disease. Although multiple staging and scoring systems exist, there is not one universally accepted classification. Furthermore, because of the geographic variation in risk factors for development of HCC, one staging system may perform better than others in certain regions.

The BCLC staging system, which includes factors related to tumor burden, liver function, and performance status, also incorporates a recommended treatment algorithm based on stage (Figure 12.1). Although treatment algorithms such as the one proposed by the BCLC are helpful for understanding options that exist for particular groups patients, it is important to recognize that indications and treatment are evolving and that individualizing treatment decisions within the context of multidisciplinary evaluation remains critical.

12.2.1 Management of early-stage HCC

For patients with early-stage HCC, potentially curative treatment options exist, including surgical resection, liver transplantation, or ablative therapies. For patients without cirrhosis, surgical resection is the preferred management [12,13]; five-year survival following resection in these patients approaches 50% [14–16]. The majority of patients (>80%), however, develop HCC within the context of cirrhosis. Resection of HCC in patients with cirrhosis requires cautious selection, taking into account tumor-related features (number and size of lesions, vascular invasion, presence of extrahepatic disease) and patient-dependent factors (liver function, performance status, medical comorbidities) [15,17–20]. Optimal outcomes following resection of HCC have been observed in patients with preserved liver function without evidence of portal hypertension, adequate hepatic reserve to tolerate resection, disease confined to the liver, and small (≤3 cm), solitary tumors without evidence of vascular invasion. There is growing evidence that laparoscopic resection of HCC can be performed safely with equivalent oncological outcomes compared with open surgery and with lower perioperative morbidity, particularly in patients with cirrhosis [21,22]. Although risk of recurrence is higher, surgery may still have a role in the management of larger, multifocal tumors and disease associated with vascular invasion [19,23,24].

The presence of lymph node metastasis in patients with HCC is a poor prognostic factor. The presence of pathologically proven lymph node metastasis in the absence of distant metastatic disease was found in one recent study to be associated with an outcome similar to locally advanced disease [25]. Other studies of patients with HCC who have undergone curative hepatic resection and lymph node resection have shown similar results [26]. However, the role and clinical impact of routine regional lymphadenectomy in patients with HCC remain under debate. For patients without cirrhosis undergoing resection of HCC, lymph node dissection can provide important staging and prognostic information. However, in patients with cirrhosis, lymph node excision can impair lymphatic drainage and increase the risk of postoperative ascites [27]. The possible benefits of lymph node excision need to be balanced against this added risk.

Among patients with HCC with advanced cirrhosis who are not candidates for resection, orthotopic liver transplantation can be considered for selected patients. The benefits of liver transplantation include the removal of both tumor and underlying diseased liver. In a landmark study by Mazzafero and colleagues, liver transplantation was associated with a four-year overall survival rate of 85% and a recurrence-free survival rate of 92% in patients with HCC and a single lesion ≤5 cm or up to three tumors, each ≤3 cm, and no evidence of vascular invasion and no nodal metastatic disease [28]. These criteria, known as the Milan criteria, have been used widely in the selection of patients for liver transplant although efforts are being made to expand the indications for transplantation.

For patients with small HCCs who are poor surgical candidates because of impaired liver function or other serious medical comorbidities, local ablative therapy with techniques including radiofrequency ablation (RFA), percutaneous ethanol injection (PEI), laser, and microwave thermal ablation can be considered. RFA has become a more widely used option since recent studies have shown superior outcome with RFA compared with PEI, particularly for tumors >2 cm [29–31]. RFA also has been compared to surgical resection for HCC in several randomized trials. The results have varied, with some studies demonstrating superior overall survival and recurrence-free survival rates for patients undergoing surgery [32] and others showing no differences in survival between the two treatment groups [33,34]. A recent meta-analysis of 10 randomized controlled trials or large cohort studies comparing percutanous ablation therapy with surgical resection for early-stage HCC demonstrated improved overall survival and recurrence-free survival with surgery [35].

12.2.1.1 Neoadjuvant and adjuvant strategies

Unfortunately, only 10–30% of patients with HCC are candidates for surgical resection at the time of diagnosis, and recurrent HCC is reported in 50–80% of patients five years after resection [12,20,36–38]. Most recurrences are intrahepatic and may reflect local recurrence or development of a second primary lesion. Neoadjuvant approaches, including regional therapy with transarterial chemoembolization (TACE), have been examined as a means to improve disease control prior to resection [39–42]. However, neoadjuvant therapy has not been associated with improvement in overall survival. Furthermore, TACE prior to surgery for resectable disease has been associated with worse survival, potentially because of a delay in surgical resection [40–43].

The benefit of adjuvant medical therapy following resection of HCC is uncertain and remains under investigation. Most HCCs are chemorefractory in nature, and thus, cytotoxic chemotherapy has no proven benefit following surgical resection. Furthermore, in patients with cirrhosis, an increase in mortality related to administration of postoperative therapy has been demonstrated [44,45].

Sorafenib, a small molecule tyrosine kinase inhibitor that blocks Raf signaling and vascular endothelial growth factor recptor (VEGFR), platelet-derived growth factor (PDGF), and c-kit, has been shown to improve overall survival in patients with advanced HCC [46–48]. Cases have been reported of significant necrosis associated with sorafenib use and subsequent ability to resect HCC [49]. However, the absence of significant tumor response decreases the likelihood of surgery for initially unresectable HCC following treatment with sorafenib. The benefit of adjuvant sorafenib was investigated in the STORM study, an international, randomized, phase III study of sorafenib versus placebo following surgical resection or local ablation of HCC. No difference in recurrence-free survival, time to recurrence or overall survival was observed with administration of adjuvant sorafenib compared with placebo [50]. Thus, there is no role for sorafenib following resection of HCC.

12.2.2 Management of intermediate-stage HCC

Transarterial chemoembolization is a widely used treatment option for patients with intermediate-stage HCC who have relatively well-preserved liver function, large (>5 cm) or multifocal tumors without main portal vein occlusion or the presence of extrahepatic disease [3,12]. A survival benefit for TACE has been demonstrated in two randomized controlled trials. In the first study, Llovet and colleagues found that TACE with doxorubicin was associated with improved overall survival compared with best supportive care in patients with unresectable HCC and Child–Pugh class A or B liver dysfunction. The one- and two-year survival probabilities were 82% and 63% in patients treated with TACE compared with 63% and 27% of patients receiving a supportive care approach [51]. Similarly, in a second study of patients with unresectable HCC, Lo and colleagues found that TACE with cisplatin and lipiodol was associated with a 57% and 31% one- and two-year survival, compared with 32% and 11% for patients receiving supportive care [52]. Despite these promising results, TACE has not been associated with improved overall survival (OS) in other randomized clinical trials [53,54]. Other embolization techniques, including drug-eluting beads TACE and yttrium-90 radioembolization, and external beam radiation have demonstrated encouraging antitumor activity in patients with unresectable, intermediate-stage HCC [55–59].

Sorafenib has also been investigated as an adjunct to chemoembolization. Post-TACE administration of sorafenib was associated with improved time to tumor progression (TTP) in a randomized phase II study of patients with hepatitis C and intermediate-stage HCC randomized to receive postprocedure sorafenib or placebo (9.2 months for sorafenib versus 4.9 months for placebo, P < 0.001) [60]. However, sorafenib following or concurrent with TACE has not demonstrated improvement in TTP in other studies [61,62]. Thus, existing studies suggest modest if any delay in disease progression with postembolization sorafenib; the survival benefit of adding sorafenib to TACE remains under investigation.

There is also a growing body of evidence that radiation therapy can provide sustained local control for HCC not suited for other locoregional treatments and for disease associated with portal vein thrombus [58,59,63,64]. A recent phase II study examining high-dose hypofractionated proton beam radiation therapy for patients with locally advanced, unresectable HCC and intrahepatic cholangiocarcinoma demonstrated a high two-year local control rate of 94.8% for patients with HCC, supporting further studies on radiation in patients with primary liver cancers [64]. Whether improved local control will translate into an improvement in overall survival still needs to be determined. Finally, the questions of which patients benefit most from radiation and where radiation fits within the spectrum of other local therapies for HCC remain under investigation.

12.2.3 Advanced-stage HCC
12.2.3.1 Systemic chemotherapy
Cytotoxic chemotherapy has modest efficacy against HCC, which has been attributed to inherent chemoresistance related to upregulation of multidrug resistance genes and drug efflux mechanisms [65–67]. Furthermore, chemotherapy may not be well tolerated in patients with significant underlying liver dysfunction because of altered drug metabolism and medical comorbidities. Finally, a benefit of therapy may be difficult to ascertain owing to the poor survival of patients related to advanced liver disease. Doxorubicin has been the most widely investigated cytotoxic chemotherapeutic agent for advanced HCC. Despite a modest objective response rate of 20% or less, two controlled trials have suggested that doxorubicin may be associated with a small survival advantage than either best supportive care alone or noletrexed, an inhibitor of thymidylate synthase [68,69].

Many other cytotoxic chemotherapy agents, including gemcitabine [70,71], irinotecan [72], paclitaxel [73], and capecitabine [74], have been tested in HCC in phase II studies. Response rates ranging from 10% to 30% have been reported, but no clear effect on survival has been identified. Combination chemotherapy, with a regimen such as cisplatin, interferon, doxorubicin, and 5-fluorouracil (PIAF), may be associated with a higher response rate and tumor control, but a benefit on overall survival has not been clearly demonstrated [75]. The combination of infusional 5-fluorouracil, leucovorin, and oxaliplatin (FOLFOX) was recently evaluated in Asian patients with HCC in a randomized trial compared with doxorubicin [76]. At the time of final analysis, there was a nonsignificant trend towards improved overall survival in patients treated with FOLFOX compared with doxorubicin (6.4 versus 4.97 months, $P = 0.07$). A post hoc analysis with longer follow-up later found that the overall survival advantage with FOLFOX was maintained. For patients with advanced HCC who experience progressive disease on sorafenib or who are intolerant of sorafenib, this study suggests that FOLFOX may provide modest benefit.

12.2.3.2 Molecularly targeted therapy

Until recently, no systemic therapies had been associated with improved overall survival in patients with advanced-

stage HCC. Because HCCs are vascular tumors with increased expression of VEGF and microvessel density, inhibition of angiogenesis has been investigated as a potential therapeutic strategy [77]. Two randomized studies have demonstrated improved overall survival in patients with advanced HCC treated with sorafenib (Table 12.1). In the phase III Sorafenib HCC Assessment Randomized Protocol (SHARP) trial, 602 patients with ECOG PS 0–2 and Child–Pugh class A liver function were randomized to receive sorafenib or a placebo [48]. Although the number of complete (0%) and partial responses (2%) to treatment was low, sorafenib was associated with improved overall survival (median OS, 10.7 months versus 7.9 months, $P < 0.001$). Furthermore, sorafenib was also associated with a delay in TTP. Similar results were seen in the phase III Asian-Pacific study of sorafenib versus placebo [78].

Other receptor tyrosine kinase inhibitors have been evaluated in patients with advanced HCC and compared directly against sorafenib (see Table 12.1). However, neither

Table 12.1 Results of selected randomized phase III clinical trials of molecularly targeted therapies for advanced HCC.

Agent	Molecular target	Line of therapy	ORR (%)	TTP (months)	Median OS (months)
Sorafenib versus placebo [48]	VEGFR, PDGFR, FLT-3, RAF	1st	2 versus 1	5.5 versus 2.8; HR 0.58 (0.45–0.74)	10.7 versus 7.9; HR 0.69 (0.55–0.87)
Sorafenib versus placebo [78]	VEGFR, PDGFR, FLT-3, RAF	1st	3.3 versus 1.3	2.8 versus 1.4; HR 0.57 (0.42–0.79)	6.5 versus 4.2; HR 0.68 (0.50–0.93)
Brivanib versus placebo [138]	VEGFR, FGFR	2nd	10 versus 2	4.2 versus 2.7; HR 0.56 (0.42–0.75)	9.4 versus 8.2; HR 0.89 (0.69–1.15)
Ramucirumab versus placebo [83]	VEGFR-2	2nd	7 versus 1	PFS: 2.8 versus 2.1; HR 0.63 (0.52–0.75)	9.2 versus 7.6; HR 0.87 (0.72–1.05)
Brivanib versus sorafenib [80]	VEGFR, FGFR	1st	12 versus 9	4.2 versus 4.1; HR 1.01 (0.88–1.16)	9.5 versus 9.9; HR 1.06 (0.93–1.22)
Sunitinib versus sorafenib [79]	VEGFR, PDGFRα/β, c-kit, FLT3, RET	1st	6.6 versus 6.1	4.1 versus 3.8, HR 1.13 (0.96–1.31)	7.9 versus 10.2; HR 1.3 (1.13–1.50)
Linifanib versus sorafenib [81]	VEGFR, PDGFR	1st	13.0 versus 6.9	5.4 versus 4.0; HR 0.76 (0.64–0.90)	9.1 versus 9.8; HR 1.05 (0.90–1.22)
Erlotinib + sorafenib versus placebo + sorafenib [82]	EGFR	1st		3.2 versus 4.0 mo; HR 1.14 (0.94–1.37)	9.5 versus 8.5; HR 0.93 (0.78–1.11)
Everolimus versus placebo [84]	mTOR	2nd	2.2 versus 1.6	3.0 versus 2.6; HR 0.93 (0.75–1.15)	7.6 versus 7.3; HR 1.05 (0.86–1.27)

EGFR, epidermal growth factor receptor; FGFR, fibroblast growth factor receptor; FLT-3, FMS-related tyrosine kinase 3; HR, hazard ratio; mTOR, mammalian target of rapamycin; ORR, overall response rate (complete response or partial response as measured by Response Evaluation Criteria in Solid Tumors [RECIST] or modified RECIST for HCC); OS, overall survival; PDGFR, platelet-derived growth factor receptor; PFS, progression-free survival; RAF, Raf kinases; RET, glial cell line-derived neurotropic factor receptor (REarranged during Transfection); VEGFR, vascular endothelial growth factor receptor.

sunitinib, brivanib, linifanib nor the combination of sorafenib plus erlotinib have demonstrated superiority or noninferiority to sorafenib [79–82]. Additionally, no significant survival advantage was observed in phase III trials of ramucirumab, a monoclonal antibody that blocks activation of VEGFR-2, or everolimus, an inhibitor of the mammalian target of rapamycin (mTOR), versus placebo and in patients with advanced HCC following first-line therapy with sorafenib [83,84].

Other agents targeting different molecular pathways involved in hepatocarcinogenesis, including hepatocyte growth factor/c-MET (tivantinib, cabozantinib) and other inhibitors of angiogenesis, remain under investigation [85,86]. Furthermore, early promising results have been demonstrated with the immune checkpoint inhibitor nivolumab, a monoclonal antibody that blocks the programmed cell death 1 (PD-1) receptor on activated T cells [87].

KEY POINTS: HEPATOCELLULAR CARCINOMA

- Hepatocellular carcinoma arises in the setting of chronic liver disease and cirrhosis in over 80% of patients. This can adversely affect overall survival, limit surgical options, and affect tolerance to systemic therapy.

- For patients with early-stage HCC, potentially curative treatment options exist.
  - For patients without advanced cirrhosis, surgical resection is the preferred management.
  - For patients with cirrhosis who are not candidates for resection, liver transplantation can be considered for patients meeting transplant criteria.
  - For patients with small HCCs who are poor surgical candidates because of impaired liver function or other serious medical comorbidities, local ablative therapy can be considered.
  - Neoadjuvant and adjuvant therapies have no proven benefit and remain under investigation.

- For patients with intermediate-stage HCC, preserved liver function, and large or multifocal tumors without main portal vein occlusion or extrahepatic metastases, hepatic artery embolization or radiation therapy can be considered.

- Cytotoxic chemotherapy has limited efficacy against HCC. Sorafenib has demonstrated an overall survival benefit for patients with advanced HCC. Other molecularly targeted agents remain under investigation.

12.3 Biliary tract cancers

Biliary tract cancers represent a heterogeneous group of malignancies that include cholangiocarcinoma and gallbladder carcinoma. Cholangiocarcinomas, primarily adenocarcinoma, arise from the epithelium of the bile ducts and are classified according to location as intrahepatic and extrahepatic cholangiocarcinoma (Figure 12.2). Extrahepatic tumors can be further subclassified into hilar carcinomas, arising at or near the junction of the left and right hepatic ducts, and distal cholangiocarcinoma. Approximately 60–70% of biliary tract cancers arise in the perihilar region (Klatskin tumors). Extrahepatic and intrahepatic cholangiocarcinomas occur in approximately 20–30% and 5–10% of patients, respectively [88]. Because most biliary tract cancers present at an advanced stage, these cancers are associated with a poor prognosis with five-year survival rates less than 5–10% [89].

12.3.1 Resected, localized biliary tract cancers: role of adjuvant therapy

Surgical resection represents the only potentially curative treatment modality, but it is estimated that less than 35%

of patients are candidates for resection owing to extent of local disease or presence of metastatic disease [90,91]. The five-year survival rates for patients with resected biliary tract cancers are in the range of 30–50% [92]. Outcomes vary depending on location and stage of the primary lesion. Distal cholangiocarcinomas have a more favorable prognosis compared with perihilar

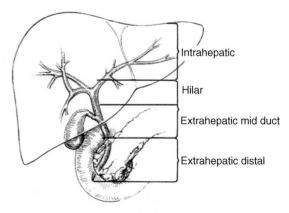

Figure 12.2 Anatomical classification of biliary tract cancers. Source: Turaga [149]. Reproduced with permission of Springer.

cholangiocarcinoma [93]. Gallbladder carcinoma, in general, is the most aggressive of the biliary tract cancers and is associated with the shortest median survival [94].

Multiple studies have demonstrated that the presence of lymph node metastases in patients with cholangiocarcinoma is a poor prognostic factor [93,95–97]. Furthermore, studies including patients with perihilar carcinoma and distal cholangiocarcinoma have demonstrated survival differences related to total lymph node count among those with pathologically node-negative disease [96,97]. This observation has raised the possibility of a therapeutic benefit for lymphadenectomy, but more likely reflects the effects of accurate staging of disease. While lymph node dissection itself may have little direct impact on survival, staging information may influence decisions regarding postsurgical treatment that potentially could affect outcome. Although regional lymphadenectomy is performed routinely for carcinomas arising from extrahepatic bile ducts, indications for lymph node dissection for intrahepatic cholangiocarcinoma remain controversial [27,98]. Nonetheless, because lymph node involvement is such an important prognostic factor, lymphadenectomy should be considered to obtain a precise stage of disease and to provide prognostic information that could influence postoperative management.

Local recurrence in the liver is the most common pattern for relapse following resection of biliary tract cancers although there is a suggestion that gallbladder cancer may also be associated with greater risk of distant metastatic spread [90,94]. Because of the high rate of recurrence, adjuvant chemotherapy and radiation have been investigated as potential strategies to improve outcome. However, most of the studies investigating the efficacy and tolerance of adjuvant therapy in this patient population have been retrospective in nature and based on small numbers of patients that include both gallbladder and bile duct cancers arising from various locations. Thus, the role of adjuvant therapy for resected biliary tract cancers remains a controversial topic, and its benefits have not been well defined.

12.3.1.1 Adjuvant chemotherapy

Although retrospective studies have suggested an advantage with adjuvant chemotherapy alone, randomized studies have not demonstrated that chemotherapy can improve survival following resection of cholangiocarcinoma. A multicenter randomized trial conducted in Japan compared postoperative chemotherapy with mitomycin C and 5-FU versus surgery alone in patients with resected pancreaticobiliary malignancies. Among patients with

resected cholangiocarcinoma, five-year OS in patients receiving chemotherapy (27%) was not significantly different to those undergoing surgery alone (24%) [99]. Furthermore, the European ESAPC-3 study randomized patients with resected periampullary malignancies to receive adjuvant 5-FU with leucovorin versus gemcitabine versus observation following surgery. Among the subset of patients with bile duct cancer, there was no improvement in median survival associated with receipt of chemotherapy. The median survival rates of patients receiving no chemotherapy, 5-FU/leucovorin, and gemcitabine were 27, 18, and 20 months, respectively [100].

12.3.1.2 Adjuvant radiation therapy

Data have been mixed regarding the benefits of adjuvant radiation therapy following complete resection of biliary tract cancers. Some retrospective studies have demonstrated improved local control and survival among patients with undergoing intraoperative and postoperative radiation therapy [101–103]. However, contrasting studies also suggest no improvement in outcome and significant side-effects [104–106]. One subgroup of patients who may benefit from postoperative radiation is those with positive resection margins. In a retrospective study of patients undergoing curative-intent surgery for extrahepatic cholangiocarcinoma, those with microscopically positive resection margins who received adjuvant radiation therapy had higher median disease-free survival rates than those who underwent surgery alone (21 months versus 10 months, respectively, P = 0.042) [107].

12.3.1.3 Adjuvant chemoradiation therapy

Several retrospective and phase II studies have suggested benefit for postoperative chemoradiation therapy in patients with completely or incompletely resected biliary tract cancers. In a retrospective analysis of patients with resected extrahepatic cholangiocarcinoma, similar survival was observed between patients with standard risk disease (R0 resection, node-negative disease) and those with high-risk disease (R1 resection, node-positive disease) who received adjuvant chemoradiation. The lack of a survival difference between the two groups suggests that patients at high risk for locoregional recurrence may benefit from adjuvant chemoradiation following surgery [108]. Similarly, in another retrospective study of patients with extrahepatic cholangiocarcioma undergoing curative-intent resection, receipt of adjuvant chemoradiation therapy was associated with improved overall survival, disease-free survival, and locoregional control compared with surgical resection alone after controlling for other prognostic factors [109]. A recent phase II study provides prospective data regarding the benefit of adjuvant chemotherapy (capecitabine plus gemcitabine) followed by 5-FU-based chemoradiation after resection of extrahepatic cholangiocarcinoma and gallbladder cancer. Promising results were demonstrated: two-year OS, DFS, and local recurrence rates were 65%, 52%, and 11% respectively, among all 79 patients treated (54 with cholangiocarcinoma, 25 with gallbladder cancer) [110].

Among more recent retrospective studies that include only patients with gallbladder carcinoma, adjuvant chemoradiation therapy following resection has been associated with improved survival after adjusting for other predictors of survival [111,112]. Similarly, a model based on treatment and outcome of patients with resected gallbladder carcinoma included in the United States National Cancer Institute SEER-Medicare database demonstrated the greatest benefit for adjuvant chemoradiation therapy among patients with node-positive disease or with tumors staged as T2 or higher [113].

A recent meta-analysis has further examined the role of adjuvant therapy in the treatment of biliary tract cancers [114]. The analysis was composed of trials of adjuvant therapy for patients undergoing adjuvant chemotherapy, radiotherapy, or both after curative-intent surgery for gallbladder and bile duct cancers and included patients who underwent surgery alone as a comparator group. In the pooled data, there was a nonsignificant improvement in OS with any adjuvant therapy compared with surgery alone (odds ratio [OR] 0.74; 95% confidence interval [CI] 0.55–1.10; P = 0.06). A nonsignificant survival benefit was also observed when patients with gallbladder and bile duct carcinomas were analyzed independently. Those receiving chemotherapy (OR 0.39; 95% CI 0.23–0.66; P < 0.001) or chemoradiation therapy (OR 0.61; 95% CI 0.38–0.99; P = 0.049) appeared to derive greater benefit than those treated with radiation alone (OR 0.98; 95% CI 0.67–1.43; P = 0.90). The greatest benefit was observed for adjuvant therapy in patients with high-risk lymph node-positive disease and those with incomplete R1 resections. These data suggest that adjuvant chemotherapy or chemoradiation therapy may improve outcome in patients with resected, high-risk gallbladder and bile duct cancers and provide support for a common practice of administering adjuvant therapy. However, prospective, randomized trials are necessary to further evaluate the benefit of postoperative therapy.

12.3.2 Locally advanced and metastatic biliary tract cancers

12.3.2.1 Radiation and chemoradiation therapy

The majority of patients with cholangiocarcinoma present with locally unresectable disease. There is limited experience with neoadjuvant therapy as a surgical conversion strategy in the management of patients with initially unresectable, locally advanced disease. However, reports have suggested a potential role for selected patients. In a retrospective report of 45 patients with resected extrahepatic cholangiocarcinoma, 12 patients were treated with neoadjuvant therapy. Of these 12 patients, 10 had disease deemed initially unresectable and two had potentially resectable disease but received neoadjuvant chemoradiation therapy owing to physician preference. Supporting the concept that neoadjuvant therapy can improve the ability to resect initially unresectable disease, three of the 12 patients who received neoadjuvant chemoradiation therapy had a complete pathological response to treatment, and 11 of the 12 patients underwent an R0 resection [115]. Additionally, in a series of patients with extrahepatic cholangiocarcinoma, three of nine patients who were treated with preoperative chemoradiation therapy had a pathological complete response to therapy. Furthermore, all nine patients who received chemoradiation therapy had negative margins at resection, compared with only half who did not receive neoadjuvant therapy [116]. Although these results are promising, particularly for patients with initially unresectable disease, additional prospective studies are needed to clarify the benefits of neoadjuvant therapy.

Although data are limited, radiation may also provide local control of disease for patients with unresectable, locally advanced disease. In a retrospective study of patients with locally advanced extrahepatic cholangiocarcinoma who were treated with external beam radiation therapy with concurrent chemotherapy and/or brachytherapy, overall survival and local control rates at one year were 59% and 90%, respectively. At the time of death, the majority of patients had local control of disease, suggesting that local effects of tumor might be effectively controlled with radiation therapy [117]. A more recent phase II study demonstrated high local control rates with high-dose hypofractionated proton beam radiation therapy for locally advanced, unresectable HCC and intrahepatic cholangiocarcinoma, supporting further investigation into the role of radiation therapy for unresectable primary liver cancers [64].

12.3.2.2 Hepatic artery-based therapy

Much of the data supporting the role of hepatic artery-based therapy for primary liver cancers is derived from series also including patients with HCC. Recent studies, however, have examined the efficacy of hepatic artery embolization, particularly radioembolization, for localized, unresectable intra-hepatic cholangiocarcinoma [118–122]. In a multi-institutional series including 198 patients with intrahepatic cholangiocarcinoma treated with chemoembolization, bland embolization or yttrium-90 radioembolization, complete or partial radiographic responses were reported in 26% of patients, while 62% had stable disease [123]. Median OS was 13.2 months and did not vary according to type of embolization technique. Randomized studies comparing the various hepatic artery-based therapies to radiation or chemotherapy are not yet available.

12.3.2.3 Chemotherapy

Systemic chemotherapy remains a cornerstone in the palliative management of patients with unresectable and metastatic biliary tract cancers. The combination of 5-FU, leucovorin, and etoposide has demonstrated an overall survival benefit compared with best supportive care in a randomized study of patients with advanced biliary tract and pancreatic cancers (median OS, six months versus 2.5 months) [124]. Furthermore, quality of life measures improved more and deteriorated less often in the patients receiving chemotherapy. Multiple phase II studies have also demonstrated activity of chemotherapy in the treatment of this disease. In a pooled analysis of 104 trials including 2810 patients with advanced biliary tract cancer, superior tumor response and control rates were observed in patients receiving chemotherapy regimens containing gemcitabine and platinum [125].

The combination of gemcitabine and cisplatin has been shown to improve overall survival in patients with advanced biliary tract cancers. In the UK ABC-02 trial, patients with advanced biliary tract cancers were randomized to receive gemcitabine and cisplatin or gemcitabine alone. OS was significantly improved in patients receiving combination therapy compared with single-agent gemcitabine (11.7 months versus 8.1 months, $P < 0.001$) [126]. The rate of tumor control, as defined by complete or partial responses and stable disease, was also higher in patients receiving gemcitabine and cisplatin (81.4% versus 71.8%, $P = 0.049$). Similarly, a randomized phase II study reported

Table 12.2 Results of selected clinical trials of molecularly targeted therapies for advanced biliary tract cancers.

Agent/target	Trial phase	Line of therapy	ORR (%)	Median PFS (months)	Median OS (months)
EGFR					
Erlotinib [139]	II	1st/2nd	8	2.6	7.5
Gemcitabine + oxaliplatin +/− erlotinib [140]	III (randomized)	1st	30 versus 16 (P = 0.005)	5.8 versus 4.2; HR 0.80 (0.61–1.03)	9.5 versus 9.5; HR 0.93 (0.69–1.25)
Gemcitabine + oxaliplatin +/− cetuximab [141]	II (randomized)	1st	24 versus 23	6.1 versus 5.5	11.0 versus 12.4
Gemcitabine + oxaliplatin + capecitabine + panitumumuab [142]	II	1st	33	8.3	9.8
VEGF					
Gemcitabine + oxaliplatin + bevacizumab [143]	II	1st	40	7.0	12.7
Sorafenib [144]	II	Any	2	2.3	4.4
Sorafenib [145]	II	1st	0	3	9
Sunitinib [146]	II	2nd	8.9	1.7	4.8
HER2					
Lapatinib [147]	II	1st/2nd	0	1.8	5.2
MEK					
Selumetinib [148]	II	2nd	12	3.7	9.8

EGFR, epidermal growth factor receptor; HER2, human epidermal growth factor receptor 2; HR, hazard ratio; MEK, mitogen-activated protein kinase; ORR, overall response rate; OS, overall survival; PFS, progression-free survival; VEGF, vascular endothelial growth factor.

by Okusaka *et al.* also showed improved outcome for patients with advanced biliary tract cancers treated with the combination of gemcitabine and cisplatin compared with gemcitabine alone [127]. Although gemcitabine plus cisplatin has been shown to be superior to gemcitabine alone, this combination has not been compared with other chemotherapy combinations. Other regimens that have demonstrated activity in advanced biliary tract cancers in phase II trials have included gemcitabine and oxaliplatin [128–130], gemcitabine and fluoropyrimidine [131–133], and fluoropyrimidine and oxaliplatin [134].

Although chemotherapy has improved outcomes for patients with advanced biliary tract cancers, prognosis for patients remains poor. Targeted therapies directed against signaling pathways in biliary tract cancers, including the epidermal growth factor receptor (EGFR), angiogenesis, and the mitogen-activated protein kinase (MEK) pathway, have been investigated with early promising results (Table 12.2). Recent studies have also identified genomic alterations in cholangiocarcinoma and gallbladder cancer involving chromatin remodeling genes and the *IDH1* and *IDH2* genes that encode metabolic enzymes [135]. Furthermore, alterations in fibroblast growth factor receptor 2 (*FGF2*), including novel gene fusions, have been identified [136,137]. These findings have the potential to translate into new targets and improvements in therapy for patients with advanced disease.

KEY POINTS: BILIARY TRACT CANCERS

- Biliary tract cancers are a heterogeneous group of tumors composed of gallbladder carcinoma, intrahepatic, perihilar, and distal cholangiocarcinoma. Most patients present at an advanced stage with unresectable disease.

- Surgical resection remains the only curative treatment modality.

- The role of adjuvant therapy for completely resected biliary tract cancers is controversial, and benefits have not been well defined.
    - In R0 resected patients, external beam radiation has not shown survival benefit. However, adjuvant radiation may benefit patients with positive resection margins.
    - Adjuvant chemoradiation therapy may have benefit for patients with high-risk disease (lymph node and/or margin positive).

- There are limited data about the role of chemoradiation therapy for patients with locally advanced disease. In selected patients, it may improve ability to resect initially unresectable tumors and improve local control. Radiation may also provide local control of disease for patients with unresectable, locally advanced disease.

- Hepatic artery-based therapies are a promising strategy for patients with unresectable locally intrahepatic cholangiocarcinoma and warrant prospective evaluation in comparison to other standards of care.

- Systemic chemotherapy with gemcitabine and cisplatin improves overall survival for patients with advanced biliary tract cancer. Other combination chemotherapy regimens are active in the treatment of patients with metastatic disease.

12.4 Conclusion

Although the management of patients with primary liver cancers remains challenging because of underlying liver dysfunction, complex molecular biology, and heterogeneity of disease, recent progress in surgical and medical therapy has improved the prognosis of patients with both early and advanced disease. Future advances, including those involving minimally invasive surgery, interventional radiology, and radiation techniques, have the potential to further improve outcomes for patients with early and intermediate-stage disease. Systemic chemotherapy can improve survival of patients with advanced disease, and hopefully the identification of novel molecular targets and predictors of response will translate into new therapeutic strategies. A multidisciplinary approach is essential to optimizing patient outcome.

References

1 Torre LA, Bray F, Siegel RL, *et al.* Global cancer statistics, 2012. CA Cancer J Clin 2015; 65(2):87–108.

2 Siegel R, Miller K, Jemal A. Cancer statistics, 2014. CA Cancer J Clin 2014; 64(1):9–29.

3 Bruix J, Sherman M. Management of hepatocellular carcinoma. Hepatology 2005; 42(5):1208–1236.

4 Forner A, Llovet JM, Bruix J. Hepatocellular carcinoma. Lancet 2012; 379(9822):1245–1255.

5 Henderson JM, Sherman M, Tavill A, *et al.* AHPBA/AJCC consensus conference on staging of hepatocellular carcinoma: consensus statement. HPB (Oxford) 2003; 5(4):243–250.

6 Edge SB, Byrd D, Compton C, *et al.* AJCC Cancer Staging Manual. New York: Springer, 2010.

7 Llovet JM, Bru C, Bruix J. Prognosis of hepatocellular carcinoma: the BCLC staging classification. Semin Liver Dis 1999; 19(3):329–338.

8 A new prognostic system for hepatocellular carcinoma: a retrospective study of 435 patients: the Cancer of the Liver Italian Program (CLIP) investigators. Hepatology 1998; 28(3):751–755.

9 Okuda K, Ohtsuki T, Obata H, *et al.* Natural history of hepatocellular carcinoma and prognosis in relation to treatment. Study of 850 patients. Cancer 1985; 56(4):918–928.

10 Kudo M, Chung H, Osaki Y. Prognostic staging system for hepatocellular carcinoma (CLIP score): its value and limitations, and a proposal for a new staging system, the Japan Integrated Staging Score (JIS score). J Gastroenterol 2003; 38(3):207–215.

11 Leung TW, Tang A, Zee B, *et al.* Construction of the Chinese University Prognostic Index for hepatocellular carcinoma and comparison with the TNM staging system, the Okuda staging system, and the Cancer of the Liver Italian Program staging system: a study based on 926 patients. Cancer 2002; 94(6):1760–1769.

12 EASL–EORTC clinical practice guidelines: management of hepatocellular carcinoma. J Hepatol 2012; 56(4):908–943.

13 Bruix J, Sherman M. Management of hepatocellular carcinoma: an update. Hepatology 2011; 53(3):1020–1022.

14 Fong Y, Sun R, Jarnagin W, *et al.* An analysis of 412 cases of hepatocellular carcinoma at a Western center. Ann Surg 1999; 229(6):790–799; discussion 799–800.

15 Nathan H, Schulick RD, Choti M, *et al.* Predictors of survival after resection of early hepatocellular carcinoma. Ann Surg 2009; 249(5):799–805.

16 Chang CH, Chau G, Lui W, *et al.* Long-term results of hepatic resection for hepatocellular carcinoma originating from the noncirrhotic liver. Arch Surg 2004; 139(3):320–325; discussion 326.

17 Bruix J, Castells A, Bosch J, *et al.* Surgical resection of hepatocellular carcinoma in cirrhotic patients: prognostic value of preoperative portal pressure. Gastroenterology 1996; 111(4):1018–1022.

18 Rahbari NN, Mehrabi A, Mollberg N, *et al.* Hepatocellular carcinoma: current management and perspectives for the future. Ann Surg 2011; 253(3):453–469.

19 Pawlik TM, Poon R, Abdalla E, *et al.* Critical appraisal of the clinical and pathologic predictors of survival after resection of large hepatocellular carcinoma. Arch Surg 2005; 140 (5):450–457; discussion 457–458.

20 Imamura H, Matsuyama Y, Tanaka E, *et al.* Risk factors contributing to early and late phase intrahepatic recurrence of hepatocellular carcinoma after hepatectomy. J Hepatol 2003; 38(2):200–207.

21 Cheung TT, Poon R, Yuen W, *et al.* Long-term survival analysis of pure laparoscopic versus open hepatectomy for hepatocellular carcinoma in patients with cirrhosis: a single-center experience. Ann Surg 2013; 257(3):506–511.

22 Zhou YM, Shao W, Zhao Y, *et al.* Meta-analysis of laparoscopic versus open resection for hepatocellular carcinoma. Dig Dis Sci 2011; 56(7):1937–1943.

23 Roayaie S, Jibara G, Taouli B, *et al.* Resection of hepatocellular carcinoma with macroscopic vascular invasion. Ann Surg Oncol 2013; 20(12):3754–3760.

24 Ishizawa T, Hasegawa K, Aoki T, *et al.* Neither multiple tumors nor portal hypertension are surgical contraindications for hepatocellular carcinoma. Gastroenterology, 2008; 134(7):1908–1916.

25 Hasegawa K, Makuuchi M, Kokudo N, *et al.* Impact of histologically confirmed lymph node metastases on patient survival after surgical resection for hepatocellular carcinoma: report of a Japanese nationwide survey. Ann Surg 2014; 259(1):166–170.

26 Xiaohong S, Huikai L, Feng W, *et al.* Clinical significance of lymph node metastasis in patients undergoing partial hepatectomy for hepatocellular carcinoma. World J Surg 2010; 34(5):1028–1033.

27 Ercolani G, Grazi GL, Ravaioli M, *et al.* The role of lymphadenectomy for liver tumors: further considerations on the appropriateness of treatment strategy. Ann Surg 2004; 239 (2):202–209.

28 Mazzaferro V, Regalia E, Doci R, *et al.* Liver transplantation for the treatment of small hepatocellular carcinomas in patients with cirrhosis. N Engl J Med 1996; 334(11):693–699.

29 Cho YK, Kim J, Kim M, *et al.* Systematic review of randomized trials for hepatocellular carcinoma treated with percutaneous ablation therapies. Hepatology 2009; 49(2):453–459.

30 Lencioni RA, Allgaier H, Cioni D, *et al.* Small hepatocellular carcinoma in cirrhosis: randomized comparison of radio–frequency thermal ablation versus percutaneous ethanol injection. Radiology 2003; 228(1):235–240.

31 Germani G, Pleguezuelo M, Gurusamy K, *et al.* Clinical outcomes of radiofrequency ablation, percutaneous alcohol and acetic acid injection for hepatocelullar carcinoma: a meta-analysis. J Hepatol 2010; 52(3):380–388.

32 Huang J, Yan L, Cheng Z, *et al.* A randomized trial comparing radiofrequency ablation and surgical resection for HCC conforming to the Milan criteria. Ann Surg 2010; 252(6):903–912.

33 Chen MS, Li J, Zheng Y, *et al.* A prospective randomized trial comparing percutaneous local ablative therapy and partial hepatectomy for small hepatocellular carcinoma. Ann Surg 2006; 243(3):321–328.

34 Feng K, Yan J, Li X, *et al.* A randomized controlled trial of radiofrequency ablation and surgical resection in the treatment of small hepatocellular carcinoma. J Hepatol 2012; 57 (4):794–802.

35 Ni JY, Xu L, Sun H, *et al.* Percutaneous ablation therapy versus surgical resection in the treatment for early-stage hepatocellular carcinoma: a meta-analysis of 21, 494 patients. J Cancer Res Clin Oncol 2013; 139(12):2021–2033.

36 Llovet JM., Schwartz M, Mazzaferro V. Resection and liver transplantation for hepatocellular carcinoma. Semin Liver Dis 2005; 25(2):181–200.

37 Portolani N, Coniglio A, Ghidoni S, *et al*. Early and late recurrence after liver resection for hepatocellular carcinoma: prognostic and therapeutic implications. Ann Surg 2006; 243(2):229–235.

38 Poon RT, Fan S, Ng I, *et al*. Different risk factors and prognosis for early and late intrahepatic recurrence after resection of hepatocellular carcinoma. Cancer 2000; 89(3):500–507.

39 Meric F, Patt Y, Curley S, *et al*. Surgery after downstaging of unresectable hepatic tumors with intra-arterial chemotherapy. Ann Surg Oncol 2000; 7(7):490–495.

40 Lee KT, Lu Y, Wang S, *et al*. The effect of preoperative transarterial chemoembolization of resectable hepatocellular carcinoma on clinical and economic outcomes. J Surg Oncol 2009; 99(6):343–350.

41 Wu CC, Ho Y, Ho W, *et al*. Preoperative transcatheter arterial chemoembolization for resectable large hepatocellular carcinoma: a reappraisal. Br J Surg 1995. 82(1):122–126.

42 Sasaki A, Iwashita Y, Shibata K, *et al*. Preoperative transcatheter arterial chemoembolization reduces long-term survival rate after hepatic resection for resectable hepatocellular carcinoma. Eur J Surg Oncol 2006; 32(7):773–779.

43 Kishi Y, Saiura A, Yamamoto J, *et al*. Preoperative transarterial chemoembolization for hepatocellular carcinoma. Hepatogastroenterology 2012; 59(119):2295–2299.

44 Yamamoto M, Arii S, Sugahara K, *et al*. Adjuvant oral chemotherapy to prevent recurrence after curative resection for hepatocellular carcinoma. Br J Surg 1996; 83(3):336–340.

45 Ono T, Yamanoi A, Nazmy El Assal O, *et al*. Adjuvant chemotherapy after resection of hepatocellular carcinoma causes deterioration of long-term prognosis in cirrhotic patients: metaanalysis of three randomized controlled trials. Cancer 2001; 91(12):2378–2385.

46 Wilhelm SM, Carter C, Tang L, *et al*. BAY 43–9006 exhibits broad spectrum oral antitumor activity and targets the RAF/MEK/ERK pathway and receptor tyrosine kinases involved in tumor progression and angiogenesis. Cancer Res 2004; 64 (19):7099–7109.

47 Liu L, Cao Y, Chen C, *et al*. Sorafenib blocks the RAF/MEK/ERK pathway, inhibits tumor angiogenesis, and induces tumor cell apoptosis in hepatocellular carcinoma model PLC/PRF/5. Cancer Res 2006; 66(24):11851–11858.

48 Llovet JM, Ricci S, Mazzaferro V, *et al*. Sorafenib in advanced hepatocellular carcinoma. N Engl J Med 2008; 359(4):378–390.

49 Barbier L, Muscari F, Le Guellec S, *et al*. Liver resection after downstaging hepatocellular carcinoma with sorafenib. Int J Hepatol 2011; 2011: 791013.

50 Bruix J, Takayama T, Mazzaferro V, *et al*. Adjuvant sorafenib for hepatocellular carcinoma after resection or ablation (STORM): a phase 3, randomised, double-blind, placebo-controlled trial. Lancet Oncol 2015; 16(13): 1344–54.

51 Llovet JM, Real MI, Montana X, *et al*. Arterial embolisation or chemoembolisation versus symptomatic treatment in patients with unresectable hepatocellular carcinoma: a randomised controlled trial. Lancet 2002; 359(9319):1734–1739.

52 Lo CM, Ngan H, Tso W, *et al*. Randomized controlled trial of transarterial lipiodol chemoembolization for unresectable hepatocellular carcinoma. Hepatology 2002; 35(5):1164–1171.

53 Doffoel M, Bonnetain F, Bouche O, *et al*. Multicentre randomised phase III trial comparing Tamoxifen alone or with Transarterial Lipiodol Chemoembolisation for unresectable hepatocellular carcinoma in cirrhotic patients (Federation Francophone de Cancerologie Digestive 9402). Eur J Cancer 2008; 44(4):528–538.

54 Groupe d'Etude et de Traitement du Carcinome Hepatocellulaire. A comparison of lipiodol chemoembolization and conservative treatment for unresectable hepatocellular carcinoma. N Engl J Med 1995; 332(19):1256–1261.

55 Lammer J, Malagari K, Vogl T, *et al*. Prospective randomized study of doxorubicin-eluting-bead embolization in the treatment of hepatocellular carcinoma: results of the PRECISION V study. Cardiovasc Intervent Radiol 2010; 33(1):41–52.

56 Varela M, Real MI, Burrel M, *et al*. Chemoembolization of hepatocellular carcinoma with drug eluting beads: efficacy and doxorubicin pharmacokinetics. J Hepatol 2007; 46 (3):474–481.

57 Salem R, Lewandowski RJ, Mulcahy M, *et al*. Radioembolization for hepatocellular carcinoma using Yttrium-90 microspheres: a comprehensive report of long-term outcomes. Gastroenterology 2010; 138(1):52–64.

58 Klein J, Dawson LA. Hepatocellular carcinoma radiation therapy: review of evidence and future opportunities. Int J Radiat Oncol Biol Phys 2013; 87(1):22–32.

59 Bujold A, Massey CA, Kim J, *et al*. Sequential phase I and II trials of stereotactic body radiotherapy for locally advanced hepatocellular carcinoma. J Clin Oncol 2013; 31(13):1631–1639.

60 Sansonno D, Lauletta G, Russi S, *et al*. Transarterial chemoembolization plus sorafenib: a sequential therapeutic scheme for HCV-related intermediate-stage hepatocellular carcinoma: a randomized clinical trial. Oncologist 2012; 17(3):359–366.

61 Kudo M, Imanaka K, Chida N, *et al*. Phase III study of sorafenib after transarterial chemoembolisation in Japanese and Korean patients with unresectable hepatocellular carcinoma. Eur J Cancer 2011; 47(14):2117–2127.

62 Lencioni RA, Llovet JM, Han G, *et al*. Sorafenib or placebo in combination with transarterial chemoembolization (TACE) with doxorubicin-eluting beads (DEBDOX) for intermediate-stage hepatocellular carcinoma (HCC): phase II, randomized, double-blind SPACE trial. J Clin Oncol 2012; 30 (suppl 4): abstr. LBA154.

63 Wahl DR, Stenmark MH, Tao Y, *et al*. Outcomes after stereotactic body radiotherapy or radiofrequency ablation for hepatocellular carcinoma. J Clin Oncol 2015 (epub ahead of print).

64 Hong TS, Wo JY, Yeap BY, *et al*. Multi-institutional phase II study of high-dose hypofractionated proton beam therapy in patients with localized, unresectable hepatocellular carcinoma and intrahepatic cholangiocarcinoma. J Clin Oncol 2015 (epub ahead of print).

65 Huang M, Liu G. The study of innate drug resistance of human hepatocellular carcinoma Bel7402 cell line. Cancer Lett 1999; 135(1):97–105.

66 Kato A, Miyazaki M, Ambiru S, *et al.* Multidrug resistance gene (MDR-1) expression as a useful prognostic factor in patients with human hepatocellular carcinoma after surgical resection. J Surg Oncol 2001; 78(2):110–115.

67 Chenivesse X, Franco D, Brechot C. MDR1 (multidrug resistance) gene expression in human primary liver cancer and cirrhosis. J Hepatol 1993; 18(2):168–172.

68 Lai CL, Wu PC, Chan G, *et al.* Doxorubicin versus no antitumor therapy in inoperable hepatocellular carcinoma. A prospective randomized trial. Cancer 1988; 62(3):479–483.

69 Gish RG, Porta C, Lazar L, *et al.* Phase III randomized controlled trial comparing the survival of patients with unresectable hepatocellular carcinoma treated with nolatrexed or doxorubicin. J Clin Oncol 2007; 25(21):3069–3075.

70 Fuchs CS, Clark JW, Ryan D, *et al.* A phase II trial of gemcitabine in patients with advanced hepatocellular carcinoma. Cancer 2002; 94(12):3186–3191.

71 Yang TS, Lin Y, Chen J, *et al.* Phase II study of gemcitabine in patients with advanced hepatocellular carcinoma. Cancer 2000; 89(4):750–756.

72 O'Reilly EM, Stuart K, Sanz-Altamira P, *et al.* A phase II study of irinotecan in patients with advanced hepatocellular carcinoma. Cancer 2001; 91(1):101–105.

73 Chao Y, Chan W, Birkhofer M, *et al.* Phase II and pharmacokinetic study of paclitaxel therapy for unresectable hepatocellular carcinoma patients. Br J Cancer 1998; 78(1):34–39.

74 Patt YZ, Hassan M, Aguayo A, *et al.* Oral capecitabine for the treatment of hepatocellular carcinoma, cholangiocarcinoma, and gallbladder carcinoma. Cancer 2004; 101(3):578–586.

75 Yeo W, Mok T, Zee B, *et al.* A randomized phase III study of doxorubicin versus cisplatin/interferon alpha02b/doxorubicin/fluorouracil (PIAF) combination chemotherapy for unresectable hepatocellular carcinoma. J Natl Cancer Inst 2005; 97(20):1532–1538.

76 Qin S, Bai Y, Lim H, *et al.* Randomized, multicenter, open-label study of oxaliplatin plus fluorouracil/leucovorin versus doxorubicin as palliative chemotherapy in patients with advanced hepatocellular carcinoma from Asia. J Clin Oncol 2013; 31(28):3501–3508.

77 Semela D, Dufour JF. Angiogenesis and hepatocellular carcinoma. J Hepatol 2004; 41(5):864–880.

78 Cheng AL, Kang Y, Chen Z, *et al.* Efficacy and safety of sorafenib in patients in the Asia-Pacific region with advanced hepatocellular carcinoma: a phase III randomised, double-blind, placebo-controlled trial. Lancet Oncol 2009; 10(1):25–34.

79 Cheng AL, Kang Y, Lin D, *et al.* Sunitinib versus sorafenib in advanced hepatocellular cancer: results of a randomized phase III trial. J Clin Oncol 2013; 31(32):4067–4075.

80 Johnson PJ, Qin S, Park J, *et al.* Brivanib versus sorafenib as first-line therapy in patients with unresectable, advanced hepatocellular carcinoma: results from the randomized phase III BRISK-FL study. J Clin Oncol 2013; 31(28):3517–3524.

81 Cainap C, Qin S, Huang W, *et al.* Phase III trial of linifanib versus sorafenib in patients with advanced hepatocellular carcinoma (HCC). J Clin Oncol 2013; 30 (suppl 34); abstr. 249.

82 Zhu AX, Rosmorduc O, Evans T, *et al.* SEARCH: a phase III, randomized, double-blind, placebo-controlled trial of sorafenib plus erlotinib in patients with hepatocellular carcinoma (HCC). Presented at the 37th Annual European Society for Medical Oncology Congress, Vienna, Austria, 2012. Abstract 917.

83 Zhu AX, Park JO, Ryoo BY, *et al.* Ramucirumab versus placebo as second-line treatment in patients with advanced hepatocellular carcinoma following first-line therapy with sorafenib (REACH): a randomised, double-blind, multicentre, phase 3 trial. Lancet Oncol 2015; 16(7):859–870.

84 Zhu AX, Kudo M, Assenat E, *et al.* Effect of everolimus on survival in advanced hepatocellular carcinoma after failure of sorafenib: the EVOLVE-1 randomized clinical trial. JAMA 2014; 312(1):57–67.

85 Finn RS. Emerging targeted strategies in advanced hepatocellular carcinoma. Semin Liver Dis 2013; 33 (suppl 1):S11–19.

86 Knox JJ, Cleary SP, Dawson LA. Localized and systemic approaches to treating hepatocellular carcinoma. J Clin Oncol 2015; 33(16):1835–1844.

87 El-Khoueiry AB, Melero I, Todd S, *et al.* Phase I/II safety and antitumor activity of nivolumab in patients with advanced hepatocellular carcinoma (HCC): CA209-040. J Clin Oncol 2015; 33(suppl): abstr LBA101.

88 Nakeeb A, Pitt H, Sohn T, *et al.* Cholangiocarcinoma. A spectrum of intrahepatic, perihilar, and distal tumors. Ann Surg 1996; 224(4):463–473; discussion 473–475.

89 Shaib YH, Davila J, McGlynn K, *et al.* Rising incidence of intrahepatic cholangiocarcinoma in the United States: a true increase? J Hepatol 2004; 40(3):472–477.

90 Endo I, Gonen M, Yopp A, *et al.* Intrahepatic cholangiocarcinoma: rising frequency, improved survival, and determinants of outcome after resection. Ann Surg 2008; 248(1):84–96.

91 Wade TP, Prasad C, Virgo K, *et al.* Experience with distal bile duct cancers in U.S. Veterans Affairs hospitals: 1987–1991. J Surg Oncol 1997; 64(3):242–245.

92 Aljiffry M, Abdulelah A, Walsh M, *et al.* Evidence-based approach to cholangiocarcinoma: a systematic review of the current literature. J Am Coll Surg 2009; 208(1):134–147.

93 DeOliveira ML, Cunningham S, Cameron J, *et al.* Cholangiocarcinoma: thirty-one-year experience with 564 patients at a single institution. Ann Surg 2007; 245(5):755–762.

94 Jarnagin WR, Ruo L, Little S, *et al.* Patterns of initial disease recurrence after resection of gallbladder carcinoma and hilar cholangiocarcinoma: implications for adjuvant therapeutic strategies. Cancer 2003; 98(8):1689–1700.

95 Kitagawa Y, Nagino M, Kamiya J, *et al.* Lymph node metastasis from hilar cholangiocarcinoma: audit of 110 patients who underwent regional and paraaortic node dissection. Ann Surg 2001; 233(3):385–392.

96 Ito K, Ito H, Allen P, *et al.* Adequate lymph node assessment for extrahepatic bile duct adenocarcinoma. Ann Surg 2010; 251(4):675–681.

97 Aoba T, Ebata T, Yokoyama Y, *et al.* Assessment of nodal status for perihilar cholangiocarcinoma: location, number, or ratio of involved nodes. Ann Surg 2013; 257(4):718–725.

98 Adachi T, Eguchi S. Lymph node dissection for intrahepatic cholangiocarcinoma: a critical review of the literature to date. J Hepatobiliary Pancreat Sci 2014; 21(3):162–168.

99 Takada T, Amano H, Yasuda H, *et al.* Is postoperative adjuvant chemotherapy useful for gallbladder carcinoma? A phase III multicenter prospective randomized controlled trial in patients with resected pancreaticobiliary carcinoma. Cancer 2002; 95(8):1685–1695.

100 Neoptolemos JP, Moore M, Cox T, *et al.* Effect of adjuvant chemotherapy with fluorouracil plus folinic acid or gemcitabine vs observation on survival in patients with resected periampullary adenocarcinoma: the ESPAC-3 periampullary cancer randomized trial. JAMA 2012; 308(2):147–156.

101 Kraybill WG, Lee H, Picus J, *et al.* Multidisciplinary treatment of biliary tract cancers. J Surg Oncol 1994; 55(4):239–245.

102 Todoroki T, Ohara K, Kawamoto T, *et al.* Benefits of adjuvant radiotherapy after radical resection of locally advanced main hepatic duct carcinoma. Int J Radiat Oncol Biol Phys 2000; 46(3):581–587.

103 Gerhards MF, van Gulik TM, Gonzalez Gonzalez D, *et al.* Results of postoperative radiotherapy for resectable hilar cholangiocarcinoma. World J Surg 2003; 27(2):173–179.

104 Pitt HA, Nakeeb A, Abrams R, *et al.* Perihilar cholangiocarcinoma. Postoperative radiotherapy does not improve survival. Ann Surg 1995; 221(6):788–797; discussion 797–798.

105 Gonzalez Gonzalez D, Gouma DJ, Rauws E, *et al.* Role of radiotherapy, in particular intraluminal brachytherapy, in the treatment of proximal bile duct carcinoma. Ann Oncol 1999; 10 (suppl 4):215–220.

106 Vern-Gross TZ, Shivnani A, Chen K, *et al.* Survival outcomes in resected extrahepatic cholangiocarcinoma: effect of adjuvant radiotherapy in a surveillance, epidemiology, and end results analysis. Int J Radiat Oncol Biol Phys 2011; 81(1):189–198.

107 Gwak HK, Kim W, Kim H, *et al.* Extrahepatic bile duct cancers: surgery alone versus surgery plus postoperative radiation therapy. Int J Radiat Oncol Biol Phys 2010; 78(1):194–198.

108 Borghero Y, Crane CH, Szklaruk J, *et al.* Extrahepatic bile duct adenocarcinoma: patients at high-risk for local recurrence treated with surgery and adjuvant chemoradiation have an equivalent overall survival to patients with standard-risk treated with surgery alone. Ann Surg Oncol 2008; 15(11):3147–3156.

109 Kim TH, Han S, Park S, *et al.* Role of adjuvant chemoradiotherapy for resected extrahepatic biliary tract cancer. Int J Radiat Oncol Biol Phys 2011; 81(5):e853–859.

110 Ben-Josef E, Guthrie KA, El-Khoueiry AB, *et al.* SWOG S0809: a phase II intergroup trial of adjuvant capecitabine and gemcitabine followed by radiotherapy and concurrent capecitabine in extrahepatic cholangiocarcinoma and gallbladder carcinoma. J Clin Oncol 2015; 33(24):2617–2622.

111 Gold DG, Miller R, Haddock M, *et al.* Adjuvant therapy for gallbladder carcinoma: the Mayo Clinic Experience. Int J Radiat Oncol Biol Phys 2009; 75(1):150–155.

112 Cho SY, Kim S, Park S, *et al.* Adjuvant chemoradiation therapy in gallbladder cancer. J Surg Oncol 2010; 102(1):87–93.

113 Wang SJ, Lemieux A, Kalpathy-Cramer J, *et al.* Nomogram for predicting the benefit of adjuvant chemoradiotherapy for resected gallbladder cancer. J Clin Oncol 2011; 29(35):4627–4632.

114 Horgan AM, Amir E, Walter T, *et al.* Adjuvant therapy in the treatment of biliary tract cancer: a systematic review and meta-analysis. J Clin Oncol 2012; 30(16):1934–1940.

115 Nelson JW, Ghafoori AP, Willett C, *et al.* Concurrent chemoradiotherapy in resected extrahepatic cholangiocarcinoma. Int J Radiat Oncol Biol Phys 2009; 73(1):148–153.

116 McMasters KM, Tuttle T, Leach S, *et al.* Neoadjuvant chemoradiation for extrahepatic cholangiocarcinoma. Am J Surg 1997; 174(6):605–608; discussion 608–609.

117 Ghafoori AP, Nelson J, Willett C, *et al.* Radiotherapy in the treatment of patients with unresectable extrahepatic cholangiocarcinoma. Int J Radiat Oncol Biol Phys 2011; 81(3):654–659.

118 Gusani NJ, Balaa FK, Steel JL, *et al.* Treatment of unresectable cholangiocarcinoma with gemcitabine-based transcatheter arterial chemoembolization (TACE): a single-institution experience. J Gastrointest Surg 2008; 12(1):129–137.

119 Vogl TJ, Naguib NN, Nour-Eldin NE, *et al.* Transarterial chemoembolization in the treatment of patients with unresectable cholangiocarcinoma: results and prognostic factors governing treatment success. Int J Cancer 2012; 131(3):733–740.

120 Saxena A, Bester L, Chua TC, *et al.* Yttrium-90 radiotherapy for unresectable intrahepatic cholangiocarcinoma: a preliminary assessment of this novel treatment option. Ann Surg Oncol 2010; 17(2):484–491.

121 Rafi S, Piduru SM, El-Rayes B, *et al.* Yttrium-90 radioembolization for unresectable standard-chemorefractory intrahepatic cholangiocarcinoma: survival, efficacy, and safety study. Cardiovasc Intervent Radiol 2013; 36(2):440–448.

122 Mouli S, Memon K, Baker T, *et al.* Yttrium-90 radioembolization for intrahepatic cholangiocarcinoma: safety, response, and survival analysis. J Vasc Interv Radiol 2013; 24(8):1227–1234.

123 Hyder O, Marsh JW, Salem R, *et al.* Intra-arterial therapy for advanced intrahepatic cholangiocarcinoma: a multi-institutional analysis. Ann Surg Oncol 2013; 20(12):3779–3786.

124 Glimelius B, Hoffman K, Sjoden P, *et al.* Chemotherapy improves survival and quality of life in advanced pancreatic and biliary cancer. Ann Oncol 1996; 7(6):593–600.

125 Eckel F, Schmid RM. Chemotherapy in advanced biliary tract carcinoma: a pooled analysis of clinical trials. Br J Cancer 2007; 96(6):896–902.

126 Valle J, Wasan H, Palmer D, *et al.* Cisplatin plus gemcitabine versus gemcitabine for biliary tract cancer. N Engl J Med 2010; 362(14):1273–1281.

127 Okusaka T, Nakachi K, Fukutomi A, *et al.* Gemcitabine alone or in combination with cisplatin in patients with biliary tract cancer: a comparative multicentre study in Japan. Br J Cancer 2010; 103(4):469–474.

128 Andre T, Tournigand C, Rosmorduc O, *et al.* Gemcitabine combined with oxaliplatin (GEMOX) in advanced biliary tract adenocarcinoma: a GERCOR study. Ann Oncol 2004; 15(9):1339–1343.

129 Andre T, Reyes-Vidal JM, Fartoux L, *et al.* Gemcitabine and oxaliplatin in advanced biliary tract carcinoma: a phase II study. Br J Cancer 2008; 99(6):862–867.

130 Manzione L, Romano R, Germano D. Chemotherapy with gemcitabine and oxaliplatin in patients with advanced biliary tract cancer: a single-institution experience. Oncology 2007; 73 (5–6):311–315.

131 Knox JJ, Hedley D, Oza A, *et al.* Combining gemcitabine and capecitabine in patients with advanced biliary cancer: a phase II trial. J Clin Oncol 2005; 23(10):2332–2338.

132 Cho JY, Paik Y, Chang Y, *et al.* Capecitabine combined with gemcitabine (CapGem) as first-line treatment in patients with advanced/metastatic biliary tract carcinoma. Cancer 2005; 104(12):2753–2758.

133 Riechelmann RP, Townsley C, Chin S, *et al.* Expanded phase II trial of gemcitabine and capecitabine for advanced biliary cancer. Cancer 2007; 110(6):1307–1312.

134 Nehls O, Oettle H, Hartmann J, *et al.* Capecitabine plus oxaliplatin as first-line treatment in patients with advanced biliary system adenocarcinoma: a prospective multicentre phase II trial. Br J Cancer 2008; 98(2):309–315.

135 Jiao Y, Pawlik T, Anders R, *et al.* Exome sequencing identifies frequent inactivating mutations in BAP1, ARID1A and PBRM1 in intrahepatic cholangiocarcinomas. Nat Genet 2013; 45(12):1470–1473.

136 Ross JS, Wang K, Gay L, *et al.* New routes to targeted therapy of intrahepatic cholangiocarcinomas revealed by next-generation sequencing. Oncologist 2014; 19(3):235–242.

137 Wu YM, Su F, Kalyana-Sundaram S, *et al.* Identification of targetable FGFR gene fusions in diverse cancers. Cancer Discov 2013; 3(6):636–647.

138 Llovet JM, Decaens T, Raoul J, *et al.* Brivanib in patients with advanced hepatocellular carcinoma who were intolerant to sorafenib or for whom sorafenib failed: results from the randomized phase III BRISK-PS study. J Clin Oncol 2013; 31(28):3509–3516.

139 Philip PA, Mahoney M, Allmer C, *et al.* Phase II study of erlotinib in patients with advanced biliary cancer. J Clin Oncol 2006; 24(19):3069–3074.

140 Lee J, Park S, Chang H, *et al.* Gemcitabine and oxaliplatin with or without erlotinib in advanced biliary-tract cancer: a multicentre, open-label, randomised, phase 3 study. Lancet Oncol 2012; 13(2):181–188.

141 Malka D, Cervera P, Foulon S, *et al.* Gemcitabine and oxaliplatin with or without cetuximab in advanced biliary-tract cancer (BINGO): a randomised, open-label, non-comparative phase 2 trial. Lancet Oncol 2014; 15(8):819–828.

142 Jensen LH, Lindebjerg J, Ploen J, *et al.* Phase II marker-driven trial of panitumumab and chemotherapy in KRAS wild-type biliary tract cancer. Ann Oncol 2012; 23(9):2341–2346.

143 Zhu AX, Meyerhardt JA, Blaszkowsky L, *et al.* Efficacy and safety of gemcitabine, oxaliplatin, and bevacizumab in advanced biliary-tract cancers and correlation of changes in 18-fluorodeoxyglucose PET with clinical outcome: a phase 2 study. Lancet Oncol 2010; 11(1):48–54.

144 Bengala C, Bertolini F, Malavasi N, *et al.* Sorafenib in patients with advanced biliary tract carcinoma: a phase II trial. Br J Cancer, 2010; 102(1):68–72.

145 El-Khoueiry AB, Rankin C, Ben-Josef E, *et al.* SWOG 0514: a phase II study of sorafenib in patients with unresectable or metastatic gallbladder carcinoma and cholangiocarcinoma. Invest New Drugs 2012; 30(4):1646–1651.

146 Yi JH, Thongprasert S, Lee J, *et al.* A phase II study of sunitinib as a second-line treatment in advanced biliary tract carcinoma: a multicentre, multinational study. Eur J Cancer 2012; 48(2):196–201.

147 Ramanathan RK, Belani C, Singh D, *et al.* A phase II study of lapatinib in patients with advanced biliary tree and hepatocellular cancer. Cancer Chemother Pharmacol 2009; 64(4):777–783.

148 Bekaii-Saab T, Phelps M, Li X, *et al.* Multi-institutional phase II study of selumetinib in patients with metastatic biliary cancers. J Clin Oncol 2011; 29(17):2357–2363.

149 Turaga KK, Tsai S, Wiebe L, *et al.* Novel multimodality treatment sequencing for extrahepatic (mid and distal) cholangiocarcinoma. Ann Surg Oncol 2013; 20(4):1230–1239.

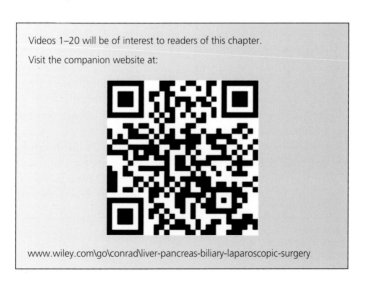

Videos 1–20 will be of interest to readers of this chapter.

Visit the companion website at:

www.wiley.com\go\conrad\liver-pancreas-biliary-laparoscopic-surgery

Oncological management of colorectal liver metastases in the era of minimal access surgery

Jennifer Chan

Department of Medical Oncology, Dana-Farber Cancer Institute, Harvard Medical School, Boston, USA

EDITOR COMMENT

This is a key chapter for laparoscopic liver surgeons because it will help to put the indications for laparoscopic resection of liver metastases from colorectal cancer into perspective and ensure that the patient will benefit from the intervention. Overall survival for patients with stage IV colon cancer has improved over the last several years as a result of the development of more effective systemic chemotherapy and molecularly targeted agents, expanding indications for resection of metastatic disease. Improvements in surgical technique have further expanded the pool of eligible patients. Greater availability of a laparoscopic approach can decrease surgical morbidity and may help to reduce time off chemotherapy. Treatment decisions regarding the optimal pre- or postoperative chemotherapy regimen, timing, and sequence of therapy require a multidisciplinary approach that takes into account patient- and disease-related factors. In patients who present with metastatic disease isolated to the liver that is deemed unresectable or borderline resectable, conversion chemotherapy can be considered with the goal of achieving sufficient downstaging to allow metastasectomy. For patients with initially resectable liver metastases, neoadjuvant chemotherapy may be particularly useful for determining disease biology for those with synchronous metastatic disease, high-risk pathological features, or disease that is technically challenging to resect. Preoperative chemotherapy, however, may not be necessary for all patients with initially resectable disease, including those with metachronous metastatic disease in a favorable location. In this chapter, Dr Chan outlines the management of patients with colorectal liver metastases, with a focus on the integration of chemotherapy and biologically targeted agents with surgical resection in order to optimize patient outcome.

Keywords: adjuvant therapy, colorectal liver metastases, conversion chemotherapy, laparoscopic resection, neoadjuvant therapy

---

13.1 Introduction

The prognosis for patients with metastatic colorectal cancer (CRC) has improved significantly over the past two decades due in part to the development of more effective systemic chemotherapy regimens, expanding indications for metastasectomy, and improvements in surgical techniques [1–4]. It is estimated that approximately 15–25% of patients have synchronous liver metastases at the time of their initial diagnosis of CRC. Furthermore, up to 25% of patients develop metachronous metastatic disease in the liver following resection of primary CRC [5–7]. Among those with liver-limited metastases, it is estimated that 10–30% of patients have potentially

resectable disease that can be treated with curative intent [2,8]. Recent series have reported five-year overall survival (OS) rates of approximately 40–50% following hepatic resection of CRC metastases, with 10-year overall survival rates ranging from 17% to 25% [1,8–11]. This is in contrast to the five-year overall survival rates of <10% in patients with unresectable metastatic disease treated with systemic therapy alone.

How to best manage patients with hepatic metastases from CRC is a complex issue requiring a multidisciplinary team approach. Patients can have variable clinical presentations. Some patients come to medical attention with synchronous liver metastases at the initial time of diagnosis, whereas others are diagnosed with metastatic

---

Laparoscopic Liver, Pancreas, and Biliary Surgery, First Edition.
Edited by Claudius Conrad and Brice Gayet.
© 2017 John Wiley & Sons, Ltd. Published 2017 by John Wiley & Sons, Ltd.

disease months to years after resection of their primary tumor and receipt of adjuvant chemotherapy. Some patients may have a solitary focus of metastatic disease while others may have multiple or bilobar sites of disease. Furthermore, some metastases may initially appear resectable, whereas others may be more technically challenging or not possible to resect owing to the involvement of biliary or vascular structures. Factors such as these must be taken into account when determining the most appropriate management strategy.

Laparoscopic hepatic resection of malignant tumors has been shown to have outcomes that are equivalent if not superior to those achieved with open resection, and it is likely that metastasectomy for CRC comprises the majority of these cases [12]. Furthermore, laparoscopic surgery has been associated with shorter recovery time and fewer postoperative complications. These advantages of minimally invasive surgery may be of particular importance in the management of patients with CRC liver metastases since perioperative complications have been associated with adverse oncological outcomes following resection of hepatic metastases from CRC [13,14]. A shorter recovery time and fewer postoperative complications may also enable more patients to receive adjuvant chemotherapy or begin the next stage of treatment at an earlier time point after surgery [15]. Additionally, selected patients who might otherwise not be candidates for an open surgical procedure because of medical comorbidities may be candidates for resection of metastatic disease via a minimally invasive strategy. In order to optimize outcome and increase the number of patients who will be candidates for potentially curative surgery, a multidisciplinary approach is critical to identify patients appropriate for resection and to determine the optimal approach, goals, timing, and sequence of surgery and chemotherapy.

13.2 Selection criteria for resection of colorectal cancer liver metastases

With the development of more effective chemotherapy agents and advanced surgical techniques, there has been an expansion in indications for metastasectomy. Selection criteria for patients who are optimal candidates for resection of CRC liver metastases are evolving. Several factors, including disease-free interval, number and size of metastases, preoperative carcinoembryonic antigen (CEA) level, and presence of extrahepatic disease, can influence prognosis [16,17]. Historically, contraindications to resection of liver metastases included more than four lesions, large size, presence of extrahepatic metastases, and the possibility of a surgical margin <1 cm [18].

Although these clinicopathological features can affect prognosis, the relevance of these factors in identifying patients appropriate for resection of metastatic disease has been challenged. For instance, in an analysis of prognostic factors after resection of liver metastases from CRC, no survival difference was found between patients who underwent resection of one to three metastases compared with four or more metastases [19]. Additionally, tumor size has not consistently been found to be predictive of adverse outcome, and response to chemotherapy may be a more important prognostic marker than original tumor size [1,20]. Furthermore, although the ability to achieve negative surgical margins is a critical factor in determining outcome following resection, margin width may not have significant impact [21,22]. As long as an R0 resection can be achieved, tumor number, size, and a predicted subcentimeter margin should not preclude potentially curative surgery, especially if there has been a response to neoadjuvant chemotherapy. Finally, although the presence of extrahepatic disease portends poor prognosis compared with liver-only disease [19], long-term survival has been reported in patients who have undergone resection of both liver and extrahepatic metastases, particularly in the lung [10,23–25]. Thus, an aggressive surgical approach may benefit a select group of patients with both hepatic and extrahepatic metastatic disease.

It is important for each member of the multidisciplinary team to be familiar with some of the more modern criteria for resection of hepatic metastases from CRC. Technical considerations include the ability to:
- achieve an R0 resection
- spare at least two, and in rare instances one, contiguous liver segments
- preserve vascular inflow and outflow and biliary drainage
- ensure adequate future liver remnant (FLR) volume, usually at least 20% of the total estimated liver volume for normal parenchyma and higher if the liver has been injured by prior chemotherapy, steatosis, hepatitis or cirrhosis [26,27].

Duration of >12 weeks of preoperative chemotherapy has been associated with increased risk of postoperative hepatic insufficiency, and FLR of >30% has been advised for patients undergoing extended hepatic resection who have received intensive preoperative chemotherapy [27]. Strategies to increase the number of patients with resectable disease include portal vein embolization to cause contralateral lobar hypertrophy and two-stage hepatectomy for patients with bilobar disease that cannot be resected in one procedure [4,28].

In addition to these technical issues, a patient's medical comorbidities and oncological factors related to disease must be taken into account when determining a strategy and sequence of treatment. Important considerations include synchronous versus metachronous presentation, disease-free interval, extent of disease, and response to prior chemotherapy. Goals of chemotherapy include conversion of initially unresectable disease to resectable; for patients with initially resectable liver metastases, chemotherapy may improve outcome by treating micrometastatic disease and also aid in patient selection for surgery by identifying those with a more aggressive biology who may have less benefit from surgery. The following sections will review the role of chemotherapy in the management of patients with CRC liver metastases.

13.3 Conversion chemotherapy for unresectable colorectal cancer liver metastases

In patients who present with metastatic disease isolated to the liver that is deemed unresectable or borderline resectable, conversion chemotherapy can be considered with the goal of achieving sufficient downstaging to allow metastasectomy. Any active chemotherapeutic regimen can be used in an attempt to achieve adequate tumor response to permit surgery. In both selected and unselected studies, there is a strong correlation between tumor response rates and resection rates [29]. 5-Fluorouracil (5-FU) alone, which has a response rate of approximately 20%, rarely provides sufficient reduction in tumor size to allow conversion of unresectable disease to resectable [30,31]. However, more active chemotherapy regimens containing irinotecan and oxaliplatin, including FOLFOX and FOLFIRI, can achieve response rates of 50–60% when used as first-line therapy [32–34]. Furthermore, the combination of 5-FU, leucovorin,

oxaliplatin, and irinotecan (FOLFOXIRI) has been associated with response rates of 60–70% [35,36].

Adam and colleagues reported the results of a large retrospective review of 1104 patients with unresectable liver metastases treated with 5-FU, leucovorin, combined with oxaliplatin (70%), irinotecan (7%), or both (4%) [8]. In this report, 12.5% of patients achieved sufficient response to allow hepatic resection after an average of 10 cycles of chemotherapy. The five-year survival of patients treated with preoperative chemotherapy who underwent resection was 33%, which approached the five-year survival rate (48%) of patients with initially resectable metastases during the same time period.

More recent clinical trials suggest that between 10% and 40% of patients with initially unresectable hepatic metastases may have sufficient objective response to chemotherapy to allow subsequent R0 resection (Table 13.1 and Table 13.2). Rates of conversion and R0 resection reported in these studies vary according to trial design, whether studies were designed specifically for patients with unresectable hepatic metastases, and criteria used to determine resectability. The optimal conversion chemotherapy regimen has not been established. However, regimens with high response rates are typically chosen given the correlation between response rate and subsequent R0 resection rate. In a phase II study of 42 patients with unresectable liver metastases, the response rate to FOLFOX was 60%, and 33% of patients were able to undergo R0 resection after a median period of six months [37]. In another study of 40 patients with unresectable liver metastases treated with FOLFIRI, the response rate to chemotherapy was 47.5%, and 33% of patients underwent R0 resection after a range of 6–12 cycles of chemotherapy [38].

Because of the high response rates seen when both oxaliplatin and irinotecan are combined with 5-FU and leucovorin, the FOLFOXIRI combination has been investigated as a potential option to further improve rates of resection of hepatic resection of CRC metastases. In a phase III study of 244 patients with metastatic CRC who were randomized to receive FOLFOXIRI or FOLFIRI, the R0 resection rate was 36% in the FOLFOXIRI arm compared with 12% in the FOLFIRI arm (P = 0.017) [35]. However, there was a higher incidence of grade 3 or 4 toxicity in the FOLFOXIRI arm. In a second randomized study investigating FOLFOXIRI compared with FOLFIRI as first-line treatment for metastatic

Table 13.1 Select trials of systemic chemotherapy reporting rates of resection of metastatic disease.

Trial	No. patients	Chemotherapy regimen	Response rate (%)	Conversion rate (%)	R0 resection rate (%)
Tournigand [34]	109	FOLFIRI → FOLFOX	56	9	NR
	111	FOLFOX → FOLFIRI	54	22	NR
Falcone [35]	122	FOLFIRI	41	NR	12*
	122	FOLFOXIRI	66	NR	36*
Souglakos [39]	146	FOLFIRI	34	2**	1**
	137	FOLFOXIRI	43	8**	7**
Masi [97]	196	FOLFOXIRI	70	24	19
Van Cutsem [98]	599	FOLFIRI	39	3.7	1.7
	599	FOLFIRI + cetuximab	47	7.0	4.8
Bokemeyer [99]	168	FOLFOX	36	NR	2.4
	169	FOLFOX + cetuximab	46	NR	4.7
Douillard [53]	325	FOLFOX + panitumumab	55	NR	8.3
	331	FOLFOX	48	NR	7.0
Saltz [48]	701	FOLFOX or capeox	47	6.1	NR
	699	FOLFOX or capeox + bevacizumab	49	8.4	NR
Kopetz [100]	43	FOLFIRI + bevacizmab	65	9	NR
Falcone [42]	508	FOLFIRI + bevacizumab	53	NR	12 (28*)
		FOFOXIRI + bevacizumab	65	NR	15 (32*)

* Results from subgroup of patients with liver metastases only.
** % of patients undergoing resection of liver metastases.
NR, not recorded.

CRC, a nonsignificant increase in the conversion rate and R0 resection rate was observed with FOLFOXIRI in comparison with FOLFIRI. Ten percent of the 137 patients treated with FOLFOXIRI underwent resection, compared with 4% of the 146 patients treated with FOLFIRI ($P = 0.08$) [39]. FOLFOXIRI has also been evaluated specifically as a conversion chemotherapy strategy in a phase II study of 34 patients with unresectable hepatic CRC

Table 13.2 Selected trials of neoadjuvant conversion chemotherapy for patients with initially unresectable CRC liver metastases.

Trial	No. patients	Chemotherapy regimen	Response rate (%)	Conversion rate (%)	R0 resection rate (%)
Alberts [37]	42	FOLFOX	60	40	33
Ho [101]	40	FOLFIRI	55	10	NR
Pozzo [102]	40	FOLFIRI	48	33	NR
Ychou [40]	34	FOLFOXIRI	71	82	27
Folprecht [52]	56	FOLFOX + cetuximab	68	NR	38
	55	FOLFIRI + cetuximab	57	NR	30
Wong [103]	46	Capeox + bevacizumab	78	40	
Masi [104]	57 (30 with liver-only metastases)	FOLFOXIRI + bevacizumab	77 (80 for liver-only metastases)	32	26 (40 for liver-only metastases)
Gruenberger [41]	41	FOLFOXIRI + bevacizumab	81	61	49
	39	FOLFOX + bevacizumab	62	49	23

NR, not recorded.

metastases. A significant proportion of patients receiving FOLFOXIRI (82%) had disease that became resectable following chemotherapy, including 27% who underwent R0 resection [40]. In another more recent phase II study including 80 patients with initially unresectable liver metastases from colorectal cancer who were randomized to receive FOLFOXIRI with bevacizumab or FOLFOX with bevacizumab, the overall resection and R0 resection rates were higher in patients receiving FOLFOXIRI bevacizumab (61% and 49%, respectively) than in those receiving FOLFOX bevacizumab (49% and 23%, respectively) [41].

However, not all data support the ability of FOL-FOXIRI to improve resection rates. In a randomized study of FOLFOXIRI with bevacizumab versus FOLFIRI with bevacizumab as first-line treatment in patients with unresectable metastatic CRC, use of FOLFOXIRI did not result in an improved R0 resection rate in the intent-to-treat population (15% versus 12%, P = 0.33) or in patients with liver-only metastatic disease (28% versus 32%, P = 0.83), and was associated with increased toxicity [42,43]. Thus, the added benefit of combining oxaliplatin and irinotecan together with 5-FU and leucovorin remains uncertain, and the added toxicity may limit its routine use in a preoperative setting before liver resection.

Although the addition of targeted therapy with anti-angiogenic agents, such as bevacizumab and aflibecept, has improved efficacy of chemotherapy for patients with metastatic CRC, the benefit of adding targeted therapies to preoperative conversion chemotherapy is not well established. Data have suggested that the addition of bevacizumab to chemotherapy regimens may improve tumor response rate [44–47]. However, in a randomized trial of FOLFOX or capecitabine and oxaliplatin with or without bevacizumab in patients with metastatic CRC, there was no improvement in tumor response rate with the addition of bevacizumab, and only a slightly higher rate of R0 resection of metastatic disease occurred with chemotherapy and bevacizumab (8.4%) compared with chemotherapy alone (6.1%) [48]. Although these data do not support the concept that bevacizumab can improve the ability to resect hepatic metastases, bevacizumab is often included in treatment plans since the subsequent ability to resect disease may be uncertain, and the addition of bevacizumab can provide effective therapy for metastatic disease. However, the added toxicity of bevacizumab must also be considered as treatment decisions are made.

The anti-EGFR antibodies cetuximab and panitumumab have improved survival for patients with KRAS wild-type tumors [49]. Two randomized studies of irinotecan- or oxaliplatin-based chemotherapy regimens with or without cetuximab as first-line therapy for patients with unresectable metastatic CRC have demonstrated improvement in tumor response rate and a modest improvement in R0 resection rates with the addition of cetuximab to chemotherapy. In the CRYSTAL trial, the addition of cetuximab to FOLFIRI significantly increased the response rate in patients whose tumors were wild-type at codons 12 and 13 of exon 2 of the KRAS gene (57% versus 40%). Furthermore, more patients with wild-type KRAS tumors receiving cetuximab were able to undergo both surgery for metastatic disease and R0 resection (surgery rate 7.9% versus 4.6%, P = 0.06; R0 resections 5.1% versus 2.0%, P = 0.03) [50]. Similarly, in the OPUS study, among patients with exon 2 KRAS wild-type tumors, the combination of cetuximab and FOLFOX was associated with an improved response rate (57% versus 34%, P = 0.0027) and ability to undergo surgery for metastatic disease compared with FOLFOX alone (12% versus 3%, P = 0.02) [51].

The phase II CELIM study has evaluated the ability of cetuximab-based chemotherapy to improve the ability to resect initially nonresectable CRC liver metastases. In this study, 114 patients with initially nonresectable CRC liver metastases were randomized to receive cetuximab in combination with either FOLFOX or FOLFIRI. High R0 resection rates were reported (38% for those receiving cetuximab + FOLFOX and 30% for those receiving cetuximab + FOLFIRI), and in a blinded, retrospective surgical review of this study, resectability rates increased from 32% (22 of 68 patients) at baseline to 60% (41 of 68) after chemotherapy (P < 0.0001). However, the lack of a group of patients in the CELIM study receiving chemotherapy alone does not allow assessment of the added benefit of cetuximab [52].

Rates of resection of metastatic disease among patients receiving the EGFR inhibitor panitumumab were reported in the PRIME trial, in which 1183 patients with unresectable metastatic CRC were randomized to receive FOLFOX versus FOLFOX with panitumumab as initial treatment. The addition of panitumumab to FOLFOX improved overall response rate (55% versus 48%, P = 0.02) and median progression-free survival (PFS) in patients with KRAS exon 2 wild-type tumors. Metastasectomy of any site was attempted in 10.5% of patients treated with panitumumab + FOLFOX4 and 9.4% of patients treated with FOLFOX4 with wild-type *KRAS* exon 2 status; complete resections were achieved in 8.3% and 7.0% of patients, respectively, suggesting a possible modest benefit for the addition of panitumumab [53].

Despite these encouraging results, somewhat conflicting evidence exists regarding the benefits of cetuximab prior to resection of CRC liver metastases. An advantage for the addition of cetuximab was suggested in a recent randomized study of 138 patients with *KRAS* wild-type unresectable CRC liver metastases randomized to receive FOLFOX or FOLFIRI with or without cetuximab [54]. The addition of cetuximab was associated with improved R0 resection rates (26% versus 7%) and prolonged survival [55]. On the other hand, the addition of cetuximab was associated with worse PFS in the new EPOC study, a randomized trial of perioperative FOLFOX with or without cetuximab for resectable or suboptimally resectable *KRAS* exon 2 wild-type CRC liver metastases [53]. Although patient selection criteria differed between the two studies, these data call into question the benefit, and suggest possible detriment, of combining cetuximab with an oxaliplatin-containing chemotherapy regimen for patients with potentially resectable liver CRC liver metastases.

A more comprehensive mutational analysis may better define patients most likely to benefit from anti-EGFR therapy. Activating mutations in exon 2 of *KRAS* (codons 12 and 13) exist in approximately 40% of patients with metastatic colorectal cancer and are associated with intrinsic resistance to anti-EGFR therapy [49,56]. More recently, mutations in exon 3 (codon 61) and exon 4 (codons 117 and 146) of *KRAS* and in exons 2, 3, and 4 of *NRAS* have also been found to be predictive of a lack of benefit with anti-EGFR therapy [57–59]. Expanded RAS mutational analysis may identify an additional 15–17% of patients with metastatic CRC who do not benefit and may have inferior outcomes with the incorporation of anti-EGFR therapy. Additional studies are warranted to identify whether there is a subgroup of patients with colorectal liver metastases who may benefit from the addition of anti-EGFR therapy.

13.3.1 Summary: conversion chemotherapy

Responses to chemotherapy can allow up to 10–40% of patients with initially unresectable hepatic metastases from CRC to undergo metastasectomy. The optimal

preoperative chemotherapy regimen has not been established, and any chemotherapeutic regimen with a high response rate can be used in an attempt to achieve adequate tumor response to allow surgery. The incremental benefit of targeted agents may be modest and must be weighed against added toxicity (see later in this chapter). Controversy exists regarding the role of anti-EGFR therapy in the management of patients with resectable liver metastases. Additionally, the duration of chemotherapy administration must be limited to minimize risk of hepatic toxicity that could preclude future surgery. Rather than continuing chemotherapy to maximal response, surgery should be considered when criteria for resection have been met. A practical example of one approach would be administration of four cycles of chemotherapy plus a targeted agent with consideration of omitting the targeted agent with the last cycle of treatment. After restaging to assess response, surgery could be undertaken five to six weeks later.

13.4 Neoadjuvant and adjuvant chemotherapy for initially resectable colorectal cancer liver metastases

Because recurrence is common following hepatectomy for CRC liver metastases, chemotherapy is often integrated into treatment with the aim of reducing risk of recurrence by eradicating occult metastatic disease. However, the optimal sequencing of surgery and chemotherapy administration for patients with initially resectable metastatic disease has not been well established. Patients with resectable liver metastases can either undergo hepatectomy first with consideration of adjuvant chemotherapy, or alternatively, they can be administered with perioperative chemotherapy before and after surgery.

13.4.1 Neoadjuvant chemotherapy

Possible advantages of neoadjuvant chemotherapy include the possibility of achieving more limited hepatectomy, earlier treatment of micrometastatic disease, and assessment of chemotherapy sensitivity of disease, which can provide prognostic information and also guide decisions regarding postoperative chemotherapy administration. However, possible disadvantages associated with neoadjuvant chemotherapy in the setting of resectable disease include the potential for disease progression that may preclude future surgery and hepatic toxicity associated with chemotherapy and targeted agents.

Several clinical trials have examined the benefit of perioperative chemotherapy for patients with resectable CRC liver metastases. The European Organization for Research and Treatment of Cancer (EORTC) randomized 364 patients with up to four liver metastases from CRC and no prior therapy with oxaliplatin to hepatectomy alone (n = 182) or to receive six cycles of FOLFOX before and after surgery (n = 182) (EORTC 40983). Complete or partial responses to chemotherapy were observed in 43% of patients receiving neoadjuvant FOLFOX. Liver resection was performed in 83% of patients randomized to receive chemotherapy, a similar rate to the 84% of patients randomized to surgery alone who underwent liver surgery [60]. Among patients receiving chemotherapy, 12 experienced disease progression during treatment, four of whom had disease subsequently rendered nonresectable on account of the appearance of new lesions and four owing to the progression of known metastases. This finding therefore suggests that only a small number of patients will experience disease progression while receiving preoperative chemotherapy and lose a window of opportunity to undergo hepatic resection. Furthermore, response to chemotherapy may identify a subset of patients with more biologically aggressive disease who may not benefit from surgery. Reversible postoperative complications, including biliary fistula, hepatic failure, wound and intra-abdominal infection, occurred at a higher rate among patients receiving perioperative chemotherapy (25% versus 16%). However, there was no increase in postoperative mortality associated with chemotherapy administration.

In an updated analysis of the EORTC 40983 study that included all randomized patients with a median follow-up of 8.5 years, there was a trend towards improved three-year PFS in patients receiving perioperative chemotherapy compared with those who underwent surgery alone (38% versus 30%, P = 0.068). The improvement in PFS was statistically significant when only eligible patients were included in the analysis. No difference in overall survival was observed with receipt of perioperative chemotherapy (five-year OS, 51% in the perioperative chemotherapy group versus 48% in the surgery only group, P = 0.34) [61].

The efficacy of cetuximab in combination with perioperative chemotherapy has been evaluated in the new EPOC trial, in which 272 patients with *KRAS* exon 2 wild-type CRC and operable liver metastases were randomized to receive FOLFOX with or without cetuximab for 12 weeks before and 12 weeks after surgery. This study was stopped early after an interim analysis demonstrated that PFS was significantly worse among patients receiving cetuximab (14.8 versus 24.2 months, P < 0.048) [55].

13.4.1.1 Summary: neoadjuvant therapy
There are advantages to administering neoadjuvant therapy for selected patients with initially resectable CRC liver metastases. Neoadjuvant therapy may be particularly useful for patients with synchronous metastatic disease, high-risk biological features, or disease more technically challenging to resect. However, for selected patients with resectable metachronous metastatic disease in a favorable location, preoperative chemotherapy may not be necessary.

13.4.2 Adjuvant chemotherapy
A theoretical advantage for the administration of postoperative chemotherapy following resection of CRC liver metastases is the ability to eradicate occult metastatic disease. Two randomized trials examining the role of adjuvant 5-FU and leucovorin following resection of CRC liver metastases have been conducted [62,63]. Both, however, closed prematurely owing to poor enrollment. A pooled analysis of both trials showed a trend toward improved PFS for patients receiving chemotherapy compared with those who underwent surgery alone (27.9 versus 18.8 months, P = 0.058) [63]. This study provides support for a possible benefit of adjuvant chemotherapy in patients who have undergone resection of liver metastases.

There are limited data from randomized trials examining the role of more modern chemotherapy regimens incorporating oxaliplatin or irinotecan following resection of CRC liver metastases. As noted above, a trial conducted by the EORTC demonstrated that compared with hepatic resection alone, perioperative FOLFOX was associated with a trend towards improved three-year PFS but had no OS advantage [61]. Furthermore, in a randomized study of patients who had undergone resection of a primary CRC tumor and R0 resection of liver metastases, disease-free survival (DFS) was not different in patients receiving postoperative FOLFIRI compared with 5-FU/LV (24.7 months for FOLFIRI versus 21.6 months for 5-FU/LV, P = 0.44) [64].

The role of biological therapy following resection of hepatic metastases also has not been well defined. As noted above, the addition of cetuximab to perioperative FOLFOX has been associated with worse PFS in patients with resectable *KRAS* exon 2 wild-type CRC liver metastases [55]. Similarly, in patients with resected stage III CRC, the addition of cetuximab to adjuvant FOLFOX did not improve DFS and was associated with worse outcomes [65]. Administration of bevacizumab also has not demonstrated improvement in DFS or OS in patients with resected stage III colon cancer, and this finding calls into question how beneficial bevacizumab may be in the postoperative therapy of patients with resected CRC liver metastases [66,67].

13.4.2.1 Summary: adjuvant therapy

There are limited data to define the benefit of postoperative chemotherapy for patients with resected CRC liver metastases. However, postoperative therapy with FOLFOX or capecitabine with oxaliplatin may be beneficial in patients who have undergone resection of synchronous metastatic disease with no, or only limited, preoperative chemotherapy or in patients with resected metachronous metastases who have not received prior adjuvant chemotherapy.

13.5 Surgical considerations related to preoperative chemotherapy

Although chemotherapy may improve outcomes and increase the number of patients who are candidates for metastasectomy, treatment can be associated with hepatic toxicity that increases the risk of postoperative complications and affects function of the remaining liver. The nature of chemotherapy-associated liver injury has been shown to be regimen specific and related to duration of therapy.

The importance of hepatic steatosis in patients undergoing liver resection has been demonstrated in several studies, including a meta-analysis demonstrating that steatosis is a risk factor for increased perioperative morbidity and mortality [68]. Although fatty infiltration can be found in nonneoplastic liver in up to 40% of patients undergoing hepatic resection for CRC metastases following downstaging by chemotherapy [8], evidence has not supported a definite increase in hepatic steatosis among patients receiving preoperative chemotherapy compared

with those who have not. In a retrospective review of nontumorous liver of patients undergoing hepatic resection for CRC metastases, patients treated with 5-FU were more likely to have steatosis involving >30% of the liver compared with patients receiving no chemotherapy (17% versus 9%) [69]. This difference, however, was not statistically significant. Additionally, in a meta-analysis of studies reporting the incidence of hepatic steatosis among patients undergoing liver resection for CRC liver metastases, there was no association between use of preoperative chemotherapy and presence of hepatic steatosis [70].

On the other hand, irinotecan-containing regimens have been shown to cause chemotherapy-associated steatohepatitis (CASH), particularly in patients with higher body mass index [69,71,72]. The development of CASH has been associated with increased risk of postoperative complications, including liver failure and increased postoperative mortality [69]. Oxalipatin-containing regimens, in contrast, have not been associated with development of steatohepatitis.

Oxaliplatin, however, has been associated with injury to endothelial cells lining the sinusoids of the liver, referred to as sinusoidal obstruction syndrome [69,73,74]. This syndrome is characterized by sinusoidal dilatation and associated hepatocyte atrophy. Later changes include perisinusoidal fibrosis and nodular regenerative hyperplasia [70]. The development of sinusoidal abnormalities has been associated with increased risk of operative bleeding but not necessarily with increased postoperative morbidity or mortality [69,74]. Although several studies have suggested that the addition of bevacizumab to oxaliplatin-containing chemotherapy regimens may reduce the severity of sinusoidal injury related to oxaliplatin, this finding requires additional study [73,75,76].

Studies suggest that the duration of preoperative chemotherapy and timing of surgery may influence postoperative outcome. In a single-institution analysis of patients who underwent liver resection for hepatic metastases from CRC, outcomes of patients who received preoperative chemotherapy were compared with the outcomes of those who did not. The risk of postoperative morbidity was correlated with the number of cycles of chemotherapy delivered preoperatively. Those receiving more than six cycles of chemotherapy had higher complication rates than those receiving five or fewer [77]. A longer duration of chemotherapy (12 or more cycles) has also been associated with longer hospitalization and higher rates of reoperation [74]. Furthermore, post-operative hepatic insufficiency has been linked to longer durations of preoperative chemotherapy without necessarily improving pathological response [74,78]. Although 20% has been defined as a minimum safe FLR in patients with normal livers undergoing extended hepatectomy, a FLR of >30% may reduce the risk of postoperative hepatic insufficiency in patients who have received more than 12 weeks of chemotherapy [27].

Thus, for patients with resectable metastases receiving neoadjuvant therapy, the duration of chemotherapy is generally limited to two to three months in order to minimize the risk of hepatotoxicity. Patients with initially unresectable or borderline resectable disease receiving conversion chemotherapy should undergo re-evaluation approximately every two months, and surgery should be performed when disease becomes resectable in order to minimize the duration of preoperative chemotherapy and risk of hepatotoxicity. For patients undergoing extended hepatectomy who have received more extensive preoperative chemotherapy (>12 weeks), a minimum FLR of >30% may ensure adequate functional reserve following surgery.

Treatment with bevacizumab has been associated with increased risk of bleeding, gastrointestinal (GI) perforation, and wound-healing complications [79,80]. Concern also exists regarding the effect of VEGF inhibition on liver regeneration. However, multiple studies have demonstrated that the addition of bevacizumab to preoperative irinotecan- and oxaliplatin-containing chemotherapy regimens does not increase postoperative complication rates [81–86]. The optimal duration of time to wait following bevacizumab administration and surgery has not been well defined. Nonetheless, because of its half-life of 20 days [87], a period of six to eight weeks from the last dose of bevacizumab and surgery is commonly recommended [88].

Finally, the optimal duration of a chemotherapy-free period prior to surgery has not been well established. A longer time interval between completion of chemotherapy and hepatic resection has been associated with reduction in surgical complications. In one study, a period of four weeks or fewer predisposed patients to a higher rate of postoperative complications [89]. Thus, many advise waiting five to six weeks after completing chemotherapy before proceeding with hepatic resection.

13.6 Future directions

As the indications for metastasectomy have expanded, efforts have also been directed towards improving prognostication systems that can identify patients most likely to benefit from resection. Radiographic and pathological responses to neoadjuvant chemotherapy have been shown to predict long-term outcome following resection of CRC metastases [90–92]. Data also suggest that the presence of somatic gene mutations may also have a prognostic role after metastasectomy. The presence of *RAS* and *BRAF* mutations has been associated with worse OS and recurrence-free survival (RFS) following resection of colorectal liver metastases [93–96]. Additionally, results of genetic profiling may predict patterns of recurrence that can influence surveillance strategies. For instance, the presence of *RAS* mutations has been associated with worse lung RFS but not worse liver RFS [95]. Integrating the results of molecular profiling may allow more individualized management by aiding the selection of patients who benefit most from an aggressive surgical approach and may allow more personalized treatment and follow-up.

13.7 Conclusion

Overall survival for patients with stage IV colon cancer has improved over the last several years thanks to the development of more effective systemic chemotherapy and molecularly targeted agents. Outcomes have also improved as a result of expanding indications for resection of metastatic disease and improvements in surgical technique. Given the complexity of issues related to determining the optimal pre- or postoperative chemotherapy regimen, timing, and sequence of therapy, a multidisciplinary approach is critical. It is clear that treatment decisions need to be highly individualized, taking into account oncological parameters such as synchronous versus metachronous presentation, disease-free interval, extent of disease, and response to prior chemotherapy. Future efforts to molecularly characterize cancers most likely to benefit from surgical resection and to define the most appropriate neoadjuvant or adjuvant therapy based on mutational status will aid further in the management of patients with CRC liver metastases.

KEY POINTS

- Overall survival for patients with stage IV colon cancer has improved owing to more effective systemic chemotherapy and molecularly targeted agents.

- In the context of novel therapeutic agents and improvements in surgical technique, the indications for resection of metastatic disease are being redefined.

- A multidisciplinary approach is critical.

- Key determinants of outcome are synchronous versus metachronous presentation, disease-free interval, extent of disease, and response to prior chemotherapy.

- Mutation status analysis of primary tumor and metastases might aid in appropriate selection of patients with CRC liver metastases.

References

1 Choti MA, Sitzmann J, Tiburi M, *et al.* Trends in long-term survival following liver resection for hepatic colorectal metastases. Ann Surg 2002; 235(6):759–766.

2 Kopetz S, Chang G, Overman M, *et al.* Improved survival in metastatic colorectal cancer is associated with adoption of hepatic resection and improved chemotherapy. J Clin Oncol 2009; 27(22):3677–3683.

3 House MG, Ito H, Gonen M, *et al.* Survival after hepatic resection for metastatic colorectal cancer: trends in outcomes for 1,600 patients during two decades at a single institution. J Am Coll Surg 2010; 210(5):744–752, 752–755.

4 Brouquet A, Abdalla E, Kopetz S, *et al.* High survival rate after two-stage resection of advanced colorectal liver metastases: response-based selection and complete resection define outcome. J Clin Oncol 2011; 29(8):1083–1090.

5 Manfredi S, Bouvier M, Lepage C, *et al.* Incidence and patterns of recurrence after resection for cure of colonic cancer in a well defined population. Br J Surg 2006; 93(9):1115–1122.

6 Manfredi S, Lepage C, Hatem C, *et al.* Epidemiology and management of liver metastases from colorectal cancer. Ann Surg 2006; 244(2):254–259.

7 Norstein J, Silen W. Natural history of liver metastases from colorectal carcinoma. J Gastrointest Surg 1997; 1(5):398–407.

8 Adam R, Delvart V, Pascal G, *et al.* Rescue surgery for unresectable colorectal liver metastases downstaged by chemotherapy: a model to predict long-term survival. Ann Surg 2004; 240(4):644–657; discussion 657–658.

9 Wei AC, Greig P, Grant D, *et al.* Survival after hepatic resection for colorectal metastases: a 10-year experience. Ann Surg Oncol 2006; 13(5):668–676.

10 Tomlinson JS, Jarnagin W, DeMatteo R, *et al.* Actual 10-year survival after resection of colorectal liver metastases defines cure. J Clin Oncol 2007; 25(29):4575–4580.

11 Rees M, Tekkis P, Welsh F, *et al.* Evaluation of long-term survival after hepatic resection for metastatic colorectal cancer: a multifactorial model of 929 patients. Ann Surg 2008; 247(1):125–135.

12 Croome KP, Yamashita MH. Laparoscopic vs open hepatic resection for benign and malignant tumors: an updated metaanalysis. Arch Surg 2010; 145(11):1109–1118.

13 Matsuda A, Matsumoto S, Seya T, *et al.* Does postoperative complication have a negative impact on long-term outcomes following hepatic resection for colorectal liver metastasis? a meta-analysis. Ann Surg Oncol 2013; 20(8):2485–2492.

14 Correa–Gallego C, Gonen M, Fischer M, *et al.* Perioperative complications influence recurrence and survival after resection of hepatic colorectal metastases. Ann Surg Oncol 2013; 20(8):2477–2484.

15 Aloia TA, Zimmitti G, Conrad C, *et al.* Return to intended oncologic treatment (RIOT): a novel metric for evaluating the quality of oncosurgical therapy for malignancy. J Surg Oncol 2014; 110(2):107–114.

16 Nordlinger B, Guiguet M, Vaillant J, *et al.* Surgical resection of colorectal carcinoma metastases to the liver. A prognostic scoring system to improve case selection, based on 1568 patients. Association Francaise de Chirurgie. Cancer 1996; 77(7):1254–1262.

17 Fong Y, Fortner J, Sun R, *et al.* Clinical score for predicting recurrence after hepatic resection for metastatic colorectal cancer: analysis of 1001 consecutive cases. Ann Surg 1999; 230(3):309–318; discussion 318–321.

18 Ekberg H, Tranberg K, Andersson R, *et al.* Determinants of survival in liver resection for colorectal secondaries. Br J Surg 1986; 73(9):727–731.

19 Altendorf–Hofmann A, Scheele J. A critical review of the major indicators of prognosis after resection of hepatic metastases from colorectal carcinoma. Surg Oncol Clin North Am 2003; 12(1):165–192, xi.

20 Pawlik TM, Abdalla E, Ellis L, *et al.* Debunking dogma: surgery for four or more colorectal liver metastases is justified. J Gastrointest Surg 2006; 10(2):240–248.

21 Pawlik TM, Scoggins C, Zorzi D, *et al.* Effect of surgical margin status on survival and site of recurrence after hepatic resection for colorectal metastases. Ann Surg 2005; 241 (5):715–722, discussion 722–724.

22 Muratore A, Ribero D, Zimmitti G, *et al.* Resection margin and recurrence-free survival after liver resection of colorectal metastases. Ann Surg Oncol 2010; 17(5):1324–1329.

23 Shah SA, Haddad R, Al-Sukhni W, *et al.* Surgical resection of hepatic and pulmonary metastases from colorectal carcinoma. J Am Coll Surg 2006; 202(3):468–475.

24 Pulitano C, Bodingbauer M, Aldrighetti L, *et al.* Liver resection for colorectal metastases in presence of extrahepatic disease: results from an international multi-institutional analysis. Ann Surg Oncol 2011; 18(5):1380–1388.

25 Brouquet A, Schulick RD, Choti MA. Improved survival after resection of liver and lung colorectal metastases compared with liver-only metastases: a study of 112 patients with limited lung metastatic disease. J Am Coll Surg 2011; 213(1):62–69; discussion 69–71.

26 Pawlik TM, Schulick RD, Choti MA. Expanding criteria for resectability of colorectal liver metastases. Oncologist 2008; 13(1):51–64.

27 Shindoh J, Tzeng C, Aloia T, *et al.* Optimal future liver remnant in patients treated with extensive preoperative chemotherapy for colorectal liver metastases. Ann Surg Oncol 2013; 20(8):2493–2500.

28 Frankel TL, d'Angelica MI. Hepatic resection for colorectal metastases. J Surg Oncol 2014; 109(1):2–7.

29 Folprecht G, Grothey A, Alberts S, *et al.* Neoadjuvant treatment of unresectable colorectal liver metastases: correlation between tumour response and resection rates. Ann Oncol 2005; 16(8):1311–1319.

30 Thirion P, Michiels S, Pignon J, *et al.* Modulation of fluorouracil by leucovorin in patients with advanced colorectal cancer: an updated meta-analysis. J Clin Oncol 2004; 22 (18):3766–3775.

31 Advanced Colorectal Cancer Meta-Analysis Project. Modulation of fluorouracil by leucovorin in patients with advanced colorectal cancer: evidence in terms of response rate. J Clin Oncol 1992; 10(6):896–903.

32 Goldberg RM, Sargent D, Morton R, *et al.* A randomized controlled trial of fluorouracil plus leucovorin, irinotecan, and oxaliplatin combinations in patients with previously untreated metastatic colorectal cancer. J Clin Oncol 2004; 22 (1):23–30.

33 De Gramont A, Figer A, Seymour M, *et al.* Leucovorin and fluorouracil with or without oxaliplatin as first-line treatment in advanced colorectal cancer. J Clin Oncol 2000; 18 (16):2938–2947.

34 Tournigand C, Andre T, Achille E, *et al.* FOLFIRI followed by FOLFOX6 or the reverse sequence in advanced colorectal cancer: a randomized GERCOR study. J Clin Oncol 2004; 22 (2):229–237.

35 Falcone A, Ricci S, Brunetti I, *et al.* Phase III trial of infusional fluorouracil, leucovorin, oxaliplatin, and irinotecan (FOLFOXIRI) compared with infusional fluorouracil, leucovorin, and irinotecan (FOLFIRI) as first-line treatment for metastatic colorectal cancer: the Gruppo Oncologico Nord Ovest. J Clin Oncol 2007; 25(13):1670–1676.

36 Masi G, Vasile E, Loupakis F, *et al.* Randomized trial of two induction chemotherapy regimens in metastatic colorectal cancer: an updated analysis. J Natl Cancer Inst 2011; 103 (1):21–30.

37 Alberts SR, Horvath W, Sternfeld W, *et al.* Oxaliplatin, fluorouracil, and leucovorin for patients with unresectable liver-only metastases from colorectal cancer: a North Central Cancer Treatment Group phase II study. J Clin Oncol 2005; 23(36):9243–9249.

38 Barone C, Nuzzo G, Cassano A, *et al.* Final analysis of colorectal cancer patients treated with irinotecan and 5-fluorouracil plus folinic acid neoadjuvant chemotherapy for unresectable liver metastases. Br J Cancer 2007; 97 (8):1035–1039.

39 Souglakos J, Androulakis N, Syrigos K, *et al.* FOLFOXIRI (folinic acid, 5-fluorouracil, oxaliplatin and irinotecan) vs FOLFIRI (folinic acid, 5-fluorouracil and irinotecan) as first-line treatment in metastatic colorectal cancer (MCC): a multicentre randomised phase III trial from the Hellenic Oncology Research Group (HORG). Br J Cancer 2006; 94 (6):798–805.

40 Ychou M, Viret F, Kramar A, *et al.* Tritherapy with fluorouracil/leucovorin, irinotecan and oxaliplatin (FOLFIRINOX): a phase II study in colorectal cancer patients with non-resectable liver metastases. Cancer Chemother Pharmacol 2008; 62(2):195–201.

41 Gruenberger T, Bridgewater J, Chau I, *et al.* Bevacizumab plus mFOLFOX-6 or FOLFOXIRI in patients with initially unresectable liver metastases from colorectal cancer: the OLIVIA multinational randomised phase II trial. Ann Oncol 2015; 26(4):702–708.

42 Falcone A, Cremolini C, Masi G, *et al.* FOLFOXIRI/bevacizumab (bev) versus FOLFIRI/bev as first-line treatment in unresectable metastatic colorectal cancer (mCRC) patients (pts): results of the phase III TRIBE trial by GONO group. J Clin Oncol 2013; 31 (suppl); abstr. 3505.

43 Loupakis F, Cremolini C, Masi G, *et al.* Initial therapy with FOLFOXIRI and bevacizumab for metastatic colorectal cancer. N Engl J Med 2014; 371(17):1609–1618.

44 Hurwitz H, Fehrenbacher L, Novotny W, *et al.* Bevacizumab plus irinotecan, fluorouracil, and leucovorin for metastatic colorectal cancer. N Engl J Med 2004; 350(23):2335–2342.

45 Giantonio BJ, Catalano PJ, Meropol N, *et al.* Bevacizumab in combination with oxaliplatin, fluorouracil, and leucovorin (FOLFOX4) for previously treated metastatic colorectal cancer: results from the Eastern Cooperative Oncology Group Study E3200. J Clin Oncol 2007; 25(12):1539–1544.

46 Hurwitz HI, Fehrenbacher L, Hainsworth J, *et al.* Bevacizumab in combination with fluorouracil and leucovorin: an active regimen for first-line metastatic colorectal cancer. J Clin Oncol 2005; 23(15):3502–3508.

47 Fuchs CS, Marshall J, Barrueco J. Randomized, controlled trial of irinotecan plus infusional, bolus, or oral fluoropyrimidines in first-line treatment of metastatic colorectal cancer: updated results from the BICC-C study. J Clin Oncol 2008; 26(4):689–690.

48 Saltz LB, Clarke S, Diaz-Rubio E, *et al.* Bevacizumab in combination with oxaliplatin-based chemotherapy as first-line therapy in metastatic colorectal cancer: a randomized phase III study. J Clin Oncol 2008; 26(12):2013–2019.

49 Karapetis CS, Khambata-Ford S, Jonker D, *et al.* K-ras mutations and benefit from cetuximab in advanced colorectal cancer. N Engl J Med 2008; 359(17):1757–1765.

50 Van Cutsem E, Kohne C, Lang I, *et al.* Cetuximab plus irinotecan, fluorouracil, and leucovorin as first-line treatment for metastatic colorectal cancer: updated analysis of overall survival according to tumor KRAS and BRAF mutation status. J Clin Oncol 2011; 29(15):2011–2019.

51 Bokemeyer C, Bondarenko I, Hartmann J, *et al.* Efficacy according to biomarker status of cetuximab plus FOLFOX-4 as first-line treatment for metastatic colorectal cancer: the OPUS study. Ann Oncol 2011; 22(7):1535–1546.

52 Folprecht G, Gruenberger T, Bechstein W, *et al.* Tumour response and secondary resectability of colorectal liver metastases following neoadjuvant chemotherapy with cetuximab: the CELIM randomised phase 2 trial. Lancet Oncol 2010; 11(1):38–47.

53 Douillard JY, Siena S, Cassidy J, *et al.* Randomized, phase III trial of panitumumab with infusional fluorouracil, leucovorin, and oxaliplatin (FOLFOX4) versus FOLFOX4 alone as first-line treatment in patients with previously untreated metastatic colorectal cancer: the PRIME study. J Clin Oncol 2010; 28(31):4697–4705.

54 Ye LC, Liu T, Ren L, *et al.* Randomized controlled trial of cetuximab plus chemotherapy for patients with KRAS wild-type unresectable colorectal liver-limited metastases. J Clin Oncol 2013; 31(16):1931–1938.

55 Primrose J, Falk S, Finch-Jones M, *et al.* Systemic chemotherapy with or without cetuximab in patients with resectable colorectal liver metastasis: the New EPOC randomised controlled trial. Lancet Oncol 2014; doi http://dx.doi.org/10.1016/S1470-2045(14)70105-6

56 Amado RG, Wolf M, Peeters M, *et al.* Wild-type KRAS is required for panitumumab efficacy in patients with metastatic colorectal cancer. J Clin Oncol 2008; 26 (10):1626–1634.

57 Douillard JY, Oliner K, Siena S, *et al.* Panitumumab-FOLFOX4 treatment and RAS mutations in colorectal cancer. N Engl J Med 2013; 369(11):1023–1034.

58 Tejpar S, Lenz H, Kohne C, *et al.* Effect of KRAS and NRAS mutations on treatment outcomes in patients with metastatic colorectal cancer (mCRC) treated first-line with cetuximab plus FOLFOX4: new results from the OPUS study. J Clin Oncol 2014; 32 (suppl 3); abstr. LBA444.

59 Ciardiello F, Lenz H, Kohne C, *et al.* Treatment outcome according to tumor RAS mutation status in CRYSTAL study patients with metastatic colorectal cancer (mCRC) randomized to FOLFIRI with/without cetuximab. J Clin Oncol 2014; 32 (5)(suppl); abstr. 3506.

60 Nordlinger B, Sorbye H, Glimelius B, *et al.* Perioperative chemotherapy with FOLFOX4 and surgery versus surgery alone for resectable liver metastases from colorectal cancer (EORTC Intergroup trial 40983): a randomised controlled trial. Lancet 2008; 371(9617):1007–1016.

61 Nordlinger B, Sorbye H, Glimelius B, *et al.* Perioperative FOLFOX4 chemotherapy and surgery versus surgery alone for resectable liver metastases from colorectal cancer (EORTC 40983): long-term results of a randomised, controlled, phase 3 trial. Lancet Oncol 2013; 14(12): 1208–1215.

62 Portier G, Elias D, Bouche O, *et al.* Multicenter randomized trial of adjuvant fluorouracil and folinic acid compared with surgery alone after resection of colorectal liver metastases: FFCD ACHBTH AURC 9002 trial. J Clin Oncol 2006; 24 (31):4976–4982.

63 Mitry E, Fields A, Bleiberg H, *et al.* Adjuvant chemotherapy after potentially curative resection of metastases from colorectal cancer: a pooled analysis of two randomized trials. J Clin Oncol 2008; 26(30):4906–4911.

64 Ychou M, Hohenberger W, Thezenas S, *et al.* A randomized phase III study comparing adjuvant 5-fluorouracil/folinic acid with FOLFIRI in patients following complete resection of liver metastases from colorectal cancer. Ann Oncol 2009; 20(12):1964–1970.

65 Alberts SR, Sargent D, Nair S, *et al.* Effect of oxaliplatin, fluorouracil, and leucovorin with or without cetuximab on survival among patients with resected stage III colon cancer: a randomized trial. JAMA 2012; 307(13):1383–1393.

66 Allegra CJ, Yothers G, O'Connell M, *et al.* Bevacizumab in stage II–III colon cancer: 5-year update of the National Surgical Adjuvant Breast and Bowel Project C-08 trial. J Clin Oncol 2013; 31(3):359–364.

67 De Gramont A, van Cutsem E, Schmoll H, *et al.* Bevacizumab plus oxaliplatin-based chemotherapy as adjuvant treatment for colon cancer (AVANT): a phase 3 randomised controlled trial. Lancet Oncol 2012; 13(12):1225–1233.

68 De Meijer VE, Kalish B, Puder M, *et al.* Systematic review and meta-analysis of steatosis as a risk factor in major hepatic resection. Br J Surg 2010; 97(9):1331–1339.

69 Vauthey JN, Pawlik T, Ribero D, *et al.* Chemotherapy regimen predicts steatohepatitis and an increase in 90-day mortality after surgery for hepatic colorectal metastases. J Clin Oncol 2006; 24(13):2065–2072.

70 Robinson SM, Wilson C, Burt A, *et al.* Chemotherapy-associated liver injury in patients with colorectal liver

metastases: a systematic review and meta-analysis. Ann Surg Oncol 2012; 19(13):4287–4299.

71 Pawlik TM, Olino K, Gleisner K, *et al.* Preoperative chemotherapy for colorectal liver metastases: impact on hepatic histology and postoperative outcome. J Gastrointest Surg 2007; 11(7):860–868.

72 Ryan P, Nanji S, Pollett A, *et al.* Chemotherapy-induced liver injury in metastatic colorectal cancer: semiquantitative histologic analysis of 334 resected liver specimens shows that vascular injury but not steatohepatitis is associated with preoperative chemotherapy. Am J Surg Pathol 2010; 34 (6):784–791.

73 Rubbia-Brandt L, Audard V, Sartoretti P, *et al.* Severe hepatic sinusoidal obstruction associated with oxaliplatin-based chemotherapy in patients with metastatic colorectal cancer. Ann Oncol 2004; 15(3):460–466.

74 Aloia T, Sebagh M, Plasse M, *et al.* Liver histology and surgical outcomes after preoperative chemotherapy with fluorouracil plus oxaliplatin in colorectal cancer liver metastases. J Clin Oncol 2006; 24(31):4983–4990.

75 Klinger M, Eipeldauer S, Hacker S, *et al.* Bevacizumab protects against sinusoidal obstruction syndrome and does not increase response rate in neoadjuvant XELOX/FOLFOX therapy of colorectal cancer liver metastases. Eur J Surg Oncol 2009; 35(5):515–520.

76 Ribero D, Wang H, Donadon M, *et al.* Bevacizumab improves pathologic response and protects against hepatic injury in patients treated with oxaliplatin-based chemotherapy for colorectal liver metastases. Cancer 2007; 110(12):2761–2767.

77 Karoui M, Penna C, Amin-Hashem M, *et al.* Influence of preoperative chemotherapy on the risk of major hepatectomy for colorectal liver metastases. Ann Surg 2006; 243 (1):1–7.

78 Kishi Y, Zorzi D, Contreras C, *et al.* Extended preoperative chemotherapy does not improve pathologic response and increases postoperative liver insufficiency after hepatic resection for colorectal liver metastases. Ann Surg Oncol 2010; 17(11):2870–2876.

79 Hochster HS, Hart L, Ramanathan R, *et al.* Safety and efficacy of oxaliplatin and fluoropyrimidine regimens with or without bevacizumab as first-line treatment of metastatic colorectal cancer: results of the TREE Study. J Clin Oncol 2008; 26(21):3523–3529.

80 Saif MW, Elfiky A, Salem RR. Gastrointestinal perforation due to bevacizumab in colorectal cancer. Ann Surg Oncol 2007; 14(6):1860–1869.

81 Kesmodel SB, Ellis L, Lin E, *et al.* Preoperative bevacizumab does not significantly increase postoperative complication rates in patients undergoing hepatic surgery for colorectal cancer liver metastases. J Clin Oncol 2008; 26 (32):5254–5260.

82 Gruenberger B, Tamandl D, Schueller J, *et al.* Bevacizumab, capecitabine, and oxaliplatin as neoadjuvant therapy for patients with potentially curable metastatic colorectal cancer. J Clin Oncol 2008; 26(11):1830–1835.

83 Okines A, Puerto O, Cunningham D, *et al.* Surgery with curative-intent in patients treated with first-line chemotherapy plus bevacizumab for metastatic colorectal cancer First BEAT and the randomised phase-III NO16966 trial. Br J Cancer 2009; 101(7):1033–1038.

84 Tamandl D, Gruenberger B, Klinger M, *et al.* Liver resection remains a safe procedure after neoadjuvant chemotherapy including bevacizumab: a case-controlled study. Ann Surg 2010; 252(1):124–130.

85 Van der Pool AE, Marsman HA, Verheij J, *et al.* Effect of bevacizumab added preoperatively to oxaliplatin on liver injury and complications after resection of colorectal liver metastases. J Surg Oncol 2012; 106(7):892–897.

86 D'Angelica M, Kornprat P, Gonen M, *et al.* Lack of evidence for increased operative morbidity after hepatectomy with perioperative use of bevacizumab: a matched case-control study. Ann Surg Oncol 2007; 14(2):759–765.

87 Gordon MS, Margolin A, Talpaz M, *et al.* Phase I safety and pharmacokinetic study of recombinant human anti-vascular endothelial growth factor in patients with advanced cancer. J Clin Oncol 2001; 19(3):843–850.

88 Ellis LM, Curley SA, Grothey A. Surgical resection after downsizing of colorectal liver metastasis in the era of bevacizumab. J Clin Oncol 2005; 23(22):4853–4855.

89 Welsh FK, Tilney H, Tekkis P, *et al.* Safe liver resection following chemotherapy for colorectal metastases is a matter of timing. Br J Cancer 2007; 96(7):1037–1042.

90 Adam R, Pascal G, Castaing D, *et al.* Tumor progression while on chemotherapy: a contraindication to liver resection for multiple colorectal metastases? Ann Surg 2004; 240 (6):1052–1061; discussion 1061–1064.

91 Blazer DG 3rd, Kishi Y, Maru D, *et al.* Pathologic response to preoperative chemotherapy: a new outcome end point after resection of hepatic colorectal metastases. J Clin Oncol 2008; 26(33):5344–5351.

92 Shindoh J, Loyer E, Kopetz S, *et al.* Optimal morphologic response to preoperative chemotherapy: an alternate outcome end point before resection of hepatic colorectal metastases. J Clin Oncol 2012; 30(36):4566–4572.

93 Nash GM, Gimbel M, Shia J, *et al.* KRAS mutation correlates with accelerated metastatic progression in patients with colorectal liver metastases. Ann Surg Oncol 2010; 17 (2):572–578.

94 Karagkounis G, Torbenson M, Daniel H, *et al.* Incidence and prognostic impact of KRAS and BRAF mutation in patients undergoing liver surgery for colorectal metastases. Cancer 2013; 119(23):4137–4144.

95 Vauthey JN, Zimmitti G, Kopetz S, *et al.* RAS mutation status predicts survival and patterns of recurrence in patients undergoing hepatectomy for colorectal liver metastases. Ann Surg 2013; 258(4):619–626; discussion 626–627.

96 Teng HW, Huang Y, Lin J, *et al.* BRAF mutation is a prognostic biomarker for colorectal liver metastasectomy. J Surg Oncol 2012; 106(2):123–129.

97 Masi G, Loupakis F, Pollina L, *et al.* Long-term outcome of initially unresectable metastatic colorectal cancer patients treated with 5-fluorouracil/leucovorin, oxaliplatin, and irinotecan (FOLFOXIRI) followed by radical surgery of metastases. Ann Surg 2009; 249(3):420–425.

98 Van Cutsem E, Kohne C, Hitre E, *et al.* Cetuximab and chemotherapy as initial treatment for metastatic colorectal cancer. N Engl J Med 2009; 360(14):1408–1417.

99 Bokemeyer C, Bondarenko I, Makhson A, *et al.* Fluorouracil, leucovorin, and oxaliplatin with and without cetuximab in the first-line treatment of metastatic colorectal cancer. J Clin Oncol 2009; 27(5):663–671.

100 Kopetz S, Hoff P, Morris J, *et al.* Phase II trial of infusional fluorouracil, irinotecan, and bevacizumab for metastatic colorectal cancer: efficacy and circulating angiogenic biomarkers associated with therapeutic resistance. J Clin Oncol 2010; 28(3):453–459.

101 Ho WM, Ma B, Mok T, *et al.* Liver resection after irinotecan, 5-fluorouracil, and folinic acid for patients with unresectable colorectal liver metastases: a multicenter phase II study by the Cancer Therapeutic Research Group. Med Oncol 2005; 22(3):303–312.

102 Pozzo C, Basso M, Cassano A, *et al.* Neoadjuvant treatment of unresectable liver disease with irinotecan and 5-fluorouracil plus folinic acid in colorectal cancer patients. Ann Oncol 2004; 15(6):933–939.

103 Wong R, Cunningham D, Barbachano Y, *et al.* A multicentre study of capecitabine, oxaliplatin plus bevacizumab as perioperative treatment of patients with poor-risk colorectal liver-only metastases not selected for upfront resection. Ann Oncol 2011; 22(9):2042–2048.

104 Masi G, Loupakis F, Salvatore L, *et al.* Bevacizumab with FOLFOXIRI (irinotecan, oxaliplatin, fluorouracil, and folinate) as first-line treatment for metastatic colorectal cancer: a phase 2 trial. Lancet Oncol 2010; 11(9):845–852.

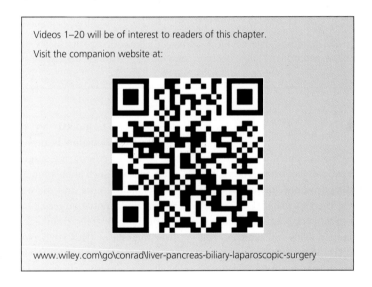

Videos 1–20 will be of interest to readers of this chapter.

Visit the companion website at:

www.wiley.com\go\conrad\liver-pancreas-biliary-laparoscopic-surgery

CHAPTER 14

Resection of noncolorectal liver metastases

Universe Leung and William R. Jarnagin

Hepatopancreatobiliary Service, Department of Surgery, Memorial Sloan-Kettering Cancer Center, New York, USA

EDITOR COMMENT

In this comprehensive and important chapter, the authors concisely describe the presentation and treatment of noncolorectal liver metastases, providing sections on noncolorectal neuroendocrine and noncolorectal nonneuroendocrine liver metastases. Ten percent to 20% of patients with neuroendocrine tumors present with limited disease, making liver-directed therapy a viable treatment option. Debulking surgery for neuroendocrine liver metastases can allow for symptomatic relief and even prolong survival in some cases. Patients with neuroendocrine liver metastases are frequently good candidates for a minimally invasive resection although greater challenges regarding ultrasound detection of all disease exist. While disease almost always recurs, many patients may be candidates for repeat liver-directed therapy, which might be facilitated by a minimally invasive approach. Only limited evidence exists for resection of noncolorectal nonneuroendocrine liver metastases. While patients with unresectable disease often have dismal prognosis, in highly selected patients surgery may result in a long-term survival rate in the order of 30% at five years. Outcome is dependent on identifying patients with favorable tumor biology, which can be achieved through neoadjuvant chemotherapy and disease stability over a defined period of time. As the authors point out, a multidisciplinary approach is essential for optimal outcome.

Keywords: ablation, breast liver metastases, germ cell liver metastases, gynecological liver metastases, melanoma liver metastases, neuroendocrine liver metastases, noncolorectal liver metastases, sarcoma liver metastases, transplantation and resection of neuroendocrine liver metastases

14.1 Introduction

With improving patient selection, operative technique, and perioperative care, hepatic resection has evolved into a safe and effective therapeutic option for primary and selected metastatic tumors. The vast majority of experience and data is drawn from colorectal cancer, a common disease where approximately 50% of patients will develop liver metastases [1]. Knowledge gained from modern studies in patients managed in a multidisciplinary setting has enabled 20–30% of patients with colorectal liver metastases (CRLM) to undergo resection, with five-year survival rates reaching 35–58% [2]. The advent of more effective systemic therapy has increased the proportion of patients eligible for resection and extended overall survival, with recent reports of five-year survival rates as high as 69% and 10-year survival of

17–36% [3–7]. Indeed, for patients with resectable CRLM, liver resection is now standard. Furthermore, the selection criteria for surgery continue to expand, with adjuncts such as ablation and portal vein embolization enabling more and more patients to benefit from potentially curative surgery.

The role of liver resection in the setting of noncolorectal liver metastases (NCLM) is more controversial, due to differing disease biology and lack of robust data. However, the lack of effective alternative therapy for many NCLM and the encouraging results for surgery in CRLM have led to increasing use of hepatic resection in selected NCLM patients. The results are highly variable and depend critically on the primary tumor type and patient selection. In this chapter, we will review the current evidence in support of liver resection for NCLM. Liver metastases from a neuroendocrine primary (NELM) warrants a

---

Laparoscopic Liver, Pancreas, and Biliary Surgery, First Edition.
Edited by Claudius Conrad and Brice Gayet.
© 2017 John Wiley & Sons, Ltd. Published 2017 by John Wiley & Sons, Ltd.

discussion on its own as it has emerged as a subgroup of NCLM with a distinct biology, a wider range of treatment options, and a more favorable outcome.

14.2 Neuroendocrine liver metastases

14.2.1 Natural history

Most neuroendocrine tumors (NET) that metastasize to the liver arise from the gastrointestinal tract. These are gastroenteropancreatic neuroendocrine tumors (GEP-NET) and include those of pancreatic (PNET) and gastrointestinal (GIC, "carcinoid") origins. There have been numerous classification systems over the years with confusing nomenclature and variable criteria for grading and staging. The European Neuroendocrine Tumor Society (ENETS) proposed a system in 2010, which is now recommended by the World Health Organization, differentiating GEP-NETs as low- (G1), intermediate- (G2), and high-grade (G3) tumors based on their mitotic rate or Ki67 proliferation index. Grades 1 and 2, which comprise well-differentiated tumors, have a relatively indolent clinical course, even after metastasis. In contrast, high-grade or poorly differentiated tumors are aggressive, metastasize widely, and are generally not candidates for liver metastasectomy [8].

Overall, 13% of GICs are associated with distant metastases at presentation, including 20–30% of small bowel carcinoids [9]. Importantly, small bowel GICs account for 75–90% of carcinoid syndrome, a debilitating condition for many patients. Carcinoid syndrome generally occurs in the presence of liver metastases due to the loss of first-pass metabolism of humoral factors released by the tumor [10].

Pancreatic neuroendocrine tumors can produce a variety of peptides including gastrin, insulin, glucagon, and vasoinhibitory peptide. They give rise to a number of clinical syndromes that compromise quality of life and may cause life-threatening hypoglycemia, gastrointestinal perforation or bleeding, and electrolyte disturbances. Approximately 60% of PNETs are associated with distant metastases at presentation [11].

Patients with unresected GEP-NET liver metastases, regardless of primary site, have a five-year survival rate ranging from 13% to 54% [12]. House *et al.* reported a median survival of 17 months in a series of patients with unresectable PNET liver metastases [13]. Approximately

50% of patients with carcinoid syndrome will have valvular heart disease, which reduces their three-year survival rate to 31%, about half that of patients without heart disease [14]. These patients require a thorough biochemical and cardiovascular work-up preoperatively and should be given a somatostatin analogue perioperatively to prevent carcinoid crisis [15].

14.2.2 Surgery

The majority of patients with NELM have diffuse disease, such that only 10–20% of patients are candidates for resection [16]. Although traditional surgical philosophy dictates that liver resection for metastasis should be attempted only if all disease can be removed, the unique biology of NELM appears to lend itself to cytoreductive surgery, defined as removal of >90% of disease [17]. NELMs are typically slow growing so even if surgery is not curative, prolonged survival may be achieved. As with CRLM, venous drainage of GEP-NETs into the liver via the portal vein indicates that metastatic spread may be relatively localized; NELMs tend not to encase major vessels or bile ducts, and therefore may be amenable to limited sacrifice of hepatic parenchyma. Furthermore, alternative medical therapies have shown limited efficacy in controlling disease progression, and endocrine symptoms are most effectively palliated by surgical intervention.

Patients are considered surgical candidates if their primary and regional disease is resectable or already resected, the disease is well differentiated, and surgery can be done with acceptable morbidity and mortality risks. Complete resection of the liver disease should be the aim, but palliative cytoreductive surgery has also been advocated [18]. The presence of right heart failure from significant valvular heart disease is a contraindication to surgery, and consideration should be given to valve replacement followed by treatment of the liver disease [19]. The role of surgery in asymptomatic, non-hormonally active disease, particularly in patients with large-volume disease, is controversial and should be individualized.

Liver resection is effective in controlling symptoms in patients with hormonally active tumors. Que *et al.* from the Mayo Clinic described the first large series of NELM with data from 74 patients who underwent resection with either curative or palliative intent, and found an overall symptomatic control rate of 90% and a mean duration of response of 19.3 months [20]. Seven out of 23 (30%) symptomatic patients treated with curative intent developed recurrent symptoms after a mean of 20.4 months, while 26 of 46 (57%) symptomatic patients treated with palliative intent developed recurrent symptoms after a mean of 11.3 months. The overall survival rate at 4 years was 73% and did not differ between the two groups. The authors concluded that even though cytoreduction is associated with shorter durable symptomatic response, overall survival is unchanged, therefore lending support to a cytoreductive approach even if complete resection is not possible.

Although there are no published studies that directly compare surgery with supportive care, a number of reports have demonstrated survival rates of 60–70% with surgery, compared to <50% without surgery historically. Sarmiento *et al.* published the extended Mayo Clinic experience in 2003 to include a total of 170 patients (44% curative, 56% palliative), and found overall five- and 10-year survival rates of 61% and 35%, respectively [21]. The recurrence rates were high: 84% at five years and 94% at 10 years. While suggestive of a benefit from resection, the selection bias associated with these retrospective studies prevents any definitive conclusions in this regard.

The largest published series to date came from an analysis by Mayo *et al.* of data from 339 patients at multiple centers in the USA and Europe [22]. Approximately 30–50% of resections were palliative, and 16% of resected patients had extrahepatic disease. A significant number of patients also underwent repeated surgery to treat recurrence. Recurrence rates were 94% at five years and 99% at 10 years; neither margin status (R0/R1 versus R2) nor presence of extrahepatic disease was associated with recurrence, reflecting the palliative nature of treatment regardless of intent. The overall survival rates from time of first liver resection were 74% at five years and 51% at 10 years (Figure 14.1). On multivariate analysis, factors associated with poorer survival were nonfunctioning NET, synchronous disease, and extrahepatic disease. Interestingly, patients with a functioning NET and R0/R1 resection fared better than those who underwent R2 resection, but for nonfunctioning NETs there was no survival difference regardless of whether gross disease was left behind.

Saxena *et al.* performed a systematic review of 29 studies with 1400 patients who underwent liver resection for NELM [23]. Overall, 65% of the operations were performed with curative intent and 35% were palliative. In the 16 studies that reported symptom response, 95% of

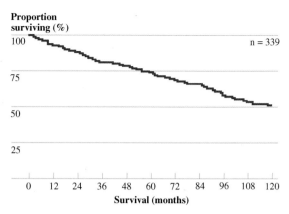

Figure 14.1 Overall survival for hepatic neuroendocrine metastasis from time of first hepatic resection. Source: Mayo *et al.* [22]. Reproduced with permission of Springer.

patients experienced relief, including 57% who had complete response. Median rates of overall survival were 70.5% at five years and 42% at 10 years, but corresponding rates of progression-free survival were only 29% and 1%. The median perioperative mortality rate was 0% (range 0–9%), and median morbidity rate was 23% (range 3–45%). Table 14.1 summarizes recent studies reporting outcomes after surgery for NELM.

Table 14.1 Selected contemporary studies of liver resection for neuroendocrine metastases.

Study	n	Symptom control	5OS
Sarmiento 2003 [21]	170	96%	61%
Osborne 2006 [73]	61	92%	43 months (median)
Hibi 2007 [74]	21	92%	41%
Eriksson 2008 [75]	42	70%	80%
Landry 2008 [76]	39	NR	75%
Kianmanesh 2008 [77]	41	NR	79%
Chambers 2008 [78]	30	75%	74%
Frilling 2009 [79]	23	NR	100%
Scigliano 2009 [80]	38	NR	79%
Mayo 2010 [22]	339	NR	74%
Glazer 2010 [81]	172	NR	77%
Saxena 2011 [82]	74	NR	63%
Gaujoux 2012 [83]	36	NR	69%

5OS, five-year overall survival; NR, not reported.

14.2.3 Laparoscopic resection

There is a paucity of data pertaining to laparoscopic resection for NELM specifically; hence, no specific recommendations can be made, although the advantages and disadvantages, perioperative care, and operative technique can be extrapolated from experience with liver resection for other indications [24]. Selection of NELM patients for laparoscopic resection is similar to that for hepatocellular carcinoma or CRLM, namely, based on size, number, and location of the metastases. In general terms, small (<5 cm) or exophytic tumors in the peripheral and anterolateral parts of the liver, away from major pedicles and veins, are suitable for resection [25]. Kandil *et al.* reported a single-institution retrospective comparison of 21 open and 15 laparoscopic resections of NELM, and found that the laparoscopic group had shorter operating times (2.7 versus 5.4 h), less blood loss, and shorter hospital stay (3.2 versus 7.5 days) [26]. Perioperative morbidity, efficacy of symptom relief, surgical margins, and three-year survival rates were comparable. However, laparoscopic major hepatectomies are technically demanding procedures and considerable experience with open resection and advanced laparoscopic techniques are required to achieve good outcomes.

14.2.4 Nonresectional therapy

A full description of the role of nonresectional management of NELM is beyond the scope of this chapter so it will be mentioned only briefly for completeness.

14.2.4.1 Ablation and embolization

In recent years, ablation (radiofrequency and microwave) has gained popularity for the treatment of small CRLM and hepatocellular carcinoma due to its relative safety, possibility of percutaneous or laparoscopic approach, and ability to spare parenchyma [27–29]. Use of ablation has been extended to NELM, but there are limited data on its efficacy. Given the multifocal and bulky nature of NELM, ablation is infrequently applicable.

Akyildiz *et al.* reported a series of 89 patients who underwent 119 laparoscopic radiofrequency ablations (LRFA) for NELMs, which were symptomatic or progressive [30]. The mean number of lesions treated at first session was six, and mean tumor size was 3.6 cm. Of the patients who were symptomatic, 97% reported symptomatic relief at one week, and the median duration of symptom control was 14 months. Morbidity rate was 6% and 30-day mortality

rate was 1%. After a median follow-up of 30 months, 22% of patients had developed recurrence (6.3% per lesion). Median survival after LRFA was six years, with a five-year survival rate of 57%.

Due to the hypervascular nature of NELMs, hepatic artery embolization with particles or chemotherapeutic agents has been used for unresectable disease. It is effective for symptom treatment, and series have shown a median survival of 18–56 months and a five-year survival rate of up to 30% [31].

14.2.4.2 Transplantation

Liver transplantation has been used in some centers to treat NELM patients with intrahepatic disease that is too extensive for resection and with no extrahepatic disease, with five-year survival rates of 30–60% reported. Mazzaferro *et al.* [32] suggested the following selection criteria for liver transplantation, extrapolated from the Milan Criteria [33] used for patients with hepatocellular carcinoma: primary tumor drained by the portal system, liver parenchymal involvement ≤50%, age ≤55 years, stable disease for at least six months, and exclusion of high-grade tumors. More recently, some authors have advocated a further expanded set of criteria to enable more patients to benefit from potentially curative transplantation. The largest series to date compiled data from 35 centers in Europe over 27 years with a total of 213 patients. Le Treut *et al.* reported a three-month mortality rate of 10%, median overall survival of 67 months, and five-year overall and disease-free survival rates of 52% and 30%, respectively [34].

14.2.4.3 Medical treatment

A number of medical treatments are available for NELM. Somatostatin analogues such as octreotide have been a mainstay for palliation of symptoms and are effective in >60% of patients. They can also temporarily stabilize tumors in 36–70% of patients with a median duration of 12 months [35,36]. α-Interferon can achieve similar results, particularly with low-proliferation tumors. Systemic therapy, such as streptozotocin-based regimens and cisplatin/etoposide combinations, has limited efficacy with response rates ranging from 10% in low-grade tumors to >50% in high-grade tumors. Conventional external beam radiotherapy is generally ineffective for NELM. Recently, there has been interest in peptide receptor radionuclide therapy (PRRT) using radioactive yttrium and lutetium attached to octreotide-based compounds (DOTATOC/

DOTATATE), with early results demonstrating tumor response rates of 20–40% [37,38].

14.2.5 Summary

Neuroendocrine liver metastases tend to be diffuse on presentation, but in 10–20% of patients the disease is more limited, and surgery with or without ablation is an increasingly accepted treatment. Resection with curative intent is ideal, but cytoreduction by removing >90% of disease appears to yield comparable results. Although there is no conclusive evidence for a survival advantage, multiple series have established good long-term survival rates after resection, of the order of 40–80% at five years, compared to historical series showing a five-year survival of around 30% with medical treatment only. In addition, for symptomatic patients, resection offers effective short-to medium-term relief. As with other malignancies of the liver, NELMs are amenable to laparoscopic resection, ablation, and regional and systemic therapies. Although the disease almost always recurs, many patients may be candidates for further liver-directed therapy, and prolonged survival can be achieved.

14.3 Noncolorectal, nonneuroendocrine liver metastases

Historically, patients with noncolorectal, nonneuroendocrine liver metastases (NCNN) were considered to have disseminated disease and were treated nonoperatively. Unlike CRLM and NELM, the majority of NCNNs do not directly drain via the portal vein into the liver, and the presence of liver metastases was taken as evidence of widespread systemic disease. The oncological justification of liver resection is therefore questionable. However, such patients are a heterogeneous group with variable outcomes, and a minority will have more favorable cancer biology, which translates to prolonged survival and, uncommonly, even cure after resection of liver metastases. The strength and breadth of evidence are not as strong as those for CRLM or NELM, but the underlying histology has emerged as a major determinant of long-term outcomes.

14.3.1 Studies with multiple tumor types

In most centers, experience with individual tumor types is very limited, and hence many reports combine tumor types to enable meaningful analysis. Studies examining the outcome of surgically treated NCNNs generally have the limitations of being retrospective, uncontrolled, and having heterogeneous populations, particularly with regard to the tumor type and use of adjuvant therapies. Table 14.2 summarizes recent studies reporting outcomes after surgery for NCNN. Overall five-year survival is approximately 25–40%, representing a highly selected group with a better prognosis. The predominant tumor types are breast, genitourinary, and sarcoma, reflecting the selection of tumors with more favorable biology. Resection for other types, particularly gastrointestinal metastases, is rarely associated with long-term survival.

Weitz et al. from the Memorial Sloan Kettering Cancer Center (MSKCC) reported a series of 141 patients with resected NCNNs and found a median survival of 35 months, and a three-year cancer-specific survival rate of 57% [39]. At the end of the study there were 24 actual five-year survivors. The predominant tumor types were breast (20%), reproductive tract (28%), and melanoma (12%). Factors associated with better survival were disease-free interval >24 months, primary tumor type (reproductive tract fared best), and margin status.

The largest study to date was performed by Adam et al., who analyzed data from 1452 patients from 41 centers [40]. The most common tumor types were breast (32%), gastrointestinal (16%), genitourinary (14%), and melanoma (10%). Sixty-day mortality was 2.3%, and major complications occurred in 21.5% of patients. Overall survival rates at five and 10 years were 36% and 23%, respectively, with a median survival of 35 months, and 46 actual 10-year survivors (Figure 14.2). Multivariate analysis showed that the following factors were associated with poorer survival: age >60, nonbreast origin or melanoma or squamous histology, disease-free interval <12 months, extrahepatic disease, R2 resection, and major hepatectomy. The authors proposed a scoring system using these factors to stratify patients into low-, mid-, and high-risk groups.

O'Rourke et al. reported a series of 114 patients from Australia and the United Kingdom and found a five-year overall survival rate of 39% and a median survival of 42 months [41]. In this study, size of the largest liver metastases (>5 cm) was associated with a >50% reduction in disease-free and overall survival. More recently, Groeschl et al. reported a series of 420 patients from four American centers [42]. Predominant tumor types were breast (27%), sarcoma (23%), and genitourinary (22%).

Table 14.2 Selected studies of noncolorectal liver metastases with at least 20 patients, excluding neuroendocrine tumors.

Study	n	5OS	Dominant pathology
Harrison 1997 [84]	96	37%	Sarcoma, GU
Elias 1998 [85]	120	36%*	Breast, GU
Lang 1999 [86]	127	16%	Breast, sarcoma, GI
Buell 2000 [87]	25	3OS 36%	GU
Hamy 2000 [88]	27	27%*	GI, sarcoma
Hemming 2000 [89]	37	45%	GU, GI, sarcoma
Laurent 2001 [90]	39	35%	GI, GU, breast
Van Ruth 2001 [91]	28	35%	GU, breast
Yamada 2001 [92]	33	12%	GI
Cordera 2005 [93]	64	30%	GU, GI, breast
Weitz 2005 [39]	141	CSS 3 y 57%	GU, breast, melanoma
Yedibela 2005 [94]	162	27%*	GI, breast, GU
Ercolani 2005 [95]	142	34%	Breast, GI, GU
Adam 2006 [40]	1452	36%	Breast, GI, GU
Earle 2006 [96]	77	31%	GU, sarcoma, GI
Lendoire 2007 [97]	106	19%	GU, sarcoma, breast
Reddy 2007 [98]	82	37%	Breast, sarcoma, GU
O'Rourke 2008 [41]	102	39%	Soft tissue, GU, GI
Ercolani 2009 [99]	134	40%	(abstract only)
Lehner 2009 [100]	242	28%	(non-English language article)
Marudanayagam 2010 [101]	65	26%	GU
Schmelze 2010 [102]	44	20%	GU, GI, breast
Duan 2011 [103]	62	30%	Breast, lung, stomach
Groeschl 2012 [42]	420	31%	Breast, sarcoma, GU
Takemura 2013 [104]	145	41%	GI, breast

*Survival figures included patients with neuroendocrine tumors.

3OS, three-year overall survival; 5OS, five-year overall survival; CSS, cancer-specific survival; GI, gastrointestinal; GU, genitourinary.

Sixty-day mortality was 1.9% and complications occurred in 20%. Overall survival rates at three and five years were 50% and 31%, respectively, with a median of 49 months. Overall recurrence rate was 66% and was similar across the various cancer types. Lymphovascular invasion and size of metastases (≥ 5 cm) predicted poorer survival, whereas type of tumor did not.

14.3.2 Studies of specific tumor types
14.3.2.1 Breast
Distant metastases occur in approximately 50% of breast cancer patients, of which the liver is involved in 6–25% cases. With supportive treatment only, median survival is <1 month. With systemic treatment using chemotherapy and/or endocrine therapy, good responders have a median survival around 13–23 months [43,44].

Most patients have disseminated disease, but about 5% have isolated liver metastases that may be amenable to surgery [45]. Adam *et al.* reported a series of 85 patients undergoing liver resection with a five-year overall survival rate of 37%, and median survival of 32 months [46]. Sixty-nine percent of patients recurred after a median of 10 months, with about half of those recurrences in the liver only. Response to chemotherapy predicted survival, as did macroscopic residual tumor. In their series of 86 patients, Abbott *et al.* found a five-year overall survival rate of 44%, and median survival of 57 months [47]. They found that estrogen receptor negativity and progression on chemotherapy were signs of poor prognosis. Table 14.3 summarizes recent studies reporting outcomes after surgery for breast cancer liver metastases.

14.3.2.2 Gastrointestinal
The majority of evidence regarding NCNN from gastrointestinal (GI) sources comes from gastric cancer series from Asia. At time of diagnosis of gastric cancer, 35% of

(a)

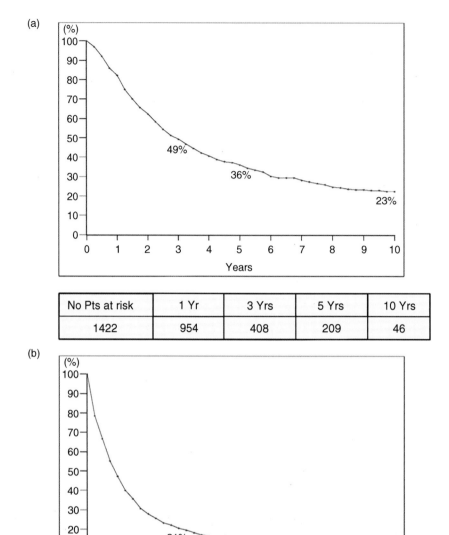

No Pts at risk	1 Yr	3 Yrs	5 Yrs	10 Yrs
1422	954	408	209	46

(b)

No Pts at risk	1 Yr	3 Yrs	5 Yrs	10 Yrs
1358	548	180	95	26

Figure 14.2 Survival curves for 1452 patients in 41 centers after hepatectomy for NCNN. (a) Overall survival. (b) Recurrence-free survival. Source: Adam *et al.* [40]. Reproduced with permission of Lippincott, Williams, & Wilkins.

Table 14.3 Selected contemporary series of breast cancer liver metastases with at least 20 patients.

Study	n	5OS	Poor prognostic factors
Yoshimoto 2000 [105]	25	27%	None
Pocard 2000 [106]	52	3OS 49%	Node-positive primary, short disease-free interval
Elias 2003 [45]	54	34%	Negative hormonal status
Adam 2006 [46]	85	37%	Poor response to pre-op chemotherapy, positive margin, repeat hepatectomy
Thelen 2008 [107]	39	42%	Positive margin
Abbott 2012 [47]	86	44%	Negative hormonal status, progression on pre-op chemotherapy
Van Walsum 2012	32	37%	>1 metastasis
Dittmar 2013 [109]	54	28%	Extrahepatic disease, HER2 positivity, age >50
Kostov 2013 [110]	42	38%	Negative hormonal status, size >4 cm, positive margin, positive portal nodes, poor response to preoperative chemotherapy

3OS, three-year overall survival; 5OS, five-year overall survival.

patients have distant metastases, and 4–14% have liver metastases. With chemotherapy only, the median survival is in the order of 7–15 months and five-year survival is rare, around 2% [48,49]. Takamura *et al.* reported the largest surgical series to date with 64 patients [50]. After resection, the overall five-year survival rate was 37%, median 34 months. Presence of metastases >5 cm and invasion of serosa by the primary tumor were indicators of poor prognosis. Table 14.4 summarizes recent studies reporting outcomes after surgery for gastric cancer liver metastases.

Data for metastatic pancreatic cancer are even more limited. A systematic review by Michalski *et al.* found 21 studies with a total of 103 patients over 15 years [51].

Median survival after surgery was only 6–14 months. Significantly, Takada *et al.* found that patients who underwent synchronous pancreaticoduodenectomy and liver resection had the same survival as patients who underwent palliative bypass only and no liver resection, reflecting the unfavorable biology of pancreatic cancer [52].

14.3.2.3 Gynecological

Most of the data on NCNN of gynecological origin are drawn from ovarian cancer. Isolated liver metastases are rare as ovarian cancer commonly spreads transperitoneally. However, the biology of this disease lends itself to cytoreductive surgery, which may include liver resection, to reduce macroscopic disease to <1 cm.

Table 14.4 Selected contemporary series of gastric cancer liver metastases.

Study	n	5OS	Poor prognostic factors
Sakamoto 2007 [111]	37	11%	Size >4 cm, bilobar metastases
Koga 2007 [112]	42	42%	>1 metastasis, T3 primary
Thelen 2008 [113]	24	10%	Positive margin
Morise 2008 [114]	18	27%	T3 primary, LVI
Makino 2010 [115]	16	37%	
Tsujimoto 2010 [116]	17	32%	Size >6 cm, D1 lymphadenectomy
Schildberg 2012 [117]	31	13%	>1 metastasis, positive margin, synchronous
Dittmar 2012 [118]	15	27%	
Takemura 2012 [50]	64	37%	Size >5 cm, T3 primary
Baek 2013 [119]	12	39%	
Qiu 2013 [120]	25	29%	>1 metastasis
Vigan 2013 [121]	14	33%	Progression on chemotherapy

5OS, five-year overall survival; LVI, lymphovascular invasion.

Table 14.5 Selected contemporary studies of liver resection for gynecological metastases.

Study	n	Outcome	Poor prognostic factors	Notes
Yoon 2003 [53]	24	Median OS 62 months		Recurrent ovarian cancers
Bosquet 2006 [122]	35	Median DFS 41 months	Residual disease (<1 cm better than >1 cm)	Recurrent ovarian cancers
Abood 2008 [123]	10	Median 33 months	Size >5 cm, positive margin	Ovarian cancers
Lim 2009 [124]	14	5OS 51%		Epithelial ovarian cancers only
Kamel 2011 [54]	52	5OS 41%		77% tumors ovarian, 17% tumors uterine
Neumann 2012 [125]	41	Median 42 months	Positive margin, ascites, bilobar metastases	Epithelial ovarian cancers only

5OS, five-year overall survival; DFS, disease-free survival; OS, overall survival.

Involvement of the liver with ovarian cancer is most commonly in the form of capsular implants and, less often, parenchymal metastases. Even in the presence of extensive disease, therefore, parenchymal-sparing resection is often possible.

Yoon *et al.* from the MSKCC reported a series of 24 patients submitted to hepatic resection, achieving a median survival of 62 months, with cancer recurring in 75% of patients [53]. The authors noted that these patients were initially chemosensitive and had experienced prolonged disease-free survival (median 36 months), highlighting the importance of selecting patients with favorable biology. Kamel *et al.* reported their series of 52 patients, resulting in a 75% recurrence rate at a median of 13 months, with an overall five-year survival rate of 41%, median 38 months [54]. Table 14.5 summarizes recent studies reporting outcomes after surgery for gynecological liver metastases.

14.3.2.4 Germ cell tumors

Chemotherapy with cisplatin-based regimens is the mainstay of treatment for metastatic germ cell tumors, with a cure rate of 60–80%. The presence of liver metastasis worsens the prognosis to a 49% five-year survival rate, and liver resection has been used as an adjunct to medical management. Rivoire *et al.* examined the outcomes of liver resection in 37 patients after chemotherapy and found an overall survival rate of 62% at five years and a median survival of 54 months [55]. These authors identified three negative prognostic factors: presence of pure embryonal carcinoma in the primary tumor, liver metastases >30 mm, and presence of viable residual disease. The authors proposed that because germ cell tumors are generally chemosensitive, liver resection should be

employed selectively. For male patients, they concluded that metastases between 10 and 29 mm should be resected, tumors ≤10 mm should be observed due to the high probability of them being necrotic, and tumors ≥30 mm are a poor prognostic group that is unlikely to benefit from surgery. Female patients fared better, leading the authors to propose that all liver metastases >10 mm should be considered for resection. Hartmann *et al.* reported a series of 43 male patients undergoing postchemotherapy liver resection with a five-year overall survival rate of 71% [56]. They found that tumors refractory to chemotherapy had a worse prognosis.

14.3.2.5 Renal cell carcinoma

Liver metastases develop in 10–20% of patients with renal cell carcinoma (RCC), of which 2–4% are amenable to hepatic resection. Without treatment, only 10% of patients survive more than 1 year. With surgery, five-year survival rates of approximately 25–60% have been reported. Thelen *et al.* reported a series of 31 patients who underwent liver resection and found an overall five-year survival rate of 39% [57]. Staehler *et al.* reported a five-year survival rate of 62%, median 142 months, in 68 resected patients, compared to 29% five-year survival and median of 27 months in 20 unresected patients [58]. Table 14.6 summarizes recent studies reporting outcomes after surgery for renal cell cancer liver metastases.

14.3.2.6 Melanoma

Liver metastases develop in 10–20% of patients with metastatic melanoma, with a dismal prognosis of from two to seven months median survival, and are generally chemo-resistant with a response rate of 10–30% [59].

Table 14.6 Selected contemporary series of liver resection for renal cell carcinoma metastases.

Study	n	5OS	Poor prognostic factors
Aloia 2006 [126]	19	26%	Size >5 cm, female sex
Thelen 2007 [57]	31	39%	Positive margin
Staehler 2010 [58]	68	62%	
Ruys 2011 [127]	29	43%	Synchronous metastases, positive margin
Langan 2012 [128]	10	33%	Synchronous metastases

5OS, five-year overall survival.

Ocular melanoma has been reported to have a particularly high propensity to spread to the liver, in up to 95% of patients [60]. In a review of 1750 melanoma patients with liver metastases presenting to the John Wayne Cancer Institute and Sydney Melanoma Unit, Rose *et al.* reported a series of 24 patients (1.4%) who underwent curative or palliative hepatectomy [61]. In this highly selected group, median survival was 28 months and the five-year overall survival rate was 29%. In comparison, 10 patients who were surgically explored but not resected had a median survival of four months. In addition, 899 patients treated nonoperatively had a median survival of six months and a five-year survival rate of 4%.

Pawlik *et al.* showed that tumor recurred after liver resection in 75% of patients at a median of eight months [59]. Ocular melanoma tended to recur more often within the liver whereas cutaneous melanoma recurred more often extrahepatically. Five-year survival rate was also better for ocular primary at 20.5%, compared to no five-year survivors in the cutaneous group. Aubin *et al.* conducted a systematic review of 22 studies involving 579 patients undergoing liver resection for metastatic melanoma and found an overall five-year survival rate of 11–36%, median 14–41 months, compared to a median survival of 4–12 months for nonoperative management [62]. The number of metastases and an R0 versus R1/R2 resection were found to be significant prognostic factors.

In recent years, a number of new agents have emerged for treatment of metastatic melanoma. The cytotoxic T lymphocyte-associated antigen-4 (CTLA-4) blocking monoclonal antibody ipilimumab has been shown in two phase III trials to improve overall survival when used alone or in combination with dacarbazine. Ipilimumab acts as an immune modulator by blocking intrinsic T-cell inhibition [63,64]. Vemurafenib and trametinib are inhibitors of the BRAF/MAP-kinase growth pathway that have been shown in phase III trials to improve overall survival [65]. They are only effective in patients with BRAF mutations, present in approximately 50% of melanomas. Finally, trials are ongoing to investigate the role of imatinib in the subset of melanoma harboring KIT mutations, with promising phase II results [66]. Through better systemic control of disease, the number of patients who become surgical candidates may expand in the future.

14.3.2.7 Sarcoma

Soft tissue sarcoma (STS) is relatively chemo-resistant. An early series from the MSKCC showed a 6% partial response rate to doxorubicin [67].

In 2001, DeMatteo *et al.* published a 19-year series of 4270 patients with STS from the MSKCC, in which 331 (7.8%) patients had liver metastases, 40% of which were gastrointestinal stromal tumors (GIST) or intestinal leiomyosarcomas [68]. Liver resection with curative intent was performed in 56 (17%) patients. There was recurrence in 84% of patients at a median of 16 months. The five-year disease-free survival rate was 30%, median 39 months, with 10 actual five-year survivors. In contrast, patients who did not undergo resection had a five-year disease-free survival rate of 4%, median 12 months. Eight patients who underwent palliative resection (R2) for relief from symptoms had no survival benefit with a median of only eight months. On multivariate analysis, the only independent predictor of outcome was time interval to liver metastasis of >2 years. Neither primary histology, number or size of metastases, extrahepatic disease, nor microscopic margin predicted survival.

The emergence of imatinib has completely changed the approach to treatment of GIST. Imatinib is a selective tyrosine kinase inhibitor that targets GISTs harboring gain-of-function mutations in cKIT and PDGFR-α proto-oncogenes, the main pathogenic mechanism in 95% of GISTs. So effective is this drug that it is now the first-line treatment for liver metastases. However, response is rarely complete, and most patients will progress after a median of two years due to acquired tumor resistance. Cytoreductive surgery has been used in addition to imatinib to delay disease progression but the evidence to support such adjuvant surgery is from retrospective analysis and prone to selection bias.

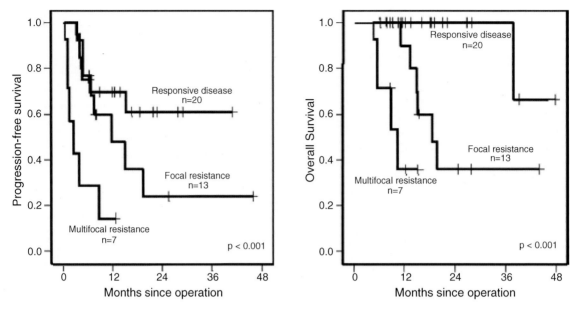

Figure 14.3 Progression-free and overall survival of patients who underwent surgery for metastatic GIST (including liver, pancreas, and peritoneal), grouped by preoperative radiological response to six months of imatinib. Source: DeMatteo *et al.* [69]. Reproduced with permission of Lippincott, Williams, & Wilkins.

Furthermore, the optimum timing of cytoreduction is unclear. DeMatteo *et al.* studied patients who underwent surgery after six months of imatinib therapy, stratified according to response [69]. Responders had a two-year overall survival rate of 100%; patients with focal resistance progressed after a median of 12 months and had an overall two-year survival of 36%; patients with multifocal resistance progressed after three months and had an overall one-year survival of 36% (Figure 14.3). The authors concluded that patients with responsive disease or focal resistance may benefit from surgery, but those with multifocal resistance do not.

An *et al.* investigated the reverse approach [70]. In 249 patients, they retrospectively compared

cytoreduction (17% of patients underwent hepatectomy) followed by imatinib with imatinib alone, and found no difference in disease progression, need for salvage surgery or overall survival. They concluded that initial or "upfront" cytoreduction, despite being effective in reducing tumor bulk, is not beneficial and hence imatinib should remain first-line therapy for metastatic GIST. Table 14.7 summarizes recent studies reporting outcomes after surgery for sarcoma liver metastases.

14.3.3 Laparoscopic resection
There are no published studies to date specifically addressing the role of laparoscopic resection for NCNN.

Table 14.7 Selected contemporary series of liver resection for metastatic sarcoma.

Study	n	5OS	Histology types	Poor prognostic factors
DeMatteo 2001 [68]	56	30%	61% GIST, 19% extraintestinal leiomyosarcoma	DFI <24 months
Pawlik 2006 [59]	66	27%	55% GIST, 27% leiomyosarcoma	
Rehders 2009 [129]	45	49%	30% leiomyosarcoma, 22% GIST	DFI <24 months

5OS, five-year overall survival; DFI, disease-free interval; GIST, gastrointestinal stromal tumor.

Table 14.8 Selected studies and prognostic factors.

Study	Disease-free interval	Largest metastasis size	R0 versus R1/R2	Primary tumor type	Other
Cordera 2005 [93]	Yes	NR	No	Yes. GI worse than non-GI	
Weitz 2005 [39]	Yes, 24 months	No	Yes	Yes. Genital better than nongenital	
Yedibela 2005 [94]	NR	NR	Yes	Yes	
Ercolani 2005 [95]	No	Yes, 5 cm	NR	Yes. GI worst, GU best	Total tumor volume
Adam 2006 [40]	Yes, 12 months	Yes	Yes	Yes. Nonbreast, squamous, and melanoma worst	Extrahepatic disease, age, ≥3 segments resected
Earle 2006 [96]	Yes, 24 months	NR	NR	Yes. GI worse than non-GI	Synchronous versus metachronous, number of metastases
Lendoire 2007 [97]	No	NR	Yes	Yes. GU and breast best	Synchronous versus metachronous
O'Rourke 2008 [41]	No	Yes, 5 cm	Yes	No	Extrahepatic nodal disease
Duan 2012 [103]	Yes, 12 months	Yes, 5 cm	NR	Yes. Breast and GU best, GI intermediate	>1 metastasis
Groeschl 2012 [42]	No	Yes, 5 cm	No	No	Primary lymphovascular invasion

GI, gastrointestinal; GU, genitourinary; NR, not reported.

A number of larger series of laparoscopic liver resection included small numbers of NCNNs in their patient cohorts [71,72]. As with NELM, selection of NCNN for laparoscopic resection is based on size, number, and location of metastases rather than histological type. There are no documented differences in the outcomes between NCNN and CRLM attributable to laparoscopic technique.

14.3.4 Patient selection for surgery

The most important factor to consider when selecting patients with NCNN for surgery is tumor biology. Most authors suggest liver resection only if all disease in the liver and extrahepatic sites can be resected and/or ablated, with the exception of gynecological metastases where cytoreduction is proven to be effective treatment, and in selected GISTs as an adjunct to imatinib to delay progression. Prognostic factors identified in various series provide some insight into which patients may benefit most from surgery: longer disease-free interval, small metastasis size, solitary metastasis, and good response to or stability with chemotherapy. Efforts to improve

selection criteria are clearly warranted (Table 14.8, Figure 14.4, Figure 14.5).

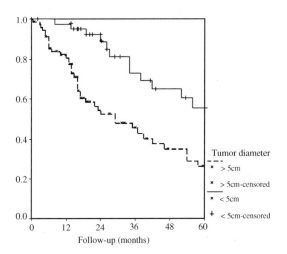

Figure 14.4 Overall survival following hepatic resection for 102 patients with NCNN, grouped by tumor size.
Source: O'Rourke *et al.* [41]. Reproduced with permission of Springer.

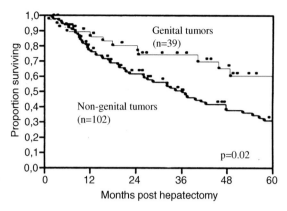

Figure 14.5 Disease-specific survival for 141 patients with NCNN, grouped by tumor type. Source: Weitz *et al.* [39]. Reproduced with permission of Lippincott, Williams, & Wilkins.

14.3.5 Summary

The management of NCNN is controversial, but may follow that of CRLM and NELM. Evidence is difficult to interpret due to small heterogeneous studies and selection bias. The majority of patients have unresectable disease and their prognosis is dismal. The proportion of patients with limited disease amenable to resection ranges from 1% (melanoma) to 17% (sarcoma). In highly selected patients, surgery may result in a long-term survival rate in the order of 30% at five years, but outcome is critically dependent on identifying patients with favorable tumor biology. It is important to recognize that most patients submitted to hepatic resection are not cured of their disease. A multidisciplinary approach is essential for optimal outcome.

KEY POINTS

Neuroendocrine liver metastases (NELM)

- About 10–20% of patients have limited disease amenable to surgery.
- Aim to completely resect all liver disease, but cytoreduction of >90% can yield similar survival and is effective for palliation of symptoms of hormonal excess.
- Disease recurs after resection in most patients.
- Overall five-year survival rates of 40–80% with surgery, compared to 30% without.

Noncolorectal, nonneuroendocrine liver metastases (NCNN)

- Most patients have disseminated disease with poor prognosis; only a small percentage of patients are candidates for liver resection.
- Careful selection of patients with limited disease and favorable cancer biology can result in five-year survival rates of 25–40%.
- Metastases arising from breast, genitourinary, and sarcoma primaries have better prognosis than those arising from gastrointestinal and melanoma primaries.
- Favorable factors to consider include smaller size (<5 cm), solitary metastasis, longer disease-free interval (>24 months), and good response to chemotherapy.

References

1 Steele G Jr, Ravikumar TS. Resection of hepatic metastases from colorectal cancer. Biologic Perspective. Ann Surg 1989; 210:127–138.

2 Adam R, Delvart V, Pascal G, *et al.* Rescue surgery for unresectable colorectal liver metastases downstaged by chemotherapy. a model to predict long-term survival. Ann Surg 2004; 240:644–658.

3 Nikfarjam M, Shereef S, Kimchi E, *et al.* Survival outcomes of patients with colorectal liver metastases following hepatic resection or ablation in the era of effective chemotherapy. Ann Surg Oncol 2009; 16:1860–1867.

4 Tomlinson J, Jarnagin W, DeMatteo R, *et al.* Actual 10-year survival after resection of colorectal liver metastases defines cure. J Clin Oncol 2007; 25:4575–4580.

5 Shimizu Y, Yasui K, Sano T, *et al.* Treatment strategy for synchronous metastases of colorectal cancer: is hepatic

resection after an observation interval appropriate? Langenbecks Arch Surg 2007; 392(5):535–538.

6 Giuliante F, Ardito F, Vellone M, *et al.* Role of the surgeon as a variable in long-term survival after liver resection for colorectal metastases. J Surg Oncol 2009; 100(7):538–545.

7 Pulitano C, Castillo F, Aldrighetti L, *et al.* What defines "cure" after liver resection for colorectal metastases? results after 10 years of follow-up. HPB 2010; 12:244–249.

8 Klimstra D, Modlin I, Coppola D, Lloyd R, Suster S. The pathological classification of neuroendocrine tumors. A review of nomenclature, grading, and staging systems. Pancreas 2010; 39:707–712.

9 Modlin I, Lye K, Kidd M. A 5-decade analysis of 13,715 carcinoid tumors. Cancer 2004; 97:934–959.

10 Feldman J. Carcinoid tumors and syndrome. Semin Oncol 1987; 14:237.

11 Yao J, Eisner M, Leary C, *et al.* Population-based study of islet cell carcinoma. Ann Surg Oncol 2007; 14(12):3492–3500.

12 Frilling A, Sotiropoulos G, Li J, Kornasiewicz O, Plockinger U. Multimodal management of neuroendocrine liver metastases. HPB 2010; 12:361–379.

13 House M, Cameron J, Lillemoe K, *et al.* Resectable versus unresectable metastases from pancreatic islet cell cancer. J Gastrointest Surg 2006; 10:138–145.

14 Fox D, Khattar S. Carcinoid heart disease: presentation, diagnosis, and management. Heart 2004; 90:1224–1228.

15 Palaniswamy C, Frishman W, Aronow W. Carcinoid heart disease. Cardiol Rev 2012; 20:167–176.

16 Reddy S, Clary B. Neuroendocrine liver metastases. Surg Clin North Am 2010; 90:853–861.

17 Sarmiento J, Que F. Hepatic surgery for metastases from neuroendocrine tumors. Surg Oncol Clin North Am 2003; 12:231–242.

18 Steinmuller T, Kianmanesh R, Falconi M, *et al.* Consensus guidelines for the management of patients with liver metastases from digestive (neuro)endocrine tumors: foregut, midgut, hindgut, and unknown primary. Neuroendocrinology 2008; 87:47–62.

19 Lillegard J, Fisher J, Mckenzie T, *et al.* Hepatic resection for the carcinoid syndrome in patients with severe carcinoid heart disease: does valve replacement permit safe hepatic resection? J Am Coll Surg 2011; 213:130–138.

20 Que F, Nagorney D, Batts K, Linz L, Kvols L. Hepatic resection for metastatic neuroendocrine carcinomas. Am J Surg 1995; 169:36–43.

21 Sarmiento J, Heywood G, Rubin J, Ilstrup D, Nagorney D, Que F. Surgical treatment of neuroendocrine metastases to the liver: a plea for resection to increase survival. J Am Coll Surg 2003; 197:29–37.

22 Mayo S, de Jong M, Pulitano C, *et al.* Surgical management of hepatic neuroendocrine tumor metastasis: results from an international multi-institutional analysis. Ann Surg Oncol 2010; 17:3129–3136.

23 Saxena A, Chua T, Perera M, Chu F, Morris D. Surgical resection of hepatic metastases from neuroendocrine neoplasms: a systematic review. Surg Oncol 2012; 21:e131–e141.

24 Abu Hilal M, di Fabio F, Salameh M, Pearce N. Oncological efficiency analysis of laparoscopic liver resection for primary and metastatic cancer. Arch Surg 2012; 147(2):42–48.

25 Buell J, Cherqui D, Geller D, *et al.* The international position on laparoscopic liver surgery. The Louisville Statement, 2008. Ann Surg 2009; 250:825–830.

26 Kandil E, Noureldine S, Koffron A, Yao L, Saggi B, Buell J. Outcomes of laparoscopic and open resection for neuroendocrine liver metastases. Surgery 2012; 152:1225–1231.

27 Wong S, Mangu P, Choti M, *et al.* American Society of Clinical Oncology 2009 clinical evidence review on radiofrequency ablation of hepatic metastases from colorectal cancer. J Clin Oncol 2010; 28:493–508.

28 Pathak S, Jones R, Tang J, *et al.* Ablative therapies for colorectal liver metastases: a systematic review. Colorectal Dis 2011; 13:252–265.

29 Karanicolas P, Jarnagin W, Gönen M, *et al.* Long-term outcomes following tumor ablation for treatment of bilateral colorectal liver metastases. JAMA Surg 2013; 148(7):597–601.

30 Akyildiz H, Mitchell J, Milas M, Siperstein A, Berber E. Laparoscopic radiofrequency thermal ablation of neuroendocrine hepatic metastases: long-term follow-up. Surgery 2010; 148:1288–1293.

31 Lee E, Pachter L, Sarpel U. Hepatic arterial embolization for the treatment of metastatic neuroendocrine tumors. Int J Hepatol 2012; rticle ID 471203.

32 Mazzaferro V, Pulvirenti A, Coppa J. Neuroendocrine tumors metastatic to the liver: how to select patients for liver transplantation? J Hepatol 2007; 47:454–475.

33 Mazzaferro V, Regalia E, Doci R, *et al.* Liver transplantation for the treatment of small hepatocellular carcinomas in patients with cirrhosis. N Engl J Med 1996; 334:693–699.

34 Le Treut Y, Gregoire E, Klempnauer J, *et al.* Liver transplantation for neuroendocrine tumors in Europe – results and trends in patient selection. A 213-case European Liver Transplant Registry study. Ann Surg 2013; 257:807–815.

35 Oberg K, Astrup L, Eriksson B, *et al.* Guidelines for the management of gastroenteropancreatic neuroendocrine tumours (including bronchopulmonary and thymic neoplasms). Acta Oncol 2004; 43:617–625.

36 Rinke A, Muller H, Schade-Brittinger C, *et al.* Placebo-controlled, double-blind, prospective, randomized study on the effect of octreotide LAR in the control of tumor growth in patients with metastatic neuroendocrine midgut tumors: a report from the PROMID Study Group. J Clin Oncol 2009; 27:4656–4663.

37 Kam B, Teunissen J, Krenning E, *et al.* Lutetium-labelled peptides for therapy of neuroendocrine tumours. Eur J Nucl Med Mol Imaging 2012; 39 (suppl 1):S103–S112.

38 Bodei L, Cremonesi M, Grana C, *et al.* Yttrium-labelled peptides for therapy of NET. Eur J Nucl Med Mol Imaging 2012; 39(suppl 1): S93–S102.

39 Weitz J, Blumgart L, Fong Y, *et al.* Partial hepatectomy for metastases from noncolorectal, nonneuroendocrine carcinoma. Ann Surg 2005; 241:269–276.

40 Adam R, Chiche L, Aloia T, *et al.* Hepatic resection for noncolorectal nonenodcrine liver metastases. Analysis of

1452 patients and development of a prognostic model. Ann Surg 2006; 24:524–535.

41 O'Rourke T, Tekkis P, Yeung S, *et al.* Long-term results of liver resection for non-colorectal non-neuroendocrine metastases. Ann Surg Oncol 2008; 15(1):207–218.

42 Groeschl R, Nachmany I, Steel J, *et al.* Hepatectomy for non-colorectal non-neuroendocrine metastatic cancer: a multi-institutional analysis. J Am Coll Surg 2012; 214:769–777.

43 Atalay G, Biganzoli L, Renard F, *et al.* Clinical outcome of breast cancer patients with liver metatases alone in the anthracycline–taxane era: a retrospective analysis of two prospective, randomised metastatic breast cancer trials. Eur J Cancer 2003; 39:2439–2449.

44 Wyld L, Gutteridge E, Sinder S, *et al.* Prognostic factors for patients with hepatic metastases from breast cancer. Br J Cancer 2003; 89:284–290.

45 Elias D, Maisonnette F, Druet-Cabanac M, *et al.* An attempt to clarify indications for hepatectomy for liver metastases from breast cancer. Am J Surg 2003; 185:158–164.

46 Adam R, Aloia T, Krissat J, *et al.* Is liver resection justified for patients with hepatic metastases from breast cancer? Ann Surg 2006; 244:897–908.

47 Abbott D, Brouquet AS, Mittendorf E, *et al.* Resection of liver metastases from breast cancer: estrogen receptor status and response to chemotherapy before metastasectomy define outcome. Surgery 2012; 151:710–716.

48 Romano F, Garancini M, Uggeri F, *et al.* Surgical treatment of liver metastases of gastric cancer: state of the art. World J Surg Oncol 2012; 10:157.

49 Yoshida M, Ohtsu A, Boku N, *et al.* Long-term survival and prognostic factors in patients with metastatic gastric cancers treated with chemotherapy in the Japan Clinical Oncology Group (JCOG) study. Jpn J Clin Oncol 2004; 34(11):654–659.

50 Takemura N, Saiura A, Koga R, *et al.* Long-term outcomes after surgical resection for gastric cancer liver metastasis: an analysis of 64 macroscopically complete resections. Langbenbecks Arch Surg 2012; 397:951–957.

51 Michalski C, Erkan M, Huser N, *et al.* Resection of primary pancreatic cancer and liver metastasis: a systematic review. Dig Surg 2008; 25:473–480.

52 Takada T, Yasuda H, Amano H, Yoshida M, Uchida T. Simultaneous hepatic resection with páncreatoduodenectomy for metastatic pancreatic head carcinoma: does it improve survival? Hepatogastroenterology 1997; 44:567–573.

53 Yoon S, Jarnagin W, Fong Y, *et al.* Resection of recurrent ovarian or fallopian tube carcinoma involving the liver. Gynecol Oncol 2003; 91:383–388.

54 Kamel S, de Jong M, Schulick R, *et al.* The role of liver-directed surgery in patients with hepatic metastasis from a gynecologic primary carcinoma. World J Surg 2011; 35:1345–1354.

55 Rivoire M, Elias D, de Cian F, Kaemmerlen P, Theodore C, Droz J. Multimodality treatment of patients with liver metastases from germ cell tumors. The role of surgery. Cancer 2001; 92:578–587.

56 Hartmann J, Rick O, Oechsle K, *et al.* Role of postchemotherapy surgery in the management of patients with liver metastases from germ cell tumors. Ann Surg 2005; 242:260–266.

57 Thelen A, Jonas S, Benckert C, *et al.* Liver resection for metastases from renal cell carcinoma. World J Surg 2007; 31:802–807.

58 Staehler M, Kruse J, Haseke N, *et al.* Liver resection for metastatic disease prolongs survival in renal cell carcinoma: 1two-year results from a retro-spective comparative analysis. World J Urol 2010; 28:543–547.

59 Pawlik T, Zorzi D, Abdall E, *et al.* Hepatic resection for metastatic melanoma: distinct patterns of recurrence and prognosis for ocular versus cutaneous disease. Ann Surg Oncol 2006; 13(5):712–720.

60 Li Y, McClay E. Systemic chemotherapy for the treatment of metastatic melanoma. Semin Oncol 2002; 29:413–426.

61 Rose D, Essner R, Hughes T, *et al.* Surgical resection for metastatic melanoma to the liver. The John Wayne Cancer Institute and Sydney Melanoma Unit experience. Arch Surg 2001; 136:950–955.

62 Aubin J, Rekman J, Vandenbroucke-Menu F, *et al.* Systematic review and meta-analysis of liver resection for metastatic melanoma. Br J Surg 2013; 100:1138–1147.

63 Hodi F, O'Day S, McDermott D, *et al.* Improved survival with ipilimumab in patients with metastatic melanoma. N Engl J Med 2010; 363:711–723.

64 Robert C, Thomas L, Bondarenko I, *et al.* Ipilimumab plus dacarbazine for previously untreated metastatic melanoma. N Engl J Med 2011; 364:2517–2526.

65 Flaherty K, Robert C, Hersey P, *et al.* Improved survival with MEK inhibition in BRAF-mutated melanoma. N Engl J Med 2012; 367:107–114.

66 Carvajal R, Antonescu C, Wolchok J, *et al.* KIT as a therapeutic target in metastatic melanoma. JAMA 2011; 305 (22):2327–2334.

67 Jaques D, Coit D, Caster E, Brennan M. Hepatic metastases from soft-tissue sarcoma. Ann Surg 1995; 221:392–397.

68 DeMatteo R, Shah A, Fong Y, Jarnagin W, Blumgart L, Brennan M. Results of hepatic resection for sarcoma metastatic to liver. Ann Surg 2001; 234:540–548.

69 DeMatteo R, Maki R, Singer S, Gönen M, Brennan M, Antonescu C. Results of tyrosine kinase inhib–itor therapy followed by surgical resection for metastatic gastrointestinal stromal tumor. Ann Surg 2007; 245:347–352.

70 An H, Rye M, Ryoo B, *et al.* The effects of surgical cytoreduction prior to imatinib therapy on the prognosis of patients with advanced GIST. Ann Surg Oncol 2013; 20:4212–4218.

71 Bryant R, Laurent A, Tayar C, Cherqui D. Laparoscopic liver resection – understanding its role in current practice. The Henri Mondor Hospital experience. Ann Surg 2009; 250:103–111.

72 Buell J, Thomas M, Rudich S, *et al.* Experience with more than 500 minimally invasive hepatic procedures. Ann Surg 2008; 248:475–486.

73 Osborne D, Zervos E, Strosberg J, *et al.* Improved outcome with cytoreduction versus embolization for symptomatic hepatic metastases of carcinoid and neuroendocrine tumors. Ann Surg Oncol 2006; 13(4):572–581.

74 Hibi T, Sano T, Sakamoto Y, *et al.* Surgery for hepatic neuroendocrine tumors: a single institutional experience in Japan. Jpn J Clin Oncol 2007; 37(2):102–107.

75 Eriksson J, Stalberg P, Nilsson A, *et al.* Surgery and radio-frequency ablation for treatment of liver metastases from midgut and foregut carcinoids and endocrine pancreatic tumors. World J Surg 2008; 32:930–938.

76 Landry C, Scoggins C, McMasters K, Martin R. Management of hepatic metastases of gastrointestinal carcinoid tumors. J Surg Oncol 2008; 97(3):253–258.

77 Kianmanesh R, Sauvanet A, Hentic O, *et al.* Two-step surgery for synchronous bilobar liver metastases from digestive endocrine tumors: a safe approach for radical resection. Ann Surg 2008; 247(4):659–665.

78 Chambers A, Pasieka J, Dixon E, Rorsrad O. The palliative benefit of aggressive surgical intervention for both hepatic and mesenteric metastases from neuroendocrine tumors. Surgery 2008; 144(4):645–651.

79 Frilling A, Li J, Malamutmann E, Schmid K, Bockisch A, Broelsch C. Treatment of liver metastases from neuro-endocrine tumours in relation to the extent of hepatic disease. Br J Surg 2009; 96:175–184.

80 Scigliano S, Lebtahi R, Maire F, *et al.* Clinical and imaging follow-up after exhaustive liver resection of endocrine metastases: a 1five-year monocentric experience. Endocr Relat Cancer 2009; 16(3):977–990.

81 Glazer E, Tseng J, Al-Refaie W, *et al.* Long-term survival after surgical managment of neuroendocrine hepatic metastases. HPB 2010; 12:427–433.

82 Saxena A, Chua T, Sarkar A, Chu F, Liauw W, Zhao J, Morris D. Progression and survival results after radical hepatic metastasectomy of indolent advanced neuroendocrine neo-plasms (NENs) supports an aggressive surgical approach. Surgery 2011; 149(2):209–220.

83 Gaujoux S, Gönen M, Tang L, *et al.* Synchronous resection of primary and liver metastases for neuroendocrine tumors. Ann Surg Oncol 2012; 19:4270–4277.

84 Harrison L, Brennan M, Newman E, *et al.* Hepatic resection for noncolorectal nonneuroendocrine metastases: a fifteen-year experience with ninety-six patients. Surgery 1997; 121:625–632.

85 Elias D, Cavalcanti de Albuquerque A, Eggenspieler P, *et al.* Resection of liver metastases from a noncolorectal primary: indications and results based on 147 monocentric patients. J Am Coll Surg 1998; 187:487–493.

86 Lang H, Nussbaum K, Weimann A, Raab R. Liver resection for non-colorectal, non-neuroendocrine hepatic metastases. Chirurg 1999; 70(4):439–446.

87 Buell J, Rosen S, Yoshida A, *et al.* Hepatic resection: effective treatment for primary and secondary tumors. Surgery 2000; 128:686–693.

88 Hamy A, Paineau J, Mirallie E, Bizouarn P, Visset J. Hepatic resections for non-colorectal metastases: forty resections in 35 patients. Hepatogastroenterology 2000; 47(34):1090–1094.

89 Hemming A, Sielaff T, Gallinger S, *et al.* Hepatic resection of non-colorectal nonneuroendocrine metastases. Liver Trans-plantation 2000; 6:97–101.

90 Laurent C, Rullier E, Feyler A, Masson B, Saric J. Resection of noncolorectal and nonneuroendocrine liver metastases: late metastases are the only chance of cure. World J Surg 2001; 25:1532–1536.

91 Van Ruth S, Mutsaerts E, Zoetmulder F, Coevorden F. Metastasectomy for liver metastases of non-colorectal pri-maries. EJSO 2001; 27:662–667.

92 Yamada H, Katoh H, Kondo S, Okushiba S, Morikawa T. Hepatectomy for metastases from non-colorectal and non-neuroendocrine tumor. Anticancer Res 2001; 21(6A): 4159–4162.

93 Cordera F, Rea D, Rodriguez-Davalos M, Hoskin T, Nagor-ney D, Que F. Hepatic resection for non-colorectal non-neuroendocrine metastases. J Gastrointest Surg 2005; 9:1361–1370.

94 Yedibela S, Gohl J, Graz V, *et al.* Changes in indication and results after resection of hepatic metastases from noncolor-ectal primary tumors: a single-institutional review. Ann Surg Oncol 2005; 12(10):778–785.

95 Ercolani G, Grazi G, Ravaioli M. The role of liver resection for noncolorectal, nonneuroendocrine metastases: experience with 142 observed cases. Ann Surg Oncol 2005; 12(6):1–8.

96 Earle S, Perez E, Gutierrez J, *et al.* Hepatectomy enables prolonged survival in select patients with isolated noncolor-ectal liver metastasis. J Am Coll Surg 2006; 203:436–446.

97 Lendoire J, Moro M, Andriani O, *et al.* Liver resection for non-colorectal, non-neuroendocrine metastases: analysis of a multicenter study from Argentina. HPB 2007; 9:435–439.

98 Reddy S, Barbas A, Marroquin C, Morse M, Kuo P, Clary B. Resection of noncolorectal nonneuroendocrine liver metas-tases: a comparative analysis. J Am Coll Surg 2007; 204 (3):372–382.

99 Ercolani G, Vetrone G, Grazi G, *et al.* The role of liver surgery in the treatment of non-colorectal non-neuroendocrine metastases (NCRNNE). Analysis of 134 resected patients. Minerva Chirurg 2009; 64(6):551–558.

100 Lehner F, Ramackers W, Bektas H, Becker T, Klempnauer J. Liver resection for non-colorectal, non-neuroendocrine liver metastases – is hepatic resection justified as part of the onco-surgical treatment? Zentralbl Chir 2009; 134(5):430–436.

101 Marudanayagam R, Sandhu B, Perera M, *et al.* Liver resec-tion for metastatic soft tissue sarcoma: an analysis of prog-nostic factors. Eur J Surg Oncol 2011; 37(1):87–92.

102 Schmelze M, Eisenberger C, am Esch J, Matthaei H, Krausch M, Knoefel W. Non-colorectal, non-neuroendocrine, and non-sarcoma metastases of the liver: resection as a promis-ing tool in the palliative management. Langenbecks Arch Surg 2010; 395(3):227–234.

103 Duan X, Dong N, Zhang T, Li Q. Comparison of surgical outcomes in patients with colorectal liver metastases versus non-colorectal liver metastases: a Chinese experience. Hep-atol Res 2012; 42:296–303.

104 Takemura N, Saiura A, Koga R, *et al.* Long-term results of hepatic resection for non-colorectal, non-neuroendocrine liver metastasis. Hepatogastroenterology 2013; 127 (60):1705–1712.

105 Yoshimoto M, Tada T, Saito M, *et al*. Surgical treatment of hepatic metastases from breast cancer. Breast Cancer Res Treat 2000; 59:177–184.

106 Pocard M, Pouillart P, Asselain B, Salmon R. Hepatic resection in metastatic breast cancer: results and prognostic factors. Eur J Surg Oncol 2000; 26(2):155–159.

107 Thelen A, Benckert C, Jonas S, *et al*. Liver resection for metastases from breast cancer. J Surg Oncol 2008; 97:25–29.

108 Van Walsum G, de Ridder J, Verhoef C, *et al*. Resection of liver metastases in patients with breast cancer: survival and prognostic factors. EJSO 2012; 38:910–917.

109 Dittmar Y, Altendorf-Hofmann A, Schule S, *et al*. Liver resection in selected patients with metastatic breast cancer: a single-centre analysis and review of literature. J Cancer Res Clin Oncol 2013; 139(8):1317–1325.

110 Kostov D, Kobakov G, Yankov D. Prognostic factors related to surgical outcome of liver metastases of breast cancer. J Breast Cancer 2013; 16(2):184–192.

111 Sakamoto Y, Sano T, Shimada K, *et al*. Favorable Indications for hepatectomy in patients with liver metastasis from gastric cancer. J Surg Oncol 2007; 95:534–539.

112 Koga R, Yamamoto J, Ohyama S, *et al*. Liver resection for metastatic gastric cancer: experience with 42 patients including eight long-term survivors. Jpn J Clin Oncol 2007; 37(11):836–842.

113 Thelen A, Jonas S, Benchert C, *et al*. Liver resection for metastatic gastric cancer. Eur J Surg Oncol 2008; 34 (12):1328–1334.

114 Morise Z, Sugioka A, Hoshimoto S, *et al*. The role of hepatectomy for patients with liver metastases of gastric cancer. Hepatogastroenterology 2008; 55(85):1238–1241.

115 Makino H, Kunisaki C, Izumisawa Y, *et al*. Indication for hepatic resection in the treatment of liver metastasis from gastric cancer. Anticancer Res 2010; 30:2367–2376.

116 Tsujimoto H, Ichikura T, Ono S, *et al*. Outcomes for patients following hepatic resection of metastatic tumors from gastric cancer. Hepatol Int 2010; 4:406–413.

117 Schildberg C, Croner R, Merkel S, *et al*. Outcome of operative therapy of hepatic metastic stomach carcinoma: a retrospective analysis. World J Surg 2012; 36(4):872–878.

118 Dittmar Y, Altendorf-Hofmann A, Rauchfuss F, *et al*. Resection of liver metastases is beneficial in patients with gastric cancer: a report on 15 cases and review of literature. Gastric Cancer 2012; 15(2):131–136.

119 Baek H, Kim S, Cho E, *et al*. Hepatic resection for hepatic metastases from gastric adenocarcinoma. J Gastric Cancer 2013; 13(2):86–92.

120 Qiu J, Deng M, Li W, *et al*. Hepatic resection for synchronous hepatic metastasis from gastric cancer. EJSO 2013; 39:694–700.

121 Vigan L, Vellone M, Ferrero A, Guiliante F, Nuzzo G, Capussotti L. Liver resection for gastric cancer metastases. Hepatogastroenterology 2013; 60(123). doi: 10.5754/hge11187.

122 Bosquet J, Merideth M, Podratz K, Nagorney D. Hepatic resection for metachronous metastases from ovarian carcinoma. HPB 2006; 8:93–96.

123 Abood G, Bowen M, Potkul R, Aranha G, Shoup M. Hepatic resection for recurrent metastatic ovarian cancer. Am J Surg 2008; 195:370–373.

124 Lim M, Kang S, Lee K, *et al*. The clinical significance of hepatic parenchymal metastasis in patients with primary epithelial ovarian cancer. Gynecol Oncol 2009; 112:28–34.

125 Neumann U, Fotopoulou C, Schmeding M, *et al*. Clinical outcome of patients with advanced ovarian cancer after resection of liver metastases. Anticancer Res 2012; 32:4517–4522.

126 Aloia T, Adam R, Azoulay D, Bismuth H, Castaing D. Outcome following hepatic resection of metastatic renal tumors: the Paul Brousse Hospital experience. HPB 2006; 8:100–105.

127 Ruys A, Tanis P, Iris N, *et al*. Surgical treatment of renal cell cancer liver metastases: a population–based study. Ann Surg Oncol 2011; 18:1932–1938.

128 Langan R, Ripley R, Davis J, *et al*. Liver directed therapy for renal cell carcinoma. J Cancer 2012; 3:184–190.

129 Rehders A, Peiper M, Stoecklein N, *et al*. Hepatic metastasectomy for soft-tissue sarcomas: is it justified? World J Surg 2009; 33:111–117.

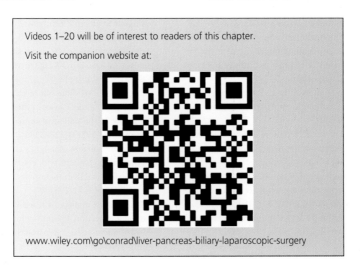

Videos 1–20 will be of interest to readers of this chapter.

Visit the companion website at:

www.wiley.com\go\conrad\liver-pancreas-biliary-laparoscopic-surgery

CHAPTER 15

Intraoperative laparoscopic ultrasound for laparoscopic hepatopancreatobiliary surgery

Kenichiro Araki[1] and Claudius Conrad[2]

[1]Department of General Surgical Science, Gunma University Graduate School of Medicine, Gunma, Japan
[2]Department of Surgical Oncology, University of Texas MD Anderson Cancer Center, Houston, USA

EDITOR COMMENT

In this chapter, we describe the critical importance of intraoperative ultrasound. A probe with at least four degrees of freedom is needed to overcome the limitations imposed by the trocar-to-target axis and to obtain optimal apposition of the probe against the target lesion. Nevertheless, trocar placement must anticipate the intraoperative use of ultrasound. Additionally, because of the limitation of the trocar-to-target axis, the laparoscopic ultrasound image might be more challenging to interpret and therefore requires practice. Frequent use of intraoperative ultrasound during laparoscopic liver surgery increases its safety through the identification of landmark structures and assessment of the relationship of lesions to critical anatomical structures. Ultrasound of the future liver remnant with and without Doppler mode excludes other lesions and ensures perfusion. Intraoperative laparoscopic ultrasound also has an important role during pancreatic surgery in nodal staging and in the identification of pancreatic neuroendocrine tumors. This chapter can help the reader to improve their ultrasound technique, while further practice is needed to optimize the skill.

Keywords: anatomical laparoscopic liver resection, contrast-enhanced laparoscopic ultrasound, intraoperative laparoscopic ultrasound

---

15.1 Introduction

Intraoperative ultrasonography (IOUS) is a critical tool for laparoscopic hepatopancreatobiliary (HPB) surgery. This technique is valuable both for the intraoperative diagnosis of liver or pancreas lesions but also for guidance of the actual resection. Especially in open and laparoscopic liver resection, laparoscopic IOUS technique is important for planning and guiding liver parenchymal transection. In our experience, the systematic use of IOUS is indispensable for both laparoscopic anatomical and nonanatomical liver resections [1]. In pancreas surgery, reports show that laparoscopic IOUS is useful for detecting tumors (especially neuroendocrine tumors) and screening for metastatic lesions. In this chapter, we describe our IOUS technique for laparoscopic HPB surgery, with a focus on laparoscopic IOUS techniques for laparoscopic liver resection.

15.2 Technical requirements for laparoscopic intraoperative ultrasonography

The patient is usually placed in a low lithotomy position, and the operating surgeon stands in the middle between the patient's legs; the ultrasound probe should be handled from this position. Five or six trocars are used in the right upper quadrant of the abdomen and maintained in position with a focus on optimal triangulation. While most trocars are 5 mm in size, we usually insert two 12 mm (or 10 mm) trocars in an axis that allows for using the ultrasound probe while maintaining an optimal view with the camera on the liver. The observed liver anatomy and target lesions should complement the mental image obtained preoperatively using multidetector computed tomography (CT) or magnetic resonance imaging (MRI).

Laparoscopic Liver, Pancreas, and Biliary Surgery, First Edition.
Edited by Claudius Conrad and Brice Gayet.

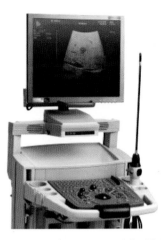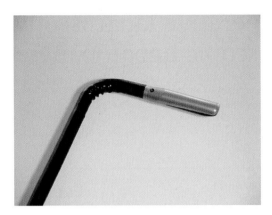

Figure 15.1 Pro Focus ultrasound system and flexible laparoscopic probe (BK Medical).

The laparoscopic ultrasound probe should have a flexible tip to allow for optimal apposition with the liver. This probe can be adjusted through an angle of up to 90° in four planes by two levers. Keeping the handle as a reference in an upright position, possible movements are up, down, left, and right as well as twisting the probe (Figure 15.1). Thus, it can be placed into the optimal relationship to the target structure to obtain a high-quality ultrasound image, despite the limitations in movements defined by the trocar–target axis.

The ultrasound monitor is optimally placed next to the laparoscopic monitor to allow for in-line working. Preferred over this approach is the "picture-in-picture" mode on the laparoscopic monitor, which allows the surgeon to see both laparoscopic and ultrasound images on one monitor, which further optimizes ergonomics. Using a remote control function of the ultrasound system optimizes team dynamics and facilitates making changes to the ultrasound settings such as changing parameters of the echo mode, measuring tumor margin, and switching Doppler blood flow mode (Figure 15.2).

15.2.1 Intraoperative ultrasonography with contrast enhancement in liver

Recent studies of intraoperative contrast-enhanced ultrasound (CEUS) with different contrast agents have shown that it is more sensitive, specific, and accurate than normal IOUS, CT, or MRI in defining resectability of liver metastases or hepatocellular carcinoma. It is now recognized that the more aggressive the adopted surgical approach, the higher the impact of intraoperative CEUS. Also, in laparoscopic procedures, intraoperative CEUS can be helpful to exclude new liver lesions not previously discovered on preoperative imaging. The new guideline for the use of CEUS was published in 2013 [2].

Contrast agents for ultrasonography are now licensed in many parts of the world. There are two vascular contrast agents: SonoVue (sulfur hexafluoride with a phospholipid shell; Bracco SpA, Milan, Italy) and Definity/Luminity (octafluoropropane [perflutren] with a lipid shell; Lantheus Medical, Billerica, MA, USA). Injections may be repeated for global assessment or to assess the arterial phase enhancement of identified lesions for their characterization. After it has disappeared from the

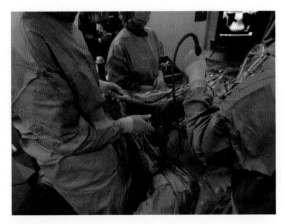

Figure 15.2 Handling the laparoscopic IOUS with a remote controller.

vascular pool, Sonazoid (perfluorobutane with a phospholipid shell: hydrogenated egg phosphatidyl serine; Daiichi-Sankyo, Tokyo, Japan) persists for several hours in liver and spleen. Sonazoid is phagocytosed by Kupffer cells, which contributes to its persistent uptake in the liver. However, this agent is licensed only in Japan and South Korea (November 2013). Using Sonazoid enhanced intraoperative ultrasound, detection of malignant focal liver lesions begins 10 minutes after injection.

15.3 Laparoscopic ultrasonography for liver resection

Laparoscopic hepatectomy is a safe procedure and has potential advantages over open surgery with respect to blood loss and postoperative hospital stay [3,4]. However, significant bleeding is more difficult to control during laparoscopic hepatectomy than during an open approach and therefore the prevention of vascular injury is crucial. This should be achieved not only through an excellent preoperative understanding of the vascular anatomy derived from preoperative imaging but also through real-time image guidance during surgery. Some procedures, such as posterosuperior segmentectomy (Sg7 or Sg8) and limited resection for deeply located liver tumors, require expert laparoscopic hepatectomy techniques. For these procedures, accurate real-time imaging of liver anatomy and a thought-out operative resection plan are necessary. In order to accomplish this, the use of

intraoperative ultrasound imaging is of the utmost importance.

The procedural steps for IOUS of hepatectomy are as follows. After screening the entire liver, we focus our attention on the future liver remnant in case of cancer surgery. It is more important to rule out any undetected lesions in the future liver remnant than to identify liver lesions in the liver to be resected. The tumor characteristics of known tumors are important as known isodense liver lesions predict a higher likelihood of missing lesions not identified on preoperative imaging. The hepatic veins and their branches and their relationship to the resection line are determined and the portal structures at the transection plane visualized. After this information has been gathered, we determine the vertical (longitudinal) and horizontal (latitudinal) lines of the parenchymal transection plane. Doppler mode is used to identify the portal pedicles, hepatic veins, and hepatic arteries if necessary.

Table 15.1 summarizes technical differences between laparoscopic and open IOUS techniques. The laparoscopic ultrasound probe position and angulation are restricted by the trocar's position, abdominal cavity, and target area of the liver. The laparoscopic liver surgeon is frequently required to place the probe at an angle different from that of an open procedure because of the laparoscopic restrictions imposed by the trocar–target axis. Thus, laparoscopic surgeons must consider the relationship between the trocar positions and liver in order to place the ultrasonic probe in such a way that the resulting image is easily

Table 15.1 Technical differences between laparoscopic and open IOUS in liver surgery.

	Laparoscopic IOUS	Open IOUS
Visualization of ultrasound view	On the monitor (PiP mode)	Direct view
Width of scan area	Good	Good
Depth of scan area	Good	Good
Freedom of ultrasound probe	Limited (need flexible probe)	Good
Direction tendency of probe	Vertical	Horizontal
Application for PS segments	Transdiaphragmatic access	Mobilization of right lobe
Additional tactile information	Poor	Good
Ultrasound-guided puncture	Difficult (biopsy attachment)	Easy
Contrast enhancement	Possible	Possible

IOUS, intraoperative ultrasonography; PiP, picture in picture; PS, posterosuperior.

interpretable. Achieving an optimal and easily interpretable ultrasound image is facilitated with a laparoscopic probe that is flexible.

An important goal of IOUS is to identify portal and hepatic vessels and their positional relationship. In major hepatectomy procedures, IOUS allows for the identification of the middle (right and left hepatectomy) or the right (central hepatectomy and extended left hepatectomy) hepatic veins as a landmark of the parenchymal transection plane and the drainage branches of the hepatic vein. The flexibility of the IOUS probe allows placement of the probe in the necessary direction. We discourage the use of fixed probes as the probe orientation is determined by the relationship of trocar to target and the most effective orientation of the probe might not be achievable. In segmentectomies, it is important to identify the vertical (longitudinal) demarcation line and IOUS allows for visualization of the hepatic vein as a vertical landmark; for example, the middle hepatic vein is between segments IV and V/VIII, and the right hepatic vein is between segments V/VIII and VI/VII. To identify the horizontal (latitudinal) demarcation line of the segment, such as that between segments V and VIII, or segments VI and VII, IOUS allows for visualization of the bifurcation of the portal pedicle as a horizontal landmark.

Below, we describe six applications of IOUS, which highlight the importance of it. The cases demonstrated in the accompanying video (Video 1) are left lateral sectionectomy, right hepatectomy, and segmentectomy VIII. We aimed to describe general principles of our IOUS technique in this video, so it can be adapted for other procedures, such as limited (wedge or partial) resection, left hepatectomy, and so on.

15.3.1 Identification of hepatic and portal vessels in left lateral sectionectomy

In left lateral sectionectomy, it is important to understand the distance between the portal pedicle and left hepatic vein along the transection plane using IOUS (Figure 15.3). The video shows identification of the portal pedicle (P2, P3) and left hepatic vein, and their subsequent safe resection. In this procedure, the middle hepatic vein also needs to be identified, because its drainage runs close to the transection plane in the upper part of the parenchymal transection plane (see Figure 15.3).

15.3.2 Visualization and dissection of branches of the hepatic vein during major hepatectomy

In major hepatectomies (e.g. right and left hepatectomy), we identify with IOUS the middle hepatic vein as the landmark vein as well as its branches (V4, V5, and V8 and the fissure veins) before commencing with the parenchymal transection. The video shows that the branches of V4, V5, and V8 are exposed during right hepatectomy (Figure 15.4) and can be safely dissected (V5 and V8) or preserved (V4). These steps described in the video for a right hepatectomy are analogous for a left hepatectomy.

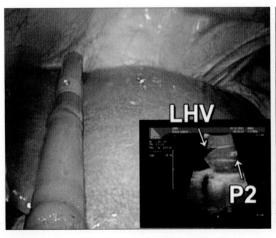 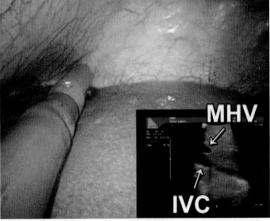

Figure 15.3 Laparoscopic IOUS in left lateral sectionectomy.

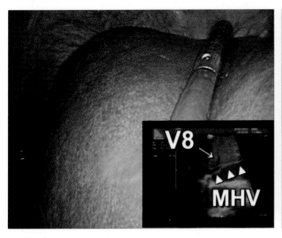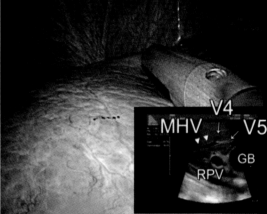

Figure 15.4 Laparoscopic IOUS in major hepatectomy.

15.3.3 Determination of the parenchymal transection plane in segmentectomy

For segmentectomies, we visualized the landmark hepatic vein as the vertical (longitudinal) demarcation line using IOUS and bifurcation of the portal pedicle as the horizontal (latitudinal) demarcation line in each procedure (Figure 15.5). In the video we demonstrate a resection of Sg8: we visualize the middle and right hepatic veins as the landmarks of the vertical line and the P8 portal pedicle as the landmark of the horizontal line (see Figure 15.5). In limited resection, accurate recognition of the hepatic vein and portal pedicle near the resected liver tumor is also important, so these steps are also important for limited (wedge or partial) resection.

15.3.4 Identification the tumor-bearing portal pedicles for segmentectomies

The tumor-bearing portal pedicle was determined with IOUS, which allowed for visualization of the portal flow and calculation of the margin. We sometimes inject dye or indocyanine green into the vein in order to visualize the true limits of the segment [5]. The video shows the Sg8 portal pedicle and measurement of the resection margin (see Figure 15.5). We used regenerated oxidized cellulose (Surgicel Fibrillar, Ethicon Inc., Somerville, NJ, USA) for hemostasis during parenchymal dissection. In addition, the echogenicity of the material is useful for visualization of the transecting line as the echo artifact can be clearly visualized in the parenchymal transection plane.

15.3.5 Ensuring intact vascularization in the remnant parenchyma

Doppler mode is useful for detecting intact vascularization in the remnant liver parenchyma. The video shows a case of segmentectomy VIII after left lateral sectionectomy and visualization of the preserved hepatic vein vascularization (V4a, V4b) in the remnant segment IV after the dissection between segments IV and VIII.

15.3.6 Visualization of the drainage of the right hepatic vein for posterosuperior segmentectomy

Posterosuperior segmentectomy (Sg7 or Sg8) is one of the most difficult procedures of laparoscopic hepatectomy. In this procedure, we used a right intercostal and transdiaphragmatic access. Transdiaphragmatic trocar placement allows for a direct approach to the drainage of the right hepatic vein. Such transdiaphragmatic trocars might facilitate accurate location of the position of the right hepatic vein and venous branches for parenchymal dissection with IOUS. In the video, using IOUS, we expose the V8 branch of the right hepatic vein (Figure 15.6), safely perform the dissection, and finally expose the roots of the middle and right hepatic veins.

15.4 Laparoscopic ultrasonography for pancreas surgery

In pancreatic surgery, laparoscopic ultrasonography provides the surgeon with an additional sensitive means of

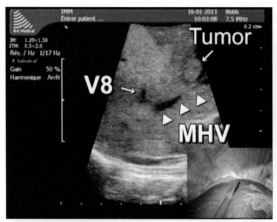

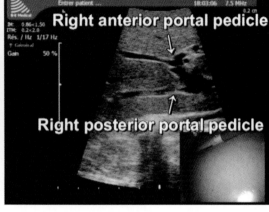

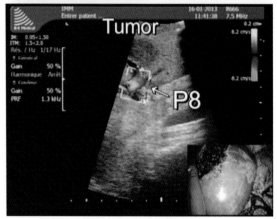

Figure 15.5 Laparoscopic IOUS in segmentectomy.

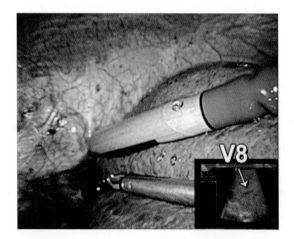

Figure 15.6 Laparoscopic IOUS in posterosuperior segmentectomy.

detecting small metastases during staging and allows for the assessment of local tumor invasion, regional nodal involvement, and distant metastatic spread to the liver [6]. Several articles have reported encouraging preliminary results with laparoscopy and laparoscopic ultrasonography in the assessment of patients with pancreatic tumors and liver metastases. We usually perform laparoscopic staging with IOUS for presumably resectable pancreatic cancer. This frequently demonstrates metastastic disease or local unresectability, which precludes curable resection. This approach reduces the rate of nontherapeutic laparotomy.

Resection for pancreatic neuroendocrine tumor requires accurate localization. However, pancreatic neuroendocrine tumors are frequently difficult to detect with the laparoscopic view only. Their localization can be greatly facilitated through the use of intraoperative ultrasound. Several articles have described the utility of laparoscopic ultrasonography for the intraoperative localization of neuroendocrine tumors [7]. Because of their hypervascularity, IOUS with contrast enhancement can be performed for selected, difficult-to-detect pancreatic neuroendocrine tumors.

15.5 Laparoscopic ultrasonography for biliary surgery

In biliary surgery, IOUS has been reported to be an effective tool not only in detecting bile duct stones but also in evaluating the biliary anatomy [8]. We routinely use laparoscopic IOUS during laparoscopic cholecystectomy to rule out the existence of common bile duct stones. Some reports suggest that routine use of IOUS reduces the need for intraoperative cholangiography during laparoscopic cholecystectomy with high sensitivity and without increased overall cost [9].

KEY POINTS

- Intraoperative laparoscopic ultrasound is crucial for operative planning, lesion detection, and ensuring perfusion of the future liver remnant.

- Contrast-enhanced laparoscopic ultrasound can facilitate lesion detection and characterization.

- Laparoscopic ultrasound can facilitate the identification of pancreatic neuroendocrine tumors.

- Advanced laparoscopic anatomical resections can only be performed if the surgeon is well versed in the use of laparoscopic ultrasound.

References

1 Araki K, Conrad C, Ogiso S, Kuwano H, Gayet B. Intraoperative ultrasonography of laparoscopic hepatectomy: key technique for safe liver transection. J Am Coll Surg 2014; 218:e37–41.

2 Claudon M, Dietrich CF, Choi BI, *et al.* Guidelines and good clinical practice recommendations for contrast enhanced ultrasound (CEUS) in the liver-update 2012. Ultraschall Med 2013; 34(1):11–29.

3 Nguyen KT, Marsh JW, Tsung A, Steel JJ, Gamblin TC, Geller DA. Comparative benefits of laparoscopic vs open hepatic resection: a critical appraisal. Arch Surg 2011; 146(3):348–356.

4 Croome KP, Yamashita MH. Laparoscopic vs open hepatic resection for benign and malignant tumors: an updated meta-analysis. Arch Surg 2010; 145(11):1109–1118.

5 Ishizawa T, Zuker NB, Kokudo N, Gayet B. Positive and negative staining of hepatic segments by use of fluorescent imaging techniques during laparoscopic hepatectomy. Arch Surg 2012; 147(4):393–394.

6 John TG, Greig JD, Carter DC, Garden OJ. Carcinoma of the pancreatic head and periampullary region. Tumor staging with laparoscopy and laparoscopic ultrasonography. Ann Surg 1995; 221(2):156–164.

7 Iihara M, Kanbe M, Okamoto T, Ito Y, Obara T. Laparoscopic ultrasonography for resection of insulinomas. Surgery 2001; 130(6):1086–1091.

8 Biffl WL, Moore EE, Offner PJ, Franciose RJ, Burch JM. Routine intraoperative laparoscopic ultrasonography with selective cholangiography reduces bile duct complications during laparoscopic cholecystectomy. J Am Coll Surg 2001; 193:272–280.

9 Machi J, Oishi AJ, Tajiri T, Murayama KM, Furumoto NL, Oishi RH. Routine laparoscopic ultrasound can significantly reduce the need for selective intraoperative cholangiography during cholecystectomy. Surg Endosc 2007; 21(2):270–274.

CHAPTER 16

Minimally invasive liver surgery: indications and contraindications

Thomas A. Aloia

Department of Surgical Oncology, University of Texas MD Anderson Cancer Center, Houston, USA

EDITOR COMMENT

This chapter describes a conceptual framework for the indications and contraindications for liver resection for achieving the healthcare goals set forth by the Institute of Medicine's publication *Safe, Effective, Patient-Centered, Timely, Efficient, and Equitable Care*. This review of the available literature indicates that the majority of minimally invasive liver resections have been minor procedures. Only a limited number of highly specialized centers have reported major minimally invasive liver resections. To us, these data indicated that there is a need for greater diffusion of surgical concepts and techniques that would allow for the safe and oncologically sound expansion of more advanced laparoscopic liver surgery – a prime impetus for creating this work. Further, the author calls for introspective professionalism, oversight, and monitoring of exact indications on a case-by-case basis to safely expand the experience to more extensive laparoscopic liver resection. These are concepts that certainly are not limited to minimally invasive liver resections, but the complex nature of advanced minimally invasive liver resection demands apprehension of a significant number of oncological, patient management, and technical concepts that have been presented to the reader throughout this work.

Keywords: indications for laparoscopic liver surgery, indications for minimally invasive liver surgery, oncological outcomes of laparoscopic liver surgery, professionalism in laparoscopic liver surgery, quality control in laparoscopic liver surgery, safety in laparoscopic liver surgery

---

16.1 Introduction

The past 20 years have seen a rapid expansion of the indications for minimally invasive approaches to liver surgery. The increased utilization of minimally invasive approaches to liver resection has paralleled improvements in open surgical technique, anesthetic management, and multidisciplinary care that have combined to greatly improve the safety of liver surgery. Given our current ability to rapidly introduce and communicate new techniques and technologies, there is no doubt that the indications for liver surgery and minimally invasive approaches will continue to evolve. As experience builds, new techniques are disseminated and new equipment is introduced, the indications for minimally invasive liver resection will undoubtedly expand, potentially mak-ing the specific content of this chapter obsolete. To reduce the chance of this occurring, this chapter intentionally avoids drawing concrete "lines in the sand" regarding the indications and contraindications to minimally invasive liver resection. Instead, it proposes a more flexible conceptual framework for evaluating resectability issues that may accommodate both predictable and unpredictable future advances in the field.

From a quality of medicine perspective, the discussion of indications and contraindications for minimally invasive liver surgery can be framed by the Institute of Medicine (IOM) healthcare goals of *Safe, Effective, Patient-Centered, Timely, Efficient, and Equitable Care* [1] (Table 16.1). Independent of advances in instrumentation, when these criteria are met, there is and will continue to be a clear indication for this approach to liver

---

Laparoscopic Liver, Pancreas, and Biliary Surgery, First Edition.
Edited by Claudius Conrad and Brice Gayet.
© 2017 John Wiley & Sons, Ltd. Published 2017 by John Wiley & Sons, Ltd.

Table 16.1 Conceptual framework of indications and contraindications for minimally invasive approaches to liver resection based on Institute of Medicine (IOM) quality of care aims.

IOM aim	Indications	Contraindications
Safe	Surgical skill in and experience with hepatobiliary and minimally invasive surgery Proper equipment and techniques that provide adequate patient positioning, exposure, and visualization of operative planes of dissection A liver transection strategy that limits bleeding and bile leaks Ability to progress through the procedure in a timely fashion, minimizing exposure to transfusion, anesthetic complications, and surgical team fatigue	Tumor locations, patient body habitus, and/or adhesions that increase the risk of injury to adjacent structures or impair the ability to obtain vascular control in case of hemorrhage
Effective	An overall patient experience that provides less pain, earlier return to normal activity, and earlier return to intended adjuvant oncological therapies	Inability to identify and/or treat all sites of disease Inability to achieve adequate oncological margins Inability to perform adequate portal lymphadenectomy
Patient centered	Ability to lessen postoperative pain In selected cases, the ability to provide a cosmetic benefit Limiting selection of benign tumor patients to those with malignant potential and/or significant symptoms Willingness to convert to hybrid or open approach surgery in cases of perceived or realized issues with patient safety and/or surgical efficacy	
Efficient	Ability to solve diagnostic dilemmas, limiting the need for subsequent follow-up and intervention	
Equitable	Ability to provide equivalent surgical efficacy with lower postoperative care costs	Dependence on expensive instrumentation that creates excessive intraoperative costs
Timely	Ability to provide surgical intervention within an oncologically appropriate time interval	

surgery. Ultimately, however, the surgical principles of resectability, and in particular the oncological principles of malignant tumor resection, will remain inviolable.

16.2 General comments

To date, the vast majority of minimally invasive liver resection cases reported in the literature have been performed for benign indications or for small peripherally located malignant liver tumors [2–4]. When outcomes for these cases are compared with the general population of patients historically and currently treated with open approach liver surgery, they are favorable [2]. In almost all of these studies, however, the median magnitude liver resection is greater in the open approach group, and it is therefore difficult to separate the morbidity contribution of case magnitude from that of the surgical approach [5–8]

(Table 16.2). For example, Cannon et al. compared 35 laparoscopic hepatectomy cases with both a historical open cohort and a contemporary open cohort. In general, the outcomes in the laparoscopic cohort were superior to those of the open cohort; however, 83% of patients in the laparoscopic cohort underwent anatomical hepatectomy along sectional planes while only 50% of those in the historical open cohort and 52% of those in the open contemporary cohort underwent anatomical hepatectomy, potentially explaining differences in blood loss, bile leak, and other complications [9].

Unfortunately, despite the 20 years that have elapsed since the introduction of minimally invasive liver surgery [10], we have failed to design and execute a scientifically valid prospective study comparing these approaches [11]. Left with retrospective comparisons between larger magnitude and more complex open surgery and smaller magnitude and more straightforward

Table 16.2 Selected reports comparing open to minimally invasive hepatectomy.

	Open group	MIS group	Transfusion	Estimated blood loss	Conversion rate	Length of stay	Morbidity	Mortality	Comments
Mala 2002 [59]	n = 14	n = 13	7.1% versus 7.6%	500 mL versus 600 mL	0%	8.5 versus 4 days	28% versus 15%	0% versus 0%	Retrospective, case matched
Morino 2003 [66]	n = 30	n = 30	6.6% versus 13%	479 mL versus 300 mL	0%	8.7 versus 6.4 days	6.6% versus 6.6%	0% versus 0%	Retrospective, case matched
Lesurtel 2003 [3]	n = 20	n = 18	15% versus 0%	429 mL versus 236 mL	11%	10 versus 8 days	15% versus 11%	0% versus 0%	Retrospective, case–control
Laurent 2003 [23]	n = 14	n = 13	28% versus 7.6%	720 mL versus 260 mL	15%	12.5 versus 8 days	50% versus 36%	14% versus 0%	Retrospective, case matched
Lee 2007 [67]	n = 25	n = 25	0% vs. 4%	100 mL versus 250 mL	8%	7 vs 4 days	5.2% versus 5.2%	0% versus 0%	Retrospective, matched pair
Cai 2008 [31]	n = 31	n = 31	Not reported	588 mL versus 503 mL	3.2%	12.2 versus 7.5 days	16% versus 0%	0% versus 0%	Retrospective, matched pair
Castaing 2009 [7]	n = 60	n = 60	36% versus 15%	Not reported	10%	10 versus 11 days	28% versus 26%	1.7% versus 1.7%	Retrospective case matched
Sarpel 2009 [68]	n = 56	n = 20	not reported	Not reported	17%	Not reported	7.1% versus 5%	Not reported	Retrospective, case matched
Dagher 2009 [28]	n = 50	n = 22	18% versus 14%	735 mL versus 519 mL	9%	12.5 versus 8.2 days	34% versus 9%	2% versus 0%	Retrospective
Belli 2009 [5]	n = 125	n = 54	25% versus 11%	580 mL versus 297 mL	7%	Not reported	36% versus 18%	2% in the laparoscopic group	Retrospective
Tranchart 2009 [8]	n = 42	n = 42	16.7% versus 9.5%	724 mL versus 364 mL	5%	9.6 versus 6.7 days	11.9% versus 9.5%	2% versus 2%	Retrospective, matched pair
Cannon 2011 [9]	n = 140	n = 35	32% versus 17%	385 mL versus 202 mL	Not reported	8.3 versus 4.8 days	49% versus 23%	1.4% versus 0%	Retrospective, case matched
Guerron 2012 [41]	n = 40	n = 40,	5% versus 20%	753 mL versus 376 mL	5%	6.5 versus 3.7 days	20% versus 15%	0% versus 0%	Retrospective, case matched
Doughtie 2013 [12]	n = 84	n = 8	31% versus 14%	400 mL versus 225 mL	0%	7 versus 3.5 days	60.5% versus 12.5%	9% versus 0%	Retrospective, case matched

MIS, minimally invasive surgery.

minimally invasive surgery, we are forced to constrain our conclusions regarding the comparative safety and efficacy of each approach [12].

However, experience with minimally invasive major hepatectomy is increasingly being reported [9,13–15], allowing a more precise comparison between outcomes that are largely dependent only on surgical approach. Most of the reports on major hepatectomy come from specialized and high-volume centers [13,14,16,17]. When considering a discussion about the indications and contraindications of these approaches, it is therefore critical to take into account the skill and experience of the operative team. One surgeon/center may be very proficient and safe at minimally invasive major liver resection while another surgeon/center would be contraindicated to perform a difficult minimally invasive liver resection based on a lack of experience, support, or equipment.

16.3 Aim 1: Safe

In determining the appropriateness of any treatment or approach, the primary consideration is patient safety. Surgical experience and skill are baseline requirements to achieve safe minimally invasive liver resections. Many have advocated that only the subset of surgeons who are dually trained in hepatobiliary surgery and minimally invasive surgery are adequately equipped to safely perform these operations [18]. However, significant numbers of hepatobiliary surgeons have successfully "retrained" in laparoscopic techniques, largely aided by a broad experience with laparoscopic cholecystectomy, to achieve an adequate level of safety with at least minor minimally invasive liver resection [19]. Given the technical rigor of these cases, one study estimated that the slope of the learning curve for minimally invasive liver surgery may not inflect until over 60 cases were performed [20], potentially limiting the indications for major laparoscopic liver surgery to a small subset of high-volume centers. Of course, it is expected that minor resections would be mastered with a lower number of cases.

The contribution of adequate equipment to the safety of minimally invasive liver surgery cannot be overestimated. As with any surgical approach, adequate exposure and visualization are paramount in performing safe minimally invasive surgery. Liver surgery poses unique challenges with regard to these two attributes. The location of

the liver in the right upper quadrant of the abdomen, with over half of the liver parenchyma below the horizon of a typical laparoscopic view, makes visualization of the relevant anatomy difficult. Both the porta hepatis and the vena cava are, likewise, obscured over the visual horizon of the colon and duodenum, creating the need to position the camera and working ports in a more cephalad/subcostal orientation than is the case in general abdominal laparoscopy. Obesity may pose additional challenges to visualization of certain tumor locations within the liver. In some cases and locations, however, visualization with angled lens laparoscopes may be superior to that with open anterior incisions. Irrespective of this variability, failure to adequately visualize the transection plane and/or critical vascular and other surrounding structures is an absolute *contraindication* to minimally invasive liver resection.

There is a growing body of literature that defines several additional factors that contribute to the safe application of minimally invasive approaches to liver surgery. With regard to patient safety, a primary objective of open and minimally invasive liver surgery is the ability to avoid hemorrhage and/or to be able to recover from a vascular injury [14]. Traditionally, with regard to bleeding, the main component of liver surgery safety has been the magnitude of resection, with larger magnitude resections engendering more risk for vascular injury. To avoid these risks, the minimally invasive liver surgeon requires the ability to expose and control adjacent vascular structures within the porta hepatis and retrohepatic/vena caval areas [21].

Even in the most skilled hands, laparoscopic approaches to liver resection may be associated with an impaired ability to recover quickly from a major vascular injury. Although conversion rates are not well documented for minimally invasive liver surgery, ranging from 0% to 15% (see Table 16.2), bleeding is clearly the most frequent *indication* for conversion [2,7,16,22,23]. Likewise, the ability to rapidly control vascular structures, particularly in teaching environments, is a perceived advantage of hybrid and hand-assisted approaches to major hepatic resection [4,24–27].

The hemostatic issues with open and minimally invasive liver surgery fall into two categories: sudden large-volume blood loss from vascular injury and general hemostasis along the cut surface of the liver. On the whole, catastrophic bleeding events have been infrequently described in minimally invasive liver surgery.

This is likely due to disincentives to self-report such complications as well as a historical avoidance of major resections that would risk significant vascular injury. As indications are extended to larger and more complex resections, however, a persistent *contraindication* to minimally invasive approaches will be tumor locations and resections that create situations with either high likelihood of vascular injury and/or limited ability to rapidly control hemorrhage.

With regard to subcatastrophic bleeding, typically from the parenchymal transection surface, both the technique of transection and the availability of topical thermal and nonthermal coagulants need to be considered. Although expensive, there are an ever increasing number of devices and agents to serve this purpose, almost all of which are only supported by preclinical evidence of efficacy. In the reported literature to date, dominated by nonchemotherapy-treated patients and minor hepatectomy procedures, rates of estimated blood loss (EBL) and perioperative transfusion in minimally invasive liver resection are low [2]. In the limited series from the most advanced centers reporting on minimally invasive major hepatectomy, the median blood transfusion rates acceptably range from 14% to 17% [6,7,13,14,28]. One point to note is that a catastrophic hemorrhage will frequently not be reflected in reported median EBL and transfusion numbers. These events in minimally invasive liver surgery are likely rare but important reminders of the narrow therapeutic index of liver resection regardless of approach [29–31].

In many cases, the size and location of the tumor may increase the risk of a vascular injury or impede access to vascular control to a degree that completely *contraindicates* a minimally invasive approach. For bulky liver tumors, a frequent issue is difficulty in laparoscopic mobilization of the liver. Unlike general abdominal laparoscopy, the ribcage does not allow the pneumoperitoneum to significantly enlarge the volume of work space for liver surgery. Although reports of minimally invasive liver resection for large liver tumors are emerging [12], bulky tumors that can be mobilized and manipulated through an open incision can at times completely obscure laparoscopic transection planes and critical structures. Visualization issues may be compounded by body habitus, adhesions, and intra-abdominal obesity. Ultimately, the safety value of the surgical principles of positioning, exposure, and lighting remain constant for minimally and maximally invasive surgery.

Another unanswered issue regarding the safety of minimally invasive liver surgery is the ability to prevent postoperative bile leak. Despite better understanding of liver anatomy and transection techniques, postoperative bile leak continues to be a frequent and significant complication in liver surgery [32]. As this is largely related to magnitude of resection, observational studies addressing mainly minor laparoscopic liver resections have reported low rates of this complication (1.4%) [2]. As minimally invasive liver surgery is expanded to more substantial resections with broad transection surface areas and division of larger bile ducts deeper within the liver parenchyma, it is anticipated that the bile leak rate would rise.

For minimally invasive major hepatectomy, most surgeons use a vessel sealing device, endovascular staplers or a combination to transect the liver parenchyma. Few reports exist comparing biliary complications after major transections using these devices and techniques [33]. In practice, the bile leak rate should be less than 5% for major resection. Given the significant impact that postoperative bile leak has on related morbidity, including venous thromboembolism, delayed discharge, delayed recovery, need for additional procedures, and costs of care, minimally invasive techniques that result in a bile leak rate in excess of this number may signal a *contraindication* to these approaches on a center-by-center basis [32,34].

16.4 Aim 2: Effective

After the safety of the operation, the efficacy of the operative approach is the next most important factor that should inform the discussion of surgical indication or contraindication. In contrast to patient safety (the avoidance of a negative outcome, typically a short-term consideration), the effectiveness or quality of liver surgery (achievement of a positive outcome) is measured on a longer time scale across several different domains.

With regard to liver resection, the most important domain of efficacy of the minimally invasive approach is freedom from recurrence of malignant disease. Intraoperative factors that directly contribute to this domain include identification and oncological resection of all tumor sites. To this end, technical ability with intraoperative ultrasound and availability of appropriate laparoscopic ultrasound probes and consoles are necessary to assist in the identification of small, previously undiagnosed tumors. Although several studies have suggested that intraoperative ultrasound may identify previously underappreciated lesions in 3–50% of patients [35,36], it is unclear what percentage of these findings were aided by liver palpation and complete visualization that subsequently directed the ultrasound to small subcapsular lesions [24,37–39]. As totally laparoscopic approaches are limited in their ability to visualize and, in particular, palpate subtle liver tumors, a higher premium must be placed on preoperative imaging and intraoperative ultrasound to detect occult disease and avoid early "recurrence" from undetected lesions after laparoscopic resection. Whenever there is concern for additional malignant disease that is not laparoscopically accessible, a conversion to open surgery is *indicated* [7].

Frequently in hepatobiliary cancer surgery, nodal recovery is critical to staging and prognosis, as well as providing the *indication* for postoperative therapies. As such, the ability to perform a minimally invasive portal, aortocaval, and celiac node dissection is often comparably as important as the ability to perform the liver tumor resection. In contrast to liver transection, which can be performed in the linear plane of the typically rigid instruments used in laparoscopic liver surgery, portal lymphadenectomy requires a perpendicular set of angles of attack with a more vertical orientation. This necessitates creativity, unique technical skills, and, at times, additional port sites and special instrumentation, all of which may be necessary to consider a laparoscopic approach *indicated* for resection of liver malignancy [40].

To date, we have few data regarding long-term oncological outcomes in patients treated with minimally invasive hepatectomy. There are several recently published studies documenting longer term survivals in patients with laparoscopically resected metastatic and primary liver malignancies that suggest acceptable midterm outcomes (Table 16.3). It should be noted that the median follow-up intervals in these reports rarely exceed 24 months, statistically limiting the validity of benchmark five-year survival estimates [6,7,16,29,41,42]. Also, none of these studies report early recurrence rates that may reflect "missed" disease in the operating room. This having been noted, there is no reason to expect that well-performed minimally invasive liver surgery for malignant indications would result in any decrement in long-term recurrence rates and overall survivals. Indeed, data regarding modulation of the immunosuppressive effects of surgery associated with minimally invasive approaches

may provide an oncological advantage to these patients [43,44]. Further correlative clinical studies are required to determine the realization of this theoretical benefit.

In the absence of data comparing long-term oncological outcomes, the only available surrogate oncological quality indicator is pathological margin status. Although the adequate oncological width of the margin of resection is debated based on tumor histology, preoperative therapy, and other anatomical and technical factors, in general it is clear that patients with metastatic disease have lower recurrence rates after R0 resection [45,46] and patients with hepatocellular carcinoma (HCC) have lower recurrence rates with anatomical resections that entirely remove the segments of liver that contain tumor [47,48]. Based on these concepts, the inability to achieve adequate oncological margins is one of the strongest *contraindications* to minimally invasive surgery.

The vast majority of minimally invasive liver resections reported in the literature are for benign indications and/or small tumors requiring minor liver resection [2,49,50]. In both of these scenarios, adequate margins are fairly simple to obtain, as reflected in the modest margin-positive rates for minimally invasive liver resection ranging from 0% to 18%, with rates of margins less than 1 cm ranging from 0% to 43% [2,11,26] (see Table 16.3). As minimally invasive approaches extend to involve larger magnitude resections, it may be anticipated that margin status will become a major focus of outcomes analyses [51]. Certainly, the long-term outcomes of minimally invasive liver surgery need to be thoroughly studied, as a marginal difference in short-term length of stay cannot be considered more valuable than a lower recurrence rate in oncological surgery.

The nature of the current instrumentation for minimally invasive liver surgery imposes some limitations to access and exposure of liver tumors, placing surgeons at higher risk of obtaining inadequate oncological margins. As almost all visualization ports are placed anterior and caudal to the liver, segments II, III, IVb, V, and VI are the most accessible for resection [26,52,53]. Segments I, IVb, VIII, and particularly segment VII are difficult to visualize adequately [38,54,55]. The fixed planar orientation of laparoscopic instruments creates further obstacles to margin-negative tumor removal in these difficult locations. When tumor location justifies an intended line of liver division on a sectional plane (i.e. right hepatectomy, left hepatectomy, left lateral bisegmentectomy), the

Table 16.3 Selected reports of oncological outcomes after minimally invasive liver resection for cancer.

	n=	Anatomical/nonanatomical	Minor/major	Margins	Recurrence	Overall survival	Follow-up
Mala 2002 [59]	21	6/15	0/21	R0=95%, 29% <1 cm	Not reported	2/21	Not reported
Gigot 2002 [69]	27	24/3	2/25	R1=7%	53% at 2 years	100% at 2 years	Mean: 14 months
Laurent 2003 [3]	13	Not reported	0/13	R0=92%, 23% <1 cm	44% at 3 years	9% at 3 years	Not reported
O'Rourke 2004 [70]	33	27/5	24/9	3.5% positive, mean 1.1 cm	9 recurred/22, 67% at 2 years	15 recurred/22, 75% at 2 years	20 months
Keneko 2005 [71]	30	10/20	0/30	Not reported	31% at 5 years	61% at 5 years	Not reported
Vibert 2006 [62]	65	Not reported	32/33	Median 5 mm (CRM), 10 mm (HCC)	51% at 3 years	87% at 3 years	Mean: 30 months (only 17 patients at risk at 3 years)
Poultsides 2007 [39]	28	Not reported	Not reported	R0=100%	13% at 2 years	61% at 2 years	Mean: 24 months
Lee 2007 [67]	19	11/16	19/0	Median 1.41 cm (0–3 cm)	DFS=24 months	2 deaths/19	11 months
Chen 2008 [72]	116	11/105	4/112	Not reported	Not reported	62% at 5 years	Mean: 94 months
Dagher 2008 [22]	32	26/6	4/28	Not reported	55% at 3 years	72% at 3 years	Mean: 26 months
Robles 2008 [38]	21	21/0	2/19	R0=100%	5 recurred/21	80% at 3 years	Mean: 32 months
Cai 2008 [31]	31	14/17	28/3	>1 cm in all patients	11 recurred/31	60% at 3 years	Mean: 30 months
Sarpel 2009 [68]	20	Not reported	Not reported	Not reported	70% at 2 years	100% at 2 years	21 months
Belli 2009 [5]	54	33/21	3/51	R0=100%	52% at 3 years	67% at 3 years	24 months
Castaing 2009 [7]	60	35/25	29/31	R0=87%	RFS: 30% at 3 years	82% at 3 years	30 months
Sasaki 2009 [42]	76	10%	76/0	R0=91%	Not reported	64% at 3 years	22 months
Nguyen 2009 [16]	109	70/39	67/42	R0=94.5%		50% at 5 years	20 months
Kazaryan 2010 [29]	139 total, 113 malignant	110/38	141/7	R0=94%	NR	46% at 5 years	19 months
Guerron 2012 [41]	40	16/24	35/5	R0=not reported Median: 1.0 cm	Median DFS: 23 months	98% at 2 years	16 months
Cannon 2012 [6]	35	29/6	19/16	R0=97%	15% at 5 years	36% at 5 years	Not reported
Doughtie 2013 [12]	8	8/0	1/7	R0=100%	DFS=14.4 months	87% at 1 year	Not reported

DFS, disease-free survival; HCC, hepatocellular carcinoma.

overlapping orientation of the transection line with the plane of the laparoscopic instruments increases the ability to achieve an oncologically effective operation, explaining the overrepresentation of these anatomical transections in reported series of minimally invasive hepatectomies (see Table 16.2) and the rapidity with which the minimally invasive approach is becoming a standard for these resections [6,9,13,56–58].

This point is highlighted in several recent multicenter reports. In one report, 210 minimally invasive major hepatectomies were described, including 114 malignant tumor resections, with the majority being solitary lesions and all treated with anatomical resections on sectional planes [14]. Only three of these were associated with a positive margin of resection (2.6%). Likewise, a comparative study that included 60 minimally invasive liver resection patients with malignant indications, with 58% treated with anatomical resections including 52% major resections, reported a microscopic margin-positive rate of only 8% [7]. Unfortunately, straightforward anatomical resections for malignant indications (where patients frequently present with bilateral, multifocal disease and/or underlying liver disease) are the exception rather than the rule. More frequently, the liver surgeon is called upon to perform resections across multiple angles and to create curvilinear planes of transection. Somewhat paradoxically, the limitations on transection curvature imposed by laparoscopic liver surgery's fixed planar angles of approach actually mandate a less parenchyma-sparing technique to achieve adequate margins in some cases [4]. In either a nonanatomical or anatomical resectional setting, when the limitations of the laparoscopic instrumentation impair the surgeon's ability to achieve an adequate margin of resection, this becomes a *contraindication* to a minimally invasive approach.

It is anticipated that future improvements in instrumentation, with the ability to angulate instruments, either manually or via robotic manipulation, will progressively overcome these barriers, making more difficult intrahepatic locations accessible and widening the ability to achieve adequate oncological margins when nonanatomical transection planes are required.

16.5 Aim 3: Patient centered

When evaluating the utility of minimally invasive liver surgery, it is critically important to objectively assess the true benefits of the approach from the patient's perspective. Early studies comparing minimally invasive and open approach liver surgery demonstrated a shorter length of hospital stay (LOS) and improvements in postoperative pain associated with the minimally invasive strategy [59,60]. Although inpatient LOS is an important indicator of recovery, more specific midterm recovery metrics may be better indicators of the quality of the surgical approach from the patient's point of view. These include the time to return to normal/baseline performance status and, very importantly for patients with hepatobiliary malignancy, the time to return to intended adjuvant oncological therapies. Also, the implementation of fast-track enhanced recovery pathways is significantly closing the gap in terms of the patient experience with recovery between minimally invasive and open approach liver surgery [61].

The other often quoted patient-centered benefit of minimally invasive approaches is cosmesis. Although this factor may play a role for a subset of younger patients, it is not consistently rated as a decision-making factor for cancer patients desiring curative resection. As surgeons, therefore, we must be careful to evaluate the approach to liver resection from the patient's point of view, choosing the best oncological operation independent of approach.

Likewise, surgeons need to maintain a patient-centered view on the issue of conversion of laparoscopic resection to open surgery whenever there is a perceived or realized safety or quality issue. Unfortunately, particularly in the United States, there is a significant stigma associated with conversion of a minimally invasive procedure to an open procedure. Many surgeons have been formally and informally "trained" to view conversion of minimally invasive to open surgery as a personal technical failure. In this setting, some surgeons may persist with unsafe laparoscopic situations, considering their own motivations and ego over the patient's best interests. From a patient-centered point of view, this must be avoided. To this end, the liver surgical community has a responsibility to de-emphasize both ends of the conversion spectrum (not overlauding reports of low conversion rates and not criminalizing reports of high conversion rates), particularly during the long learning phase of acquisition of competency [14].

It has been well documented that the early era of minimally invasive surgery was characterized by an overrepresentation of benign tumor resections [2]. Despite benign tumors accounting for less than 20% of indications for liver resection overall, only recently have large series begun to report on histological distributions with less than 50% of the minimally invasive resections done for benign indications [14,17,39,42,62]. Clearly, patients with symptomatic benign tumors and those at risk for malignant degeneration or rupture benefit from minimally invasive surgical approaches. Although the question of whether the ability to perform minimally invasive liver resection should expand the indications for benign tumor resection was initially debated, there is currently clear consensus that this should not be done [18,63,64].

However, there is certainly a subset of patients who present with indeterminate or minimally suspicious liver tumor imaging findings that, prior to the availability of minimally invasive liver surgery, would have been recommended for observation instead of incurring the risks and disability of open surgery but who now are *indicated* for minimally invasive diagnostic/therapeutic procedures [63]. Given the advances in imaging accuracy, these cases are becoming more rare, but as discussed below, the ability of minimally invasive liver resection to resolve diagnostic dilemmas should be considered an *indication* for this approach.

16.6 Aim 4: Efficient

In terms of the IOM aim of efficiency, the ability to obtain a definitive diagnosis of indeterminate liver pathology lends a significant *indication* to minimally invasive approaches to liver surgery. Simultaneous increases in the number and type of abdominal imaging procedures have improved the detection of indeterminate and incidental liver lesions. Although the accuracy of computed tomography (CT) and magnetic resonance imaging (MRI) has improved, the sensitivity of lesion detection has outpaced the specificity of lesion characterization, leaving a small number of patients with radiological diagnoses of indeterminate or atypical lesions. These lesions are frequently difficult to biopsy and/or the amount of pathological material available via fine needle or core biopsy is inadequate to provide a definitive diagnosis.

Previously, these patients had two choices: observation, with multiple subsequent scans and a possibility of disease progression in the rare case of unrecognized malignancy, or open surgical incisional or excisional biopsy, which in most cases was overly invasive given the likelihood of a benign diagnosis. The advent of minimally invasive liver surgery has provided an alternative option that is significantly more efficient [62,63]. The ability to obtain adequate tissue for diagnosis, with

minimal physiological impact to the patient, and the potential freedom from anxiety-producing and time-consuming subsequent imaging and follow-up make these cases a prime *indication* for minimally invasive liver surgery.

16.7 Aim 5: Equitable

In the current healthcare environment, on a population basis, liver surgeons do need to be sensitive to cost issues. Unfortunately, the lack of head-to-head comparisons of laparoscopic versus open liver resection clinical outcomes has impeded determination of the comparative cost-effectiveness of these approaches. In general, the cost structure of minimally invasive liver surgery is thought to parallel the paradigm of other minimally invasive approaches, where there are more charges incurred in the operating room compared with those incurred in open techniques [17,65]. This differential is largely attributed to the need for additional expensive and mainly disposable instruments and to longer operative times. Similar to other areas within minimally invasive surgery, these additional intraoperative costs may be counterbalanced by lower postoperative care charges, mainly related to shorter length of inpatient hospitalization [65]. However, few cost comparison studies have been able to control well for case magnitude. With enhanced recovery and other perioperative initiatives lowering all liver surgical LOS numbers, the validity of future cost analyses will be heavily dependent on separately comparing minor open resection to minor minimally invasive resection and major open hepatectomy to major minimally invasive hepatectomy.

16.8 Aim 6: Timely

Of course, the availability of minimally invasive surgery within a region or an individual hospital should be time sensitive. Particularly for patients with malignant diagnoses, access to expeditious operative therapy is important and should not be delayed based on a lack of availability of a certain approach, piece of equipment or technique. Likewise, with increasing numbers of patients benefiting from multimodality approaches to their tumors, appropriate timing of surgical intervention within the larger treatment strategy should not be sacrificed for surgical approach considerations. Continued careful and responsible training and dissemination of laparoscopic techniques are anticipated to make these approaches more widely available over time.

16.9 Conclusion

This chapter describes a conceptual framework for the indications and contraindications for minimally invasive approaches to liver resection. Critical review of the literature indicates that the majority of minimally invasive liver resections that have been successfully performed have been for solitary tumors in anterior segments of the liver with either wedge resection or resection on sectional planes. In general, the reported outcomes for these procedures demonstrate safety and efficacy. Only a handful of highly specialized centers have reported success with minimally invasive atypical, major, and/or radical resections. Based on these data, this chapter emphasizes the need for safe and oncologically sound operations, regardless of approach. Also, patient-centered, efficient, equitable, and timely care may variably support or contraindicate the expansion of indications for minimally invasive approaches. It is hoped that this conceptual framework will serve to establish standards across a highly variable set of procedures, surgical skill sets, and technological advances. Ultimately, it will require introspective professionalism and oversight to carefully monitor exact indications on a case-by-case basis.

KEY POINTS

- Reported outcomes demonstrate that laparoscopic liver surgery as practiced today is safe and effective.

- Quality control is important to ensure safe expansion of minimally invasive liver resection to more advanced resection.

- The goals of advanced laparoscopic liver resection align with the Institute of Medicine healthcare goals of *Safe, Effective, Patient-Centered, Timely, Efficient, and Equitable Care.*

- Most resections today are performed for solitary tumors in anterior segments of the liver with either wedge resection or resection on sectional planes, with only a handful of highly specialized centers performing advanced resections.

- Introspective professionalism and oversight to carefully monitor exact indications on a case-by-case basis are needed to safely expand advanced minimally invasive liver surgery.

References

1 Institute of Medicine. Crossing the Quality Chasm: A New Health System for the 21st Century. Washington, DC: National Academies Press, 2001.

2 Nguyen KT, Gamblin TC, Geller DA. World review of laparoscopic liver resection–2,804 patients. Ann Surg 2009; 250 (5):831–841.

3 Lesurtel M, Cherqui D, Laurent A, Tayar C, Fagniez PL. Laparoscopic versus open left lateral hepatic lobectomy: a case-control study. J Am Coll Surg 2003; 196(2):236–242.

4 Buell JF, Koffron AJ, Thomas MJ, Rudich S, Abecassis M, Woodle ES. Laparoscopic liver resection. J Am Coll Surg 2005; 200(3):472–480.

5 Belli G, Limongelli P, Fantini C, *et al.* Laparoscopic and open treatment of hepatocellular carcinoma in patients with cirrhosis. Br J Surg 2009; 96(9):1041–1048.

6 Cannon RM, Scoggins CR, Callender GG, McMasters KM, Martin RC 2nd. Laparoscopic versus open resection of hepatic colorectal metastases. Surgery 2012; 152(4):567–573; discussion 573–574.

7 Castaing D, Vibert E, Ricca L, Azoulay D, Adam R, Gayet B. Oncologic results of laparoscopic versus open hepatectomy for colorectal liver metastases in two specialized centers. Ann Surg 2009; 250(5):849–855.

8 Tranchart H, di Giuro G, Lainas P, *et al.* Laparoscopic resection for hepatocellular carcinoma: a matched-pair comparative study. Surg Endosc 2010; 24(5):1170–1176.

9 Cannon RM, Brock GN, Marvin MR, Buell JF. Laparoscopic liver resection: an examination of our first 300 patients. J Am Coll Surg 2011; 213(4):501–507.

10 Gagner M, Rhealt M, Dubue J. Laparoscopic partial hepatectomy for liver tumor. Surg Endosc 1992; 6: 97–98.

11 Rao A, Rao G, Ahmed I. Laparoscopic or open liver resection? Let systematic review decide it. Am J Surg 2012; 204(2):222–231.

12 Doughtie CA, Egger ME, Cannon RM, Martin RC, McMasters KM, Scoggins CR. Laparoscopic hepatectomy is a safe and effective approach for resecting large colorectal liver metastases. Am Surg 2013; 79(6):566–571.

13 Gayet B, Cavaliere D, Vibert E, *et al.* Totally laparoscopic right hepatectomy. Am J Surg 2007; 194(5):685–689.

14 Dagher I, O'Rourke N, Geller DA, *et al.* Laparoscopic major hepatectomy: an evolution in standard of care. Ann Surg 2009; 250(5):856–860.

15 Koffron AJ, Auffenberg G, Kung R, Abecassis M. Evaluation of 300 minimally invasive liver resections at a single

institution: less is more. Ann Surg 2007; 246(3):385–392; discussion 392–394.

16 Nguyen KT, Laurent A, Dagher I, *et al*. Minimally invasive liver resection for metastatic colorectal cancer: a multi-institutional, international report of safety, feasibility, and early outcomes. Ann Surg 2009; 250(5):842–848.

17 Buell JF, Thomas MT, Rudich S, *et al*. Experience with more than 500 minimally invasive hepatic procedures. Ann Surg 2008; 248(3):475–486.

18 Buell JF, Cherqui D, Geller DA, *et al*. The international position on laparoscopic liver surgery: the Louisville Statement, 2008. Ann Surg 2009; 250(5):825–830.

19 Gagner M, Rogula T, Selzer D. Laparoscopic liver resection: benefits and controversies. Surg Clin North Am 2004; 84 (2):451–462.

20 Vigano L, Laurent A, Tayar C, Tomatis M, Ponti A, Cherqui D. The learning curve in laparoscopic liver resection: improved feasibility and reproducibility. Ann Surg 2009; 250(5):772–782.

21 Honda G, Kurata M, Okuda Y, *et al*. Totally laparoscopic hepatectomy exposing the major vessels. J Hepato-Biliary-Pancreat Sci 2013; 20(4):435–440.

22 Dagher I, Lainas P, Carloni A, *et al*. Laparoscopic liver resection for hepatocellular carcinoma. Surg Endosc 2008; 22(2):372–378.

23 Laurent A, Cherqui D, Lesurtel M, Brunetti F, Tayar C, Fagniez PL. Laparoscopic liver resection for subcapsular hepatocellular carcinoma complicating chronic liver disease. Arch Surg 2003; 138(7):763–769; discussion 769.

24 Fong Y, Jarnagin W, Conlon KC, DeMatteo R, Dougherty E, Blumgart LH. Hand-assisted laparoscopic liver resection: lessons from an initial experience. Arch Surg 2000; 135(7):854–859.

25 Huang MT, Wei PL, Wang W, Li CJ, Lee YC, Wu CH. A series of laparoscopic liver resections with or without HALS in patients with hepatic tumors. J Gastrointest Surg 2009; 13(5):896–906.

26 Mala T, Edwin B. Role and limitations of laparoscopic liver resection of colorectal metastases. Digest Dis 2005; 23(2): 142–150.

27 Koffron AJ, Kung RD, Auffenberg GB, Abecassis MM. Laparoscopic liver surgery for everyone: the hybrid method. Surgery 2007; 142(4):463–468; discussion 468 e1–2.

28 Dagher I, di Giuro G, Dubrez J, Lainas P, Smadja C, Franco D. Laparoscopic versus open right hepatectomy: a comparative study. Am J Surg 2009; 198(2):173–177.

29 Kazaryan AM, Pavlik Marangos I, *et al*. Laparoscopic liver resection for malignant and benign lesions: ten-year Norwegian single-center experience. Arch Surg 2010; 145(1):34–40.

30 Buell JF, Thomas MJ, Doty TC, *et al*. An initial experience and evolution of laparoscopic hepatic resectional surgery. Surgery 2004; 136(4):804–811.

31 Cai XJ, Yang J, Yu H, *et al*. Clinical study of laparoscopic versus open hepatectomy for malignant liver tumors. Surg Endosc 2008; 22(11):2350–2356.

32 Zimmitti G, Roses RE, Andreou A, *et al*. Greater complexity of liver surgery is not associated with an increased incidence of liver-related complications except for bile leak: an experience with 2,628 consecutive resections. J Gastrointest Surg 2013; 17(1):57–64; discussion 64–65.

33 Buell JF, Gayet B, Han HS, *et al*. Evaluation of stapler hepatectomy during a laparoscopic liver resection. HPB (Oxford) 2013; 15(11):845–850.

34 Tzeng CW, Katz MH, Fleming JB, *et al*. Risk of venous thromboembolism outweighs post-hepatectomy bleeding complications: analysis of 5651 National Surgical Quality Improvement Program patients. HPB (Oxford) 2012 Aug; 14(8):506–513.

35 Parker GA, Lawrence W Jr, Horsley JS 3rd, *et al*. Intraoperative ultrasound of the liver affects operative decision making. Ann Surg 1989; 209(5):569–576; discussion 576–577.

36 Wagnetz U, Atri M, Massey C, Wei AC, Metser U. Intraoperative ultrasound of the liver in primary and secondary hepatic malignancies: comparison with preoperative 1.5-T MRI and 64-MDCT. Am J Roentgenol 2011; 196(3):562–568.

37 Hsu TC. Intra-abdominal lesions could be missed by inadequate laparoscopy. Am Surg 2008; 74(9):824–826; discussion 827–828.

38 Robles R, Marin C, Abellan B, Lopez A, Pastor P, Parrilla P. A new approach to hand-assisted laparoscopic liver surgery. Surg Endosc 2008; 22(11):2357–2364.

39 Poultsides G, Brown M, Orlando R 3rd. Hand-assisted laparoscopic management of liver tumors. Surg Endosc 2007; 21 (8):1275–1279.

40 Satoh S, Okabe H, Kondo K, *et al*. Video. A novel laparoscopic approach for safe and simplified suprapancreatic lymph node dissection of gastric cancer. Surg Endosc 2009; 23 (2):436–437.

41 Guerron AD, Aliyev S, Agcaoglu O, *et al*. Laparoscopic versus open resection of colorectal liver metastasis. Surg Endosc 2013; 27(4):1138–1143.

42 Sasaki A, Nitta H, Otsuka K, Takahara T, Nishizuka S, Wakabayashi G. Ten-year experience of totally laparoscopic liver resection in a single institution. Br J Surg 2009; 96 (3):274–279.

43 Tsamis D, Theodoropoulos G, Stamopoulos P, *et al*. Systemic inflammatory response after laparoscopic and conventional colectomy for cancer: a matched case-control study. Surg Endosc 2012; 26(5):1436–1443.

44 Lee SW, Whelan RL. Immunologic and oncologic implications of laparoscopic surgery: what is the latest? Clin Colon Rectal Surg 2006; 19(1):5–12.

45 Pawlik TM, Scoggins CR, Zorzi D, *et al*. Effect of surgical margin status on survival and site of recurrence after hepatic resection for colorectal metastases. Ann Surg 2005; 241 (5):715–722.

46 Andreou A, Aloia TA, Brouquet A, *et al*. Margin status remains an important determinant of survival after surgical resection of colorectal liver metastases in the era of modern chemotherapy. Ann Surg 2013 19; 257(6):1079–1088.

47 Hasegawa K, Kokudo N, Imamura H, *et al*. Prognostic impact of anatomic resection for hepatocellular carcinoma. Ann Surg 2005; 242(2):252–259.

48 Kokudo N, Tada K, Seki M, *et al*. Anatomical major resection versus nonanatomical limited resection for liver metastases from colorectal carcinoma. Am J Surg 2001; 181(2):153–159.

49 Andreou A, Vauthey JN, Cherqui D, *et al.* Improved long-term survival after major resection for hepatocellular carcinoma: a multicenter analysis based on a new definition of major hepatectomy. J Gastrointest Surg 2013; 17(1):66–77; discussion 77.

50 Reddy SK, Barbas AS, Turley RS, *et al.* A standard definition of major hepatectomy: resection of four or more liver segments. HPB (Oxford) 2011; 13(7):494–502.

51 Postriganova N, Kazaryan AM, Rosok BI, Fretland AA, Barkhatov L, Edwin B. Margin status after laparoscopic resection of colorectal liver metastases: does a narrow resection margin have an influence on survival and local recurrence? HPB (Oxford) 2014; 16(9):822–829.

52 Cherqui D, Husson E, Hammoud R, *et al.* Laparoscopic liver resections: a feasibility study in 30 patients. Ann Surg 2000; 232(6):753–762.

53 Nguyen KT, Geller DA. Outcomes of laparoscopic hepatic resection for colorectal cancer metastases. J Surg Oncol 2010; 102(8):975–977.

54 Cho JY, Han HS, Yoon YS, Shin SH. Feasibility of laparoscopic liver resection for tumors located in the posterosuperior segments of the liver, with a special reference to overcoming current limitations on tumor location. Surgery 2008; 144(1):32–38.

55 Costi R, Capelluto E, Sperduto N, Bruyns J, Himpens J, Cadiere GB. Laparoscopic right posterior hepatic bisegmentectomy (Segments VII–VIII). Surg Endosc 2003; 17(1):162.

56 Gumbs AA, Gayet B. Totally laparoscopic left hepatectomy. Surg Endosc 2007; 21(7):1221.

57 Chang S, Laurent A, Tayar C, Karoui M, Cherqui D. Laparoscopy as a routine approach for left lateral sectionectomy. Br J Surg 2007; 94(1):58–63.

58 Belli G, Gayet B, Han HS, *et al.* Laparoscopic left hemihepatectomy a consideration for acceptance as standard of care. Surg Endosc 2013; 27(8):2721–2726.

59 Mala T, Edwin B, Gladhaug I, *et al.* A comparative study of the short-term outcome following open and laparoscopic liver resection of colorectal metastases. Surg Endosc 2002; 16 (7):1059–1063.

60 Farges O, Jagot P, Kirstetter P, Marty J, Belghiti J. Prospective assessment of the safety and benefit of laparoscopic liver resections. J Hepatobiliary Pancreat Surg 2002; 9(2):242–248.

61 Schultz NA, Larsen PN, Klarskov B, *et al.* Evaluation of a fast-track programme for patients undergoing liver resection. Br J Surg 2013; 100(1):138–143.

62 Vibert E, Perniceni T, Levard H, Denet C, Shahri NK, Gayet B. Laparoscopic liver resection. Br J Surg 2006; 93(1):67–72.

63 Koffron A, Geller D, Gamblin TC, Abecassis M. Laparoscopic liver surgery: shifting the management of liver tumors. Hepatology 2006; 44(6):1694–1700.

64 Ardito F, Tayar C, Laurent A, Karoui M, Loriau J, Cherqui D. Laparoscopic liver resection for benign disease. Arch Surg 2007; 142(12):1188–1193; discussion 93.

65 Vanounou T, Steel JL, Nguyen KT, *et al.* Comparing the clinical and economic impact of laparoscopic versus open liver resection. Ann Surg Oncol 2010; 17(4):998–1009.

66 Morino M, Morra I, Rosso E, Miglietta C, Garrone C. Laparoscopic vs open hepatic resection: a comparative study. Surg Endosc 2003; 17(12):1914–1918.

67 Lee KF, Cheung YS, Chong CN, *et al.* Laparoscopic versus open hepatectomy for liver tumours: a case control study. Hong Kong Med J 2007; 13(6):442–448.

68 Sarpel U, Hefti MM, Wisnievsky JP, Roayaie S, Schwartz ME, Labow DM. Outcome for patients treated with laparoscopic versus open resection of hepatocellular carcinoma: case-matched analysis. Ann Surg Oncol 2009; 16(6):1572–1577.

69 Gigot JF, Glineur D, Santiago Azagra J, *et al.* Laparoscopic liver resection for malignant liver tumors: preliminary results of a multicenter European study. Ann Surg 2002; 236(1):90–97.

70 O'Rourke N, Shaw I, Nathanson L, Martin I, Fielding G. Laparoscopic resection of hepatic colorectal metastases. HPB (Oxford) 2004; 6(4):230–235.

71 Kaneko H, Takagi S, Otsuka Y, *et al.* Laparoscopic liver resection of hepatocellular carcinoma. Am J Surg 2005; 189(2):190–194.

72 Chen HY, Juan CC, Ker CG. Laparoscopic liver surgery for patients with hepatocellular carcinoma. Ann Surg Oncol 2008; 15(3):800–806.

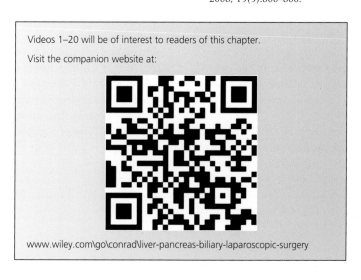

Videos 1–20 will be of interest to readers of this chapter.

Visit the companion website at:

www.wiley.com\go\conrad\liver-pancreas-biliary-laparoscopic-surgery

CHAPTER 17

Laparoscopy (hybrid) and hand-assisted laparoscopy in liver surgery: why, when, and how?

Yasushi Hasegawa[1] and Go Wakabayashi[2]

[1]*Department of Surgery, Iwate Medical University School of Medicine, Morioka, Japan*
[2]*Department of Surgery, Ageo Central General Hospital, Ageo City, Japan*

EDITOR COMMENT

This chapter, by expert laparoscopic liver surgeons, allows the reader to learn the important indications for hybrid and hand-assisted approaches to advanced laparoscopic liver resection. We believe that there are important yet selected indications with clear advantages of a hybrid technique. These include the beginning of a surgical experience where placement of a surgical laparotomy pad inside the abdomen early in the case allows for manual compression with the pad in case of bleeding and subsequent safe conversion to open surgery. Hand-assisted approaches can be important when preoperative imaging and intraoperative ultrasound are not sufficient to ensure complete tumor removal and palpation of the liver is required. When a hand-assisted approach is performed, placement of the assistant's hand rather than the operating surgeon's hand in the abdomen can improve ergonomics and facilitate graduation to a purely laparoscopic approach. Another important indication for hand-assisted or hybrid approaches are patients with significant abdominal adhesions. The placement of a hand-assist access port allows for the creation of a working space through this access port from which the remainder of the case can be performed purely laparoscopically.

Keywords: hand-assisted laparoscopic liver surgery, hybrid laparoscopic liver surgery

17.1 Introduction

Laparoscopic liver resection was first reported in the 1990s and since then, laparoscopic liver resection has been established as a safe and feasible treatment option for both benign and malignant liver tumors [1–4]. Despite the clinical benefits of laparoscopic liver resection (e.g. reduced blood loss, pain, and analgesic requirements; shorter hospital stays; and improved cosmetic results), its application remains limited because of insufficient hepatic and laparoscopic surgical experience among surgeons.

Laparoscopic liver resection can be divided into pure laparoscopy, hand-assisted laparoscopy, and the hybrid technique [2]. In the pure laparoscopic procedure, the entire resection of the liver is completed through laparoscopic ports; hand-assisted laparoscopy is defined by the placement of a hand port to facilitate the procedure; and the hybrid technique is defined as a procedure that is started as a pure or hand-assisted laparoscopy but in which the final resection is performed through a mini-laparotomy incision.

There is no evidence that any of these three approaches is superior to the others; however, hand-assisted laparoscopy and the hybrid technique may help overcome certain difficulties associated with pure laparoscopy, and may be less invasive than open laparotomy [3].

The role of these two methods compared with pure laparoscopy and open laparotomy is discussed in this chapter.

Laparoscopic Liver, Pancreas, and Biliary Surgery, First Edition.
Edited by Claudius Conrad and Brice Gayet.
© 2017 John Wiley & Sons, Ltd. Published 2017 by John Wiley & Sons, Ltd.

17.2 The hybrid technique (laparoscopy-assisted method)

As mentioned earlier, the hybrid technique consists of two parts: it has an initial component in which limited laparoscopic skills are required (usually liver mobilization) and a subsequent part that is technically more challenging and performed open through a mini-laparotomy (the actual liver resection) [2]. The hybrid technique is also frequently called the "laparoscopy-assisted" method. The main feature of this method is that the only laparoscopic skill required is liver mobilization, and it can thus be relatively easily performed by most liver surgeons [5,6].

17.2.1 Surgical procedure

There are two stages to the hybrid technique: first, the liver mobilization is performed through a laparoscope, followed by parenchymal transection being performed through a small laparotomy incision.

The patient is fixed in a semi-left lateral decubitus position that allows an intraoperative change from the supine to the left lateral position by rotating the operative table. A laparoscopic trocar is inserted from the umbilicus in an open procedure and an expected small incision line of up to 12 cm is drawn at the upper midline or right subcostal region. The trocar position is shown in Figure 17.1.

First, the liver is mobilized using the laparoscopic technique. When right liver mobilization is performed, the operating table is rotated to have the patient in the left lateral position. Sufficient mobilization of the liver ensures the safety of the subsequent hepatic parenchymal transection through a smaller incision.

After the mobilization is completed, a minimal incision is made along the expected line in the upper midline or right subcostal region. A wound protector is used, and retraction is performed at the incision site in the cranial direction with a Kent retractor.

The liver hanging maneuver is an essential procedure that allows handling through the smaller surgical incision to be performed safely [6,7]. For the liver hanging maneuver through a small incision, the authors prefer the use of Nitta forceps (commercially available forceps with a long, blunt, highly curved tip) (Figure 17.2). To perform the liver hanging maneuver, the tissue between the middle hepatic vein and the right hepatic vein is dissected. The Nitta forceps are inserted beginning at the 11 o'clock position on the inferior vena cava (IVC) and are used to carefully dissect the tissue between the liver and the anterior surface of the IVC. When the tissue between the IVC and liver is passed through, a Penrose drain is clamped with the Nitta forceps and placed there for the liver hanging maneuver.

Hepatic parenchymal transection through a small incision can be performed with the same procedures by open laparotomy. Various devices are available for hepatic parenchymal transection, and a surgeon may choose devices that are suitable to his/her preferred method (Figure 17.3).

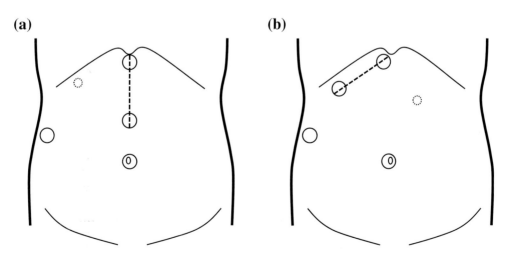

(a)   **(b)**

Figure 17.1 (a,b) Trocar placement and incision for laparoscopy-assisted liver resection.

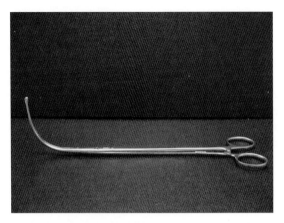

Figure 17.2 Nitta forceps for liver hanging maneuver with long blunt, highly curved tip.

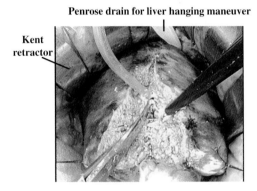

Figure 17.3 Liver parenchymal transection in laparoscopy-assisted liver resection.

17.2.2 Advantages of the hybrid technique

The biggest advantage of the hybrid technique is the smaller incision compared with open laparotomy. In open hepatectomy, a subcostal incision with midline incision, i.e. reversed T incision or reversed L incision, is usually needed to mobilize the liver, because the liver is fixed by ligaments behind the ribcage. However, if the mobilization is performed by laparoscopy, a large incision is not needed. Some studies have reported that laparoscopic liver resection is associated with less pain and fewer analgesic requirements than open surgery. Smaller incisions should theoretically result in less pain, so the hybrid technique thus also contributes to reducing patient morbidity and enhancing their well-being post-operatively, when compared with open laparotomy.

When liver mobilization is performed laparoscopically, not only the operator but also the assistants have the opportunity to obtain a clear view of the posterior side of the liver, owing to laparoscopic magnification. This view can assist the surgeons in mobilizing the right liver more safely.

Transection of the liver parenchyma, dividing of the hepatic hilum, and dissection of the hepatic vein are performed though the mini-laparotomy incision under direct vision. These procedures are typically more challenging to perform using pure laparoscopy to the requirement for advanced laparoscopic skills. In particular, the liver parenchymal transection has the potential to prolong the operation time when performed laparoscopically. When using the hybrid technique, this subset of challenging procedures is carried out using standard open laparotomy techniques, which may be easier for many liver surgeons.

In addition, the hybrid technique is also useful for cases requiring reconstruction of the biliary tract, such as hilar cholangiocarcinomas. Reconstruction of the biliary tract under pure laparoscopy is very difficult and highly technical, whereas under mini-laparotomy, it is much more easily achieved.

17.2.3 Disadvantages of the hybrid technique

The principal difference between pure laparoscopy and the hybrid technique is the method of liver parenchymal transection. The pneumoperitoneum induced during laparoscopic surgery has a tendency to reduce bleeding at the surgical site. Because the hybrid technique does not allow for peritoneal insufflation, the benefits of pneumoperitoneum-induced reduction in hepatic venous back bleeding are not present in the hybrid technique.

In addition, the patient's body habitus has a larger effect on the difficulty of surgery in the hybrid technique compared with pure laparoscopy. When a patient's anterior–posterior trunk diameter is long, the operative field becomes difficult to see, and the technique is associated with an increased risk of hemorrhage deep in the abdominal cavity (i.e. of the IVC or hepatic vein).

17.2.4 Why and when?

The hybrid technique has some advantages over pure laparoscopy, but we believe that these advantages diminish when surgeons overcome the difficulties in pure laparoscopic procedure with proper laparoscopic training [3,8]. There are two main motives for selecting the hybrid technique over a full laparoscopic procedure.

The first reason, as noted above, is when a surgeon has insufficient experience in performing the full laparoscopic procedure available. Laparoscopic liver parenchymal transection commonly takes a great deal of investment in both effort and education, in order to be able to perform the procedure effectively. However, having experience in liver mobilization in laparoscopy-assisted hepatectomy is helpful for learning how to perform it stepwise.

The other main motive for using the hybrid technique is for biliary reconstruction (i.e. choledochojejunostomy). While this procedure can be done using the full laparoscopic procedure, the level of mastery for this procedure, including the reconstruction using a pure laparoscopic technique, requires a great deal of experience and time investment by the surgeon. Particularly in facilities where this procedure is done infrequently, it is preferable to use the hybrid method, to allow as many advantages as possible from the laparoscopic technique, while assuring that the more complex aspects of the surgery are managed in a safe and oncologically sound way.

17.3 Hand-assisted laparoscopy

In the Louisville Statement, hand-assisted laparoscopy was defined as the elective placement of a hand port during laparoscopic liver resection to facilitate the procedure, and this technique is frequently called hand-assisted laparoscopic surgery (HALS) [2,9,10]. The main feature of this method is that the surgeon's hand is in the abdominal cavity, as for open laparotomy, and this is associated with a number of both advantages and disadvantages.

17.3.1 Surgical procedure

There are two main positions for inserting the hand during the procedure. One is the right lateral abdomen of the patient and the other is the upper midline abdominal area. In the former method, the operator inserts the hand into the abdominal cavity and uses it for liver parenchymal transection, whereas in the latter method, the assistant inserts the hand and uses it for liver mobilization. Moreover, the upper midline abdominal incision

can also be used in the hybrid technique (laparoscopy-assisted liver resection). In this section, the former method is described, which is useful mainly in cases of tumors located in the right liver, especially in segments VII or VIII.

In HALS, for ergonomic reasons, it is important to correctly position the surgeon (i.e. on the left side of the patient, between the patient's legs, or on the right side of the patient), the hand-access device, and the trocars. There is no definite "right way" to do this, and the positions are decided on a case-by-case basis according to the operator's preferences. If the correct setting is misjudged when placing the hand-assist access port, the surgeon is forced to remain in a nonergonomic position during the entire operation, which can contribute to operator fatigue.

A laparoscopic trocar is inserted at the umbilicus in an open fashion. A small incision (5–8 cm, depending on the surgeon's hand size), which is where the hand is inserted in hand-assisted situations, is marked out at the right lateral abdominal region. Two 12 mm trocars are inserted at both ends of this expected small midline incision, and two more trocars are inserted at the epigastric region and right subcostal region (Figure 17.4).

The right liver mobilization is usually performed by the pure laparoscopic technique, and the parenchymal transection is performed by HALS. After the mobilization is completed, a small incision along the previously

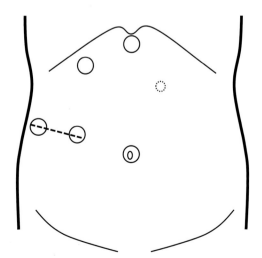

Figure 17.4 Trocar placement and incision for hand-assisted liver resection.

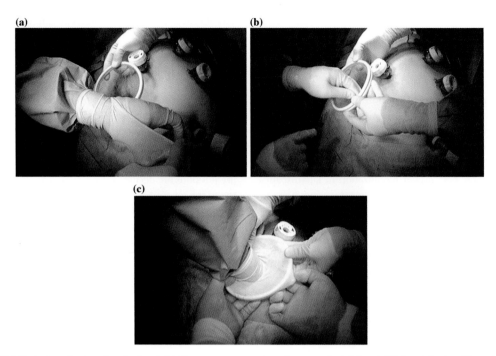

Figure 17.5 Technique for inserting the hand. (a) The surgeon wears two gloves on the left hand. (b) Insert the hand into abdomen through the wound retractor. (c) Loop the outside glove around the wound retractor.

marked line in right lateral abdominal region is created. A hand-port device or wound retractor with double surgical groves is used, and the operator's left hand is inserted into the abdominal cavity (Figure 17.5). During the parenchymal transection, the hand can be used for retracting and moving the liver, and the fingers can be used for opening the liver cut surface (Figure 17.6). Aside from the advantage of palpation and tactile feedback, the parenchymal transection is carried out in a similar manner to pure laparoscopic liver resection.

17.3.2 Advantages of HALS

A disadvantage of laparoscopic surgery is the restriction of movement, and HALS is helpful in avoiding this problem. Additionally, HALS can facilitate the retraction and moving of the liver. Moving the liver using a hand can help in various stages of a liver resection such as during parenchymal transection, mobilization, and dissecting vessels.

During the laparoscopic parenchymal transection of the liver, there can be some difficulty in directing the transection plane towards the operating surgeon, because

the trocar position is fixed. However, this can be overcome by repositioning the liver using the hand to allow for an optimal orientation of the parenchymal transection line towards the surgeon's instruments. To dissect the liver parenchyma effectively, tension created by counter-traction plays an important role. During HALS, tension on the cut surface is created not only by laparoscopic forceps but also by the surgeon's fingers through the HALS port.

During liver surgery there is the risk of significant blood loss. To control bleeding requires compression of the bleeding point. Intra-abdominally, the surgeon's hand can compress the bleeding point more easily and sometimes more effectively than is possible using only laparoscopic instruments. Once the bleeding point is found, it can be stopped by an energy device or by suturing. Furthermore, continuous bleeding from the liver parenchyma can be controlled by raising the liver with the hand, when the HALS method is used. To accomplish this, the right or middle hepatic vein is raised, resulting in the intrahepatic venous pressure being reduced, thereby lessening the bleeding from the hepatic vein. This technique is easier in HALS than in pure laparoscopy, where

(a)

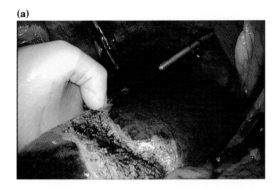

(b)

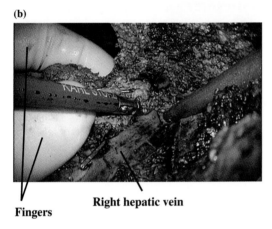

Fingers   **Right hepatic vein**

Figure 17.6 (a,b) Hand-assisted extended posterior sectionectomy.

all movement must be accomplished using only the laparoscopic forceps.

Pneumoperitoneum is an advantage of laparoscopic surgery, compared with the hybrid technique or open surgery. Bleeding from the hepatic vein is decreased by the pressure of the pneumoperitoneum, and because HALS uses a port that seals the abdominal cavity, allowing for insufflation, HALS is thus associated with less potential blood loss than the hybrid technique or open laparotomy method during parenchymal transection.

Good tactile feedback is another advantage of HALS, with direct palpation of tumors being possible. It is crucial to achieve negative surgical margins for the resection of malignancies, and concerns have been raised about the positive margin rate observed in laparoscopic surgery potentially being higher than with the other techniques. Tactile feedback aids in the identification of tumor margins and of the correct direction in parenchymal transection.

17.3.3 Disadvantages of HALS

Hand-assisted laparoscopic surgery has some crucial disadvantages. First, the surgeon's hand sometimes interferes with the view of the surgical field provided by the laparoscopic camera. The hand takes up a very large space in the abdominal cavity, in comparison with other laparoscopic instruments, and this can impede visibility if the positioning of the camera trocar is not managed effectively.

The second concern is one of ergonomics. Because the operator's hand is confined in position by the HALS port, the operator can experience poor body positioning, resulting in muscle ache and increased risk of operator fatigue, especially when the surgical time is prolonged. Additionally, special care should be taken to be sufficiently careful and gentle with activities undertaken within the abdominal cavity through the HALS port, as the procedure of hand-assisted liver resection can be less refined than that of pure laparoscopy, which tends to allow small and delicate movements through the abdominal field.

17.3.4 Why and when?

The pros and cons of HALS are described above. The advantages of HALS may be overcome by proper training in the pure laparoscopic technique, and HALS can function as a bridge to pure laparoscopic liver resection [3]. For surgeons training in laparoscopic hepatectomy, HALS may be helpful, especially during posterior sectionectomy and wedge resection for tumors located at segment VII or VIII. Moreover, cirrhotic livers are hard to move and lift, so HALS may be useful for these cases. When there is delayed or little progress in obtaining adequate hemostasis, conversion to HALS from pure laparoscopy may be an answer.

17.4 Conclusion

We believe that, although most liver resections can be successfully performed by pure laparoscopy, both the hybrid technique and HALS play important roles in minimal invasive hepatectomy. The appropriate procedure should be selected depending on the experience of the surgeon, the tumor location, and the quality of the underlying liver parenchyma.

KEY POINTS

- There are important yet selected indications with advantages of a hybrid technique.

- Manual compression with a laparotomy pad through a hand port in case of bleeding and subsequent safe conversion to open surgery can be life saving.

- Specific oncological cases might demand manual palpation of the liver.

- The placement of a hand-assist access port allows for the creation of a working space through the port from which the remainder of the case can be performed purely laparoscopically.

References

1 Gagner M, Rheault M, Dubuc J. Laparoscopic partial hepatectomy for liver tumor. Surg Endosc 1992; 6:97–98.

2 Buell JF, Cherqui D, Geller DA, *et al.* The international position on laparoscopic liver surgery: the Louisville Statement, 2008. Ann Surg 2009; 250:825–830.

3 Wakabayashi G, Cherqui D, Geller DA, *et al.* Recommendation for laparoscopic liver resection: a report from the second international consensus conference held in Morioka. Ann Surg 2015; 261:619–629.

4 Lin NC, Nitta H, Wakabayashi G. Laparoscopic major hepatectomy: a systematic literature review and comparison of 3 techniques. Ann Surg 2013; 257:205–213.

5 Koffron AJ, Kung RD, Auffenberg GB, *et al.* Laparoscopic liver surgery for everyone: the hybrid method. Surgery 2007; 142:463–468.

6 Nitta H, Sasaki A, Fujita T, *et al.* Laparoscopy-assisted major liver resections employing a hanging technique: the original procedure. Ann Surg 2010; 251:450–453.

7 Wakabayashi G. Laparoscopy-assisted donor right hepatectomy employing a hanging technique. In: Asbun H, Geller D (eds) ACS Multimedia Atlas of Surgery: Liver Volume. Chicago: American College of Surgeons, 2014.

8 Takahara T, Wakabayashi G, Hasegawa Y, *et al.* Minimally invasive donor hepatectomy: evolution from hybrid to pure laparoscopic techniques. Ann Surg 2015; 26 (1):e3–4.

9 Fong Y, Jarnagin W, Conlon KC, *et al.* Hand-assisted laparoscopic liver resection: lessons from an initial experience. Arch Surg 2000; 135 (7): 854–859.

10 Cuschieri A. Laparoscopic hand-assisted surgery for hepatic and pancreatic disease. Surg Endosc 2000; 14 (11): 991–996.

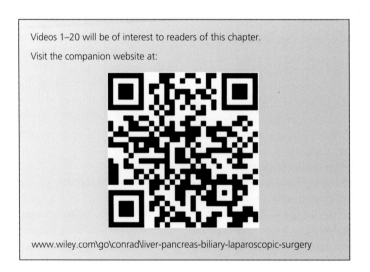

Videos 1–20 will be of interest to readers of this chapter.

Visit the companion website at:

www.wiley.com\go\conrad\liver-pancreas-biliary-laparoscopic-surgery

CHAPTER 18

Ablation strategies for tumors of the liver and pancreas

Danielle K. DePeralta and Kenneth K. Tanabe

Division of Surgical Oncology, Harvard Medical School, Massachusetts General Hospital, Boston, Massachusetts, USA

EDITOR COMMENT

In this very comprehensive chapter on nonresective approaches to hepatocellular carcinoma and secondary liver cancers, the authors explain the technical aspects, indications, and expected outcomes for common liver-directed therapies. These include radiofrequency ablation, microwave ablation, irreversible electroporation, cryoablation, and transarterial chemoembolization. The authors further detail key considerations for the ablation of hepatocellular carcinoma, colorectal, neuroendocrine, and breast liver metastases. Advantages and disadvantages of the various approaches such as percutaneous, open or laparoscopic are explained. Laparoscopic ablation probe placement has become more precise with advances in intraoperative ultrasound and ablation probe placement.

While RFA is the standard of care for small unresectable HCCs, with greater experience in the minimally invasive resection of hepatocellular carcinoma in cirrhotic livers, it has become an option that combines the benefits of ablation and resection. A laparoscopic resection of early HCC can be performed with the low morbidity of ablation, but tumor removal allows for assessment of the most important predictor of oncological outcome in HCC: vascular invasion.

Among the newer ablation technologies, irreversible electroporation is a nonthermal ablation that spares surrounding vasculature and bile ducts and may even be an option for some patients with locally advanced pancreatic cancer.

This chapter on liver-directed strategies is important for all advanced minimally invasive hepatopancreatobiliary surgeons treating a wide spectrum of patients with early and advanced, primary and secondary liver cancer.

Keywords: ablation of hepatocellular carcinoma, ablation of of liver metastases, cryoablation, irreversible electroporation, liver ablation, microwave ablation, postembolization syndrome radiofrequency ablation, transarterial chemoembolization

---

Surgical extirpation, via either hepatic resection or transplantation, remains the best option for potentially curable liver tumors. However, since many patients are not candidates for surgical resection or transplantation, there has been increasing focus on locoregional therapies, which generally include transarterial and ablative strategies, as both palliative and in some cases curative techniques. In this chapter, we will focus on local ablative strategies (Box 1) for hepatocellular carcinoma (HCC), metastatic liver tumors, and to a lesser extent pancreatic cancers.

18.1 Overview of modalities

The options for local ablation have grown in recent years and while radiofrequency ablation remains the most clinically useful, the surgeon must have a thorough understanding of the therapeutic options. Each of the strategies discussed below may be performed percutaneously, laparoscopically, or during an open operation, depending on both patient functional status and tumor characteristics. We focus on the most relevant techniques here.

Laparoscopic Liver, Pancreas, and Biliary Surgery, First Edition.
Edited by Claudius Conrad and Brice Gayet.
© 2017 John Wiley & Sons, Ltd. Published 2017 by John Wiley & Sons, Ltd.

18.1.1 Radiofrequency ablation (RFA)

Jacques-Arsène d'Arsonval first described the thermal effects of radiofrequency (RF) energy on tissue in 1891 [1] and in 1928 the Bovie knife, a crude monopolar RF electrode, was incorporated into the surgical repertoire [2]. After gaining experience in animal models, RFA was first performed in patients with liver tumors in the early 1990s, initially in Europe and later in the United States [3]. No other locoregional therapy has gained the same acceptance among surgeons or interventional radiologists, or has been as well studied.

Radiofrequency ablation induces cell death by coagulative necrosis. A simple circuit is created using an RF generator, grounding pad, and the interstitial electrode(s) placed within the liver tumor. Electrode(s) are carefully positioned within the tumor under direct visualization or with image guidance, and rapidly alternating RF current leads to ion agitation and heat generation at the site of the electrode, with subsequent coagulation necrosis (Figure 18.1). The greatest heat is generated at the site of the electrode and extends peripherally by thermal conduction.

Irreversible cellular injury and death occur as tissues are heated beyond 60 °C. Most current systems can reliably generate a 3 cm ablation zone. For larger tumors, the electrode can be repeatedly repositioned to generate an approximately 1 cm margin around the tumor.

Radiofrequency electrodes (Figure 18.2) are commercially available with expandable multitined, clustered, and straight insulated needles with a metallic tip.

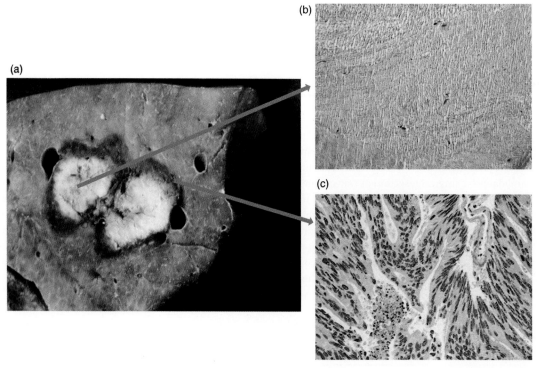

Figure 18.1 (a) Explanted liver resected immediately following radiofrequency ablation. (b) Central area of coagulation necrosis. (c) Surrounding margin of incompletely ablated liver with a majority of cells that are histologically abnormal and would undergo apoptosis if left in situ.

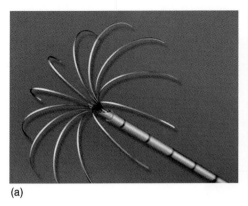 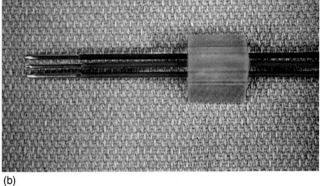

(a) (b)

Figure 18.2 Radiofrequency electrodes. (a) Expandable multitined probe. (b) Cluster of three straight electrodes spaced optimally by a plastic guide.

Multitined electrodes allow for increased spatial distribution of heat and can create larger ablation zones. Internally cooled electrodes aim to prevent desiccation (charring) at the electrode–tissue interface, which disrupts energy transfer to deeper tissues. Traditionally, monopolar systems have been used, but bipolar and multipolar systems are also now available. A bipolar circuit is completed with a second interstitial electrode and obviates the need for a skin surface grounding pad, while multipolar systems allow the operator to transition between sets of bipolar electrodes on a single needle. These strategies can generally produce larger ablative volumes.

There is a small risk of thermal injury at the site of the grounding pads, which warrants careful temperature monitoring. Strategies such as pad cooling and the use of multiple pads to increase surface area are possible in the setting of high pad temperatures and impedance.

Even as new technologies are developed, RFA remains the most widely used of all ablative techniques within the liver.

18.1.2 Microwave ablation

Microwave ablation (MWA) generates heat through dielectric hysteresis. Polar molecules, such as water, present within the liver are subjected to a rapidly oscillating electromagnetic field, and when they fail to align with the field, some of the applied energy is converted to heat with subsequent cytotoxic effects on adjacent tumor tissue. A basic MWA set-up requires a generator (magnetron or solid state), a coaxial cable with inner and outer conductors for power distribution, and MWA antennas for

energy transfer to tissue (Figure 18.2). In contrast to RF electrodes, MWA antennas unload energy as a propagating field, not an electric current. Thus, they can create large zones of active heating without the need for a grounding pad or additional electrodes to complete a bipolar circuit. The specific design of individual MWA antennas can alter the shape and depth of ablative zones and cooling systems can minimize collateral damage along the insertion track of a long probe needed for deeper lesions [4]. Cooling also helps protect skin at the insertion site during percutaneous and laparoscopic procedures; it can be achieved with either gas or water cooling systems.

Microwave ablation is frequently used for hepatic tumor ablation in China and Japan and is gaining interest within Europe and the United States. This technique holds promise as an alternative to RFA, particularly for large tumors, because it is capable of performing multiple ablations at the same time (multiple antennas powered simultaneously by a single generator), generates higher temperatures and heats tissue more efficiently (Figure 18.3). This theoretically translates into larger ablation volumes produced more rapidly (Figure 18.4).

18.1.3 Irreversible electroporation

Irreversible electroporation (IRE) is a new nonthermal ablation technology that uses high-voltage pulses of electrical current to create permanent nanopores in cells that ultimately result in irreversible membrane damage and cell death by apoptosis. Voltages as high as 1500 volts/cm are used with electrical pulses gated to

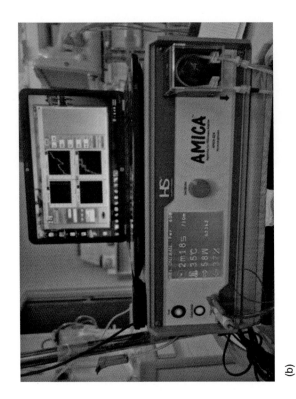

(b)

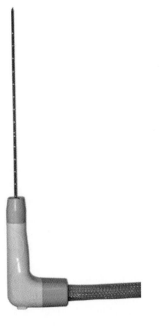

(a)

Figure 18.3 Microwave ablation instruments. (a) Cooled shaft AMICA probe. (b) Generator. (c) Schematic of electrode from (a), with accompanying intraprocedural imaging: CT-guided ablation of a lung tumor (*left*) and ultrasound-guided ablation of liver tumor (*right*). Source: HS Hospital Services SpA, Rome, Italy. Reproduced with permission.

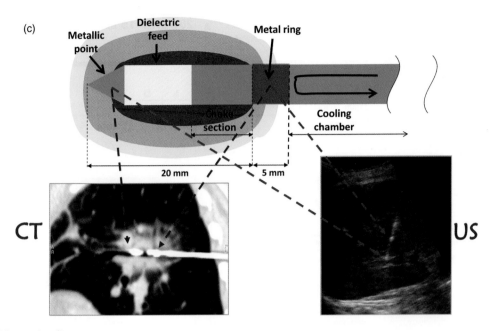

Figure 18.3 (*Continued*)

the cardiac cycle to minimize the risk of generating an arrhythmia. Complete muscle paralysis is required during treatment. Very early data suggest that IRE is a more precise and complete method of tumor ablation, with possibilities in both the liver and pancreas. IRE generates permanent nanopores within cell membranes but does not affect noncellular structures, such as basement membranes, lamina propria, and adventitia. It thereby preserves vital vascular and ductal structures within the ablation zone [5]. Furthermore, it avoids the heat or cold sink effects of neighboring vessels with the potential to create a more complete ablation, thereby reducing the risk of local recurrence in tumors adjacent to hepatic and pancreatic vasculature. Since tumor ablation is not induced by thermal energy, many of the limitations of RFA and MWA are avoided. Well-demarcated margins are produced with IRE, compared to larger gray zones with both RFA and MWA that have some viable parenchymal and cancer cells mixed within a generally necrotic region. Ablation times are even shorter with IRE than MWA, with 90 pulses needed to ablate a 3 cm tumor complete within one minute [6]. As a result of cell death by apoptosis instead of coagulation necrosis, the ablation zone resolves relatively quickly.

This cutting-edge technology has only recently been applied in patients and reported in small-scale studies [7,8]. Limitations include the necessity of extremely precise applicator positioning, which adds time to an otherwise short ablative approach. All patients must receive muscle relaxants for these cases as the IRE pulses can trigger muscle twitches. Cardiac arrhythmias are also a concern owing to alterations in ion transport initiated by electrical current. This procedure should not be performed in close proximity to the heart or in the absence of an experienced anesthesiologist. The safety and efficacy of IRE are yet to be confirmed in larger studies, and this approach is still in its infancy.

18.1.4 Cryoablation

Though once in widespread use, most surgeons no longer perform cryotherapy because it is associated with significant start-up costs and high morbidity compared with other options. Bleeding is among the most notable complications, but patients are also at risk of "cracking" the iceball formed during ablation, fracture of the liver surface, and myoglobinuria, with the potential for acute renal failure. Unlike other modalities, cryotherapy generally requires laparotomy.

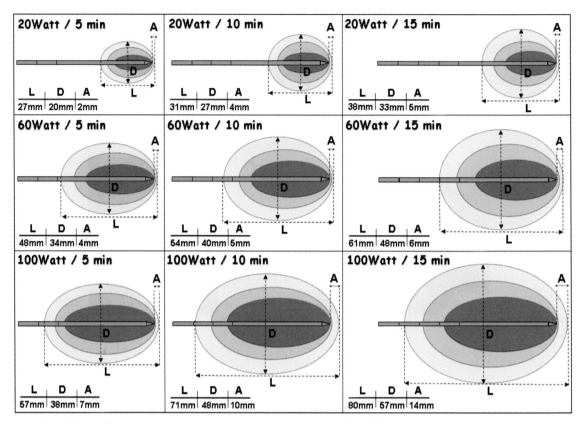

Figure 18.4 Table of ablation zones. Approximate ablation zone sizes generated by MWA based on power setting and duration. Source: HS Hospital Services SpA, Rome, Italy. Reproduced with permission.

18.1.5 Chemical ablation

Prior to the development of RFA, ethanol injection was the most commonly employed means of ablation for liver tumors. It was primarily used for HCC within a cirrhotic liver because these tumors tend to be softer compared with metastatic disease and the cirrhotic parenchyma provided a barrier to ethanol diffusion outside the tumor. The superiority of RFA over ethanol injection has subsequently been demonstrated by multiple randomized trials, as well as two large meta-analyses [9–13]. Patients treated with RFA have improved local recurrence rates, cancer-free survival at three years, and overall survival [7]. Ethanol ablation seems to have similar efficacy when compared with RFA for small solitary HCCs ≤2 cm [14,15]. However, its utility is limited by patient discomfort and the need for multiple visits for recurring injections.

In countries with resources sufficient to support the expenses of RFA, perhaps the only role for ethanol

ablation is in small tumors that are not amenable to thermal ablation because of their proximity to major vasculature, the hepatic hilum, or the gallbladder. It is generally agreed that in skilled hands, RFA can be safely performed on tumors of the dome adjacent to the diaphragm. Ethanol ablation may also be a reasonable alternative in resource-poor settings owing to its lower cost, minimal complications, and need for relatively simple equipment.

Acetic acid injection is another option for chemical ablation, which appears to have comparable efficacy and fewer adverse effects [16].

18.2 Ablation of hepatocellular carcinoma

Hepatocellular carcinoma is distinguished from other liver cancers by the increased prevalence of a cirrhotic liver parenchyma. While patients with a normal surrounding liver can tolerate resection of 70–80% of their liver volume, cirrhotics can only tolerate resections in the 40–50% range. Even if the size of the functional liver remnant (FLR) is sufficient, there is a dramatic increase in perioperative mortality as cirrhosis progresses. An inadequate FLR or advanced cirrhosis, as well as invasion of major hepatic vasculature and extrahepatic disease, may deem a patient unresectable. In contrast to resection, RFA is improved by a cirrhotic liver because of the "oven effect," whereby the surrounding cirrhotic liver traps heat within the tumor and promotes more effective ablation.

18.2.1 Small unresectable HCCs

Radiofrequency ablation alone is potentially curative for small, limited HCCs and should be considered first-line treatment when a patient with reasonably preserved liver function (Childs A or B) and good functional reserve presents with an unresectable tumor and is not a candidate for transplantation. Specifically, patients with up to three tumors ≤3 cm each who are otherwise unresectable should be treated with RFA unless tumor is not safely accessible or other contraindications are present [17,18].

Efficacy should be assessed one month following tumor ablation with contrast-enhanced computed tomography (CT) or magnetic resonance imaging (MRI). Loss of contrast enhancement within the tumor indicates successful ablation.

18.2.2 Small resectable HCCs

Though more controversial, there may be a role for RFA in patients with limited resectable disease. Three randomized trials and a meta-analysis compare RFA with hepatic resection for the treatment of small resectable HCCs. The largest trial randomized patients who fell within the Milan criteria (single tumor <5 cm; three or fewer tumors, each ≤3 cm) to undergo resection or RFA, and resected patients enjoyed a clear advantage in survival, disease-free survival, and local recurrence rates [19]. The two remaining randomized trials [20,21] and the meta-analysis [22] suggested no difference between RFA and surgical resection, particularly for small tumors ≤3 cm. Despite these provocative findings, most experienced centers continue to favor surgical resection whenever feasible. In cases of small tumors where tumor, liver, or patient-related factors tip the balance towards RFA, it is a reasonable treatment option. In some cases, RFA may be

preceded by transarterial chemoembolization as the combination has been demonstrated to increase ablation sizes and potentially decrease recurrence (see later in this chapter).

18.2.3 Ablation of bulky unresectable disease

As technology advances, there may be an expanding role for tumor ablation, both alone and in combination with other locoregional and surgical therapies, in the management of larger or multifocal tumors that would otherwise be considered nonoperable. Traditionally, management of intermediate to large tumors has relied most heavily on transarterial approaches.

18.2.4 Multipolar RFA

The efficacy of monopolar RF techniques falls off after tumors exceed 3 cm in diameter. Complete ablation often requires multiple repositionings of monopolar devices, which may increase procedure times and complications and decrease efficacy, even in experienced hands. In addition, ultrasound becomes a less reliable guidance modality as the ablative process continues and progressive tissue water vaporization causes transient hyperechogenicity in the heated tissue because of the formation of microbubbles. This makes accurate placement of additional probes difficult.

Most multipolar RFA systems consist of three bipolar electrodes, which are positioned no more than 3 cm apart and can generate 15 sequentially activated RF combinations. Ablation zones of 6 cm can be reliably produced with the need for probe repositioning. After the first round of ablation, one or two probes can be repositioned to expand the ablative margin as necessary. Clusters of four probes are also available. These techniques have shown promise in animal models and small patient series [23] but implementation has been limited because of complex equipment and high costs.

A separable clustered electrode known as the Octopus (Taewoong Medical, Goyang, Republic of Korea) used in conjunction with a multichannel generator was recently compared with traditional RFA clusters (three electrodes on a single fixed body with a fixed 5 mm interelectrode distance) in a porcine model using an open approach [24]. Unlike other systems, Octopus electrodes can be used either simultaneously in monopolar mode or in the switching monopolar mode and may be a reasonable option for tumors >5 mm in the future.

18.2.5 Microwave ablation

As discussed above, microwave ablation holds promise for large tumors. It penetrates charred or desiccated tissue, and multiple antennas may be employed simultaneously to generate larger ablative volumes as well as greater temperatures compared with RFA. In preclinical models, ablation zones up to 6.5 cm are reliably and rapidly created using three 17 gauge antennas simultaneously powered by a single generator [25]. Furthermore, mounting evidence shows that MWA is less susceptible to the heat sink effect of neighboring hepatic vasculature, which is known to increase local recurrence rates in tumors treated with RFA. Preclinical evidence suggests that MWA is effective for tumors adjacent to vessels measuring up to 10 mm [26,27], while RFA is limited by hepatic vessels greater than 3 mm [28]. Furthermore, MWA times, often in the 2–10 minute range, are much shorter than those needed for RFA [29]. This certainly has implications for efficiently treating larger and multiple unresectable tumors. Though the modality seems promising, particularly for the ablation of large and multiple tumors, more convincing long-term clinical evidence will be forthcoming as MWA gains greater acceptance among hepatobiliary surgeons.

18.2.6 Pre-RFA transarterial embolization

In patients with Childs A or B cirrhosis and large or multifocal tumors who are not candidates for surgical resection or transplantation, combined ablation and transarterial methods may also be considered. Transarterial chemoembolization (TACE) has become the default therapy for patients with intermediate size (>4–5 cm) or multifocal HCC. It combines the cytotoxic effects of targeted chemotherapy administration to the hepatic arterial circulation supplying the tumor and induces ischemic necrosis by arterial embolization. When combined with RFA, TACE diminishes the heat sink effect of the surrounding vasculature and allows for ablation of larger areas [30]. In addition, the effect of chemotherapeutic agents on the cancer cell microenvironment may attenuate its susceptibility to hyperthermia and promote additional coagulative necrosis [31]. TACE may also disrupt intratumoral septa that, when present, limit the efficacy of RFA. Although combination therapy with TACE and RFA is the most well studied, other transarterial and ablative combinations can also be considered on a case-by-case basis. Mounting data in the form of meta-analyses [32] and randomized trials support combination

therapy as a regional approach [33], especially for intermediate-stage tumors [34,35]. The morbidity associated with a combined approach must be carefully weighed by the multidisciplinary treatment team.

18.2.7 Tumor ablation as a bridge to transplant

The scarcity of transplantable livers has prompted most centers to consider locoregional or surgical therapies as a bridge to liver transplant for patients expected to have prolonged wait times, generally greater than six months [36]. Bridging treatments are pursued with the hope of containing tumor progression and decreasing the risk of "drop-off" from waiting lists. High-quality data in the form of prospective randomized trials are lacking, but pretransplant RFA is widely accepted as a safe approach that may allow patients to be maintained on waitlists for longer periods [37,38].

18.3 Ablation of liver metastases

As with HCC, resection is the treatment of choice for isolated liver metastases whenever feasible. Although superimposed cirrhosis is rarely present, the majority of patients with liver metastases are still not candidates for resection owing to tumor size, location, mutifocality, or the presence of significant co-morbidities. In contrast to patients with HCC, patients with metastatic liver tumors are almost never candidates for transplantation, which increases the relevance of RFA (or resection plus RFA) for bilobar disease. In the absence of extrahepatic metastases, some of these patients are candidates for tumor ablation as a potentially curative therapy.

18.3.1 Colorectal cancer

Compared with other malignancies, isolated hepatic metastases are relatively common in patients with colorectal cancer and the survival benefits associated with surgical resection are well documented. Ablation for colorectal metastases is generally reserved for patients who are poor surgical candidates. Currently, no randomized trials have addressed whether tumor ablation affords similar overall survival, progression-free survival, or local recurrences rates, though the majority of retrospective data suggest that resection is superior [39,40]. Based on the available data, it would be inappropriate to pursue ablation over resection in patients who are operative candidates outside a clinical trial [41].

18.3.2 Breast cancer

As many as one in five deaths from breast cancer result from liver failure in the setting of metastatic disease [42]. In the vast majority of these patients, metastatic disease is not limited to the liver and systemic therapy is the first-line treatment. Patients with isolated liver metastases that are stable or decrease while on appropriate chemo-therapeutic regimens may obtain some benefit when treated with RFA. The use of RFA in breast cancer patients with isolated hepatic metastases is limited to relatively small case series, and though reasonable in select patients, its role remains unclear.

18.3.3 Neuroendocrine tumors

As with other metastatic hepatic tumors, hepatic resection is the treatment of choice for patients with neuro-endocrine tumors who are optimal surgical candidates. Many patients with metastatic neuroendocrine disease will go on to live for several years and control of hormone hypersecretion is of tremendous value. Accordingly,

ablation of hepatic metastases can be helpful even in the presence of small-volume extrahepatic disease. Symptomatic control from excess hormone release can immediately and dramatically improve quality of life.

18.4 Postablation follow-up

All ablation strategies require postprocedural imaging to assess the completeness of ablation and for thermal modalities, to ensure an adequate 5–10 mm circumfer-ential margin (Figure 18.5). Successful ablation is indi-cated by the absence of contrast enhancement and, over time, the formation of a contracted and fibrotic scar. Even in the setting of an entirely necrotic ablation zone with adequate margins, patients are at risk for local recurrence, as well as new primary HCC or meta-static tumors. While a positron emission tomography (PET) scan may be helpful to detect local recurrence, it is subject to false-positive interpretation as a result of fluo-rodeoxyglucose (FDG) uptake in inflammatory cells. As with postresection surveillance, current National Compre-hensive Cancer Network (NCCN) guidelines recommend

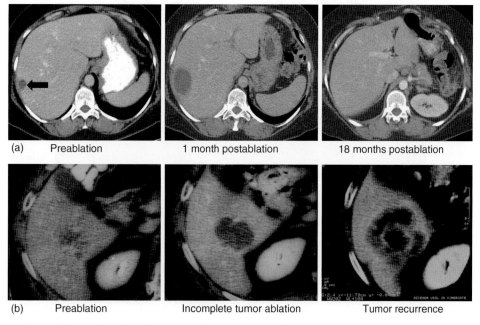

(a)   Preablation   1 month postablation   18 months postablation

(b)   Preablation   Incomplete tumor ablation   Tumor recurrence

Figure 18.5 (a) Successful RFA of a colorectal carcinoma liver metastases with CT imaging prior to ablation, one month following ablation, and 18 months following ablation. (b) Incomplete ablation leads to local recurrence. Figure shows preablation CT, postoperative CT revealing contour of ablation affected by blood vessels, and ultimately tumor recurrence resulting from incomplete ablation.

imaging every 3–6 months for the first two years following ablation and then annually [43].

18.5 Treatment approach: percutaneous, laparoscopic or open?

Most ablation modalities can be performed with open, laparoscopic, or percutaneous approaches. Each approach comes with specific risks and benefits and it is crucial that the choice be tailored to the individual patient. In this section we focus on advances in the laparoscopic approach after discussing a few key general points.

18.5.1 Percutaneous tumor ablation

The percutaneous approach (Figure 18.6a) is beneficial in that it is the least invasive and can often be completed on an outpatient basis without the need for general anesthesia. It is the preferred option for patients with

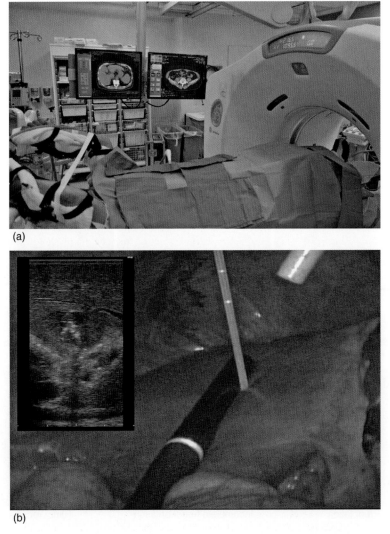

(a)

(b)

Figure 18.6 Microwave ablation. (a) Set-up for CT-guided percutaneous MWA of HCC in a poor surgical candidate. (b) MWA of hepatic tumor via a laparoscopic approach with accompanying ultrasound-guided imaging. Intraoperative ultrasound demonstrates hypoechogenic tumor with typical intraprocedural hyperechoic ablation artifacts. Source: Dr R. Santambrogio, San Paolo Hospital, University of Milan, Italy. Reproduced with permission.

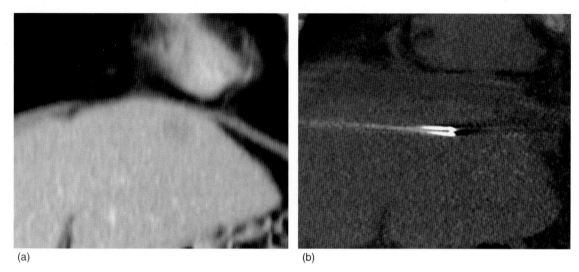

(a)   (b)

Figure 18.7 Hydrodissection to protect neighboring structures from thermal injury during percutaneous ablation. (a) HCC in the dome of the liver in close proximity to the diaphragm and heart. (b) Saline percutaneously injected into potential space between liver and hemidiaphragm to create an insulating barrier, effectively protecting the heart from thermal injury.

small tumors located in easily accessible regions. Guidance of electrodes with CT or MRI is generally better than with intraoperative ultrasound. Percutaneous ablation of tumors in the dome of the liver should be attempted with great caution on account of the risk of diaphragmatic injury (Figure 18.7a). The same is true for tumors along the inferior edge of the liver adjacent to the stomach, duodenum, or colon. These structures can be protected from thermal injury by hydrodissection, a technique that involves instillation of saline to separate the structure from the ablation zone (Figure 18.7b).

18.5.2 Open tumor ablation

Open tumor ablation provides the best hepatic exposure and allows for a thorough inspection of the peritoneum for concomitant extrahepatic metastases. It is ideally suited for patients who require laparotomy for another reason, such as combined hepatic resection and RFA, or colon resection for a primary colorectal tumor. It is also ideal for tumors in difficult locations in which care must be taken to avoid injury to adjacent viscera or vasculature. A surgical approach also allows for a Pringle maneuver to temporarily interrupt hepatic inflow to decrease the effects of heat sink when ablating large hypervascular tumors or tumors adjacent to major vasculature. Finally, high-resolution intraoperative ultrasound can be conducted with relative ease and is better suited to detect occult hepatic metastases.

18.5.3 Laparoscopic tumor ablation

Many believe that laparoscopy should be the first-line approach for thermal ablation of potentially curable tumors [44] (Figure 18.6b). In skilled hands, laparoscopy combines many of the benefits of percutaneous and open resection. The procedure is minimally invasive, yet affords the surgeon the opportunity to assess for disseminated disease, effectively protect adjacent organs, and take advantage of high-quality intraoperative ultrasonography. Hepatic or colon resections may also be performed under the same anesthesia.

Experience with laparoscopic ultrasound and ultrasound-guided needle placement is crucial as precise probe placement optimizes the chances for complete ablation with a clear margin. This aspect of the operation is particularly crucial when treating difficult-to-access deep or posterior tumors or tumors adjacent to major vasculature. Despite the aforementioned drawbacks, intraoperative ultrasound can be used in real time and is more readily available and cost-effective when compared with other imaging modalities, such as CT or MRI.

Advances in three-dimensional (3D) ultrasound probes and the use of contrast-enhanced ultrasound have improved intraoperative tumor identification and effective probe placement. Data suggest that contrast-enhanced 3D ultrasound (CE-3DUS) rivals CT and MRI in sensitivity and accuracy [45]. Contrast enhancement can also help distinguish viable tumor regions when ablating large tumors or managing a recurrence. Currently available software can accurately measure tumor dimensions, which is useful in selecting the optimal RFA probes for a given tumor. CE-3DUS can also measure the extent of coagulation necrosis approximately 10 minutes after ablation, with complete ablation marked by the absence of tumor enhancement [46].

In an attempt to streamline optimal placement of RF probes, a pilot study [47] reported a novel 3D laparoscopic magnetic ultrasound image guidance technique used in a preclinical in vitro model. Magnetic sensors were embedded into a 3D laparoscopic ultrasound transducer and a needle. Creation of an electromagnetic field allowed for real-time image guidance on a stereoscopic monitor and enabled both novices and expert hepatobiliary surgeons to accurately target 100% (44/44) of 5 mm lesions. This compared with hit rates of 0% and 59%, for novices and experts

respectively, using a traditional approach. Though still under development, such technology could dramatically improve intraoperative targeting for tumor ablation, especially for tumors in deep or complex locations.

18.6 Ablation of pancreatic tumors

The implications for tumor ablation are different in patients with liver and pancreatic tumors. Patients with liver cancer typically die of liver-specific complications, while patients with pancreatic cancer die of disseminated disease. As such, it is generally inappropriate to pursue ablation with curative intent in patients with locally advanced pancreatic cancer, while this may be possible in patients with unresectable hepatic disease. These organs are also quite distinct with respect to the safety of ablation. It is feasible to ablate somewhat large regions of hepatic parenchyma without compromising neighboring organs or vascular and ductal structures. This is nearly impossible within the pancreas.

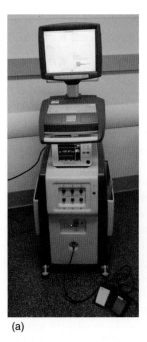
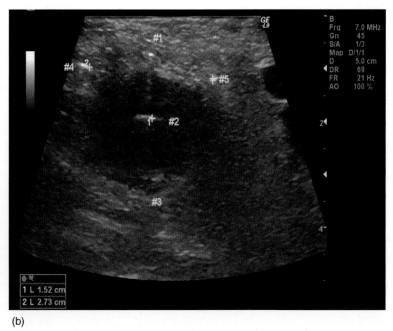

(a)   (b)

Figure 18.8 Irreversible electroporation. (a) IRE generator. (b) Intraoperative ultrasound-guided placement of IRE electrodes. (c) Cross-sectional location of the first five IRE probes relative to tumor target area (shown in yellow). (d) Voltage and current measurements across IRE electrode numbers 2 and 4 during treatment. (e) CT imaging prior to IRE showing tumor in uncinate process of pancreas (transaxial top, coronal bottom). (f) CT imaging three months post IRE (transaxial top, coronal bottom).

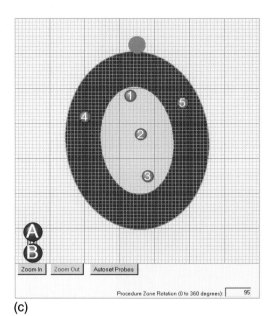

(c)

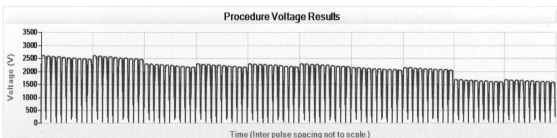

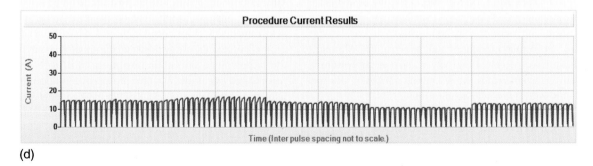

(d)

Figure 18.8 (*Continued*)

18.6.1 Thermal ablation

Although some groups consider RFA or MWA for unresectable pancreatic tumors, the majority of centers do not offer thermal ablation because of unacceptable risks in the setting of low efficacy [48]. Unlike many unresectable liver tumors, unresectable pancreatic tumors are, by definition, in close relation to adjacent organs, major vasculature, or pancreatic ductal tissue. The necessity

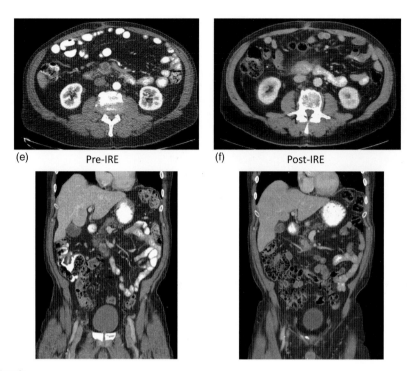

(e)   Pre-IRE   (f)   Post-IRE

Figure 18.8 (*Continued*)

of 1 cm margins to increase the likelihood of complete ablation increases the risk of damage to surrounding viscera and uncontrolled hemorrhage, as well as the risk of fistula formation and pancreatitis. Although some have suggested that lower ablation temperatures may be as efficacious, while limiting morbidity, this has not been convincingly demonstrated.

18.6.2 Irreversible electroporation

Use of IRE, a nonthermal technique, may allow precise and complete ablation as a palliative modality for locally advanced pancreatic tumors (Figure 18.8). Current evidence supports IRE as an approach for the ablation of large tumors even in close proximity to vascular or ductal structures [49]. Preclinical animal models have demonstrated rapid resolution of pancreatic inflammation [50].

Furthermore, it is also feasible to treat through blood vessels or adjacent biliopancreatic ducts. Because the vessel and duct walls are not compromised by IRE, bleeding and bile leakage are avoided and the apoptosed cells of the intima/media/adventitia or mucosa/muscularis are repopulated over time. A recent prospective multicenter pilot study [7] evaluated palliative IRE in 27 patients with locally advanced disease, defined as arterial encasement of the celiac axis or superior mesenteric artery or both. The authors reported complete ablation in all patients and no evidence of local recurrence after 90 days. No patients developed clinical pancreatitis or pancreatic fistulas. While more evidence is needed, these preliminary data suggest that IRE may play a role in ablation of locally advanced disease or in conjunction with pancreatic resection for margin control.

KEY POINTS

- Thermal ablation techniques, including RFA, MWA, and cryoablation, use different methods to induce coagulation necrosis.

- RFA is the standard of care for small unresectable HCCs.

- Laparoscopy combines many of the benefits of percutaneous and open ablation approaches.

- Advances in intraoperative ultrasound and ablation probe placement enhance the precision of laparoscopic thermal ablation and decrease the chances of local recurrence.

- IRE is an emerging nonthermal technique for tumor ablation that spares surrounding vasculature and ductal structures and may be an option for patients with locally advanced pancreatic cancer.

References

1 d'Arsonval MA. Action physiologique des courants alternatives. C R Soc Biol 1891; 43:283–286.

2 Hong K, Georgiades C. Radiofrequency ablation: mechanism of action and devices. J Vasc Interv Radiol 2010; 21: S179–S186.

3 Tanabe KK, Curley SA, Dodd GD, Siperstein AE, Goldberg SN. Radiofrequency ablation: the experts weigh in. Cancer 2003; 100(3):641–650.

4 Brace CL. Microwave ablation technology: What every user should know. Curr Probl Diagn Radiol 2009; 38(2):61–67.

5 Lee EW, Chen C, Prieto VE, Dry SM, Loh CT, Kee ST. Advanced hepatic ablation technique for creating complete cell death: irreversible electroporation. Radiology 2010; 255:426–433.

6 Lee EW, Thai S, Kee ST. Irreversible electroporation: a novel image-guided cancer therapy. Gut Liver 2010; 4(suppl 1): S99–S104.

7 Thomson KR, Cheung W, Ellis SJ, et al. Investigation of the safety of irreversible electroporation in humans. J Vasc Interv Radiol 2011; 22(5):611–621.

8 Martin RC, Mcfarland K, Ellis S, et al. Irreversible electroporation therapy in the management of locally advanced pancreatic adenocarcinoma. J Am Coll Surg 2012; 215(3):361–369.

9 Shiina S, Teratani T, Obi S, et al. A randomized controlled trial of radiofrequency ablation with ethanol injection for small hepatocellular carcinoma. Gastroenterology 2005; 129(1):122.

10 Lin SM, Lin CJ, Lin CC, et al. Radiofrequency ablation improves prognosis compared with ethanol injection for hepatocellular carcinoma<or = 4 cm. Gastroenterology 2004; 127(6):1714.

11 Ohnishi K, Yoshioka H, Ito S, et al. Prospective randomized controlled trial comparing percutaneous acetic acid injection and percutaneous ethanol injection for small hepatocellular carcinoma. Hepatology 1998; 27(1):67.

12 Cho YK, Kim JK, Kim MY, et al. Systematic review of randomized trials for hepatocellular carcinoma treated with percutaneous ablation therapies. Hepatology 2009; 49(2):453.

13 Orlando A, Leandro G, Olivo M, et al. Radiofrequency thermal ablation vs. percutaneous ethanol injection for small hepatocellular carcinoma in cirrhosis: meta-analysis of randomized controlled trials. Am J Gastroenterol 2009; 104(2):514.

14 Brunello F, Veltri A, Carucci P, et al. Radiofrequency ablation versus ethanol injection for early hepatocellular carcinoma: a randomized controlled trial. Scand J Gastroenterol 2008; 43 (6):727.

15 Lencioni RA, Allgaier HP, Cioni D, et al. Small hepatocellular carcinoma in cirrhosis: randomized comparison of radiofrequency thermal ablation versus percutaneous ethanol injection. Radiology 2003; 228(1):235.

16 Germani G, Pleguezuelo, Gurusamy K, et al. Clinical outcomes of radiofrequency ablation, percutaneous alcohol and acetic acid injection for hepatocellular carcinoma: a meta-analysis. J Hepatol 2010; 52(3):380.

17 Bruix J, Sherman M. Management of hepatocellular carcinoma. Hepatology 2005; 42:1208–1236.

18 Bruix J, Sherman M. Management of hepatocellular carcinoma: an update. Hepatology 2011; 53(3):1020–1022.

19 Huang J, Yan L, Cheng Z, et al. A randomized trial comparing radiofrequency ablation and surgical resection for HCC conforming to the Milan criteria. Ann Surg 2010; 252(6):903.

20 Chen MS, Li JQ, Zheng Y, et al. A prospective randomized trial comparing percutaneous local ablative therapy and partial hepatectomy for small hepatocellular carcinoma. Ann Surg 2006; 243(3):321.

21 Lü MD, Kuang M, Liang LJ, et al. Surgical resection versus percutaneous thermal ablation for early-stage hepatocellular carcinoma: a randomized clinical trial. Zhonghua Yi Xue Za Zhi 2006; 86(12):801.

22 Zhou Y, Zhao Y, Li B, et al. Meta-analysis of radiofrequency ablation versus hepatic resection for small hepatocellular carcinoma. BMC Gastroenterol 2010; 10:78.

23 Seror O, Knotchou G, Ibraheem M, et al. Large (≥5 cm) HCCs: multipolar RF ablation with three internally cooled bipolar electrodes – initial experience in 26 patients. J Vasc Interv Radiol 2008; 248(1):288–296.

24 Lee ES, Lee JM, Kim WS, et al. Multiple-electrode radiofrequency ablations using Octopus® electrodes in an

in vivo porcine liver model. Br J Radiol 2012; 85(1017): e609–e615.

25 Brace CL, Laeseke PF, Sampson LA, *et al.* Microwave ablation with multiple simultaneously powered small-gauge triaxial antennas: results from an in vivo swine liver model. Radiology 2007; 244(1):151–156.

26 Shibata T, Iimuro Y, Yamamoto Y, *et al.* Small hepatocellular carcinoma: comparison of radio-frequency ablation and percutaneous microwave coagulation therapy. Radiology 2002; 223(2):331–337.

27 Wang Y, Sun Y, Feng L, Gao Y, Ni X, Liang P. Internally cooled antenna for microwave ablation: results in ex vivo and in vivo porcine livers. Eur J Radiol 2008; 67(2):357–361.

28 Lu DS, Raman SS, Limanond P, *et al.* Influence of large peritumoral vessels on outcome of radiofrequency ablation of liver tumors. J Vasc Interv Radiol 2003; 14(10):1267–1274.

29 Lubner MG, Brace CL, Hinshaw JL, Lee FT. Microwave tumor ablation: mechanism of action, clinical results and devices. J Vasc Interv Radiol 2010; 21(8 suppl):S192–S203.

30 Morimoto M, Numata K, Kondou M, *et al.* Midterm outcomes in patients with intermediate-sized hepatocellular carcinoma: a randomized controlled trial for determining the efficacy of radiofrequency ablation combined with transarterial chemoembolization. Cancer 2010; 116:5452–5460.

31 Goldberg SN, Hahn PF, Tanabe KK, *et al.* Percutaneous radiofrequency ablation: does perfusion mediated tissue cooling limit coagulation necrosis? J Vasc Interv Radiol 1998; 9:101–111.

32 Lu Z, Wen F, Guo Q, Liang H, Mao X, Sun H. Radiofrequency ablation plus chemoembolization versus radiofrequency ablation alone for hepatocellular carcinoma: a meta-analysis of randomized controlled trials. Eur J Gastroenterol Hepatol 2013; 25:187–194.

33 Aikata H, Shirakawa H, Takaki S, *et al.* Radiofrequency ablation combined with transcatheter arterial chemoembolization for small hepatocellular carcinoma. Hepatology 2006; 44:A487.

34 Chen BQ, Jia CQ, Liu CT, *et al.* Chemoembolization combined with radiofrequency ablation for patients with hepatocellular carcinoma larger than 3 cm: a randomized controlled trial. JAMA 2008; 299:1669–1677.

35 Peng ZW, Zhang YJ, Chen MS, *et al.* Radiofrequency ablation with or without transcatheter chemoembolization in the treatment of hepatocellular carcinoma: a prospective randomized trial. J Clin Oncol 2013; 31(4):426–432.

36 Clavien PA, Lesurtel M, Bossuyt PM, et al, for HCC Consensus Group. Recommendations for liver transplantation for hepatocellular carcinoma: an international consensus conference report. Lancet Oncol 2012; 13(1):e11–22.

37 DuBay DA, Sandroussi C, Kachura JR, *et al.* Radiofrequency ablation of hepatocellular carcinoma as a bridge to liver transplantation. HPB 2011; 13(1):24–32.

38 Cescon M, Cucchetti A, Ravaioli M, Pinna AD. Hepatocellular carcinoma locoregional therapies for patients in the waiting list. Impact on transplantability and recurrence rate. J Hepatol 2013; 58:609–618.

39 Abdalla EK, Vauthey JN, Ellis LM, *et al.* Recurrence and outcomes following hepatic resection, radiofrequency ablation, and combined resection/ablation for colorectal liver metastases. Ann Surg 2004; 239(6):818.

40 Lee WS, Yun SH, Chun HK, *et al.* Clinical outcomes of hepatic resection and radiofrequency ablation in patients with solitary colorectal liver metastasis. J Clin Gastroenterol 2008; 42 (8):945.

41 Wong SL, Mangu PB, Choti MA, *et al.* American Society of Clinical Oncology 2009 clinical evidence review on radiofrequency ablation of hepatic metastases from colorectal cancer. J Clin Oncol 2010; 28(3):493.

42 Gunabushanam G, Sharma S, Thulkar S, *et al.* Radiofrequecy ablation of liver metastases from breat cancer: results in 14 patients. J Vasc Interv Radiol 2007; 18:67–72.

43 National Comprehensive Cancer Network (NCCN) guidelines. Available online at www.nccn.org

44 Poon RT, Fan ST, Tsang FH, Wong J. Locoregional therapies for hepatoceullar carcinoma: a critical view from the surgeon's perspective. Ann Surg 2002; 235(4):466–486.

45 Leen E, Ceccotti P, Moug SJ, *et al.* Potential value of contrast-enhanced intraoperative ultrasonography during partial hepatectomy for metastases: an essential investigation before resection? Ann Surg 2006; 243:236–240.

46 Künzli BM, Abitabile P, Maurer CA. Radiofrequency ablation of liver tumors: actual limitations and potential solutions in the future. World J Hepatol 2011; 3(1):8–14.

47 Sindram D, McKillop IH, Martinie JB, Iannitti DA. Novel 3-D laparoscopic magnetic ultrasound image guidance for lesion targeting. HPB 2010; 12:709–716.

48 Pezzilli R, Ricci C, Serra C, *et al.* The problems of radiofrequency ablation as an approach for advanced unresectable ductal pancreatic carcinoma. Cancers (Basel) 2010; 2(3): 1419–1431.

49 Davalos RV, Mir IL, Rubinsky B. Tissue ablation with irreversible electroporation. Ann Biomed Eng 2005; 33:223–231.

50 Bower M, Sherwood L, Li Y, Martin R. Irreversible electroporation of the pancreas: definitive local therapy without systemic effects. J Surg Oncol 2011; 104:22–28.

CHAPTER 19

Technical considerations for advanced laparoscopic liver resection

Ho-Seong Han

Department of Surgery, Seoul National University College of Medicine, Gyeonggi-do, Korea

---

EDITOR COMMENT

In this chapter, expert laparoscopic surgeon Professor Han from Seoul National University provides a comprehensive overview on technical aspects of laparoscopic liver resection as well as surgical liver anatomy. The chapter highlights the indications and technical challenges for a Glissonian approach to laparoscopic anatomical liver resection with special consideration given to each segment. With his large experience in performing laparoscopic liver resection for HCC in cirrhotic patients, Professor Han covers key considerations regarding adequate future liver remnant and limited resections. This chapter will stimulate the appetite of the reader for the video atlas portion of this book.

Keywords: advanced laparoscopic liver surgery, Glissonian approach, indications and contraindications to advanced laparoscopic liver surgery, laparoscopic liver surgery in cirrhotic patients

---

19.1 Introduction

With many reports on encouraging outcomes, laparoscopic liver resection has been accepted as an attractive alternative to open liver resection. However, there are still several limitations in the indications of laparoscopic liver resection that are important to recognize and that we are in the process of overcoming. First, in most centers, laparoscopic liver resection has been limited to easily accessible lesions. Second, a laparoscopic approach has been considered not well suited when the tumor is close to a major vascular structure such as the hepatic veins or inferior vena cava (IVC). Third, this laparoscopic approach to liver resection still has limited indications in very large tumors. However, as the experience with advanced laparoscopic liver surgery grows, its prior and current indications and contraindications will change and expand.

Traditionally in Korea and other parts of the world, indications for laparoscopic liver resection have been limited to tumors in the peripheral portion of the

anterolateral segments of the liver (segments II, III, V, VI, and the inferior part of IV according to the classification of Couinaud). In contrast, lesions in the posterior or superior part of the liver (segments I, VII, VIII, and the superior part of IV) are considered poor indications for laparoscopic liver resection. However, over time, flexible laparoscopic cameras, high-definition imaging, and various advanced energy devices for parenchymal transection have been introduced for clinical use. These technical advances help overcome inadequate exposure with a greater diffusion of advanced laparoscopic liver surgery throughout Korea, Asia, and the rest of the world. Intraoperative ultrasonography is routinely used to locate lesions and guide the resection plane even for deeply located and invisible lesions.

When the tumor is centrally located (close to major hepatic veins or the IVC), laparoscopic liver resection has been considered a contraindication because of the risk of major hemorrhage and concerns for adequately controlling bleeding. While these concerns are valid, recent developments in instrumentation for parenchymal

---

Laparoscopic Liver, Pancreas, and Biliary Surgery, First Edition.
Edited by Claudius Conrad and Brice Gayet.
© 2017 John Wiley & Sons, Ltd. Published 2017 by John Wiley & Sons, Ltd.

dissection have made laparoscopic liver resection safer and more refined than before. These instruments include the laparoscopic Cavitron ultrasonic surgical aspirator (CUSA; Valleylab, Inc., Boulder, Colorado) which, similar to open liver surgery, allows safe liver resection close to the portal pedicle, major hepatic veins, or IVC. As for the current limitations on tumor size, these may change as a result of growing experience with advanced laparoscopic liver resection and the ongoing development of laparoscopic devices. However, the incision required to remove large tumors and prevention of tumor spillage through rupture will remain key considerations for laparoscopic liver surgeons.

The type of resection may also depend on the remaining liver's functional capacity. Patients with hepatocellular carcinoma (HCC) usually have poor liver function as a result of chronic liver disease or liver cirrhosis. Therefore, it is recommended to spare as much future liver remnant as possible without jeopardizing oncological safety. Anatomical liver resection may be advantageous in preserving the future liver remnant while also achieving long-term control of the cancer in some cases.

Several approaches for anatomical liver resection are available today. The Glissonian pedicle approach is one of the most important concepts for anatomical liver resection. Here, we describe technical points for performing advanced anatomical laparoscopic liver resection.

19.2 General considerations

The indications for laparoscopic liver resection are similar to open liver resection in terms of the preoperative assessment of liver function, type of liver resection, and postoperative care. For patients with HCC, absence of severe portal hypertension and adequate hepatic reserve are prerequisites for surgery. For metastatic liver tumors from colorectal cancer, liver resection is indicated in most cases when there is no evidence of extrahepatic disease and all known disease can be resected. A simultaneous laparoscopic liver resection of metastatic disease and minimally invasive colorectal resection can achieve potential cure with minimal morbidity.

Deeply seated tumors located more than 3 cm from the liver surface are usually best resected with anatomical liver resection rather than nonanatomical tumorectomy. Up to 3 cm from the liver surface, major hepatic vein branches and the hepatic veins themselves are rarely

encountered. Especially in Asia, it is thought that complete tumor clearance (especially HCC) and a safe tumor margin can be best achieved with an anatomical resection, described below.

19.3 Operative technique

Patient positioning, trocar placement, and the type of resection should be decided prior to surgery according to tumor location and surgical approach. It is our technique to establish pneumoperitoneum through a 10 mm umbilical port and maintain abdominal pressure below 12 mmHg to reduce the potential risk of CO_2 embolism. Other advanced laparoscopic liver surgeons have experimented with raising the abdominal pressure above 15 mmHg and even higher to achieve a "Pringle" effect with the aid of the pneumoperitoneum. An infraumbilical access is used in cirrhotic patients to avoid injury to a recannulated umbilical vein. A 30° laparoscope or flexible laparoscope is employed. Laparoscopic ultrasonography is used for precise localization of the tumor, for demonstrating a satellite nodule of HCC, and for achieving an adequate tumor-free margin.

For the superficial hepatic parenchymal transection, we use energy devices such as the Harmonic Scalpel (Ethicon Endo-Surgery, Inc., Cincinnati, Ohio) or a Sono-Surg (Olympus Inc., Japan), and for the deeper portion of the parenchyma, laparoscopic CUSA. Once the specimen has been completely detached from the rest of the liver, it is inserted into a protective vinyl endoscopic retrieval bag. We usually extract small specimens by extending the epigastric or umbilical port site, especially for limited resections such as tumorectomy specimens. Especially large hemihepatectomy specimens in younger patients are removed through a suprapubic transverse incision. At our institution, we apply a fibrin glue sealant (Greenplast, Green Cross Corporation, Seoul, Korea) to the raw surface after hemostasis has been achieved. After irrigating the surgical field, a silastic drain is inserted in some cases and the wound is closed in layers.

19.3.1 Glissonian approach
The Glissonian sheath is a fibrous envelope encircling the portal triad from the hepatoduodenal ligament to its segmental pedicles in the liver. By controlling the Glissonian pedicle, a precise anatomical liver resection can be performed. The Glissonian approach is an important

strategy for both minor and major anatomical liver resection through controlling inflow to the liver area to be resected. This approach was first described by Takasaki in 1998 for open liver surgery and in 2005, we applied such a Glissonian approach to a laparoscopic anatomical resection of the right posterior section.

19.3.2 Operative technique for major liver resection

Typically, for a right hemihepatectomy or right posterior sectionectomy, the liver is fully mobilized off the IVC and multiple small hepatic veins are clipped and divided. The portal pedicles are dissected outside the liver parenchyma for individual ligation. In our approach, following isolation of the Glissonian pedicle, the portal, arterial, and bile duct pedicles are controlled separately. After opening the Glissonian sheath, the arterial and portal branches can be clipped and divided. When the portal branch is too large to apply clips, it is divided with a linear stapler.

When the Glissonian approach is applied to right-sided resection, the hilar dissection is performed first to isolate the right Glissonian pedicles at the inferior surface of the quadrate lobe (area of the liver between the gallbladder fossa and the umbilical vein behind the porta hepatis). When performing a right posterior sectionectomy, the right Glissonian pedicle is followed to its division into the anterior and posterior Glissonian pedicles. Each of these two pedicles is isolated and then the posterior Glissonian pedicle is divided using a linear stapler.

19.3.3 Laparoscopic segmental liver resection

19.3.3.1 Segment I (see Video 4)

Resection of the caudate lobe is one of the most challenging procedures in liver surgery, both open and laparoscopic, because of its deep location and position close to the IVC. Although a true anatomical caudate lobectomy is a challenging technical procedure, a laparoscopic non-anatomical and even anatomical segmentectomy I is feasible in selected patients. Tumor location in the Spiegelian lobe facilitates a laparoscopic approach.

For caudate resection, the patient is placed in the 30° reverse Trendelenburg position with the lower limbs apart. The operator stands between the legs of the patient. The procedure begins with mobilization of the left liver. Then the caudate lobe is retracted anteriorly off the IVC. Next, small hepatic veins off the caudate lobe to the IVC are isolated and divided. After completely mobilizing the

caudate lobe, the parenchymal transection is performed while maintaining medial traction of the caudate lobe. The small, vascular or biliary tributaries to the caudate lobe of the main left and right portal pedicle are isolated, clipped, and divided.

19.3.3.2 Segments II and III (see Videos 2 and 3)

At most centers, a laparoscopic approach to left lateral sectionectomy is usually the first attempt at performing an anatomical liver resection.

The operative procedure is performed with the patient placed in a supine position and 30° reverse Trendelenburg. The operator stands at the right side of the patient. The vascular and biliary structures can be controlled before or during parenchymal transection. With lateral traction of the divided round ligament, parenchymal transection just left of the falciform ligament is performed cephalad using an energy device. Other groups leave the round and falciform ligaments intact for countertraction without the need to use an instrument. The Glissonian pedicles to segments II and III can be isolated separately by an extrahepatic or intrahepatic approach. For intraparenchymal control of the pedicles to segments II and III, a small portion of the parenchymal transection is begun. Once the main left portal pedicle is approached, the Glisson's pedicles to the left lateral section can be controlled using a linear stapler. An additional firing of the stapler is used for division of the left hepatic vein. By isolating Glissonian pedicles of segments II or III, an anatomical segmentectomy of segment II or segment III is possible.

19.3.3.3 Segment IV (see Videos 5, 6, and 7)

Tumorectomy is a feasible and safe resection for a relatively small tumor located in the superficial and inferior part of segment IV. However, when a tumor is located in the superior part or is deeply buried in the liver parenchyma, left hemihepatectomy is the preferred approach. Tumorectomy of a small tumor located in the superior part of segment IV is feasible but significantly more challenging, because the transection line may encounter two main hepatic veins.

Anatomical segmentectomy IV is also feasible, although this procedure is technically demanding. The Glissonian pedicle, which usually consists of several branches, needs to be isolated and controlled. Typically a segmentectomy IV is begun at the medial side of segment IV just medial to the falciform ligament. As the dissection is deepened towards the left Glissonian pedicle, the Glissonian branches to segment IV can be identified. Then, after temporary clamping of Glissonian branches to segment IV, the ischemic demarcation delineates the borders between the left lateral and right anterior section.

19.3.3.4 Segments V and VI (see Videos 8, 9, 13, and 16)

Segments V and VI are easily accessible for laparoscopic liver resection. Cholecystectomy and full liver mobilization are usually not necessary for tumorectomy or segmentectomy for a small superficial tumor. However, a deeply located or large tumor in segment VI requires right posterior sectionectomy or right hemihepatectomy, depending on the specific location or the distance of the tumor from the right hepatic vein. For a deep or large tumor in segment V, right hemihepatectomy will be the resection of choice, although right anterior sectionectomy can be considered in experienced hands. However, anatomical right anterior or posterior sectionectomy should only be attempted if the patient has an adequate future liver remnant in case conversion to a right hepatectomy is necessary. Anatomical V and VI bisegmentectomy is also feasible.

For anatomical resection of segment V, the Glissonian branch to segment V is isolated. First, the right anterior branch of the Glissonian pedicle is isolated, and then the branch to segment V is further dissected and isolated. Typically, segment V has more than one Glissonian pedicle. With clamping of the isolated branches, demarcation of segment V is achieved. Following the demarcation line, anatomical segment V segmentectomy can be performed.

Anatomical segment VI segmentectomy starts with isolation of the Glissonian branch or branches to segment VI. After careful dissection of the right posterior Glissonian pedicle, the surgeons progress peripherally to reach the branch to segment VI which can then be isolated. By clamping the Glissonian pedicle to segment VI, an anatomical segment VI segmentectomy can be performed.

19.3.3.5 Segments VII and VIII (see Videos 10, 11, 13, and 16)

Segments VII and VIII are difficult locations to access via laparoscopy because of the limited visualization that can be achieved via a purely transabdominal laparoscopic approach. It is also difficult to control bleeding should it occur. Therefore, for safe resection of tumors in this location, a flexible laparoscope can help overcome the limited visualization. Alternatively, or in addition, a transthoracic approach can be performed as published by the editors. A laparoscopic CUSA can be very useful for meticulous parenchymal transection to reduce bleeding from major vessels. It is critical that the main working port is placed as close as possible to the costal margin to minimize the distance between port and target. For tall or obese patients, even with the ports placed close to the costal margin, instruments cannot reach the dome of the liver, in which case, an extra-long or thoracoscopic approach may be required.

Poor visualization of the operative field at the dome and the intricate transection needed to create a curved or angulated transection line can make deeper lesions at the dome particularly difficult to resect. Caudal traction of the liver after releasing the right triangular ligament may facilitate exposure and transection. For those lesions, ultrasound-guided outlining of the transection line may be needed as a Glissonian approach can be challenging. At our institution, we consider even limited liver resections in segment VII or VIII as difficult and major resections. Vascular control techniques such as Pringle's maneuver may reduce blood loss during tumorectomy.

For deep-seated large tumors in segment VII, a right posterior sectionectomy can be preferable over a complicated isolated anatomical resection of segment VII or right hepatectomy.

Compared with a right hepatectomy for segment VII lesions, a posterior sectionectomy preserves the liver volume of the anterior section. Nevertheless, a posterior sectionectomy may be technically very demanding. The main problem during a right posterior sectionectomy is the difficulty of performing the parenchymal transection. Injury of major branches of the right hepatic vein or the right hepatic vein itself can lead to massive bleeding that can be very difficult to control laparoscopically.

For a deep-seated large tumor in segment VIII, a right hepatectomy can be chosen for anatomical liver resection. This is only possible, of course, if the future liver remnant has been calculated to be adequate. However, for severely cirrhotic patients with an insufficient hepatic reserve, a limited resection may be the best approach for tumors located in segment VII or VIII.

When the lesion encompasses segment VIII or IV, the challenging central bisectionectomy can be performed. The Glissonian pedicle to segment IV and the right anterior Glissonian pedicle are isolated to confirm the area of segment IV and right anterior section. After the ischemic demarcation line is drawn, the parenchymal transaction is performed in the usual manner.

19.4 Conclusion

With the improvement of laparoscopic techniques and the development of new technologies, the limitations of laparoscopic liver resection regarding tumor location are gradually being overcome. In the near future, tumor location per se might no longer be a contraindication for a laparoscopic liver resection. However, to achieve safe laparoscopic liver resection, each surgical technique must be individualized according to patient factors, future liver remnant, and tumor location with its relationship to major hepatic vessels.

> **KEY POINTS**
>
> - General considerations regarding the safety of patients undergoing laparoscopic liver resections, such as adequate future liver remnant, apply to a laparoscopic approach.
> - Anatomical liver resections via the Glissonian approach require optimal technology and surgical technique to perform safely.
> - Left lateral sectionectomy might be the optimal procedure to gain experience with anatomical laparoscopic liver resection.
> - The overview on anatomical segmental resection given in this chapter will enhance the understanding of the video atlas portion of this book.

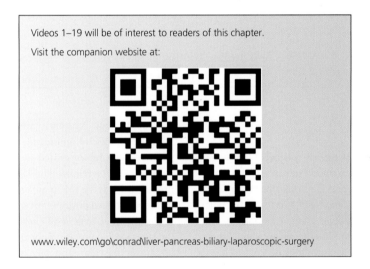

Videos 1–19 will be of interest to readers of this chapter.
Visit the companion website at:

www.wiley.com\go\conrad\liver-pancreas-biliary-laparoscopic-surgery

CHAPTER 20

Laparoscopic left lateral sectionectomy and left hepatectomy for living donation

Claire Goumard and Olivier Scatton

Department of Hepatobiliary Surgery and Liver Transplantation, Hôpital Pitié-Salpêtrière, Assistance Publique-Hôpitaux de Paris, Paris, France

---

EDITOR COMMENT

In this chapter, the authors share their experience with laparoscopic living donor liver transplantation. The key message of the chapter is that every measure should be taken to ensure donor safety during laparoscopic graft harvest. With one of the largest experiences in living donor liver transplantation, the authors share key steps and technical tricks to ensure donor safety, successfully complete the procedure laparoscopically, and optimize graft function. These include an extensive work-up of the donor's health and liver function, assessment of anatomical variations, a two-surgeon technique with alternation between the two experienced transplant surgeons, predefined criteria for conversion, and checklisting of key operative steps. The authors further share tips to minimize warm ischemia time during laparoscopic graft removal. While in this chapter and the excellent educational accompanying video, left lateral and left donor hepatectomy are described, the future of laparoscopic living donor graft harvest might include laparoscopic left hepatectomy including the middle hepatic vein and laparoscopic right hepatectomy.

Keywords: future procedures in living donor liver transplantation, laparoscopic living donor liver transplantation, left hepatectomy for living donation, left lateral sectionectomy for living donation

---

20.1 Introduction

Living donor liver transplantation has become a widely accepted alternative to cadaveric transplantation [1,2]. Such living donor grafts provide similar or better short-term graft function and long-term survival rates when compared with cadaveric liver grafts, especially in children [3–5]. Living donation has the advantages of shortening waiting list times and minimizing cold ischemia time. While significant benefits for the recipients exist, the surgical risk for donors remains the main limiting factor for a wider application of living donation [5].

Limited resection tries to reduce the risk to the donor. Therefore, open left lateral sectionectomy is a well-accepted and standardized procedure, associated with low rates of complications and mortality in living donor transplantation [6–9].

A laparoscopic approach was first proposed in 2002 with the premise of optimizing donor safety [6]; a comparative study demonstrated its safety and reproducibility in 2006 [7]. The reason why laparoscopic resection was propagated was the major advantages for the donor, that included reduced postoperative pain and shortened hospital stay [9,10]. In general, the left liver is more favorable for laparoscopic procurement than the right liver: there are fewer vascular and biliary anatomical variations, there is adequate length of extrahepatic vessels that allows easy control, and its anterior position gives access with minimal mobilization. Further, modern imaging allows an accurate and reliable assessment of both vascular and biliary anatomy. With growing experience and technical innovations, left living donor liver transplantation has evolved from an innovative procedure initially described in 2002 to the standardized procedure we

---

Laparoscopic Liver, Pancreas, and Biliary Surgery, First Edition.
Edited by Claudius Conrad and Brice Gayet.
© 2017 John Wiley & Sons, Ltd. Published 2017 by John Wiley & Sons, Ltd.

perform today. In France, more than 70 laparoscopic graft harvests have been performed [11].

20.2 Donor evaluation process

The selection of an eligible donor involves the evaluation of both technical feasibility and operative risk for the donor. Both issues mandate an extensive work-up, including an extensive search for any medical contraindications, donor psychological assessment, and evaluation of the suitability of the intended graft in terms of anatomy, volume, and function.

Currently, there is no consensus for donor age, and we rely more on physiological age than chronological age. However, an upper age limit is arbitrarily set at 55 in many centers. In our center, the oldest donor so far has been 56 years old. Every eligible donor has to be thoroughly informed about the risks involved, not only for the donor operation but also the recipient mortality (5%), together with donor mortality (0.2–1%) and morbidity rates (15–40%). Left living donor liver transplantation is favored at many centers because the mortality and morbidity rates are significantly lower for left than for right hepatectomy.

An extensive medical history should be conducted, including personal and/or familial history of diabetes mellitus, cardiovascular disease, pulmonary disease, malignancy, psychological disorders, alcohol consumption and smoking, and deep vein thrombosis risk factors (oral contraception use for women). This must be augmented by a complete physical examination with body mass index (BMI), which also includes arterial blood pressure measurements. Biological tests include classic blood hematology and biochemistry, complete glycemic and lipid profile, common viral serology screening (human immunodeficiency virus [HIV], hepatitis B and C, cytomegalovirus [CMV], varicella zoster virus [VZV]), and, in our center, extensive research on coagulation disorders (factor V Leiden, factor II, antithrombin III, antiphospholipid antibodies, protein C, protein S). Specific markers for malignancy can be added in case of any clinical suspicion.

A psychiatrist should conduct a complete psychological evaluation, and the donor case should be presented for approval by an ethics committee. All donors must give their informed consent. According to the French law "Loi Bioéthique" (1994), which was modified in 2004 and

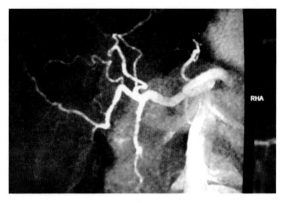

Figure 20.1 CT scan 3D arterial reconstruction.

2012, a judge of the civilian court records the donor's written consent.

The graft assessment work-up includes multiple imaging evaluations by a combination of ultrasound, computed tomograhy (CT) scan and magnetic resonance imaging (MRI) cholangiography. CT scan with three-dimensional (3D) vascular reconstruction is mandatory for arterial mapping (Figure 20.1). The course and size of the hepatic artery, and detection of anatomical variations such as a right hepatic artery arising from the superior mesenteric artery or left hepatic artery arising from the left gastric artery, are noted. The origin of the segment IV hepatic artery should be outlined (from the left or right hepatic artery). Portal venous anatomy is also assessed (Figure 20.2), in order to identify division abnormalities (i.e. portal trifurcation). Particular attention is paid to hepatic venous drainage, especially the course of the

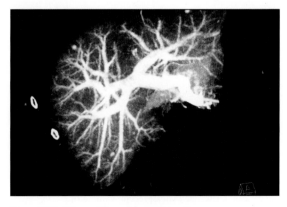

Figure 20.2 CT scan 3D portal reconstruction.

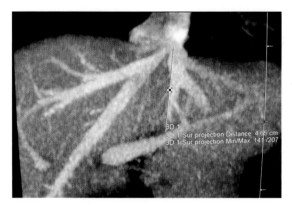

Figure 20.3 CT scan hepatic venous drainage mapping.

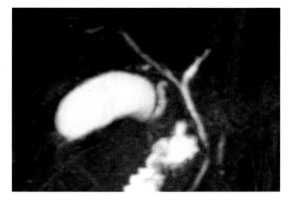

Figure 20.5 Preoperative MR cholangiography.

segment IV drainage vein in case of left donor hepatectomy (Figure 20.3).

Computed tomography volumetric measurement of the liver remnant and the intended graft should be performed (Figure 20.4) in order to obtain a safety limit for donor remnant volume of 30–35% and to ensure the 0.8% graft to body weight ratio considered a safe volume to weight ratio for the recipient [12–15].

At our center, we then perform an MR cholangiography, which is currently the best way to detect biliary anatomy abnormalities (Figure 20.5). This investigation is fundamental to search for variations, such as a right posterior or anterior sectorial duct joining the left hepatic duct; such a situation represents a formal contraindication to the intervention. The position of the left hepatic duct division and site of segment IV duct joining should also be documented.

We do not routinely perform liver biopsy, endoscopic retrograde cholangiopancreatography (ERCP), or arteriography.

Finally, the decision to perform a living donor left lateral sectionectomy is validated by a multidisciplinary review committee, where all potential medical contraindications are considered and suitability of the intended graft in terms of anatomy and volume is closely examined. It should be highlighted that there are very few anatomical contraindications for left liver graft harvesting compared with the right liver. The two absolute contraindications are existence of an exclusive right hepatic artery arising from the mesenteric artery (around 9% of cases) and/or the absence of portal bifurcation (less than 1%).

20.3 Surgical technique

To enhance donor safety, this intervention should ideally be performed by two senior surgeons. Any incident that might compromise donor safety or graft integrity should lead to prompt conversion from the laparoscopic procedure to an open procedure. In our team, we defined these events or criteria of conversion as: significant bleeding, failure to accurately recognize bile duct anatomy, any vessel injury, and inadequate exposure of the surgical site, leading to failure or slow progression during parenchymal transection.

The operation is divided into three steps: left pedicle dissection, parenchymal transection including left bile duct division, and graft extraction. Usually, these steps are performed in rotation between the two surgeons, one

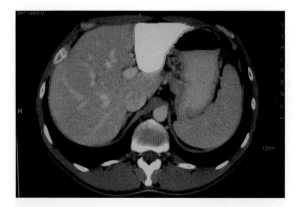

Figure 20.4 CT scan left lateral section volumetric measurement.

performing the pedicle dissection and the other doing the parenchymal transection and graft removal.

20.3.1 Preparation

The donor is placed in the supine position, legs apart (French position). Devices to prevent hypothermia (warming coverage) and deep vein thrombosis (compression stockings) are routinely used. Two monitors are placed above the patient's left and right shoulders.

A carbon dioxide pneumoperitoneum is created and maintained at 12 mmHg pressure. Five trocars, three of 12 mm diameter and two of 5 mm diameter, are inserted (Versastep Plus, Tyco Healthcare, Norwalk, Connecticut), as shown in Figure 20.6. The middle trocar is placed 2–3 cm above the umbilicus to avoid any tangential vision to the whole left lateral section.

A 30° laparoscope is useful to obtain an optimal visual field of every region of the abdominal cavity, to facilitate visualization of the hepatic vein, and to avoid forcing the operating surgeon into an unnatural viewing angle in case of a tangential dissection plane.

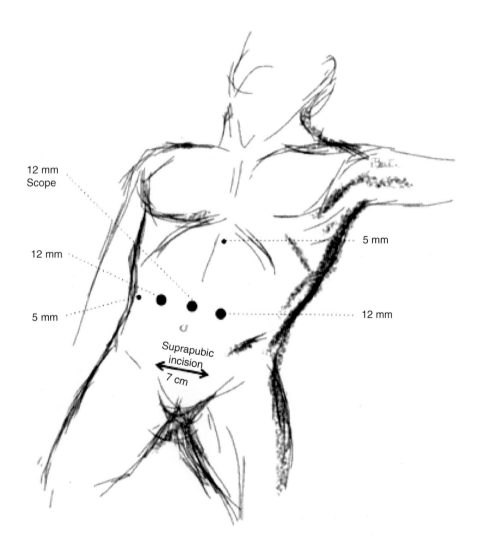

Figure 20.6 Donor position and trocar placement.

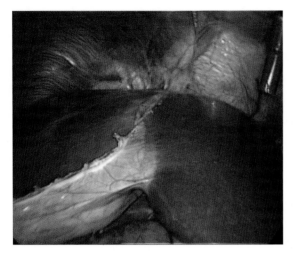

Figure 20.7 Access and mobilization of the left lateral section.

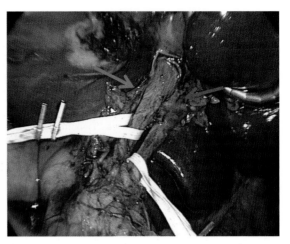

Figure 20.8 Left pedicle dissection. Left hepatic artery (*red arrow*) and left portal (*blue arrow*) branches are dissected and taped.

20.3.2 Access and mobilization of the left lateral section

After a general inspection of the liver and the abdominal cavity, the left lateral section is mobilized by first dividing the round and falciform ligaments (Figure 20.7); the lesser omentum is opened, and the left triangular ligament is divided. The dissection of the falciform ligament is continued to the level of the insertion of the hepatic veins. This first mobilization step is preferentially performed with the Harmonic Scalpel (Ethicon Endo-Surgery Inc., Cincinnati, Ohio), which offers the advantage of simultaneous cutting and coagulating of the surgical site. Alternatively, the procedure may be completed using bipolar forceps and scissors.

20.3.3 Left pedicle preparation

The left arterial and portal branches are dissected free and taped (Figure 20.8). A left hepatic artery, arising from the left gastric artery, is isolated as well. Arterial and portal branches to segment I are divided, either between clips or using the Harmonic Scalpel, depending to the vessel diameter (Figure 20.9); this also facilitates control of the left hepatic artery and portal vein by gaining length. This step of the pedicle dissection should be performed in such a way that it facilitates the future implantation of the left pedicle when the graft is transplanted into the recipient.

20.3.4 Parenchymal transection

The parenchymal transection is performed along the right side of the falciform ligament, in contrast to the conventional left lateral sectionectomy, which is typically performed to the left of the falciform ligament. Posteriorly, the transection line follows the ligament of Arantius.

Exposure during transection is maintained by traction of the round ligament and left lateral segment with an atraumatic retractor.

We use the Harmonic Scalpel for incision of the liver capsule and the superficial part of the transection (no more than 1 cm deep in the parenchyma). We prefer the ultrasonic dissector for deeper transection (Figure 20.10). The parenchyma is thus divided step by step and the encountered pedicles are identified before dividing and clipping. Vessels larger than 2 mm, such as portal pedicles to segment IV, are dissected free using the ultrasonic dissector and taped using polytetrafluoroethylene (PTFE) tapes. This is done to clearly expose both sides of the pedicle to be transected. The pedicle is then clipped,

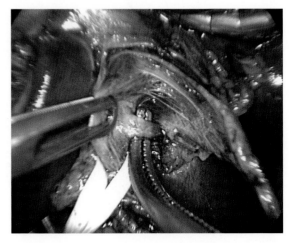

Figure 20.9 Dissection of a segment I portal branch.

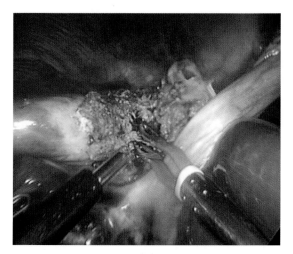

Figure 20.10 Parenchymal transection using ultrasonic dissector and bipolar coagulation simultaneously.

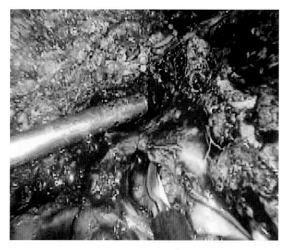

Figure 20.12 Left bile duct division with scissors.

using secured Hem-o-lok clips (Teleflex Medical, Morrisville, North Carolina), and divided (Figure 20.11).

Bleeding is controlled using bipolar cautery for minor vessels and clips for larger vascular structures. No inflow control is used to minimize ischemic damage to both donor liver and graft. A transient increase in pneumoperitoneum pressure up to 16 mmHg can be applied, if well tolerated by the donor, to improve bleeding control.

20.3.5 Left bile duct division
Once the liver transection has reached the hilar plate, the left bile duct is divided with scissors (Figure 20.12). To avoid injuring it, the left portal vein is pulled downwards using tape. This maneuver allows the surgeon to safely

divide the bile duct and may improve visualization of the hilar plate. Moreover, no electric cautery should be applied at this stage to avoid thermal injury of the bile duct and the hilar plate. The distal stump of the bile duct is closed using a secured Hem-o-lok clip (Figure 20.13). We prefer these locking clips at our center after we experienced one case of bile leakage after dislodgment of a regular titanium clip.

20.3.6 End of transection and control of the left hepatic vein
After bile duct division, the transection progresses along Arantius's line towards the left hepatic vein, which is then

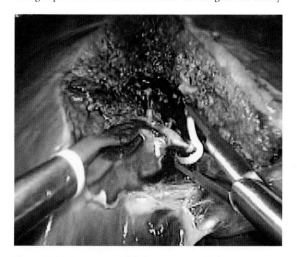

Figure 20.11 Segment IV pedicle exposure and clipping.

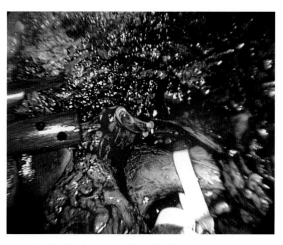

Figure 20.13 Distal stumps of the left bile duct closed with a secure clip.

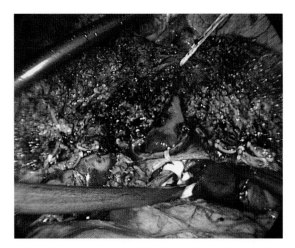

Figure 20.14 Left lateral graft ready for harvesting. Left hepatic vein, left portal branch, and left hepatic artery are taped.

dissected free, controlled, and encircled with tape. At this stage, the graft is only attached by its vessels (Figure 20.14).

20.3.7 Graft harvesting

A 7–8 cm suprapubic incision without muscular division is performed. A 15 mm port is inserted to introduce a large extraction bag (Endocatch, Tyco Healthcare, Norwalk, Connecticut). After the bag has been introduced, first the left hepatic artery is clipped and divided. The proximal end of the left arterial branch (donor side) is closed with a locking clip while the distal end (graft side) is left free without any clipping or clamping to avoid arterial damage.

The left portal branch is transected using a unilateral linear stapling device (EndoTA 30, Tyco Healthcare, Norwalk Connecticut). Clocking of warm ischemia time begins with this step. The left hepatic vein is then stapled with the same stapler. Finally, the left portal branch and left hepatic vein are divided using scissors.

The graft is rapidly inserted into the bag. CO_2 insufflation is stopped and the fascia is incised to allow externalization of the bag.

The graft is immediately weighed and perfused with a cold preservation solution through the left portal vein. This marks the end of the warm ischemia period, which is typically less than 10 minutes; clocking of cold ischemia time begins with the introduction of the cold preservation solution. The bile ducts of the graft are flushed out with the same preservation solution.

Concurrently, peritoneal reinsufflation is re-established in the donor. Hemostasis and biliostasis are

confirmed. No drain is used. CO_2 pneumoperitoneum is evacuated completely to reduce postoperative pain.

The fascias of port sites greater than 5 mm are carefully closed with absorbable suture material.

20.3.8 Special considerations for left living donor hepatectomy (see Video 19)

The operative time for a living donor left hepatectomy is similar to that of left lateral sectionectomy. Below we outline some specific technical aspects of living donor left hepatectomy.

After liver mobilization, the preparation of the portal pedicle starts with a cholecystectomy, followed by dissection and encircling of the structure of the portal pedicle with tape as described previously.

The parenchymal transection starts in the middle of the gallbladder bed, and follows the left side of the middle hepatic vein to reach the left hepatic vein origin. The middle hepatic vein could be left with the right liver of the donor, and it should be nicely exposed throughout the transection. Nevertheless, ultrasonography is mandatory to check its position during the parenchymal transection.

Particular attention should be paid to the venous drainage of segment IV during preoperative evaluation when a left hepatectomy is considered. The course of the segment IV drainage vein and its main tributaries should be extensively mapped and classified into the following three main types: majority/exclusive from left vein, majority/exclusive from middle vein, or shared left and middle vein tributary segment IV drainage. In the same manner, the origin of the segment IV hepatic artery should be preoperatively outlined. The preoperative vascular mapping helps to identify patients at risk for vascular complications involving segment IV congestion and/or necrosis; these patients may benefit from a planned peroperative segment IV removal to avoid potential severe complications. The surgical team needs to consider this latter point preoperatively.

20.4 Postoperative care

Prevention of deep vein thrombosis by use of prophylactically dosed low molecular weight heparin and compression stockings is routine from postoperative day 1. Proton pump inhibitors are used routinely to prevent gastric ulcer. No postoperative gastric tube is retained.

Oral intake is allowed in the evening of the procedure, and early mobilization is encouraged on postoperative day 1. Particular attention is paid to postoperative pain and appropriate pain medication is prescribed; their efficiency and necessity are re-evaluated daily.

Clinical features and biological tests are closely monitored every day; particular attention is paid to pulmonary examination, and any sign of pulmonary embolism is promptly addressed. Biological liver function is assessed by daily biochemical tests, including prothrombin time and serum bilirubin. Any clinical or biological sign of general or liver-related complication is documented in the patient's postoperative record and promptly addressed.

20.5 Conclusion and future perspectives

Laparoscopic right liver hepatectomy and left liver hepatectomy with the middle hepatic vein for adult living-related transplantation are still at the developmental stage but may be a promising approach in the future for living donor liver transplantation [16]. Laparoscopic living donor left liver hepatectomy will continue to be an important option in liver transplantation. However, aside from the risk for the donor, this procedure is challenging laparoscopically because of an oblique transection plane which can prevent an optimal view onto the operative site. Optimizing trocar

positioning, e.g. further to the right of the abdomen than for standard left and left lateral hepatectomy, and some mobilization of the right liver could aid in performing laparoscopic left liver living donation. While mobilization of the right liver would allow better exposure, it has the potential to jeopardize donor liver integrity. A future development may be to perform the operation in a supine rather than left lateral position. Tilting the table could optimize the operative field, an approach that is performed for tumor left lateral liver resection by some centers today.

To conclude, laparoscopic left lateral sectionectomy is a safe and reproducible procedure for living donor liver transplantation; however, donor safety is critical and therefore this approach requires experienced surgeons. A steep learning curve exists and should be flattened through the close collaboration between two experienced liver transplant surgeons.

Laparoscopic right and left liver hepatectomy (including the middle hepatic vein) may increase graft volume and function for adult living-related transplantation, but before this can be performed routinely, the technique has to be standardized and all possible measures taken to ensure donor safety.

Liver transplant surgeons should always keep in mind that donor safety is paramount, since the donors are, prior to the donation, disease-free volunteers.

Key points and technical tips

KEY POINTS

- Appropriate patient selection is key.

- Perform the steps of the hepatectomy alternating between the two experienced liver surgeons (one performing the pedicle dissection, the other the parenchymal transection).

- As a team, define preoperatively the criteria for conversion.

- As a team, define a "checklist" of key maneuvers to be validated step by step by both surgeons during the intervention (the most important steps being the left bile duct section and the left vessels stapling).

TECHNICAL TIPS

- At the level of the hilar plate, pull downwards on the portal vein using the tape in order to avoid vascular injury and to obtain an optimal exposure.

- Avoid thermal injuries close to the bile ducts.

- Locking clips rather than titanium clips minimize the risk of a bile duct stump leak.

- Anticipate the very last step of graft harvest to shorten warm ischemia time: open the endoscopic retrieval bag in the peritoneal cavity beforehand and confirm team readiness to receive the graft before staple dividing inflow.

- Anticoagulation should be discussed before vessel division. Today there is no consensus on an optimal regimen.

References

1 Raia S, Nery J, Mies S. Liver transplantation from live donors. Lancet 1989; 2:497.

2 Strong RW, Lynch SV, Ong TH, Matsunami H, Koido Y, Balderson GA. Successful liver transplantation from a living donor to her son. N Engl J Med 1990; 322:1505–1507.

3 Lo CM. Complications and long-term outcome of living liver donors: a survey of 1,508 cases in five Asian centers. Transplantation 2003; 75(3 suppl):S12–15.

4 Iida T, Ogura Y, Oike F, et al. Surgery-related morbidity in living donors for liver transplantation. Transplantation 2010; 89(10):1276–1282.

5 Cheah YL, Simpson MA, Pomposelli JJ, Pomfret EA. The incidence of death and potentially life-threatening "near miss" events in living donor hepatic lobectomy: a worldwide survey. Liver Transplant 2013; 19:499–506.

6 Cherqui D, Soubrane O, Husson E, et al. Laparoscopic living donor hepatectomy for liver transplantation in children. Lancet 2002; 359(9304):392–396.

7 Soubrane O, Cherqui D, Scatton O, et al. Laparoscopic left lateral sectionectomy in living donors: safety and reproducibility of the technique in a single center. Ann Surg 2006; 244 (5):815–820.

8 Chang S, Laurent A, Tayar C, Karoui M, Cherqui D. Laparoscopy as a routine approach for left lateral sectionectomy. Br J Surg 2007; 94(1):58–63.

9 Kim KH, Jung DH, Park KM, et al. Comparison of open and laparoscopic live donor left lateral sectionectomy. Br J Surg 2011; 98(9):1302–1308.

10 Carswell KA, Sagias FG, Murgatroyd B, Rela M, Heaton N, Patel AG. Laparoscopic versus open left lateral segmentectomy. BMC Surg 2009; 9:14.

11 Scatton O, Katsanos G, Boillot O, et al. Pure laparoscopic left lateral sectionectomy in living donor: from innovation to development in France. Ann Surg 2015; 261(3):506–512.

12 Redvanly RD, Nelson RC, Stieber AC, Dodd GD 3rd. Imaging in the preoperative evaluation of adult liver transplant candidates: goals, merits of various procedures, and recommendations. Am J Roentgenol 1995; 164:611–617.

13 Lo CM, Fan ST, Liu CL, et al. Minimum graft size for sucessful living donor liver tranplantation. Transplantation 1999; 68:1112–1116.

14 Kiuchi T, Kasahara M, Uryuhara K, et al. Impact of graft size mismatching on graft prognosis in liver transplantation from living donors. Transplantation 1999; 67:321–327.

15 Sakamoto S, Uemoto S, Uryuhara K, et al. Graft size assessment and analysis of donors for living donor liver transplantation using right lobe. Transplantation 2001; 71:1407–1413.

16 Soubrane O, Perdigao Cotta F, Scatton O. Pure laparoscopic right hepatectomy in a living donor. Am J Transplant 2013; 13(9):2467–2471.

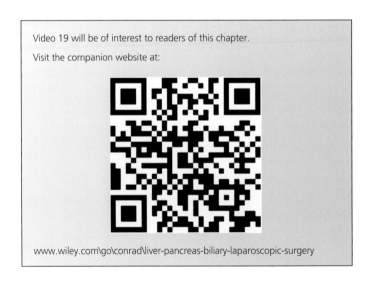

Video 19 will be of interest to readers of this chapter.

Visit the companion website at:

www.wiley.com\go\conrad\liver-pancreas-biliary-laparoscopic-surgery

CHAPTER 21

Pancreatic anatomy in the era of extensive and less invasive surgery

Yoshihiro Sakamoto, Yoshihiro Mise, and Norihiro Kokudo

Hepatobiliary Pancreatic Surgery Division, Department of Surgery, Graduate School of Medicine, University of Tokyo, Tokyo, Japan

---

EDITOR COMMENT

This chapter is critical for achieving an advanced understanding of pancreatic anatomy, which is fundamental to performing safe and oncological laparoscopic pancreatic resections. Expert pancreatic surgeons and anatomists detail the arterial as well as venous anatomy of the pancreas and expand on the importance of the celiac and superior mesenteric artery plexus in oncological pancreatic surgery. The authors highlight relevant peripancreatic lymph node stations and describe the key anatomy for an Appleby's procedure. Additionally, pancreatic embryological development is clearly outlined, providing a basis for understanding organ-preserving resections such as duodenum-preserving pancreatic head resection, pancreatic head-preserving duodenectomy, and segmental pancreas resection. The educational pictures of the intricate pancreatic anatomy will help the reader minimize the morbidity of pancreatic surgery and perform complete oncological resections. Ultimately, a detailed anatomical understanding is the basis for advanced laparoscopic pancreatic surgery.

Keywords: Appleby's procedure, arterial pancreatic anatomy, celiac and superior artery nerve plexus, duodenum-preserving pancreatic head resection, pancreatic embryology, pancreatic head-preserving duodenectomy, pancreatic lymph node station, pancreatic segmental resection, venous pancreatic anatomy

---

21.1 Introduction

Increasing numbers of laparoscopic and robotic pancreatic surgeries are being performed all over the world. Distal pancreatectomy (DP) is the most frequently performed pancreatic resection and recommended for resection of borderline malignancies or well-selected ductal adenocarcinomas located in the body or tail of the pancreas. A recent meta-analysis comparing laparoscopic with open pancreatectomy showed that laparoscopic distal pancreatectomy was associated with better short-term outcomes; that is, earlier oral intake, lower incidence of operative morbidity, and shorter hospital stay [1].

In contrast to the more widespread laparoscopic DP, laparoscopic pancreaticoduodenectomy (PD) is still technically very demanding. The challenging nature of a laparoscopic PD stems in part from the complex anatomy of the pancreatic head. An excellent understanding of the anatomy is required to safely perform a laparoscopic approach to pancreatic surgery in general and particularly in the treatment of invasive pancreatic cancer. Pancreatic cancer resection often entails extensive resections of peripancreatic tissue that includes lymph nodes, nerve

---

plexus, portal vein, and sometimes even arteries. Despite advances in our knowledge of pancreatic anatomy, critical anatomical concepts for extensive pancreatic surgery are still at a developmental stage.

Minimally invasive or less invasive pancreatic surgery has also shown considerable promise in the quest for "organ-preserving surgery." PD is one of the most invasive surgeries in the epigastrium, and a variety of organ-preserving surgeries have been reported, aiming to preserve the pancreas or the duodenum. An even more detailed anatomical knowledge is required to safely accomplish these organ-preserving surgeries.

In this chapter, we provide important information on the pancreatic anatomy required for both extensive and minimally invasive pancreatic surgery.

21.2 Basic vascular anatomy for pancreatectomy (see Videos 20–26)

21.2.1 Arterial anatomy

The superior mesenteric artery (SMA) and celiac artery (CeA) are the two major branches from the aorta. These, in turn, give off important branches to the pancreatic head. The branches off the SMA and CeA form the anterior and posterior pancreatic arterial arcades.

21.2.1.1 Superior mesenteric artery

The SMA has several important branches that are critical for surgery at the level of the pancreatic head. These include the inferior pancreaticoduodenal artery (IPDA), jejunal arteries, transverse pancreatic artery, and aberrant hepatic arteries. Among these, the key arteries affected during pancreatectomy will be the IPDA, some of the aberrant hepatic arteries, and the transverse pancreatic artery, as we will demonstrate below.

Inferior pancreaticoduodenal artery

Understanding the branching of the IPDA and its specific anatomical location is important not only for safe resection of the pancreatic head but also for oncological reasons. In advanced cases, invasive pancreatic head cancer may spread to nodal stations along the route of the IPDA [2]. It is vital to remember that transsection of the pancreatic head along the SMA involves dissection of the nerve plexus around the SMA, as well as division of the IPDA. The communication between the IPDA and

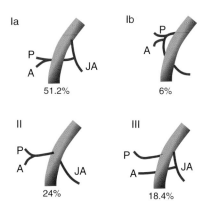

Figure 21.1 The branches off the superior mesenteric artery. *Type I (58%)*. (Ia) The inferior pancreaticoduodenal artery (IPDA) has a common trunk with the first jejunal artery (JA) at the left side of the superior mesenteric artery (SMA). This type accounts for 51% including minor variations. (Ib) The anterior IPDA (AIPDA: A) and the posterior IPDA (PIPDA: P) branch off from the JA independently at the right side of the SMA. This type accounts for 6%. *Type II (24%)*. The IPDA and JA run independently off the SMA. *Type III (18%)*. The anterior and posterior IPDA run independently off the JA behind the SMA.

the first jejunal artery (JA) has several variations (Figure 21.1). The most frequent variation is that the IPDA has a common trunk with the JA. In this case, the root of the common trunk may be located at the left dorsal aspect of the SMA (type Ia, 51.2%) or at the right side of the SMA (type Ib, 6%) [3]. A frequent variation is the individual branching of the IPDA and the JA off the SMA.

A second type of IPDA anatomy is where the IPDA has two dominant branches: (i) the anterior–inferior pancreaticoduodenal artery (AIPDA) and (ii) the posterior–inferior pancreaticoduodenal artery (PIPDA) (type II, 24%). A third variation of the IPDA is when the JA runs by itself behind the SMA (type III, 18.44%). The AIPDA often runs along the anterior aspect of the duodenum behind the inferior portion of the pancreatic head (Figure 21.2a), toward the major papilla. In most of these cases, the PIPDA runs behind the pancreatic head, giving off small branches toward the pancreas and duodenum (Figure 21.2b).

It is possible to identify the JA, IPDA, AIPIDA, and PIPDA intraoperatively (Figure 21.3), and early ligation of the inflow artery to the pancreatic head, i.e. the "artery first" approach, is reported to reduce blood loss during

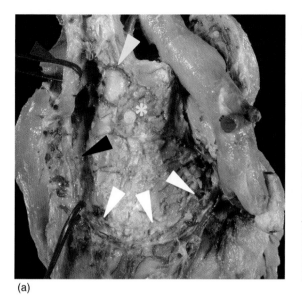

(a)

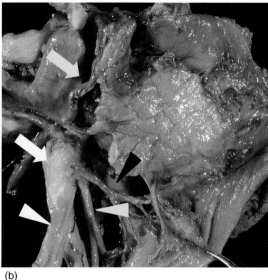

(b)

Figure 21.2 View of autopsy cases after injection of three colors of dye into the vessels and ducts. (a) Anterior–inferior pancreaticoduodenal artery (AIPDA). Anterior view of the fixed pancreatic head obtained from an autopsy case. The embryologically dorsal primordium (anterior segment) has been removed along the embryological fusion plane. Following anterior segmentectomy, the intrapancreatic bile duct (*yellow arrowhead*), the duct of Wirsung (*asterisk*), and the posterior segment (embryologically ventral primordium) have been preserved. The anterior arcade of the pancreatic head consists of the gastroduodenal artery (GDA, *red arrowhead*), the anterior–superior pancreaticoduodenal artery (ASPDA, *black arrowhead*), and the anterior–inferior pancreaticoduodenal artery (AIPDA, *white arrowheads*). (b) Posterior–inferior pancreaticoduodenal artery (PIPDA). Posterior view of the fixed pancreatic head obtained from an autopsy case. There are four branches of the superior mesenteric artery (SMA, *white arrow*): the first jejunal artery (*white arrowhead*), the anterior–inferior pancreaticoduodenal artery (AIPDA, *yellow arrowhead*), the posterior–superior pancreaticoduodenal artery (PSPDS, *yellow arrow*) and the posterior–inferior pancreaticoduodenal artery (PIPDA, *black arrowhead*). In this case, the four arteries branched off the SMA independently.

PD [4]. The artery first approach has been described for laparoscopic PD and entails early dissection and assessment of the tissue adjacent to the SMA. This approach is facilitated by the laparoscopic view below the head of the pancreas after kocherization. To minimize blood loss and risk for postoperative bleeding, it is important that pancreatic surgeons identify and control the inflow arteries to the pancreatic head coming off the SMA, as mentioned earlier.

Another important factor in the arterial anatomy of the pancreas is that there is always a small branch from the SMA to the body of the pancreas. This pancreatic body artery must be divided to remove the left side of the pancreas at the level of the portal vein. In the majority of cases, this arterial branch becomes the transverse pancreatic artery [5]. A possible variation is a communication of this artery with the dorsal pancreatic artery (DPA).

Aberrant hepatic arteries from the SMA

Aberrant right hepatic artery (RHA) from the SMA is reported in 15–25% of patients [6,7]. Aberrant RHA consists of replaced RHA (singular artery from the SMA) and accessory RHA (an additional RHA coming off the SMA). A replaced RHA often travels behind the portal vein and the pancreatic head through Calot's triangle. Any anatomical variation in the hepatoduodenal ligament should be carefully evaluated before surgery. The most dangerous variation would be a case in which the RHA is a replaced artery coming off the gastroduodenal artery (GDA), where the GDA cannot be divided at the typical location close to the common hepatic artery (CHA).

21.2.1.2 Celiac axis

The celiac axis has several branches, including the bilateral phrenic arteries, left gastric artery (LGA), splenic

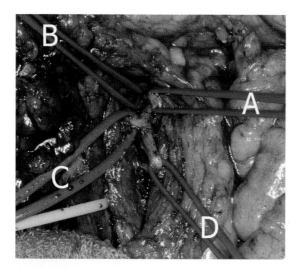

Figure 21.3 Intraoperative identification of the branches from the superior mesenteric artery (SMA). After division of the right side of the nerve plexus of the SMA, the inferior pancreaticoduodenal artery (IPDA, A), the posterior–inferior pancreaticoduodenal artery (PIPDA, B), the anterior–inferior pancreaticoduodenal artery (AIPDA, C), and the first jejunal artery (D) were taped. In the "artery first" approach, the IPDA and the first jejunal artery should be ligated, which will decrease the blood supply to the pancreatic head.

artery (SpA), common hepatic artery (CHA), dorsal pancreatic artery (DPA), aberrant hepatic artery, inferior phrenic arteries, and others.

The CeA is surrounded by the celiac nerve plexus, which in case of tumor infiltration can be the source of significant cancer-related pain. The root of the DPA can be the trunk of the CeA, CHA or SpA [5]. The first major branch of the CHA is usually the GDA, at which point the CHA becomes the proper hepatic artery (PHA). The GDA branches off the right gastroepiploic artery (RGA). After this branching, the GDA becomes the anterior–superior pancreaticoduodenal artery (ASPDA), which has a communication with the IPDA. This arterial communication creates an anterior pancreatic arcade (see Figure 21.2a). The origin of the posterior–superior pancreaticoduodenal artery (PSPDA) can be the GDA or PHA, or it may be an aberrant hepatic artery. The PSPDA travels behind the pancreatic head toward the major papilla, and it may give off additional small branches to the duodenum. The communication of the PSPDA and PIPDA creates a posterior pancreatic arcade (see Figure 21.2b). In patients

with median arcuate ligament syndrome, the root of the CeA is compressed by the ligament. This can be a critical finding when performing a pancreaticoduodenectomy since in these cases the hepatic arterial flow might be insufficient after resection of the pancreatic head. Division of the arcuate ligament will restore the flow of the CeA [8].

Maintenance of hepatic arterial inflow during distal pancreatectomy with en bloc celiac axis resection (DP-CAR) (see Videos 24 and 25)

Surgical resection of pancreatic cancer involving the celiac axis is controversial. However, recent reports have shown a five-year survival rate of 42% in patients with pancreatic invasive cancer undergoing DP-CAR, a modified Appleby's procedure [9]. In gastric cancer surgery, it had been known that total gastrectomy combined with en bloc resection of the celiac axis enables complete cancer removal with the so-called Appleby's procedure [10]. Application of Appleby's procedure to pancreatic cancer should be done only in select circumstances, because of the higher morbidity and mortality rate in comparison with conventional DP [11].

During DP-CAR, the roots of the SMA and CeA should be identified. After clamping the celiac axis from the SMA via the pancreatic head arcades, hepatic arterial flow should be confirmed before resection of the CeA (Figure 21.4a). After completion of DP-CAR, the nerve plexus of SMA is dissected, while the stump of the CeA is exposed on the dissecting plane (Figure 21.4b).

21.2.2 Venous anatomy

The venous anatomy of the pancreatic head may vary widely from patient to patient. However, there are certain common features and variations that are more likely to occur. The major portal venous tributaries to the portal system consist of the portal vein (PV), superior mesenteric vein (SMV), splenic vein (SpV), superior mesenteric vein (SPV), Henle's gastrocolic trunk (GCT), middle colic vein (MCV), inferior mesenteric vein (IMV), jejunal veins, left gastric vein (coronary vein), and right gastric vein. The venous drainage of the pancreatic head runs partly independent from the arterial tributaries. For further reading, Douglass *et al.* nicely summarize the detailed anatomy of the pancreatic venous tributaries [12].

The key branches are the PV, SpV, and SMV, and the most frequent anatomical variations are as follows.

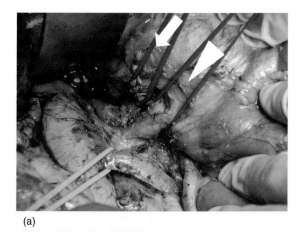

(a)

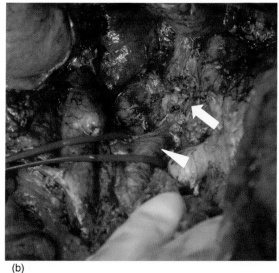

(b)

Figure 21.4 Distal pancreatectomy with en bloc celiac axis resection (DP-CAR). (a) The roots of the superior mesenteric artery (SMA, *white arrowhead*) and the celiac axis (*white arrow*) are secured at the beginning of surgery. (b) After completion of DP-CAR, the stump of the celiac axis (*white arrow*) is exposed on the dissecting plane, while the SMA (*white arrowhead*) is preserved.

21.2.2.1 PV

The noteworthy branches of the PV are the posterior–superior pancreaticoduodenal vein (PSPDV), left gastric vein, and right gastric vein. In a cadaveric study by Mourad *et al.*, the authors report that the PSPDV was absent in only one of the 45 specimens studied [13]. The PSPDV is the most dominant branch off the PV and is

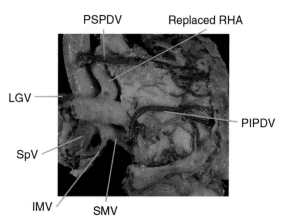

Figure 21.5 Posterior view of the autopsy cases after injection of three colors of dye into the vessels and ducts. The posterior–superior pancreaticoduodenal vein (PSPDV) joins the posterior wall of the portal vein, and the posterior–inferior pancreaticoduodenal vein (PIPDV) joins the posterior wall of the superior mesenteric vein (SMV). The boundary between the drainage area of the PSPDV and the PIPDV is the major papilla. IMV, inferior mesenteric vein; LGV, left gastric vein; replaced RHA, replaced right hepatic artery; SpV, splenic vein.

usually located on the right posterior aspect of the PV at the superior edge of the pancreas. The PSPDV drains the posterior–superior area of the pancreas and the duodenum. The PSPDV and PIPDV may in some cases form the posterior arcade at the back of the pancreatic head, although the communication between the two veins close to the major papilla is sometimes not well developed (Figure 21.5) [14,15]. There is some disagreement whether the ASPDV and AIPDV form the anterior arcade on the ventral side of the pancreatic head [14,16]. The left gastric vein (LGV), i.e. coronary vein, branches from the junction between the PV and SpV (type I, 58.9%), the PV (type II, 24.4%), and the SpV (type III, 16.7%) [12] (Figure 21.6). The right gastric vein originates in the lower portion of the lesser curvature of the stomach [12]. This vein sometimes has a common trunk with tributaries from the superior edge of the pancreas, which must be controlled carefully when performing the retropancreatic "tunneling" during a PD [17].

21.2.2.2 SpV

The noteworthy tributaries of the SpV are the LGV and inferior mesenteric vein (IMV). As described in the

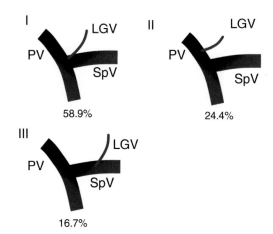

Figure 21.6 Schematic drawings of the left gastric vein in relation to the portal vein (PV) and splenic vein (SpV). Type I (58.9%): left gastric vein joins the junction between the PV and the SPV. Type II (24.4%): left gastric vein joins the PV. Type III (16.7%): left gastric vein joins the SpV.

previous section, the LGV drains into the portal venous confluence or the superior aspect of the SpV in 76% of patients (see Figure 21.6). The IMV drains into the portal venous confluence or the inferior aspect of the SpV in 72% of patients (Figure 21.7).

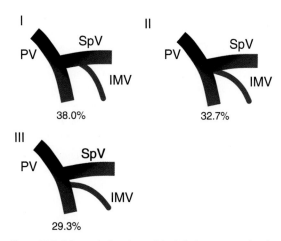

Figure 21.7 Schematic drawings of the inferior mesenteric vein (IMV) in relation to the portal vein (PV) and splenic vein (SpV). Type I (38.0%): the IMV joins the junction of the SpV. Type II (32.7%): the IMV joins the junction between the PV and SpV. Type III (29.3%): the IMV joins the PV.

21.2.2.3 SMV

The major tributaries of the SMV are the right gastro-epiploic trunk (Henle's trunk), the IMV, and the middle colic vein. Zhang *et al.* studied 50 cases with special reference to the branching of Henle's trunk [18]. They found that Henle's trunk has 2–4 of the following veins: the right gastroepiploic (100%), the superior right colic (59.3%), the superior pancreaticoduodenal (85.2%), the anterior–inferior pancreaticoduodenal (16.7%), and other colic veins (middle right, transverse).

The main trunk of the SMV arises from the confluence of the two first-order branches of the SMV: the jejunal and ileal branches. The jejunal branch runs behind the SMA in 80% of cases [19]. Katz *et al.* described that in PD, one of the jejunal or ileal veins can be sacrificed without the need for venous reconstruction, if at least one of these venous branches is preserved [19]. In addition, they propose that the preservation of the ileal vein is preferred over the jejunal vein. Falconer *et al.* demonstrated that when the jejunal branch crosses anterior to the SMA, the SMA appears between the two equally thick veins [15]. Sacrificing the left limb of the SMV, usually the jejunal vein, can be considered according to the size of the remaining venous limb.

21.2.3 Peripancreatic nerve plexus

The peripancreatic nerves impact both the sympathetic and parasympathetic autonomic nervous systems. The major ganglia are the celiac and superior mesenteric ganglia with their branches to the greater or lesser splanchnic nerves and vagus nerves.

The innervations of the pancreatic head can be classified into two parts: (i) plexus pancreaticus capitalis 1 and 2 [20], which accounts for the nerve plexus of the SMA and celiac axis, and (ii) plexus splenicus innervating the pancreatic body and tail. The neural plexi around the SMA are most likely to be involved when cancer includes perineural invasion, thus dissection of these plexi has been advocated in the treatment of invasive pancreatic cancer [21,22]. It has been reported that lymphatic vessels are present along the SMA within the SMA plexus [23], which supports systematic dissection of the nerve plexus along the SMA in patients with pancreatic cancer close to the SMA.

21.2.3.1 Nerve plexus of the SMA

The SMA is surrounded by a thick nerve plexus, and the IPDA and jejunal arteries run inside and outside the nerve

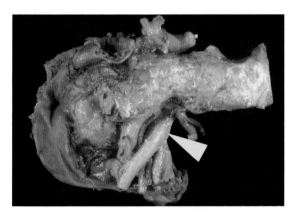

Figure 21.8 View of the pancreatic head and body in a fixed specimen. The superior mesenteric artery (SMA) is covered by the thick nerve plexus (*yellow arrowhead*), but the superior mesenteric vein is not.

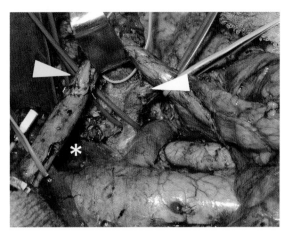

Figure 21.10 View after pancreaticoduodenectomy for invasive pancreatic cancer. After pancreaticoduodenectomy for invasive pancreatic cancer, the right half of the nerve plexus of the superior mesenteric artery (SMA, *white arrowhead*) is removed, exposing the aorta (aorta, *white asterisk*) and the left renal vein. The wall of the portal vein is reconstructed using a patch graft from bilateral ovarian veins (*yellow arrowhead*).

plexus (Figure 21.8). Pancreatic cancer often involves the nerve plexus of the SMA around the IPDA (Figure 21.9). The branches of the IPDA or jejunal artery often run within the right half of the nerve plexus of the SMA. Therefore, dissection of the right half of the plexus involves ligation or sealing of these thin arterial branches. In the left half of the plexus, no major arterial branch runs through the plexus itself, with the exception of the arterial branch to the body of the pancreas, which runs along the inferior border of the pancreas.

During PD for pancreatic invasive cancer, the right half of the SMA nerve plexus should be dissected for a complete radical resection (Figure 21.10). During a DP for pancreatic cancer involving the left-side nerve plexus of SMA, the nerve plexus should be removed for a radical resection (Figure 21.11). Extensive resection of the nerve

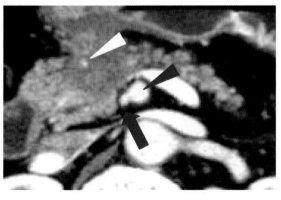

Figure 21.9 Pancreatic cancer involving the nerve plexus of the superior mesenteric artery (SMA). The pancreatic cancer involves the gastroduodenal artery (*white arrowhead*) and the distal portion of the stomach, and invades the nerve plexus of the SMA (*red arrowhead*) via the inferior pancreaticoduodenal artery (IPDA, *red arrow*).

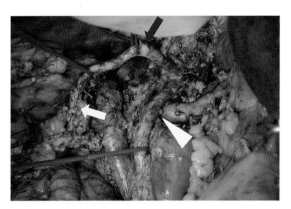

Figure 21.11 View after distal pancreatectomy for invasive pancreatic cancer. After distal pancreatectomy for invasive cancer, the left half of the nerve plexus of the superior mesenteric artery (SMA, *white arrowhead,* pancreatic head, *white arrow,* ligated gastroduodenal artery, *red arrow*).

plexus around the SMA can induce severe diarrhea and disturbance of digestion and absorption, which should be avoided to maintain optimal quality of life of patients undergoing PD for invasive cancer.

21.2.3.2 Nerve plexus of CeA and CHA

In patients with pancreatic body cancer with invasion into the nerve plexus around the CeA and the left side of the nerve plexus of the SMA, these nerve plexi need to be removed as part of a radical resection. The CeA, CHA, and the left half of the SMA wall are exposed after complete dissection of the nerve plexus (see Figure 21.11).

21.2.4 Peripancreatic nodal stations

The nodal distribution of peripancreatic regions has been well classified in the *General Rules for the Study of Pancreatic Cancer* [24] (Figure 21.12). Although a clinical impact of extensive nodal dissection in patients with invasive ductal carcinoma of the pancreas has not been proven in randomized clinical trials, at least standard nodal

dissection is necessary for accurate staging. To perform an accurate nodal dissection with a high lymph node yield, the surgeon requires an excellent understanding of the relevant nodal stations. The peripancreatic lymph node stations have been numbered based on their locations (Table 21.1). The most frequent metastatic nodal stations in pancreatic cancer are numbers 13, 16, and 17 [25].

21.3 Pancreatic anatomy for organ-preserving peripancreatic resection

Laparoscopic surgery, compared with open resection, has the potential to reduce morbidity. Pancreas head resection that preserves a significant amount of pancreas tissue has been reported, and Beger has proposed such procedures for pancreatitis [26]. These include duodenum-preserving pancreas head resection (DPPHR), inferior

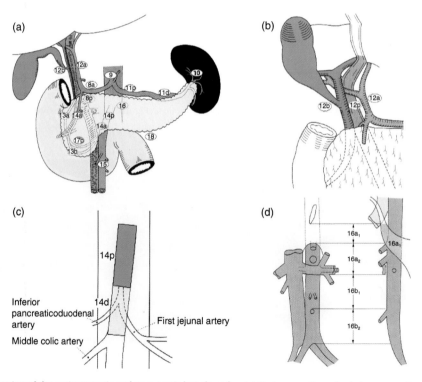

Figure 21.12 Mapping of the peripancreatic and para-aortic lymph nodes. (a) Peripancreatic nodes between no. 9 and no. 18. (b) Lymph nodes at the hepatoduodenal ligaments. (c) Lymph nodes along the superior mesenteric artery. (d) Para-aortic lymph nodes. Source: Nakao [24]. Reproduced with permission of Lippencott, Williams, & Wilkins.

Table 21.1 Numbers of peripancreatic lymph node stations.

Lymph node station number	Anatomical location
1	Right cardia
2	Left cardia
3	Lesser curvature of the stomach
4	Greater curvature of the stomach
5	Suprapyloric
6	Infrapyloric
7	Left gastric artery
8a	Common hepatic artery, anterior–superior
8p	Common hepatic artery, posterior
9	Celiac trunk
10	Splenic hilum
11p	Splenic artery, proximal
11d	Splenic artery, distal
12a	Hepatic artery
12b	Bile duct
12p	Portal vein
13a	Pancreatic head, posterior–superior
13b	Pancreatic head, posterior–inferior
14p	Superior mesenteric artery, proximal
14d	Superior mesenteric artery, distal
15	Middle colic artery
16a1	Para-aortic, superior to celiac artery
16a2	Para-aortic, between celiac artery and superior mesenteric artery
16b1	Para-aortic, between left renal vein and inferior mesenteric artery
16b2	Para-aortic, inferior to inferior mesenteric artery
17a	Pancreatic head, superior–anterior
17b	Pancreatic head, inferior–anterior
18	Pancreatic body and tail, inferior

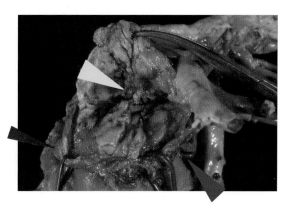

Figure 21.13 The embryological anatomy of the pancreatic head. The pancreatic head can be divided into two parts: the anterior segment (embryologically dorsal primordia) and the posterior segment (embryologically ventral primordia). The duct of Wirsung (*yellow arrowhead*) penetrates the two buds and joins the duct of Santorini, making the main pancreatic duct. The anterior–inferior pancreaticoduodenal artery (*red arrowhead*) and vein (*blue arrowhead*) can be recognized. The common bile duct and the duct of Wirsung are included in the posterior segment.

pancreatic head resection, ventral pancreatectomy, and so on. In addition, a variety of pancreas-sparing duodenectomy (PSD) with and without reconstruction of the major papilla has been reported.

21.3.1 Anatomical segmentectomy of the pancreatic head (see Video 26)

To understand the pancreatic and peripancreatic anatomy for organ-preserving surgery, it is important to consider the embryonic origin of the pancreatic dorsal and ventral buds. The fetal pancreas is composed of the ventral and dorsal anlage derived from the midgut, and the two buds fuse at week 7 or 8 of gestation, forming the pancreas. The bile duct and the duct of Wirsung originate from the ventral bud, while the duct of Santorini arises from the dorsal bud. The two buds fuse, rotating 270° from their initial position, so that the ventral bud is located behind the dorsal bud in the adult pancreas.

On fixed casts of the pancreatic head obtained from cadavers, anatomical segmentectomy of the pancreatic head along the embryological fusion plane is feasible, preserving the embryological ventral primordium containing the common bile duct (Figure 21.13) [27]. It is therefore theoretically feasible to perform anatomical anterior segmentectomy of the pancreatic head for intraductal papillary mucinous neoplasm (IPMN) in the embryological dorsal pancreas, dividing the fusion plane between the dorsal and ventral primordia [28]. However, a significant pancreatic fistula from the wide dissection plane and reconstruction of the main pancreatic duct carry a high risk of significant morbidity [29]. In addition, anatomical resection of the embryological ventral bud involves resection of the lower bile duct. Subsequently, reconstruction of the main pancreatic duct, as well as the bile duct, is required (Figure 21.14). The benefit of preserving the anterior bud of the patients tends to be very limited and therefore in most cases, PD is preferable for patients with neoplasm limited to the ventral bud.

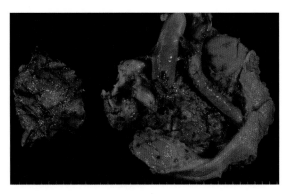

Figure 21.14 Resection of the embryologically ventral primordium. After resection of the embryologically ventral primordium, the lower bile duct, which is originally buried in the ventral primordium, was exposed on the dissecting plane. The plane coincides with the embryological fusion between the ventral and dorsal buds.

21.3.2 Pancreas-sparing duodenectomy

In patients with duodenal gastrointestinal stromal tumor (GIST) or familial adenomatous polyposis of the duodenum, resection of the duodenum while preserving the pancreas may be an indication for PSD. During PSD, the major/minor papilla, branches from the anterior–inferior pancreaticoduodenal arteries and veins, and the posterior–superior and –inferior pancreaticoduodenal arteries and veins are divided. PSD might be indicated in patients with duodenal GIST, which has a negligible risk of nodal metastasis or direct invasion to adjacent organs [30], or in very select patients with preinvasive or very early duodenal cancer [31]. The long-term prognosis of PSD for GIST is reported to be satisfactory [32].

KEY POINTS

- The arterial tributaries to the pancreas originate from either the celiac artery or the superior mesenteric artery. There are several variations of the communication between the inferior pancreaticoduodenal artery and the first jejunal artery. It is essential to safely control these arteries early during PD in order to minimize blood flow to the pancreatic head during the resection.

- There are several variations of the communication between the splenic vein, inferior mesenteric vein, the superior mesenteric vein, and the portal vein. The posterior pancreaticoduodenal veins provide drainage of the posterior pancreatic head to the portal system.

- In the treatment of invasive pancreatic cancer, partial resection of nerve plexus of the celiac artery and the superior mesenteric artery, and a peripancreatic lymph node dissection is required for oncological reasons.

- The pancreatic head can be divided into two parts along the embryological primordia: the dorsal bud and the ventral bud. Anatomical segmentectomy is theoretically possible, but practically it may be too complicated.

- Pancreas-sparing duodenectomy or duodenum-preserving pancreatic head resection requires excellent knowledge of the peripancreatic anatomy.

References

1 Nakamura M, Nakashima H. Laparoscopic distal pancreatectomy and pancreatoduodenectomy: is it worthwhile? A meta-analysis of laparoscopic pancreatectomy. J Hepatobiliary Pancreat Sci 2013; 20(4):421–428.

2 Noto M, Miwa K, Kitagawa H, et al. Pancreas head carcinoma. Frequency of invasion to soft tissue adherent to the superior mesenteric artery. Am J Surg Pathol 2005; 29:1056–1061.

3 Takamuro T, Murakami G, Hirata K. Arterial supply of the first, third and fourth portion of the duodenum. An anatomical study with special reference to the minimal invasive pancreaticoduodenectomy. Jpn J Gastroenterol Surg 1998; 31:825–835.

4 Sanjay P, Takaori K, Govil S, Shrikhande SV, Windsor JA. 'Artery-first' approaches to pancreatoduodenectomy. Br J Surg 2012; 99:1027–1035.

5 Woodburne RT, Olsen LL. The arteries of the pancreas. Anat Rec 1951; 111:255–270.

6 Michels NA. Newer anatomy of the liver and its variant blood supply and collateral circulation. Am J Surg 1962; 112:337–347.

7 Hiatt JR, Gabbay J, Busuttil RW. Surgical anatomy of the hepatic arteries in 1000 cases. Ann Surg 1994; 220:50–52.

8 Nara S, Sakamoto Y, Shimada K, et al. Arterial reconstruction during pancreatoduodenectomy in patients with celiac axis

stenosis – utility of Doppler ultrasonography. World J Surg 2005; 29:885–889.

9 Hirano S, Kondo S, Hara T, *et al.* Distal pancreatectomy with en bloc celiac axis resection for locally advanced pancreatic cancer: long-term results. Ann Surg 2007; 246:46–51.

10 Appleby L. The celiac axis in the expansion of the operation for gastric carcinoma. Cancer 1953; 6:704–707.

11 Yamamoto Y, Sakamoto Y, Ban D, *et al.* Is celiac axis resection justified for T4 pancreatic body cancer? Surgery 2012; 151:61–69.

12 Douglass BE, Baggenstoss AH, Hollinshead WH. The anatomy of the portal vein and its tributaries. Surg Gynecol Obstet 1950; 91:562–576.

13 Mourad N, Zhang J, Rath AM, Chevrel JP. The venous drainage of the pancreas. Surg Radiol Anat 1994; 16:37–45.

14 Kimura W, Nagai H. Study of surgical anatomy for duodenum-preserving resection of the head of the pancreas. Ann Surg 1995; 221:359–363.

15 Falconer WA, Griffiths E. The anatomy of the blood-vessels in the region of the pancreas. Br J Surg 1950; 37:334–344.

16 Skandalakis JL, Rowe JS, Gray SW, Skandalakis JE. Surgical embryology and anatomy of the pancreas. Surg Clin North Am 1993; 73:661–697.

17 Sakamoto Y, Nagai M, Tanaka N, *et al.* Anterior tributaries of the portal vein at the superior margin of the pancreas: is "tunneling" procedure safe during pancreatic surgery? Int J Pancreatol 2000; 28:77–80.

18 Zhang I, Rath AM, Boyer JC, *et al.* Radioanatomic study of the gastrocolic venous trunk. Surg Radiol Anat 1994; 16:413–418.

19 Katz MHM, Fleming JB, Pisters PW, Lee JE, Evans DB. Anatomy of the superior mesenteric vein with special reference to the surgical management of first-order branch involvement at pancreaticoduodenectomy. Ann Surg 2008; 248:1098–1102.

20 Yoshioka H, Wakabayashi T. Therapeutic neurotomy on head of pancreas for relief of pain due to chronic pancreatitis: a new technical procedure and its result. AMA Arch Surg 1958; 83:223–226.

21 Yi SQ, Miwa K, Ohta T, *et al.* Innervation of the pancreas from the perspective of perineural invasion of pancreatic cancer. Pancreas 2003; 27:225–229.

22 Hirai I, Kimura W, Ozawa K, *et al.* Perineural invasion in pancreatic cancer. Pancreas 2002; 24:15–25.

23 Jin G, Sugiyama M, Tuo H, *et al.* Distribution of lymphatic vessels in the neural plexuses surrounding the superior mesenteric artery. Pancreas 2006; 32:62–66.

24 Nakao A. General Rules for the Study of Pancreatic Cancer, 6th edn. Tokyo: Kenehara, 2009.

25 Nimura Y, Nagino M, Takao S, *et al.* Standard versus extended lymphadenectomy in radical pancreatoduodenectomy for ductal adenocarcinoma of the head of the pancreas. J Hepatobiliary Pancreat Sci 2012; 19:230–241.

26 Beger H, Buchler M, Bittner R, *et al.* Duodenum-preserving resection of the head of the pancreas in severe chronic pancreatitis. Early and late results. Ann Surg 1989; 209(3):273–278.

27 Sakamoto Y, Nagai M, Tanaka N, *et al.* Anatomical segmentectomy of the head of the pancreas along the embryological fusion plane: a feasible procedure? Surgery 2000; 128:822–831.

28 Seyama Y, Sakamoto Y, Sano K, *et al.* Anatomical segmentectomy of the pancreas head: can this procedure be curatively applied to intraductal papillary mucinous tumors? Pancreas 2003; 27:270–272.

29 Sakamoto Y, Tanaka N, Nagai M, *et al.* Anterior segmentectomy of the pancreatic head for islet cell tumors. Pancreas 2002; 24:317–319.

30 Asakawa M, Sakamoto Y, Kajiwara T, *et al.* Simple segmental resection of the second portion of the duodenum for the treatment of gastrointestinal tumors. Langenbeck Arch Surg 2008; 393:605–609.

31 Yamashita S, Sakamoto Y, Saiura A, *et al.* Pancreas-sparing duodenectomy for gastrointestinal tumors. Am J Surg 2014; 207:578–583.

32 Yamashita S, Sakamoto Y, Kaneko J, *et al.* Resection of the second portion of the duodenum sacrificing the minor papilla but preserving the pancreas for a recurrent duodenal adenocarcinoma: report of a case. Biosci Trends 2012; 6:44–47.

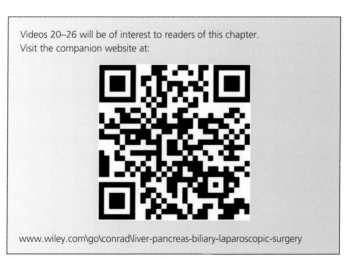

Videos 20–26 will be of interest to readers of this chapter. Visit the companion website at:

www.wiley.com\go\conrad\liver-pancreas-biliary-laparoscopic-surgery

CHAPTER 22

Management of solid and cystic lesions of the pancreas

David Fogelman and Robert A. Wolff

Department of Gastrointestinal Medical Oncology, University of Texas MD Anderson Cancer Center, Houston, USA

EDITOR COMMENT

This comprehensive chapter on pancreatic tumors discusses multidisciplinary management of pancreatic adenocarcinoma, pancreatic neuroendocrine tumors, and pancreatic cystic neoplasms as well as less often encountered pathologies such as metastases to the pancreas and lymphoepithelial cysts. While pancreatic resection in general has become safer, the advent of advanced laparoscopic pancreatectomy might contribute to reducing operative morbidity further. Pancreatic cancer therapy today requires a multidisciplinary approach, and this chapter by expert pancreas medical oncologists allows surgeons to put pancreas cancer surgery into the context of chemotherapy and/or radiation therapy.

With the widespread use of axial abdominal imaging, there has been a significant increase in the detection of pancreatic cystic lesions. The minimally invasive pancreatic surgeon will frequently be asked to manage these patients because removal of potentially premalignant or early-malignant cystic lesions with prophylactic intent makes these operations well suited for the lesser morbidities associated with a minimally invasive approach. Therefore, it is critical that the surgeon becomes very familiar with the work-up, indications for resection, and surgical approaches to managing these cystic lesions.

Keywords: borderline resectable pancreatic cancer, cystic tumor of the pancreas, diagnosis of cystic lesions of the pancreas, intraductal papillary mucinous neoplasm, lymphoepithelial cyst, metastases to the pancreas, mucinous cystic neoplasm, neoadjuvant therapy for pancreatic cancer, pancreatic adenocarcinoma, pancreatic neuroendocrine tumor, serous cystic neoplasm, solid pseudopapillary tumors of the pancreas, solid tumor of the pancreas

---

22.1 Introduction

Pancreatic adenocarcinoma is by far the most common malignancy in patients discovered to have a solid lesion in the pancreas, and in the United States, the incidence of pancreatic adenocarcinoma has increased from approximately 32 000 cases per year a decade ago to over 46 000 currently [1,2]. Similarly, pancreatic neuroendocrine carcinomas, the second most common malignant histology, also appear to be rising in incidence [3]. Furthermore, with the widespread use of cross-sectional imaging (computed tomography [CT] and magnetic resonance [MR]), a growing number of people are being found to have cystic lesions within the pancreas, many of which represent intraductal papillary mucinous neoplasms (IPMNs) of the pancreas.

This chapter will focus on the diagnostic work-up, staging, and subsequent management of patients with solid and cystic pancreatic lesions.

22.2 Solid tumors of the pancreas

In general, curative treatment of solid neoplasms of the pancreas requires complete resection of the tumor mass, and in the case of pancreatic adenocarcinoma, the delivery of adjuvant therapy has a modest impact on overall survival for patients undergoing curative

---

Laparoscopic Liver, Pancreas, and Biliary Surgery, First Edition.
Edited by Claudius Conrad and Brice Gayet.
© 2017 John Wiley & Sons, Ltd. Published 2017 by John Wiley & Sons, Ltd.

resection. For cystic lesions, treatment strategies usually require careful characterization as to the nature of the cyst and its potential for malignancy or malignant transformation. Treatment may range from no further intervention to surveillance with serial imaging or surgical resection. A critical component in all diagnostic and treatment planning is the requirement for collaboration among members of a multidisciplinary team that includes surgeons, gastroenterologists, radiologists, interventional radiologists, medical oncologist, radiotherapists, and pathologists.

During the last 10–20 years, such multidisciplinary involvement has facilitated the development of strict radiographic criteria for classifying pancreatic lesions (biopsy proven or not) into degrees of resectability, identifying criteria for resection of pancreatic neuroendocrine tumors, and selecting patients with IPMN or other cystic lesions for continued observation or resection. The overall management of each of these is discussed in this chapter with emphasis on localized lesions considered for surgical resection.

22.2.1 Management of adenocarcinoma of the pancreas

22.2.1.1 Risk factors

Several risk factors for pancreatic adenocarcinoma are fairly well established [4]. A history of tobacco smoking unequivocally increases the risk of pancreatic cancer. Some studies also suggest increased risk with use of smokeless tobacco products [5] or exposure to second-hand smoke. Type 2 diabetes mellitus, obesity, and metabolic syndrome have all been associated with an increased risk of pancreatic adenocarcinoma. Of note, recent evidence has demonstrated a potential protective effect for diabetics whose blood glucose is controlled using metformin compared with an increased risk for diabetics managed with sulfonylureas or insulin [6–9].

Other risk factors include hepatitis B virus infection, any form of chronic pancreatitis, or a history of gastric bypass surgery. Lastly, a growing number of inherited cancer syndromes put carriers at increased risk for pancreatic cancer. These include BRCA1, BRCA2, Peutz–Jeghers syndrome, germline p16 mutations (seen in familial atypical mole and melanoma), PALB-2 mutations [10], and those identified as having documented genetic mutations seen in hereditary nonpolyposis colon cancer (HNPCC) [11].

22.2.1.2 Presenting signs and symptoms

With the exception of obstructive jaundice, which is a common presenting symptom of patients with adenocarcinoma in the head of the pancreas, symptoms of pancreatic cancer are often nonspecific and include vague or poorly characterized abdominal pain or back pain. Both of these are often attributed to other causes such as gallbladder disease, peptic ulcer disease or acid reflux, or to musculoskeletal problems. Other potential signs of pancreatic cancer include unexplained venous thromboembolism, steatorrhea, weight loss, or night sweats; the latter are usually harbingers of advanced disease.

22.2.1.3 Imaging studies

Given the current rates of microscopically positive surgical margins in pancreatic cancer resections (>40%), high-quality cross-sectional CT or MR imaging must be a component of clinical staging [12].

Importantly, for patients who present with obstructive jaundice, biliary decompression with a percutaneous transhepatic catheter (PTC) or endobiliary stent should ideally be performed after acquisition of dynamic phase thin-cut helical imaging. Preprocedure imaging will avoid inflammatory changes that could result from instrumentation [13].

Adequate imaging is imperative to understand the relationship between a tumor and the mesenteric vasculature. Currently, CT scanners of various resolutions remain in use, many of which use a slice thickness of 5 mm. Our current standard for pancreatic imaging is to use slices no farther apart than 2.5 mm, and preferably as thin as 0.6 mm. Another nuance of CT imaging is the appropriate timing of contrast dye to obtain arterial and venous images; this is easily mistimed. It is our experience that the use of narrow cuts on CT scan will find potential metastases that have been missed on scans with lower resolution. A frequent difficulty is the assessment of indeterminate potential metastases in the lungs or liver. While MRI may occasionally identify these as benign or malignant, even this tool is imperfect.

Imaging may also offer clues to the underlying tumor histology. Ductal adenocarcinomas are usually poorly demarcated, low-density lesions with minimal peripheral enhancement. They can be associated with evidence of pancreatic ductal obstruction with or without upstream pancreatic atrophy, and in general, regional adenopathy is prominent but not typically bulky. In pancreatic neuroendocrine tumors (pNETs), the tumor mass may be

Table 22.1 Comparison of survival in patients with positive and negative surgical margins.

Author	Year	Overall survival (months) R0	R1
Milikan [102]	1999	17	8
Sohn [16]	2000	19	12
Benassai [103]	2000	26	9
Neoptolemos [19]	2001	17	11
Takai [20]	2003	23	8

fairly bulky and somewhat better delineated and have more enhancement than most adenocarcinomas. pNETs are not associated with pancreatic ductal obstruction and do not cause pancreatic atrophy. However, lymph node metastases are often bulky and can also show evidence of enhancement, particularly on the arterial phase of the scan. Similarly, acinar cell carcinomas are generally more enhancing and associated with bulky adenopathy. In addition, they can appear more heterogeneous than either adenocarcinoma or pNETs.

22.2.1.4 Staging of pancreatic cancer: the emergence of "borderline resectable" disease

Pancreatic adenocarcinoma is notorious for local invasion and metastatic spread to other organs at the time of diagnosis in the majority of patients (>80%). Even patients whose tumors have been discovered with no

visible metastases still have a high likelihood of recurrence after surgery. The two largest pitfalls have been surgery that results in positive margins and the development of distant metastases. Even the most recent studies demonstrate recurrence rates of over 70% within three years in resected pancreatic cancer patients [14].

How, then, does one avoid this outcome? The importance of achieving negative margins as a result of surgery cannot be overstated. In multiple prior series, patient survival was uniformly longer in those patients achieving a negative margin. These are noted in Table 22.1 [15–20]. Our observation is that patients who have undergone an R1 resection recur fairly rapidly and are often too debilitated after surgery to take effective chemotherapy. For this reason, we have tried to identify patients at higher risk for positive margins and recurrence, labeling them "borderline resectable" [21].

There is no broad consensus definition of borderline resectable disease, and at present, multiple sets of criteria have been suggested (Table 22.2). The minimal disease activity (MDA) criteria also include patients with suspected extrapancreatic disease ("borderline group B") or comorbid conditions ("borderline group C") that would increase the risk of surgery (Box 22.1; Figure 22.1, Figure 22.2, Figure 22.3, Figure 22.4, and Figure 22.5). Katz and others have previously assessed the prevalence of borderline resectable pancreatic cancer. In a review of 2454 patients evaluated between 1999 and 2006, 160 (7%) patients were classified as borderline resectable [22].

The National Comprehensive Cancer Network's (NCCN) expert panel on pancreatic cancer is in general

Table 22.2 Comparison of borderline resectable pancreatic cancer among different organizations.

	AHPBA-SSAT-SSO	MD Anderson	NCCN	Intergroup (Alliance A021101)
SMV-PV	Abutment, encasement or occlusion	Occlusion	Abutment with impingement or narrowing	Interface between tumor and vessel measuring >180° of the vessel circumference or reconstructable occlusion or both
SMA	Abutment	Abutment	Abutment	Interface between tumor and vessel measuring <180° of the circumference of the vessel wall
CHA	Abutment or short-segment encasement	Abutment or short-segment encasement	Abutment or short-segment encasement	Reconstructable, short-segment interface between tumor and vessel of any degree
Celiac trunk	No abutment or encasement	Abutment	No abutment or encasement	Interface between tumor and vessel measuring <180° of the circumference of the vessel wall

CHA, common hepatic artery; PV, portal vein; SMA, superior mesenteric artery; SMV, superior mesenteric vein.

Box 22.1 M.D. Anderson criteria for borderline resectable pancreatic cancer, with examples

> Borderline group A: anatomical criteria
>> Abutment or encasement of a short segment of the hepatic artery w/o celiac artery involved
>> Abutment of the SMA by <180°
>> Short segment occlusion of the SMV, PV or SMV/PV confluence
>> Celiac trunk abutment (includes GDA involvement with hepatic artery extension)
> Borderline group B: suspected extrapancreatic disease
>> Lymph node involvement on imaging
>> CA 19-9 >1000 in the absence of biliary obstruction
> Borderline group C: anatomically resectable with comorbid disease
>> ECOG 3 performance status
>> Significant comorbid conditions
>
> ECOG, European Cooperative Oncology Group; GDA, gastroduodenal artery; PV, portal vein; SMA, superior mesenteric artery; SMV, superior mesenteric vein.

agreement with preoperative therapy for borderline resectable patients; however, there is no consensus on what should qualify as standard treatment. Retrospective data accumulated at the MD Anderson Cancer Center suggest that a sequence of chemotherapy followed by chemoradiation, and ultimately resection, may be appropriate for patients with borderline resectable pancreatic cancer. One example of a patient successfully treated in this fashion is given in Figure 22.6. A retrospective study of 84 patients with category A borderline resectable disease found that 32 were ultimately able to undergo resection after initial chemotherapy and/or radiation. All

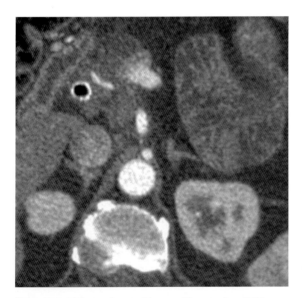

Figure 22.1 CT image from a 56-year-old man whose CHA arose off the SMA and was encased by tumor (shown). After neoadjuvant FOLFIRINOX and chemoradiation, the tumor was smaller. He was taken to the OR after six months of neoadjuvant therapy. The tumor was noted to still be at the CHA, which was resected and replaced by a graft. Three months later a local recurrence and liver metastases were noted.

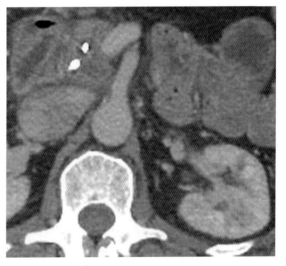

Figure 22.2 CT image from a different 56-year-old man whose tumor was noted to contact the SMA (shown) by 180°. After neoadjuvant chemotherapy only a partial response was seen. He then proceeded to radiation.

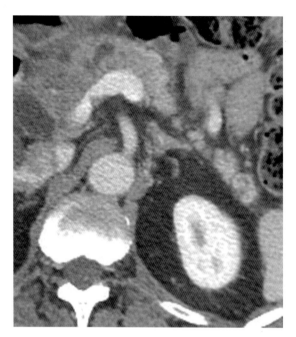

Figure 22.3 CT image from a 65-year-old man who presented with a 4.8 cm tumor encircling the SMV and narrowing the splenoportal confluence (shown). His tumor progressed through chemotherapy with subsequent complete venous occlusion seen four months after starting therapy, with collateral formation and ascites requiring paracentesis.

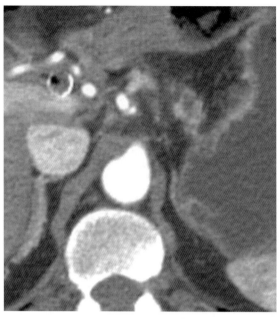

Figure 22.4 CT image from a 52-year-old man with a 4.4 cm mass at the pancreatic head, abutting the PV, PV/SMV confluence, and encasing the gastroduodenal artery (shown). He responded to FOLFIRINOX and then underwent chemoradiation. At surgery, tumor extended to the portal vein, duodenal wall, and bile duct. He remains free of visible disease one year postoperatively.

but one patient had an R0 resection. Overall median survival of the entire group was 21 months, and the survival of those patients whose neoadjuvant treatment allowed surgery was 40 months [23]. Takahashi and colleagues also found that they were able to get a significant number of patients (43 of 80) with anatomically borderline PC to the operating room with the use of gemcitabine-based chemoradiation [24]. All but one had a margin negative resection; the five-year survival rate of this group was 34%.

In another example, Kim *et al.* treated 39 borderline resectable pancreatic cancer (PC) patients with gemcitabine and oxaliplatin along with chemoradiation [25]. Of these 39, 30 completed treatment and 24 underwent resection. The median survival for this group as a whole was 18.4 months; the 24 patients who ultimately underwent resection survived a median of 25.4 months. By comparison, survival of a simultaneous cohort of resectable patients was 26.5 months for all patients and

44.7 months for those patients who ultimately underwent resection.

Our current work with borderline PC patients revolves around the FOLFIRINOX regimen, pioneered by Conroy and others in the metastatic setting [26]. In its initial phase III trial, this regimen offered a superior response rate and superior overall survival time when compared with gemcitabine. Given its promise (albeit also its toxicity), we have begun a phase II study at the MD Anderson Cancer Center offering initial FOLFIRINOX followed by chemoradiation. A parallel multicenter trial is now under way. However, unanswered questions remain: is this too toxic for patients looking to undergo surgery? Will there be an unacceptable risk of infection in patients with biliary stent? Would a more tolerable regimen, such as gemcitabine with nab-paclitaxel [27], offer a better outcome in the long term? Ongoing clinical trials will help define the best strategy for such patients.

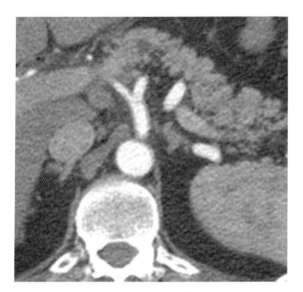

Figure 22.5 CT image from a 58-year-old man with a 3.1 cm mass at the head of the pancreas, with enlarged nodes in the hepatic arterial station (shown). The primary tumor improved with FOLFIRINOX; the nodes remained stable. He completed radiation and underwent surgery six months after diagnosis. He later developed a recurrence with malignant ascites.

22.2.1.5 Preoperative prognostication of pancreatic adenocarcinoma

While there are some patients whose medical condition encourages or demands early surgery (e.g. gastric outlet obstruction, biliary obstruction not amenable to stent placement), these patients are generally in worse shape than nonurgent patients. In one small series, these patients generally had more anorexia and weight loss, more fatigue, and a higher rate of infections than those patients sufficiently healthy to delay chemotherapy in favor of neoadjuvant chemoradiation [28]. In this group, only 61% of patients went on to adjuvant chemotherapy, as opposed to 84% of patients with good Eastern Cooperative Oncology Group (ECOG) performance status (PS) (ECOG 0–1) who began neoadjuvant chemoradiation in a nonurgent fashion. We observed that patients with ECOG PS 2–3 had, on average, longer hospital stays (24 vs 11 days, P = 0.002) than the ECOG 1–2 patients, largely because of complications. This group was also less likely than healthier patients to begin adjuvant treatment because of poor performance status (22% vs 84%).

The carbohydrate antigen (CA) 19-9 tumor marker may also serve as a tool for preoperative prognostication.

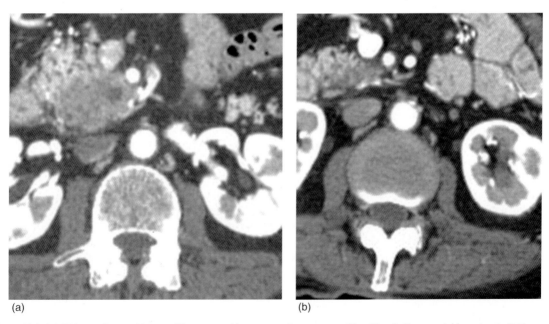

(a)   (b)

Figure 22.6 (a) CT image from a 66-year-old woman with a pancreatic cancer considered borderline resectable owing to SMA involvement. (b) The same patient after three months of FOLFIRINOX chemotherapy, with regression. She is now planned for surgery.

In the RTOG 9704 study [29], a baseline CA 19-9 of >90 suggested a shorter median survival than those patients lower than this cut-off (10- vs 21-month median survival). A smaller study of 111 patients using a CA 19-9 cut-off of 120 U/mL likewise found better survival among patients with lower preoperative values (35.6 vs 17.4 months, P = 0.044) [30]. It is important to note that CA 19-9 will be unreliable in the setting of elevated bilirubin, though corrective formulas have been proposed. Additionally, undetectable CA 19-9 levels are found in patients who lack the Lewis (a) blood antigen, and likewise may not be helpful in prognostication in these patients [31].

DPC4/SMAD4 status may also suggest prognosis: in one rapid autopsy series of 76 patients, only two of nine (22%) nonmetastatic patients had loss of DPC4 staining, compared with 16 of 22 (78%) with widely metastatic disease [32]. A second series of pancreas cancer patients likewise found that SMAD4 is lost in 70% of PC specimens and that such patients are more likely to develop metastases in the first year after surgery (51.4% vs 13%) [33]. This group found that SMAD4 status was similar in preoperative and postoperative samples, suggesting that it may be used as a predictive marker. Recent work in our own group likewise demonstrates that 73% of intact localized cancer patients had positive DPC4/SMAD4 staining, while 71% of patients with distant spread had loss of DPC4/SMAD4 [34]. It is our opinion that DPC/SMAD4 testing remains an underutilized prognostic factor in such patients.

Pancreatic tumors frequently demonstrate activation of the JAK/STAT pathway, resulting in interleukin (IL)-6 production and systemic inflammation. The modified Glasgow Prognostic Score (mGPS) is one marker of such inflammation. One point each is assigned for elevated C-reactive protein (>10 mg/L) and hypoalbuminemia (<3.5 g/dL). In one early study, an elevated GPS – on multivariate analysis with age and tumor stage – was found to be associated with poor survival [35]. When studied in a population of potentially resectable pancreatic cancer patients, median survival decreases with increasing mGPS score. Scores of 0, 1, and 2 were associated with survival durations of 37.2, 11.5, and 7.3 months, respectively. This effect was independent of age, stage, nodal status, and margin status [36]. Jamieson et al. had similar observations evaluating a different cohort of patients undergoing surgery for pancreatic ductal adenocarcinoma, finding that an elevated GPS was associated with lower survival (hazard ratio [HR] 2.26) [37].

A consensus statement of pancreatic surgeons has observed that the GPS has now been validated in more than 60 studies of organ-specific cancers, involving more than 30 000 patients from 13 different countries, and endorses its use to obtain further validation on its potential benefit for survival with surgery, although not for prediction of resectability [38]. We do note that the GPS parallels our own observation of low albumin as a poor prognostic marker and a means of categorizing patients into borderline group C.

22.2.1.6 Adjuvant trials in pancreatic adenocarcinoma

For over 25 years, solid lesions of the pancreas have generally been managed with upfront surgical resection. This has often been done when there has been a suspicion of adenocarcinoma without biopsy confirmation. What can be learned from a number of adjuvant trials and single institutional reports with upfront surgical resection of adenocarcinoma of the pancreas is briefly summarized below.

- Six months of systemic chemotherapy with either gemcitabine or fluorouracil/folinic acid (leucovorin) modestly improves median survival and five-year survival compared with observation alone.
- Chemoradiation has often been a component of adjuvant therapy, particularly in North America, but there are no definitive randomized data to support its use as a necessary component of adjuvant therapy.
- Although data are limited, perhaps as many as 40–50% of patients taken to the operating room for resection of pancreatic cancer do not undergo adjuvant therapy, based on discovery of radiographically occult metastases, an unresectable tumor, or poor recovery from surgery.
- Margin-positive resections are associated with worse survival than R0 resections.
- Elevated CA 19-9 levels postoperatively confer a poor prognosis.
- No meaningful improvement in survival has been observed in median or overall survival with an upfront surgical approach to pancreatic adenocarcinoma.

For a review of this subject, see the paper by Wolff et al. [39].

Even after successful surgery, pancreatic cancer patients suffer a high rate of relapse and death.

Randomized studies from the last decade (Table 22.3) demonstrate that the median survival of patients treated

Table 22.3 Survival among pancreatic adenocarcinoma patients after adjuvant chemotherapy.

Study	Author	Chemotherapy	# Pt	Median survival (months)	Three-year survival	Five-year overall survival
ESPAC-1	Neoptolemos [40]	5-FU	147	20.1	26%	21%
		Observation	142	15.5	13%	8%
CONKO-001	Oettle [14]	Gemcitabine	179	22.8	38%*	21%
		Observation	175	20.2	18%*	10%
ESPAC-3	Neoptolemos [41]	Fluorouracil	551	23	20%	3%
		Gemcitabine	537	23.6	19%	2%
RTOG 9704	Regine [42]	Gem/RT/Gem	221	20.5**	25%	10%
		FU/RT/FU	230	16.9**	21%	7%
JSAP-02	Ueno [43]	Gemcitabine	58	22.3	29%	24%
		Observation	60	18.4	23%	11%

FU, fluorouracil; RT, radiation therapy.

with chemotherapy, even under the best of circumstances, is generally no better than 24 months. Five-year survival after surgery approximates 25% and often less [14,40–43]. The use of adjuvant chemotherapy has generally been shown to have a small but beneficial effect. A recently published meta-analysis of adjuvant chemotherapy and chemoradiation studies to date has shown improvements in survival for those patients treated with fluorouracil and gemcitabine, with hazard ratios of 0.65 and 0.59 respectively when compared with observation alone [44]. Chemoradiation resulted in worsened survival than fluorouracil or gemcitabine (HR 1.69, 1.86 respectively). Major limitations in interpreting these studies include the heterogeneity of patients included for selection and the absence of uniform criteria for surgical resection prior to enrollment into these adjuvant studies.

22.2.1.7 Neoadjuvant trials in pancreatic adenocarcinomas

Similar to other solid tumors, to include breast, esophageal, and rectal cancer, several institutions began investigating the role of preoperative or neoadjuvant therapy for the treatment of potentially resectable pancreatic cancer. Given the biology of pancreatic cancer, such a strategy has sound logic. First, it provides for delivery of cytotoxic therapy (historically as fluorouracil [5-FU]-based chemoradiation) to an intact and relatively well-perfused tumor and surrounding microenvironment. Second, it provides for early treatment of microscopic metastatic disease, almost certainly present for the

majority of patients who present with a radiographically resectable tumor. Third, it provides a relevant time period to observe underlying tumor biology, and with restaging studies performed after preoperative therapy, a subset of patients will be discovered to have interval development of metastatic disease. Fourth, it facilitates careful observation of the patient proceeding through a course of anticancer therapy. Patients with pancreatic cancer are often older (peak age of onset 60–70 years), and they may have other comorbidities or generalized deconditioning that is not apparent on initial surgical evaluation. Chemotherapy or chemoradiation offers a selection mechanism to better identify patients who may not be able to tolerate a pancreaticoduodenectomy, or other pancreatic cancer resections.

A sequential series of preoperative therapy trials performed at the MD Anderson Cancer Center coupled with reports from other trials have provided valuable information as to the potential merits of preoperative therapy.

- Approximately 15% of patients treated with preoperative therapy will develop radiographic evidence of metastatic disease within 6–12 weeks of presentation with resectable disease. This spares one in seven potential surgical patients from a morbid surgical procedure.
- An additional 10% of patients will have radiographically occult metastatic disease found at the time of staging laparoscopy or laparotomy after neoadjuvant treatment.
- Roughly 5% of patients who embark on preoperative therapy will be considered to have unacceptable

surgical risk based on clinical observations made during preoperative treatment.

- R0 resection rates are generally higher with the use of preoperative therapy compared with upfront surgical resections performed at the same institutions [45].
- Radiation may also reduce the incidence of fistula formation after surgery [46].
- An undisturbed blood supply offers the theoretical advantage of better distribution of chemotherapy to the tumor, and less hypoxia (with attendant HIF expression) may result in less chemoresistance [47].

A rigorous application of this approach was conducted at the MD Anderson Cancer Center [48]. This study is noteworthy in that the investigators applied a specific definition of potentially resectable disease. Patients were included if there was no evidence of extrapancreatic disease; if there was no evidence of tumor extension to the superior mesenteric artery (SMA) or celiac axis; and if there was no evidence of occlusion of the superior mesenteric vein (SMV) or SMV-portal vein (PV) confluence. Tumor abutment and encasement of the SMV, in the absence of vessel occlusion or extension to the SMA, was considered resectable. Treatment included weekly gemcitabine at a dose of 400 mg/m^2 for a total of seven doses. Radiation was given over a 10-day course at a dose of 3 Gy/day. A total of 86 patients were treated; 74 were found to be resectable, among whom nine patients had metastases; an additional patient dropped out. The remaining 64 underwent surgery. The median survival of all patients was 22.7 months, but it reached 34 months for those patients who ultimately did undergo surgery. The five-year survival for these patients was 36%, which equates to 27% for the whole group. This compares favorably with any of the studies of adjuvant chemotherapy presented in Table 22.2 and has the added advantage of having prevented unhelpful surgery in a sizeable minority of patients.

The same investigators also asked whether the sequence of chemotherapy, chemoradiation, and surgery would be valuable to potentially resectable patients [49]. Here, gemcitabine and cisplatin were given every other week for four doses prior to the initiation of chemoradiation. In this study, 90 patients were enrolled, 79 completed neoadjuvant treatment, and 52 ultimately underwent resection. The median survival of resected patients was 31 months, but survival of all patients was only 17.9 months. Although the study enrolled a separate population from the earlier study, the authors concluded that the additional chemotherapy did not add to the effect of chemoradiation.

Our current approach to patients with potentially resectable PC is a course of neoadjuvant chemoradiation followed by surgery. We believe that the strategy allows the identification of distant metastases, while not compromising care of the primary tumor itself. As evidence of this, we observe that only one patient of the 176 in the two aforementioned studies actually had progression of the primary tumor precluding resection; the other patients were all excluded from surgery because of metastatic disease.

22.2.1.8 Approach to patients with presumed adenocarcinoma of the pancreas

In patients discovered to have a solid lesion involving the pancreas, dual-phase helical CT or contrast-enhanced MR of the abdomen and pelvis should be obtained. In addition, NCCN guidelines recommend plain chest X-ray or CT imaging of the chest. Laboratory studies should include a measurement of serum CA 19-9 level. For those patients with lesions in the liver, lung, or peritoneum suspicious for metastatic spread, biopsy of a metastatic site is preferred to determine histology and confirm the presence of metastatic disease. In the absence of metastatic disease, many centers still perform image-guided biopsy of the pancreatic lesion as part of diagnosis and staging, preferably utilizing endoscopic ultrasonography with fine needle aspiration to minimize the risk of peritoneal seeding or needle tract seeding that is more likely with percutaneous biopsy. However, in some centers, when high-quality imaging demonstrates a clearly resectable solid lesion of the pancreas without evidence of metastatic spread, surgical resection without prior biopsy is often recommended.

Laparoscopy remains an additional tool to rule out occult peritoneal metastatic disease not identified on cross-sectional imaging. Recent studies comparing laparoscopy to high-resolution CT imaging have been reported. In one example of 136 patients where the greater sac was inspected laparoscopically, with no mobilization of viscera, three (2%) had radiographically occult disease [50]. Subsequent laparotomy identified an additional 12 patients (9%), occurring at the posterior liver, lesser sac, retroperitoneum, and proximal jejunal mesentery. In a second group of 138 patients undergoing open staging, 15 had radiographically occult metastases. Of these, six would have been hidden from sight with standard staging laparoscopy, had it been performed. The investigators do note that a more extensive laparoscopic evaluation would have found the majority of these metastases. Other investigators have similarly noted that the sensitivity of CT for peritoneal and liver surface metastases may be as low as 42% [51], but have also noted that an elevated CA 19-9 may accompany such findings. In our own practice, we tend to reserve laparotomy for patients who have elevated CA 19-9, who have a mediocre performance status, or who are otherwise deemed at higher surgical risk.

The current standard of care for solid lesions that meet radiographic criteria for surgical resectability with no evidence of metastasis is an attempt at upfront surgical resection. In the case of pancreatic head lesions, inking of the SMA or uncinate margin is a critical component of pathological staging. While preoperative therapy for resectable pancreatic adenocarcinoma has shown promising results, neoadjuvant chemotherapy, chemoradiation, or both are still considered investigational and should preferably be delivered in the context of a clinical trial. Importantly, for those patients being considered for preoperative treatment, biopsy confirmation of malignancy is advised. As noted above, for patients who present with equivocal evidence of metastatic disease to the liver or peritoneum, or for patients who have a CA 19-9 over 500–1000 (with normal bilirubin level), staging laparoscopy prior to laparotomy is advised. However, in borderline pancreatic cancer (whether for anatomical reasons, suspected metastases, or poor performance status), biopsy confirmation is recommended. If adenocarcinoma is confirmed, preoperative treatment should be considered in most situations irrespective of the availability of a clinical trial.

There has been recent interest in the use of laparoscopic resection of pancreas body and tail lesions. There is yet relatively little literature comparing these with formal open resection. While there are no randomized trials, a number of retrospective studies have evaluated laparoscopic resection with open resection. The largest such comparison evaluated 212 patients who underwent distal pancreatectomy; 11% of these had been laparoscopic resections. These investigators noted less blood loss (790 vs 422 mL) and shorter length of stay (11 vs 7 days). R1 margin rates were similar between the groups (27% vs 26%) though the tumors in the laparoscopic group tended to be smaller (4.5 vs 3.5 cm, P = ns). Fewer patients in the laparoscopic group underwent adjuvant

chemotherapy though reasons for this are not given. As expected, absence of adjuvant chemotherapy, positive margins, and involved nodes correlated with worsened survival; the type of resection did not, with similar survival regardless of surgery type.

This study's findings are similar to a later one again retrospectively comparing outcomes of patients treated laparoscopically (n = 8) with open surgery (n = 22); this was not a randomized comparison [52]. In this smaller cohort, R0 margins were achieved in seven of eight laparoscopically treated patients and in 12 of 14 patients treated with open surgery. A longer operative time was noted in the laparoscopic group, but hospital stay was shorter (8 vs 12 days). Three-year survival was similar between the groups. These data suggest that laparoscopic surgery may be appropriate for carefully selected patients, though a randomized study (not yet performed) would be valuable information.

22.2.2 Management of pancreatic neuroendocrine tumors

Neuroendocrine tumors (NETs) represent only 3% of pancreatic cancers; however, they are important to recognize. A number of fundamental differences between pancreatic adenocarcinomas and neuroendocrine tumors lead physicians to take a different surgical and medical approach to these cancers. There are differences in prognostic factors between NETs and adenocarcinomas, differences in staging and biomarker availability, in the use of radioimaging to define tumor extent, and in the role of neoadjuvant chemotherapy and metastatectomy. Unlike adenocarcinomas, some of these tumors are metabolically active, producing hormones such as gastrin, insulin or glucagon, while others are nonfunctional.

22.2.2.1 Risk factors

Neuroendocrine tumors can arise from a number of different sites, including the foregut (lungs, stomach, pancreas), midgut (jejunum, ileum, appendix), and hindgut (distal colon) [53]. One retrospective study at a large academic medical center found a slight male predominance (55% vs 45%); this was also seen in evaluation of the SEER database [3]. Unlike patients with adenocarcinoma, cigarette smoking, BMI, and alcohol consumption were not found to be significant risk factors for NET. There was an increased incidence of diabetes mellitus in these patients (odds ratio [OR]

2.8); however, many of these were diagnosed with diabetes around the time of their cancer diagnosis.

There are some inheritable predispositions for pancreatic NET. While uncommon, the most frequent of these aberrations is MEN1 syndrome [54]. This is an autosomal dominant syndrome resulting in pituitary adenomas, parathyroid hyperplasia, and pancreatic neuroendocrine tumors; however, multiple mutations have been identified that may result in this syndrome. Other associated syndromes (also rare) include von Hippel–Lindau syndrome [55], von Recklinghausen disease, neurofibromatosis type 1, and tuberous sclerosis (TSC); this last gene was found to be mutated in roughly 9% of pancreatic NETs.

22.2.2.2 Signs and symptoms of pancreatic NETs
Pancreatic neuroendocrine tumors may be either functional (i.e. hormone producing) or nonfunctional. Fully 40% of patients are diagnosed incidentally. Both may cause symptoms resulting from the local effect of the tumor – abdominal or back pain (typically T10 level), early satiety, and duodenal obstruction. They may cause jaundice if obstructing the bile duct. Functional tumors may cause specific effects related to the hormone produced. Insulinomas may cause episodic hypoglycemia, often with confusion, palpitations, or tremulousness. Conversely, glucagonomas may cause diabetes mellitus, anemia, weight loss, diarrhea, chelitis, and necrolytic migratory erythema. Gastrinomas arising from the pancreas may result in peptic ulcer disease, and VIPomas may cause watery diarrhea, weight loss, and hypokalemia.

22.2.2.3 Diagnosis and staging
A growing recognition of the different biology of pNET and adenocarcinoma prompted alternative classification schemes. An early version of this was put forward by the World Health Organization [56,57], which classified tumors into benign, indeterminate, and malignant behavior. Each of these classifications was based on tumor size, mitoses per high power field (HPF), KI-67, perineural or vascular invasion. More recently, both the European Neuroendocrine Tumor Society (ENETS) and the American Joint Committee on Cancer (AJCC) have proposed more detailed staging systems. The purpose of both staging systems is to offer prognostic information to patients and clinicians specific to pancreatic endocrine tumors as a distinct entity from the more broad classification of carcinoid tumors as well as from exocrine

pancreatic tumor (e.g. adenocarcinomas). The ENETS staging system [58], published in 2006, was derived from a consensus conference and stages patients into a TNM system. In this system, T1 tumors are those <2 cm, T2 range from 2 to 4 cm, T3 tumors exceed 4 cm or invade the duodenum or bile duct, and T4 tumors are those that invade adjacent organs or blood vessels. Overall stage progresses from stage I (T1N0) to stage IIIA (T4N0). Lymph node-positive tumors (N1) are designated as stage IIIB, and the presence of metastases defines stage IV.

The AJCC system is based on the exocrine pancreas staging system and differs from the ENETS system as more broadly including resectable cancer as stage I, while designating tumor abutting the celiac axis or SMA without involved nodes as stage IIB. Stage III in the ENETS system includes all patients with node-positive disease, while the AJCC system lists T1–T3/N1 tumors as stage IIB [59]. They are both prognostic for relapse: five-year relapse-free survival rates for stages I–III respectively were 90%, 73%, and 66% using the AJCC system, and 100%, 84%, and 75% using the ENETS system. There is no current consensus in favor of one over the other.

Both systems also differ from the previous WHO classification by excluding reference to the proliferation rate of the tumors. However, this does remain of prognostic importance. Two separate means of testing this aspect of cell biology are KI-67 immunolabeling and counting of mitoses on slides. These two methods have recently been compared [60], with the finding that there can be discordance between the two systems. One third of tumors deemed to be grade 1 on mitotic rate alone (<2 mitoses/10 HPF) were actually grade 2 by KI-67 analysis (3–20% KI-67 positive cells). These tumors were larger and more aggressive than those found to be grade 1 on both measures. In a smaller number of tumors, the opposite (grade 1 KI-67/grade 2 WHO) was true; these tumors did not differ histologically from uniform grade 1 tumors. Ellison *et al.* have offered a point system to combine the ENETS/AJCC staging with proliferation index, patient age, and sex into a prediction of patient survival [61].

22.2.2.4 Imaging studies
Pancreatic NETs may have characteristic imaging features on CT [62]. Smaller tumors tend to be more homogeneous, while larger tumors may be more heterogeneous, with areas of cystic change, necrosis, and calcification. Well-differentiated pNETs tend to be well circumscribed, particularly compared with the more amorphous

pancreatic adenocarcinomas. They tend to displace rather than invade nearby structures. A key feature is that they have a rich capillary network, resulting in hyperattenuation with contrast on arterial and venous phase images. Cystic NETs may have a hypervascular rim, allowing them to be distinguished from more cystic neoplasms. Poorly differentiated NETs, conversely, tend to have ill-defined borders and internal necrosis. Liver and lymph node metastases may also be hypervascular and may be more prominent on arterial phase images.

Magnetic resonance imaging can also be used to image pNETs. They appear relatively hypointense on T1-weighted images, with higher signal intensity on T2-weighted images. Abundant collagen may reduce the signal intensity. Liver metastases are likewise hyperintense on T2 imaging. In one (small) study comparing CT and MRI imaging in a group of 51 patients, both modalities had similar accuracy in assessing size, margins, pancreatic duct involvement, involvement of adjacent organs, and lymph node involvement. CT was superior only in assessing the infiltration of peritumoral vessels [63]. A separate study demonstrated a sensitivity of 93% and a specificity of 77% in the ability of MRI to diagnose pancreatic NETs [64]. Diffusion-weighted imaging may also be useful for distinguishing NET from accessory splenic tissue [65].

Endoscopic ultrasound (EUS) can also be helpful in diagnosing pNETs by confirming the size and characteristics of these tumors and by offering an opportunity to biopsy these lesions. One review of patients at the MD Anderson Cancer Center correctly confirmed a pNET in 73 of 81 patients for an accuracy rate of 90% as a diagnostic tool [66]. In this study, 75 patients underwent biopsy; in six patients this was not attempted due largely to blood vessels in the path of the needle. Of the 75, 73 had a diagnosis of pNET. Additionally, EUS was able to demonstrate multiple lesions in eight cases.

One tool available for pancreatic NET is nuclear imaging with somatostatin analogues [67]. The most frequently used technique employs octreotide labeled with indium 111. Sensitivity will vary by size and tumor type. Gastrinomas are highly likely to demonstrate somatostatin uptake; this modality is able to pick up most tumors greater than 2 cm and 35–70% of tumors smaller than 1 cm. Insulinomas, conversely, tend to express fewer octreotide receptors and are imaged by somatostatin in fewer than 70%. Generally, octreoscan may be less sensitive in tumors smaller than 2 cm.

In one series of 40 patients, octreoscan was positive in 28 (70%). Its role may complement that of CT and MRI by enhancing recognition of metastatic sites or, in the case of a negative study, suggesting the presence of a poorly differentiated tumor or another histology altogether.

22.2.2.5 Adjuvant therapy

In considering patients for resection with pancreatic neuroendocrine tumors, the histological grade of the tumor may play a larger role in determining survival than margin status. This also represents a difference from adenocarcinomas. In a case series, Fischer *et al.* demonstrated that survival in patients undergoing R0 resection was no better than those undergoing R1 or R2 resection [68]. However, tumor grade was relevant: patients with poorly differentiated tumors had a median survival of 11.7 months, and none lived five years. By comparison, those patients with well-differentiated carcinomas had a median survival of 41 months. Patients with functional tumors had a generally worse prognosis (HR 2.79, $P = 0.037$).

The relatively long natural history of patients with lower grade tumors makes the conduct of randomized prospective adjuvant studies very difficult. In one retrospective analysis of 46 patients with close surgical margins, the use of radiation (n = 16) did not lead to improved overall survival, with five-year survivals of 74% in the nonradiated group compared with 28% in the group who did receive radiation [69]. Local recurrences were similar in both groups, which the authors took as a favorable sign given the larger median tumor size and increased number of positive lymph nodes in the irradiated patients. A second series from Duke compared 16 patients treated with surgery alone with 17 patients treated with additional radiation [70]. These investigators found that the majority of relapses occurred distantly, with similar two-year local control between the two groups.

An exception is made for high-grade neuroendocrine tumors. In these patients, surgery alone is rarely curative [71]; consensus guidelines from the North American Neuroendocrine Tumor Society (NANETS) suggest the use of adjuvant cisplatin and etoposide [72].

22.2.2.6 Neoadjuvant therapy

Other differences between neuroendocrine and adenocarcinomas include the ability to use radionucleotide imaging diagnostically to stage patients and therapeutically to downstage them. Barber and colleagues used luteum bound to octreotide to downstage tumors in five unresectable patients [73]. Four patients demonstrated improvements in the tumor; one underwent potentially curative surgery. Sowa-Staszczak reported that this technique reduced the mean size of tumors from 6.9 cm to 5.4 cm, enabling two patients of six to undergo surgery [74]. Ezziddin reported another such case with a recurrence-free survival of 22 months [75].

Chemotherapy can likewise assist in getting unresectable patients to surgery. The FAS regimen (fluorouracil, adriamycin, streptozocin) has proven capable of eliciting responses in 39% of patients with pancreatic endocrine tumors [76]. One example of the potential benefit of FAS is shown in Figure 22.7. The combination of capecitabine and temozolomide has also been reported to downstage a patient [77] though it is uncertain how this regimen compares with FAS, which we perceive to be the more potent combination.

Even in patients with distant metastases, resection of pNET may be possible and may result in some improvement in survival. Norton et al. reported on a series in which patients with distant metastases (particularly liver) had their disease surgically removed; half of these patients experienced a relapse (not necessarily symptomatic) by 30 months of follow-up [78]. Of five patients whose disease was incompletely removed, two patients progressed rapidly. Cusati et al. also reported a series of patients treated for either cure (R0) or palliation (R1 with 90% debulking) [79]. One-year progression-free survival (PFS) was 54% and 58% respectively, and five-year PFS was 11% and 4% respectively. Overall survival was 97%, 60%, and 45% at one, five, and 10 years. Finally, a case series from UCLA demonstrated a five-year survival of 77%, also suggesting a benefit from an aggressive approach towards surgical treatment [80].

22.2.3 Management of pancreatic cancer with unusual histology

A number of unusual histological types may be determined on tissue analysis. Solid pseudopapillary tumors have been described increasingly since 1959 [81]; they may represent somewhere between 0.1% and 2.7% of pancreatic tumors. They generally affect young (<50 years) women, do not carry KRAS or p53 mutations, and are less prone to metastasizing. Surgical resection may result in cure for 95% of patients. Acinar cancers, which account for 1–2% of pancreatic tumors, are more aggressive. Metastatic disease is seen in 50% of patients at presentation, and their prognosis is only slightly better than pancreatic ductal adenocarcinomas. Lipase hypersecretion is found in 15% of patients and results in subcutaneous nodules, eosinophilia, and arthralgias. Primary pancreatic lymphomas have also been described, but are exceedingly rare. These are typically treated with

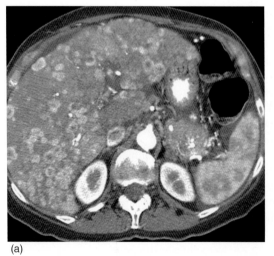
(a)

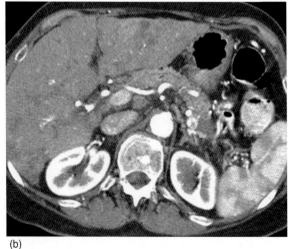
(b)

Figure 22.7 (a) CT image from a 63-year-old woman with a pancreatic neuroendocrine tumor with diffuse liver metastases. (b) CT image from the same patient, after one year of chemotherapy, demonstrating marked improvement in her disease.

chemotherapy. Finally, metastatic renal cell and colon cancers to the pancreas have been described.

22.3 Cystic lesions of the pancreas

Cystic lesions of the pancreas represent a heterogeneous spectrum of fluid-filled lesions ranging from benign serous lesions having virtually no malignant potential, to mucinous premalignant neoplasms to invasive neoplasms that are primary to the pancreas or metastatic from another site. As with solid masses of the pancreas, multidisciplinary collaboration, albeit with a more limited group of specialists (surgeons, gastroenterologists, radiologists, and pathologists), is necessary for optimal workup, longitudinal follow-up, and, on occasion, surgical intervention. In cases where invasive malignant disease is established, input from medical oncologists and radiotherapists is indicated.

The actual prevalence of cystic lesions of the pancreas is not well quantified but it is estimated that cystic abnormalities of the pancreas are now seen in up to 1–3% of CT or MR scans of the abdomen [82,83]. The incidence of reported cystic lesions is increasing and is likely based on the improving quality of cross-sectional abdominal imaging, the aging population, and the widespread use of CT and MR for surveillance of nonpancreatic malignant disease, emergent evaluations for blunt abdominal trauma, or as a component of diagnostic evaluation for back, flank, or abdominal pain.

Cystic lesions of the pancreas can be divided into distinct groups – serous neoplasms, premalignant mucinous neoplasms that can undergo malignant transformation, and invasive neoplasms (primary or metastatic) that may be predominantly solid or cystic – and often have components of both.

It is difficult to know the exact proportion of the various subtypes of cystic lesions from currently available literature. Limited data from surgically resected lesions suggest some differences in the incidence of subtypes based on a symptomatic presentation versus an incidental finding in an asymptomatic patient (Table 22.4) [84].

22.3.1 Serous cystic lesions of the pancreas
22.3.1.1 Serous cystadenoma
Serous lesions of the pancreas are common, with serous cystadenomas accounting for approximately 30% of all

Table 22.4 Incidence of various pancreatic cystic lesions from resected specimens in asymptomatic and symptomatic patients.

Type of cystic lesion resected	Incidence asymptomatic patients	Incidence symptomatic patients
Serous cystadenoma	17%	7%
Mucinous cystic neoplasms	28%	16%
Pseudocyst	4%	19%
IPMN	27%	40%
Ductal adenocarcinoma	2.5%	9%
Others/unknown	22%	9%

IPMN, intraductal papillary mucinous neoplasm.

types of cystic neoplasms found within the pancreatic parenchyma. These are often an incidental finding on abdominal imaging obtained for other reasons. However, cysts larger than 4 cm are more often associated with symptoms that can be sufficiently concerning to trigger a diagnostic evaluation with CT or MR of the abdomen [85]. Serous cystadenomas are generally found in people in their 60s and over, with women being more likely to develop these neoplasms than men. Serous cystadenomas are frequently asymptomatic and typically slow-growing. Small serous cystadenomas have an indolent growth rate of 1–2 mm per year. However, a serous cystadenoma greater than 4 cm may grow more rapidly with a rate closer to 2 cm per year.

Serous cystadenomas fall into two broad categories: microcystic and macrocystic. Microcystic cystadenomas are composed of innumerable small septations within a larger thin-walled, well-circumscribed cystic structure. On CT imaging, they have a granular, "starburst," or honeycomb appearance that is pathognomonic for microcystic cystadenoma. Macrocystic lesions have fewer large, loculated cystic areas within the primary cyst.

The histopathology of serous cystadenomas (micro- or macrocystic) is that of a multiloculated thin-walled cystic structure lined by bland cuboidal epithelium without dysplastic features. The fluid contained within a serous cystadenoma is nonviscous colloid with proteinaceous debris. Fluid analysis may also be helpful to distinguish a serous lesion from a mucinous cyst or a pseudocyst. Aspirated fluid is negative for mucin on mucicarmine

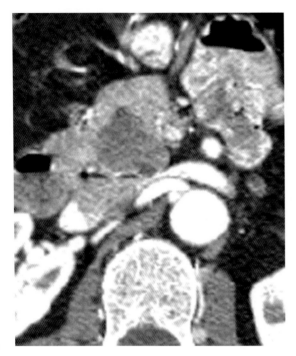

Figure 22.8 CT image of a microcystic serous cystadenoma with very thin-walled and granular appearing intracystic contents. Courtesy of Eric Tamm, University of Texas MD Anderson Cancer Center.

stains, with relatively low amylase and CEA levels favoring a benign serous lesion rather than a mucinous neoplasm or a pseudocyst. Although malignant serous cystadenocarcinoma has been reported in the literature, this is an exceedingly rare entity and requires the presence of extrapancreatic metastases (synchronous or metachronous) to firmly establish that a serous cyst has undergone malignant degeneration (Figure 22.8).

22.3.1.2 Pancreatic pseudocyst

As the name suggests, pseudocysts are not technically cysts but rather represent a residual inflammatory fluid-filled structure that develops as acute pancreatitis resolves or as a sequela of chronic pancreatitis. Unlike true pancreatic cysts, they do not have an epithelial lining and their walls consist of fibrous or granulation tissue. Pseudocysts can vary in size from a few centimeters up to 20 cm in diameter. They are generally distinguished from other cystic lesions of the pancreas by their peripheral location within the pancreas, unilocular appearance, and

an antecedent history of acute or chronic pancreatitis. Fluid aspirated from a pseudocyst typically has markedly elevated amylase levels with scattered acute and inflammatory cells seen on cytology. In asymptomatic patients, these lesions are managed conservatively. Larger pseudocysts may lead to symptoms and occasionally require resection or drainage.

22.3.2 Mucinous cystic lesions of the pancreas

Mucinous lesions of the pancreas are generally divided into mucinous cystic neoplasms (MCNs) and intraductal papillary mucinous neoplasms (IPMNs). Both are premalignant lesions that may transform to invasive adenocarcinoma. Of note, the cellular components of MCNs and IPMNs are different, with MCNs having a characteristic subendothelial architecture similar to ovarian stroma, whereas IPMNs are composed of mucin-secreting proliferative epithelium with intraductal papillary projections. Of further note, there are differences between MCNs and IPMNs in regard to gender, age of onset, and location within the pancreas.

22.3.2.1 Mucinous cystic neoplasms

Mucinous cystic neoplasms of the pancreas are distinct from other cystic lesions. First, they are found almost exclusively in women and are typically diagnosed between 30 and 50 years of age. Second, their distribution within the pancreas is generally limited to the parenchyma of the pancreatic body or tail. Third, in contrast to IPMNs, they are not associated with involvement of the pancreatic ductal system. Fourth, they are characterized by a columnar, mucinous epithelium with subendothelial stroma having similar morphology to ovarian stroma. They often stain positive for estrogen receptors (ER) and progesterone receptors (PR). Although they can be discovered incidentally in an asymptomatic woman, they are often diagnosed with abdominal imaging obtained to evaluate abdominal pain, bloating, or other GI symptoms. Radiographically, these lesions are usually round, low-density masses of varying size with a thick, enhancing wall. Risk of malignancy (invasive mucinous cystadenocarcinoma) rises for lesions greater than 3 cm in size. Given their malignant potential and development in relatively young women, surgical resection is generally the preferred treatment. An example is seen in Figure 22.9.

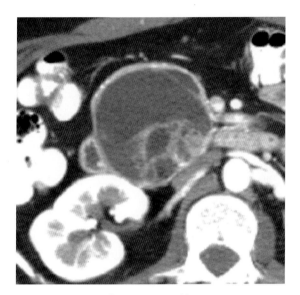

Figure 22.9 CT image from a 44-year-old woman demonstrating a mucinous cystadenoma with thick, enhancing wall. Final surgical pathology demonstrated a 7 cm lesion confined to the pancreas with low-grade epithelial dysplasia and exuberant ovarian stroma that was ER and PR positive.

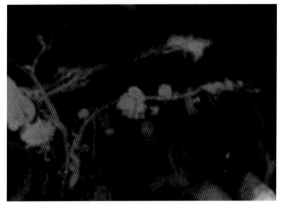

Figure 22.10 MRCP image from a 78-year-old man followed for three years with asymptomatic multifocal BD-IMPNs.

22.3.2.2 Intraductal papillary mucinous neoplasms

Intraductal papillary mucinous neoplasms are proliferative cystic dilatations of the pancreatic ductal system lined by an epithelium with papillary projections and excessive mucin production. They can arise from a side-branch pancreatic duct (also known as branch duct [BD]) or from the main pancreatic duct (MD); mixed lesions have also been reported. IPMNs are increasing recognized as a significant risk factor for the subsequent development of ductal adenocarcinoma of the pancreas, with MD-IPMNs putting patients at higher risk compared with BD. BD-IPMNs represent about 80% of IPMNs; 20% are either MD-IPMNs or mixed BD and MD-IPMNs.

Based on research from Klibansky *et al.*, it appears that the incidence of IPMN is increasing. These investigators looked at the incidence of IPMNs in Olmsted County, Minnesota, from 1985 to 2005 [86]. Although the age- and sex-adjusted incidence of IPMNs rose dramatically during that time, from 0.31 to 4.35 per 100 000 persons, the mortality attributed to adenocarcinoma of the pancreas did not increase (11/100 000). This suggests the rise in incidence is related to improvements in diagnosis rather than an actual increase in incidence. Nevertheless, as the population of the United States ages, the overall incidence and prevalence of IPMNs will likely increase.

Risk factors for IPMN have not been as well studied compared with risk factors for ductal adenocarcinoma. In a case-control study conducted in Italy, a family history of pancreatic cancer (but not other cancers), a history of chronic pancreatitis, and diabetes were all observed with higher frequency in the cases than the controls [87]. Furthermore, insulin use was even more strongly associated with the risk of IPMN by sixfold. Of note, tobacco use was not a risk factor for IPMN. In this study, median age at diagnosis was 67 years.

Radiographically, IPMNs appear as mono- or more complex polycystic mass lesions and are often associated with dilatation of the main pancreatic duct or side-branches. The walls of the cyst can be either thickened and irregular or relatively thin and homogeneous, the former being more concerning for malignancy. IPMNs can be located in any portion of the pancreatic gland, with 50% located in the head. Multifocal disease is not uncommon (Figure 22.10).

22.3.3 Solid pseudopapillary tumors of the pancreas

Solid pseudopapillary tumors (SPPT) are rare tumors usually found in women of young age (20–40 years); they have also been discovered in very young children. These tumors can be quite large, encapsulated lesions having both solid and cystic areas. Symptoms of pain or abdominal bloating are often present at diagnosis.

Although these tumors generally have slow growth and rarely metastasize, surgical resection is advised to prevent local tumor growth, minimize symptoms, and prevent metastatic spread. These neoplasms often have imaging features that are typical (encapsulated, thick-walled, with internal hemorrhage or cystic degeneration), and when found in a young female patient, they are diagnostic for SPPT. However, SPPTs can share features suggestive of pancreatic neuroendocrine tumors that have cystic components, and in cases where surgical resection may be technically challenging, preoperative biopsy may be indicated since pNETs may be sensitive to chemotherapy as a component of preoperative therapy whereas SPPTs are not. SPPTs stain positive for β-catenin, whereas pNETs have positive staining for chromogranin or synaptophysin. Radionuclide scanning with radiolabeled octreotide may also distinguish a pNET from a SPPT. Radionuclide uptake within the tumor is indicative of a pNET, while a negative study is nondiagnostic.

22.3.4 Lymphoepithelial cysts

Lymphoepithelial cysts are relatively rare neoplasms that are typically seen in older men in their 60 s to 80 s. Approximately half the time, they are an incidental finding. These lesions can be located in the head, body or tail of the pancreas, usually just below the surface of the gland, and often have an exophytic component. They are thin-walled and can be either uni- or multi-loculated, with some having a solid component. On MR, the keratin content of these cysts leads to intense T1 signal and they are hypointense on T2. This may aid in diagnosis, but such signal characteristics are not pathognomonic. In the appropriate clinical context, these cystic lesions do not require further diagnostic evaluation. If resected, pathological findings show a cyst lined with squamous epithelium with an underlying layer of lymphoid tissue. In most cases, resection is not necessary and these cysts do not carry the risk of malignant transformation.

22.3.5 Other primary or metastatic lesions to the pancreas

On occasion, other primary tumors of the pancreas can present with a cystic appearance, most notably pNETs. These tumors can be quite large and generally have a thick-walled appearance, often with enhancement and mural nodularity (Figure 22.11). Cyst aspiration

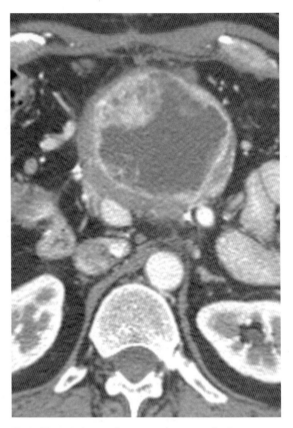

Figure 22.11 CT image of a pancreatic neuroendocrine tumor exhibiting a cystic appearance on imaging.

generally reveals low amylase and CEA levels with cytology, cell block preparations, or both, confirming a diagnosis of pNET in 86% of cases [88]. Rare primary tumors of the pancreas that may present with cystic degeneration include acinar cell carcinoma, squamous cell carcinoma, and osteoclast-like giant cell tumors of the pancreas [89–91]. On occasion, metastatic disease may involve the pancreas, most commonly from renal cell carcinoma, melanoma, and lung cancer; these are typically solid lesions. However, metastatic disease to the pancreas may manifest with cystic characteristics. An antecedent history of malignancy or radiographic evidence of a primary tumor elsewhere should prompt the clinical team to consider metastatic disease to the pancreas in the differential. Such cystic metastases have been reported in lung cancer and Merkel cell carcinoma [92,93]. Resection may be appropriate if a given patient's tumor suggests indolent biology.

22.3.6 Diagnostic evaluation of cystic pancreatic lesions

For patients being evaluated in the setting of a newly diagnosed cystic pancreatic abnormality, symptomatic or otherwise, basic personal data (age and gender) coupled with a thorough history and physical should be obtained to elicit a history, signs or symptoms that may suggest an inflammatory process based on a history of gallstones, alcohol use or pancreatitis, which may increase the chances that a pseudocyst is the likely abnormality. More worrisome symptoms, including anorexia, weight loss, jaundice, new-onset diabetes, or worsening glucose control in a known diabetic should raise concern for an underlying malignant process. In virtually all cases, a contrast-enhanced CT scan performed with thin slices as a pancreatic protocol scan should be obtained. Those lesions having a typical serous appearance and present in the appropriate clinical setting require no further diagnostic evaluation. For an excellent review, see Katz *et al.* [94].

Lesions that are not clearly serous and do not fit a clinical picture of a pseudocyst should undergo further diagnostic work-up. Some experts would recommend MRI to better delineate the presence or absence of fine internal septa which characterize serous cystic adenomas, mural nodules, and with the addition of magnetic resonance cholangiopancreatography (MRCP), may distinguish MD-IMPN from BD-IPMN [95]. Whether MRI is acquired or not, equivocal cystic abnormalities of the pancreas should undergo further evaluation with endoscopic ultrasound and, in most cases, fine needle aspiration of cyst content for fluid analysis and cytology. Any lesions with a solid component should also undergo separate fine needle aspiration for cytology. Aspiration of fluid for amylase, CEA, and assessment for the presence of mucin (either by string sign or immunohistochemical stains) is recommended (Table 22.5).

22.3.7 Clinical management of cystic pancreatic lesions

The clinical management of cystic pancreatic lesions, particularly MCNs and IPMNs, continues to evolve. Consensus guidelines from an international panel of experts who assembled in Sendai, Japan, were initially published in 2006 and subsequently updated in 2012 to better delineate high-risk features for malignancy [96,97]. These high-risk stigmata included obstructive jaundice in a patient with a cystic lesion in the head of the pancreas or an enhancing solid component within a cyst or main duct dilatation >10 mm in diameter. Worrisome features included a cyst size >3 cm, main duct 5–9 mm in diameter, a nonenhancing mural nodule, or an abrupt change in the caliber of the main duct with distal pancreatic atrophy. The updated guidelines also included an algorithm for clinical management [97].

In general, management decisions about most cystic abnormalities should be based on multidisciplinary input using a wide variety of information to include patient history and symptoms, CT or MR imaging with attention to the largest cyst diameter, main or branch duct involvement, mural nodularity or wall thickening, cyst fluid analysis and cytology, and the patient's surgical risk based on age and comorbidities. IPMNs in particular pose a management challenge since they are typically found in older patients, who may have generalized frailty or comorbidities that make surgical resection a less attractive therapeutic intervention. In addition, IPMNs can be multifocal, and it is necessary to decide on a case-by-case basis whether to perform extended pancreatic resection to remove all abnormal components of the gland or to limit the resection to the lesion at highest risk of harboring malignant epithelium or transforming to an invasive neoplasm.

Recently, efforts have been made to create algorithms and guidelines for the management of cystic lesions of the pancreas [94,98,99]. Some general principles are outlined below.

- Serous cystadenomas that are small and asymptomatic require initial short-term surveillance (one year) to ensure slow growth and minimal risk of significant progression with continued observation. Longer intervals between imaging studies may be appropriate thereafter. Larger asymptomatic lesions may require surgical intervention before they progress to the point of unresectability.
- Symptomatic serous cystadenomas in low-risk surgical patients should be considered for surgical resection.
- Mucinous cystic neoplasms should be considered for surgical resection irrespective of symptoms, given the relatively young age of the patients at risk.
- MD-IPMNs should undergo surgical resection if not medically contraindicated.
- BD-IPMNs may be followed expectantly if less than 3 cm in maximal diameter provided there are no other high-risk features on imaging or cytology.

Table 22.5 Features of various subtypes of pancreatic cystic lesions.

Pancreatic cyst subtype	Population at risk	Location at risk	Imaging characteristics	Fluid analysis	Epithelial layer and sublayers
Micro- or macrocystic serous cystadenoma	Women and men aged 60–80 M:F 1:2–3	Entire gland	Thin-walled with innumerable septa, granular or honeycombed	Low amylase High CEA - String sign and - Mucin stains	Bland cuboidal epithelium
Pseudocyst	H/O acute or chronic pancreatitis M:F 1:1	Entire gland	Macrocyst with uni- or multiloculations	High amylase Low CEA	Cytology shows inflammatory cells. No epithelial layer
Mucinous cystic neoplasm	Women aged 30–50 M:F 1:9	Body or tail	Enhancing, thick-walled cyst with or without mural nodules	Low amylase High CEA + String sign or + Mucin stains	Columnar epithelium with ovarian stroma +ER/PR
IPMN	Men and women aged 60–80 M:F 1–2:1	Head > body or tail Often multifocal	Well-circumscribed, in communication with branch ducts or main duct. Multifocal	Low amylase High CEA + String sign or + Mucin stains	Mucinous epithelium with papillary projections into ductal system
Pseudopapillary tumor	Women aged 20–40 M:F 1:1	Head	Solid and cystic components, heterogeneous	Low amylase Low CEA	Low-grade malignant epithelium + β-catenin
Cystic neuroendocrine tumor	Men and women aged 40–80 M:F 3:2	Entire gland	Thick-walled enhancing cystic mass +/- solid components	Low amylase Low CEA - String sign - Mucin stains	Malignant epithelium + chromogranin
Lymphoepithelial cyst	Men aged 60–80 M:F 4:1	Entire gland	Encapsulated, subcapsular location, exophytic component	Low amylase Low CEA - String sign - Mucin stains	Squamous epithelium

CEA, carcinoembryonic antigen; ER, estrogen receptor; H/O, history of; IPMN, intraductal papillary mucinous neoplasm; PR, progesterone receptor.

Of note, while larger trials with longer follow-up are required, there has been some investigation of non-surgical interventions to ablate cystic lesions of the pancreas. Most efforts have focused on cyst fluid aspiration followed by alcohol lavage. A small randomized trial has demonstrated that alcohol is more likely to lead to resolution compared with use of saline lavage [100]. A review of a small cohort of patients undergoing alcohol lavage for a variety of cystic lesions of the pancreas showed that for those lesions with resolution post procedure, nine of 12 patients showed continued resolution on repeat imaging for a median of 26 months post procedure (three other patients were lost to follow-up) [101].

In summary, cystic lesions of the pancreas represent a broad spectrum of clinicopathological entities which may be benign or harbor invasive disease. A multidisciplinary approach is required for initial diagnosis, therapeutic intervention, and long-term surveillance.

KEY POINTS

- Multidisciplinary management of pancreatic adenocarcinoma, pancreatic neuroendocrine tumors, and pancreatic cystic neoplasms, as well as less frequently encountered pathologies such as metastases to the pancreas and lymphoepithelial cysts, is key.

- The surgical management of pancreatic neuroendocrine tumors requires a multidisciplinary team approach to ensure that resection of primary and potentially liver metastasis is well timed with respect to tumor biology.

- Patients with potentially resectable pancreatic adenocarcinoma may benefit from a course of neoadjuvant chemoradiation followed by surgery. This strategy might allow the identification of distant metastases, while not compromising care of the primary tumor itself.

- Axial abdominal imaging has significantly increased the detection of pancreatic cystic lesions. The surgeon must be very familiar with the work-up, indications for resection, and surgical approaches to managing these cystic lesions.

References

1 Jemal A, Tiwari RC, Murray T, *et al.* Cancer statistics, 2004. CA 2004; 54(1):8–29.

2 Siegel R, Ma J, Zou Z, Jemal A. Cancer statistics, 2014. CA 2014; 64(1):9–29.

3 Yao JC, Hassan M, Phan A, *et al.* One hundred years after "carcinoid": epidemiology of and prognostic factors for neuroendocrine tumors in 35,825 cases in the United States. J Clin Oncol 2008; 26(18): 3063–3072.

4 Becker AE, Hernandez YG, Frucht H, Lucas AL. Pancreatic ductal adenocarcinoma: risk factors, screening, and early detection. World J Gastroenterol 2014; 20(32): 11182–11198.

5 Ray CS. Health consequences of smokeless tobacco use. Indian J Cancer 2012; 49(4):448.

6 Wang Z, Lai ST, Xie L, *et al.* Metformin is associated with reduced risk of pancreatic cancer in patients with type 2 diabetes mellitus: a systematic review and meta-analysis. Diabetes Res Clin Pract 2014; 106(1): 19–26.

7 Walker EJ, Ko AH, Holly EA, Bracci PM. Metformin use among type 2 diabetics and risk of pancreatic cancer in a clinic-based case–control study. Int J Cancer 2015; 136(6): E646–653.

8 Li D, Yeung SC, Hassan MM, Konopleva M, Abbruzzese JL. Antidiabetic therapies affect risk of pancreatic cancer. Gastroenterology 2009; 137(2):482–488.

9 Sadeghi N, Abbruzzese JL, Yeung SC, Hassan M, Li D. Metformin use is associated with better survival of diabetic patients with pancreatic cancer. Clin Cancer Res 2012; 18(10): 2905–2912.

10 Blanco A, de la Hoya M, Osorio A, *et al.* Analysis of PALB2 gene in BRCA1/BRCA2 negative Spanish hereditary breast/ovarian cancer families with pancreatic cancer cases. PloS One 2013; 8(7):e67538.

11 Mastoraki A, Chatzimavridou-Grigoriadou V, Chatzipetrou V, *et al.* Familial pancreatic cancer: challenging diagnostic approach and therapeutic management. J Gastrointest Cancer 2014; 45(3):256–261.

12 Bronstein YL, Loyer EM, Kaur H, *et al.* Detection of small pancreatic tumors with multiphasic helical CT. Am J Roentgenol 2004; 182(3):619–623.

13 Dunkin BJ, Marks JM, Singh J, Lash RH, Ponsky JL. Short-term endobiliary stenting results in chronic inflammation of the porcine extrahepatic biliary system. Surg Laparosc Endosc Percutan Techn 2000; 10(5):275–277.

14 Oettle H, Neuhaus P, Hochhaus A, *et al.* Adjuvant chemotherapy with gemcitabine and long-term outcomes among patients with resected pancreatic cancer: the CONKO-001 randomized trial. JAMA 2013; 310(14):1473–1481.

15 Millikan KW, Deziel DJ, Silverstein JC, *et al.* Prognostic factors associated with resectable adenocarcinoma of the head of the pancreas. Am Surg 1999; 65(7):618–623; discussion 623–624.

16 Sohn TA, Yeo CJ, Cameron JL, *et al.* Resected adenocarcinoma of the pancreas – 616 patients: results, outcomes, and prognostic indicators. J Gastrointest Surg 2000; 4(6): 567–579.

17 Benassai G, Mastrorilli M, Quarto G, Cappiello A, Giani U, Mosella G. Survival after pancreaticoduodenectomy for ductal adenocarcinoma of the head of the pancreas. Chirurg Ital 2000; 52(3):263–270.

18 Benassai G, Mastrorilli M, Quarto G, *et al.* Factors influencing survival after resection for ductal adenocarcinoma of the head of the pancreas. J Surg Oncol 2000; 73(4):212–218.

19 Neoptolemos JP, Dunn JA, Stocken DD, *et al.* Adjuvant chemoradiotherapy and chemotherapy in resectable pancreatic cancer: a randomised controlled trial. Lancet 2001; 358(9293):1576–1585.

20 Takai S, Satoi S, Toyokawa H, *et al.* Clinicopathologic evaluation after resection for ductal adenocarcinoma of the pancreas: a retrospective, single-institution experience. Pancreas 2003; 26(3):243–249.

21 Varadhachary GR, Tamm EP, Abbruzzese JL, *et al.* Borderline resectable pancreatic cancer: definitions, management, and role of preoperative therapy. Ann Surg Oncol 2006; 13 (8):1035–1046.

22 Katz MH, Pisters PW, Evans DB, *et al.* Borderline resectable pancreatic cancer: the importance of this emerging stage of disease. J Am Coll Surg 2008; 206(5):833–846; discussion 846–848.

23 Katz MH, Crane CH, Varadhachary G. Management of borderline resectable pancreatic cancer. Semin Radiat Oncol 2014; 24(2):105–112.

24 Takahashi H, Ohigashi H, Gotoh K, *et al.* Preoperative gemcitabine-based chemoradiation therapy for resectable and borderline resectable pancreatic cancer. Ann Surg 2013; 258 (6):1040–1050.

25 Kim EJ, Ben-Josef E, Herman JM, *et al.* A multi-institutional phase 2 study of neoadjuvant gemcitabine and oxaliplatin with radiation therapy in patients with pancreatic cancer. Cancer 2013; 119(15):2692–2700.

26 Conroy T, Desseigne F, Ychou M, *et al.* FOLFIRINOX versus gemcitabine for metastatic pancreatic cancer. N Engl J Med 2011; 364(19):1817–1825.

27 Von Hoff DD, Ervin T, Arena FP, *et al.* Increased survival in pancreatic cancer with nab-paclitaxel plus gemcitabine. N Engl J Med 2013; 369(18):1691–1703.

28 Aloia TA, Lee JE, Vauthey JN, *et al.* Delayed recovery after pancreaticoduodenectomy: a major factor impairing the delivery of adjuvant therapy? J Am Coll Surg 2007; 204 (3):347–355.

29 Berger AC, Winter K, Hoffman JP, *et al.* Five year results of US intergroup/RTOG 9704 with postoperative CA 19-9 </=90 U/mL and comparison to the CONKO-001 trial. Int J Radiat Oncol Biol Phys 2012; 84(3):e291–297.

30 Humphris JL, Chang DK, Johns AL, *et al.* The prognostic and predictive value of serum CA19.9 in pancreatic cancer. Ann Oncol 2012; 23(7):1713–1722.

31 Tempero MA, Uchida E, Takasaki H, Burnett DA, Steplewski Z, Pour PM. Relationship of carbohydrate antigen 19-9 and Lewis antigens in pancreatic cancer. Cancer Res 1987; 47(20):5501–5503.

32 Iacobuzio-Donahue CA, Fu B, Yachida S, *et al.* DPC4 gene status of the primary carcinoma correlates with patterns of failure in patients with pancreatic cancer. J Clin Oncol 2009; 27(11):1806–1813.

33 Boone BA, Sabbaghian S, Zenati M, *et al.* Loss of SMAD4 staining in pre-operative cell blocks is associated with distant metastases following pancreaticoduodenectomy with venous resection for pancreatic cancer. J Surg Oncol 2014; 110(2):171–175.

34 Crane CH, Varadhachary GR, Yordy JS, *et al.* Phase II trial of cetuximab, gemcitabine, and oxaliplatin followed by chemoradiation with cetuximab for locally advanced (T4) pancreatic adenocarcinoma: correlation of Smad4(Dpc4) immunostaining with pattern of disease progression. J Clin Oncol 2011; 29(22):3037–3043.

35 Glen P, Jamieson NB, McMillan DC, Carter R, Imrie CW, McKay CJ. Evaluation of an inflammation-based prognostic score in patients with inoperable pancreatic cancer. Pancreatology 2006; 6(5):450–453.

36 La Torre M, Nigri G, Cavallini M, Mercantini P, Ziparo V, Ramacciato G. The glasgow Prognostic Score as a predictor of survival in patients with potentially resectable pancreatic adenocarcinoma. Ann Surg Oncol 2012; 19 (9):2917–2923.

37 Jamieson NB, Denley SM, Logue J, *et al.* A prospective comparison of the prognostic value of tumor- and patient-related factors in patients undergoing potentially curative surgery for pancreatic ductal adenocarcinoma. Ann Surg Oncol 2011; 18(8):2318–2328.

38 Bockhorn M, Uzunoglu FG, Adham M, *et al.* Borderline resectable pancreatic cancer: a consensus statement by the International Study Group of Pancreatic Surgery (ISGPS). Surgery 2014; 155(6):977–988.

39 Wolff RA, Varadhachary GR, Evans DB. Adjuvant therapy for adenocarcinoma of the pancreas: analysis of reported trials and recommendations for future progress. Ann Surg Oncol 2008; 15(10):2773–2786.

40 Neoptolemos JP, Stocken DD, Friess H, *et al.* A randomized trial of chemoradiotherapy and chemotherapy after resection of pancreatic cancer. N Engl J Med 2004; 350(12): 1200–1210.

41 Neoptolemos JP, Stocken DD, Bassi C, *et al.* Adjuvant chemotherapy with fluorouracil plus folinic acid vs gemcitabine following pancreatic cancer resection: a randomized controlled trial. JAMA 2010; 304(10):1073–1081.

42 Regine WF, Winter KA, Abrams RA, *et al*. Fluorouracil vs gemcitabine chemotherapy before and after fluorouracil-based chemoradiation following resection of pancreatic adenocarcinoma: a randomized controlled trial. JAMA 2008; 299(9):1019–1026.

43 Ueno H, Kosuge T, Matsuyama Y, *et al*. A randomised phase III trial comparing gemcitabine with surgery-only in patients with resected pancreatic cancer: Japanese Study Group of Adjuvant Therapy for Pancreatic Cancer. Br J Cancer 2009; 101(6):908–915.

44 Liao WC, Chien KL, Lin YL, *et al*. Adjuvant treatments for resected pancreatic adenocarcinoma: a systematic review and network meta-analysis. Lancet Oncol 2013; 14(11): 1095–1103.

45 Crane CH, Varadhachary G, Wolff RA, Pisters PW, Evans DB. The argument for pre-operative chemoradiation for localized, radiographically resectable pancreatic cancer. Best Pract Res Clin Gastroenterol 2006; 20(2):365–382.

46 Ishikawa O, Ohigashi H, Imaoka S, *et al*. Concomitant benefit of preoperative irradiation in preventing pancreas fistula formation after pancreatoduodenectomy. Arch Surg 1991; 126(7):885–889.

47 Cheng ZX, Wang DW, Liu T, *et al*. Effects of the HIF-1alpha and NF-kappaB loop on epithelial-mesenchymal transition and chemoresistance induced by hypoxia in pancreatic cancer cells. Oncol Rep 2014; 31(4):1891–1898.

48 Evans DB, Varadhachary GR, Crane CH, *et al*. Preoperative gemcitabine-based chemoradiation for patients with resectable adenocarcinoma of the pancreatic head. J Clin Oncol 2008; 26(21):3496–3502.

49 Varadhachary GR, Wolff RA, Crane CH, *et al*. Preoperative gemcitabine and cisplatin followed by gemcitabine-based chemoradiation for resectable adenocarcinoma of the pancreatic head. J Clin Oncol 2008; 26(21):3487–3495.

50 Jayakrishnan TT, Nadeem H, Groeschl RT, *et al*. Diagnostic laparoscopy should be performed before definitive resection for pancreatic cancer: a financial argument. HPB 2015; 17(2):131–139.

51 Alexakis N, Gomatos IP, Sbarounis S, *et al*. High serum CA 19-9 but not tumor size should select patients for staging laparoscopy in radiological resectable pancreas head and peri-ampullary cancer. Eur J Surg Oncol 2015; 41(2):265–269.

52 Rehman S, John SK, Lochan R, *et al*. Oncological feasibility of laparoscopic distal pancreatectomy for adenocarcinoma: a single-institution comparative study. World J Surg 2014; 38(2):476–483.

53 Nilsson O, van Cutsem E, delle Fave G, *et al*. Poorly differentiated carcinomas of the foregut (gastric, duodenal and pancreatic). Neuroendocrinology 2006; 84(3):212–215.

54 Hassan MM, Phan A, Li D, Dagohoy CG, Leary C, Yao JC. Family history of cancer and associated risk of developing neuroendocrine tumors: a case–control study. Cancer Epidemiol Biomarkers Prev 2008; 17(4):959–965.

55 Zhang J, Francois R, Iyer R, Seshadri M, Zajac-Kaye M, Hochwald SN. Current understanding of the molecular biology of pancreatic neuroendocrine tumors. J Natl Cancer Inst 2013; 105(14):1005–1017.

56 Capella C, Heitz PU, Hofler H, Solcia E, Kloppel G. Revised classification of neuroendocrine tumours of the lung, pancreas and gut. Virchows Arch 1995; 425(6): 547–560.

57 Kloppel G, Heitz PU, Capella C, Solcia E. Pathology and nomenclature of human gastrointestinal neuroendocrine (carcinoid) tumors and related lesions. World J Surg 1996; 20(2):132–141.

58 Rindi G, Kloppel G, Alhman H, *et al*. TNM staging of foregut (neuro)endocrine tumors: a consensus proposal including a grading system. Virchows Arch 2006; 449(4):395–401.

59 Strosberg JR, Cheema A, Weber JM, *et al*. Relapse-free survival in patients with nonmetastatic, surgically resected pancreatic neuroendocrine tumors: an analysis of the AJCC and ENETS staging classifications. Ann Surg 2012; 256(2): 321–325.

60 McCall CM, Shi C, Cornish TC, *et al*. Grading of well-differentiated pancreatic neuroendocrine tumors is improved by the inclusion of both Ki67 proliferative index and mitotic rate. Am J Surg Pathol 2013; 37(11):1671–1677.

61 Ellison TA, Wolfgang CL, Shi C, *et al*. A single institution's 26-year experience with nonfunctional pancreatic neuroendocrine tumors: a validation of current staging systems and a new prognostic nomogram. Ann Surg 2014; 259(2): 204–212.

62 Lewis RB, Lattin GE Jr, Paal E. Pancreatic endocrine tumors: radiologic-clinicopathologic correlation. Radiographics 2010; 30(6):1445–1464.

63 Foti G, Boninsegna L, Falconi M, Mucelli RP. Preoperative assessment of nonfunctioning pancreatic endocrine tumours: role of MDCT and MRI. Radiol Med 2013; 118(7): 1082–1101.

64 Manfredi R, Bonatti M, Mantovani W, *et al*. Non-hyper-functioning neuroendocrine tumours of the pancreas: MR imaging appearance and correlation with their biological behaviour. Eur Radiol 2013; 23(11):3029–3039.

65 Kang BK, Kim JH, Byun JH, *et al*. Diffusion-weighted MRI: usefulness for differentiating intrapancreatic accessory spleen and small hypervascular neuroendocrine tumor of the pancreas. Acta Radiol 2014; 55(10):1157–1165.

66 Atiq M, Bhutani MS, Bektas M, *et al*. EUS-FNA for pancreatic neuroendocrine tumors: a tertiary cancer center experience. Dig Dis Sci 2012; 57(3):791–800.

67 Rufini V, Calcagni ML, Baum RP. Imaging of neuroendocrine tumors. Semin Nucl Med 2006; 36(3):228–247.

68 Fischer L, Kleeff J, Esposito I, *et al*. Clinical outcome and long-term survival in 118 consecutive patients with neuroendocrine tumours of the pancreas. Br J Surg 2008; 95(5): 627–635.

69 Arvold ND, Willett CG, Fernandez-del Castillo C, *et al*. Pancreatic neuroendocrine tumors with involved surgical margins: prognostic factors and the role of adjuvant radiotherapy. Int J Radiat Oncol Biol Phys 2012; 83(3): e337–343.

70 Zagar TM, White RR, Willett CG, *et al*. Resected pancreatic neuroendocrine tumors: patterns of failure and disease-related outcomes with or without radiotherapy. Int J Radiat Oncol Biol Phys 2012; 83(4):1126–1131.

71 Brenner B, Shah MA, Gonen M, Klimstra DS, Shia J, Kelsen DP. Small-cell carcinoma of the gastrointestinal tract: a retrospective study of 64 cases. Br J Cancer 2004; 90 (9):1720–1726.

72 Strosberg JR, Coppola D, Klimstra DS, *et al*. The NANETS consensus guidelines for the diagnosis and management of poorly differentiated (high-grade) extrapulmonary neuroendocrine carcinomas. Pancreas 2010; 39(6): 799–800.

73 Barber TW, Hofman MS, Thomson BN, Hicks RJ. The potential for induction peptide receptor chemoradionuclide therapy to render inoperable pancreatic and duodenal neuroendocrine tumours resectable. Eur J Surg Oncol 2012; 38(1):64–71.

74 Sowa-Staszczak A, Pach D, Chrzan R, *et al*. Peptide receptor radionuclide therapy as a potential tool for neoadjuvant therapy in patients with inoperable neuroendocrine tumours (NETs). Eur J Nucl Med Molec Imag 2011; 38 (9):1669–1674.

75 Ezziddin S, Lauschke H, Schaefers M, *et al*. Neoadjuvant downsizing by internal radiation: a case for preoperative peptide receptor radionuclide therapy in patients with pancreatic neuroendocrine tumors. Clin Nucl Med 2012; 37(1): 102–104.

76 Kouvaraki MA, Ajani JA, Hoff P, *et al*. Fluorouracil, doxorubicin, and streptozocin in the treatment of patients with locally advanced and metastatic pancreatic endocrine carcinomas. J Clin Oncol 2004; 22(23):4762–4771.

77 Devata S, Kim EJ. Neoadjuvant chemotherapy with capecitabine and temozolomide for unresectable pancreatic neuroendocrine tumor. Case Rep Oncol 2012; 5(3):622–626.

78 Norton JA, Kivlen M, Li M, Schneider D, Chuter T, Jensen RT. Morbidity and mortality of aggressive resection in patients with advanced neuroendocrine tumors. Arch Surg 2003; 138(8):859–866.

79 Cusati D, Zhang L, Harmsen WS, *et al*. Metastatic nonfunctioning pancreatic neuroendocrine carcinoma to liver: surgical treatment and outcomes. J Am Coll Surg 2012; 215(1):117–124; discussion 124–125.

80 Kazanjian KK, Reber HA, Hines OJ. Resection of pancreatic neuroendocrine tumors: results of 70 cases. Arch Surg 2006; 141(8):765–769; discussion 769–770.

81 Mortenson MM, Katz MH, Tamm EP, *et al*. Current diagnosis and management of unusual pancreatic tumors. Am J Surg 2008; 196(1):100–113.

82 Laffan TA, Horton KM, Klein AP, *et al*. Prevalence of unsuspected pancreatic cysts on MDCT. Am J Roentgenol 2008; 191(3):802–807.

83 De Jong K, Nio CY, Hermans JJ, *et al*. High prevalence of pancreatic cysts detected by screening magnetic resonance imaging examinations. Clin Gastroenterol Hepatol 2010; 8(9):806–811.

84 Fernandez-del Castillo C, Targarona J, Thayer SP, Rattner DW, Brugge WR, Warshaw AL. Incidental pancreatic cysts: clinicopathologic characteristics and comparison with symptomatic patients. Arch Surg 2003; 138(4):427–423; discussion 433–434.

85 Tseng JF, Warshaw AL, Sahani DV, Lauwers GY, Rattner DW, Fernandez-del Castillo C. Serous cystadenoma of the pancreas: tumor growth rates and recommendations for treatment. Ann Surg 2005; 242(3):413–419; discussion 419–421.

86 Klibansky D, Reid-Lombardo K, Gordon S, Gardner T. The clinical relevance of the increasing incidence of intraductal papillary mucinous neoplasm. Clin Gastroenterol Hepatol 2012; 10(5):555–558.

87 Capurso G, Boccia S, Salvia R, *et al*. Risk factors for intraductal papillary mucinous neoplasm (IPMN) of the pancreas: a multicentre case–control study. Am J Gastroenterol 2013; 108(6):1003–1009.

88 Morales-Oyarvide V, Yoon WJ, Ingkakul T, *et al*. Cystic pancreatic neuroendocrine tumors: the value of cytology in preoperative diagnosis. Cancer Cytopathol 2014; 122(6): 435–444.

89 Liu K, Peng W, Zhou Z. The CT findings of pancreatic acinar cell carcinoma in five cases. Clin Imag 2013; 37(2):302–307.

90 Colarian J, Fowler D, Schor J, Poolos S. Squamous cell carcinoma of the pancreas with cystic degeneration. South Med J 2000; 93(8):821–822.

91 Scott R, Jersky J, Hariparsad G. Case report: malignant giant cell tumour of the pancreas presenting as a large pancreatic cyst. Br J Radiol 1993; 66(791): 1055–1057.

92 Ramirez Plaza CP, Suarez Munoz MA, Santoyo Santoyo J, *et al*. [Pancreatic cystic metastasis from pulmonary carcinoma. Report of a case]. Ann Ital Chirurg 2001; 72(1): 95–99.

93 Bachmeyer C, Alovor G, Chatelain D, *et al*. Cystic metastasis of the pancreas indicating relapse of Merkel cell carcinoma. Pancreas 2002; 24(1):103–105.

94 Katz MH, Mortenson MM, Wang H, *et al*. Diagnosis and management of cystic neoplasms of the pancreas: an evidence-based approach. J Am Coll Surg 2008; 207(1): 106–120.

95 Tirkes T, Aisen AM, Cramer HM, Zyromski NJ, Sandrasegaran K, Akisik F. Cystic neoplasms of the pancreas; findings on magnetic resonance imaging with pathological, surgical, and clinical correlation. Abdom Imag 2014; 39(5): 1088–1101.

96 Tanaka M, Chari S, Adsay V, *et al.* International consensus guidelines for management of intraductal papillary mucinous neoplasms and mucinous cystic neoplasms of the pancreas. Pancreatology 2006; 6 (1–2): 17–32.

97 Tanaka M, Fernandez-del Castillo C, Adsay V, *et al.* International consensus guidelines 2012 for the management of IPMN and MCN of the pancreas. Pancreatology 2012; 12(3):183–197.

98 Law JK, Hruban RH, Lennon AM. Management of pancreatic cysts: a multidisciplinary approach. Curr Opin Gastroenterol 2013; 29(5):509–516.

99 Enestvedt BK, Ahmad N. To cease or 'de-cyst'? The evaluation and management of pancreatic cystic lesions. Curr Gastroenterol Rep 2013; 15(10):348.

100 DeWitt J, McGreevy K, Schmidt CM, Brugge WR. EUS-guided ethanol versus saline solution lavage for pancreatic cysts: a randomized, double-blind study. Gastrointest Endosc 2009; 70(4):710–723.

101 DeWitt J, DiMaio CJ, Brugge WR. Long-term follow-up of pancreatic cysts that resolve radiologically after EUS-guided ethanol ablation. Gastrointest Endosc 2010; 72(4):862–866.

102 Millikan KW, Deziel DJ, Silverstein JC, *et al.* Prognostic factors associated with resectable adenocarcinoma of the head of the pancreas. Am Surg 1999; 65: 618–624.

103 Benassai G, Mastrorilli M, Quarto G, Cappiello A, Giani U, Mosella G. Survival after pancreaticoduodenectomy for ductal adenocarcinoma of the head of the pancreas. Chir Ital 2000; 52: 263–270.

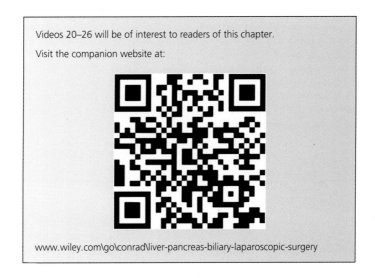

Videos 20–26 will be of interest to readers of this chapter.

Visit the companion website at:

www.wiley.com\go\conrad\liver-pancreas-biliary-laparoscopic-surgery

CHAPTER 23

Laparoscopic pancreatic surgery

Daniel Richard Rutz and David A. Kooby

Department of Surgery, Emory University School of Medicine, Atlanta, USA

EDITOR COMMENT

In this chapter, the authors summarize the results of the most commonly performed pancreatic resections: enucleation, distal pancreatectomy, and pancreaticoduodenectomy. Expected outcomes and technical considerations are discussed. Based on the presented data, distal pancreatectomy can provide comparable oncological outcomes with fewer complications, lower blood loss, and shorter hospital stay compared with open surgery for cancers of similar complexity. Laparoscopic enucleation is less commonly performed but has a role in the management of indolent small tumors not involving or approaching the main pancreatic duct. This especially includes pancreatic neuroendocrine tumors. While randomized controlled prospective data comparing laparoscopic with open pancreatic surgery are not available, the retrospective data presented by the authors are reassuring. While desirable, prospective data are difficult to obtain because of differences in technique, application of perioperative chemotherapy and chemoradiation, patient selection, surgeon and patient bias, and availability of experienced laparoscopic surgeons. Finally, the authors present the available data on laparoscopic pancreaticoduodenectomy. It indicates that this procedure is still in the developmental phase and practiced by a limited number of surgeons in selected centers. Laparoscopic pancreatic surgeons should be very familiar with the data presented in this chapter in order to put their own results into the perspective of the current outcome benchmarks for advanced laparoscopic pancreatic surgery.

Keywords: distal pancreatectomy, laparoscopic pancreas resection, pancreatic enucleation, pancreatic neoplasm, pancreaticoduodenectomy

---

23.1 Introduction

Since the first laparoscopic cholecystectomy in 1985, minimally invasive techniques have been adopted for many abdominal surgical procedures [1]. Through the use of smaller incisions and pneumoperitoneum, the laparoscopic approach results in improved cosmesis, reduced postoperative pain, and quicker recovery for many patients [2]. There appear to be immunological benefits associated with minimally invasive procedures through stress reduction and perhaps attenuation of tumor growth in the experimental setting [3]. Because of the longer learning curves and higher morbidity inherently associated with pancreatic surgery, the surgical community has adopted minimally invasive approaches to pancreatic resection more slowly than with many other organ sites. Pancreatic resections require accessing the retroperitoneum, dissecting around delicate vascula-

ture, and manipulating a soft, sensitive organ with both exocrine and endocrine function. With increased surgical experience and improvements in instrumentation, laparoscopic pancreatic resections have surged at high-volume centers for treatment of both benign and, increasingly, malignant disease. Emerging data from various reports demonstrate that laparoscopic pancreatic resections are both safe and effective compared with traditional open procedures. This review will highlight existing data and recent advances in the subject of laparoscopic pancreatic resection. Robotic pancreatectomy will be discussed elsewhere.

23.2 Laparoscopic distal pancreatectomy

Laparoscopic distal pancreatectomy (LDP) is the most commonly performed minimally invasive resection

---

Laparoscopic Liver, Pancreas, and Biliary Surgery, First Edition.
Edited by Claudius Conrad and Brice Gayet.
© 2017 John Wiley & Sons, Ltd. Published 2017 by John Wiley & Sons, Ltd.

involving the pancreas [4]. While it typically requires no anastomosis and is usually less technically demanding than laparoscopic pancreaticoduodenectomy, LDP still involves complex retroperitoneal access, careful dissection, and avoidance of injury to critical surrounding structures. The complexity of this operation varies tremendously with patient body habitus, tumor type, and tumor location within the gland.

23.2.1 Patient selection

Laparoscopic distal pancreatectomy is appropriate for benign and malignant pancreatic lesions located to the left of or overlying the superior mesenteric vein (SMV) in the pancreatic body or tail that are amenable to resection. Ideal candidates for this approach are those patients diagnosed with benign behaving disease requiring resection or those with pancreatic malignancies without substantial invasion of surrounding organs, major vessels (common hepatic artery, superior mesenteric artery [SMA], celiac axis, or portal vein) or distant metastases (with some exceptions) [5]. See Figure 23.1.

Malignant cases requiring combined venous resection or removal of adjacent organs such as left adrenal gland, portion of stomach, transverse colon, and left kidney that can result in R0 resection may be appropriate for a laparoscopic approach [6]. With greater experience,

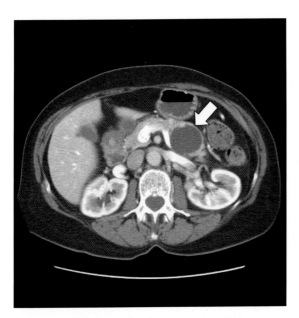

Figure 23.1 Axial CT scan showing pancreatic cystic tumor with mural nodule (*arrow*).

surgeon selection criteria have widened to include patients with increased comorbidities (Charlson score >2 40.9% vs 16.7%, P = 0.003) and larger, more medial tumors (specimen length 10.6 cm vs 8.3 cm, P < 0.001) and more proximal tumor location (74.2% vs 26.2%, P < 0.001) without significant increase in morbidity [7]. Careful selection of eligible patients is advised to limit the need for conversion to open resection, as intraoperative conversion may be associated with increased morbidity (36% vs 20%, P = 0.008) and a higher incidence of postoperative pancreatic fistula (POPF) (27% vs 13%, P = 0.03) compared with performing the case open from the start [8]. Patients undergoing planned splenectomy should be immunized against encapsulated bacterial organisms 14 days prior to surgery. If this is not possible, immunizations can be given after postoperative day 14 as opsonophagocytic function of antibodies is enhanced after this time [9].

23.2.2 Technical considerations

Common variations of LDP technique include LDP with splenectomy, spleen-preserving LDP, and radical antegrade modular pancreatectomy. Technical details of each can be found elsewhere in the literature [5,10–13]. Briefly, depending on the indication, the patient is positioned either supine or in a "lazy" right-lateral decubitus position (authors' preferred approach), and the abdomen is entered with 3–5 ports placed in various positions in the mid-left abdomen (Figure 23.2).

The peritoneal cavity is assessed for possible metastases. The stomach is retracted cephalad or towards the right and the splenic flexure of the colon is dropped, and the pancreas thus exposed and assessed with ultrasonography if necessary. The gland is mobilized from medial to lateral or vice versa, and the splenic vasculature is divided with surgical staplers (or preserved if desired and appropriate), followed by gland transection in the appropriate location. If the spleen is to be removed, it is mobilized and placed in a sac for subsequent removal en bloc or morselized separately.

Splenic conservation, when possible, may provide long-term immunological benefit for the patient. This is accomplished in two ways. The Warshaw technique involves ligating and dividing the splenic vessels at the pancreatic neck and near the splenic pedicle and removing them with the distal pancreas, leaving short gastric and left gastroepiploic vessels to perfuse the spleen [14]. While easier to perform, this technique compromises

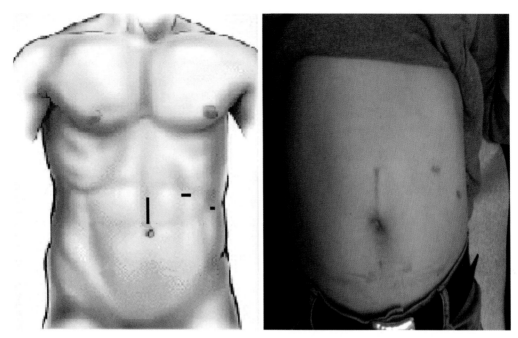

Figure 23.2 Laparoscopic distal pancreatectomy port sites. Right panel demonstrates the schematic port placement and left panel shows a patient 3 weeks after distal pancreatectomy for an 8 cm neuroendocrine tumor of the pancreatic body with splenic vein obstruction and bleeding gastric varices.

blood flow to the spleen and has been associated with splenic infarction and abscess [15]. The other method of splenic preservation involves careful dissection of the pancreatic tail away from the splenic vessels and preservation of the splenic artery and vein (Kimura method). This technique is ideal for asthenic patients with nonmalignant tumors and accessible vessels, as there is wide anatomical variability. A recent comparative analysis of LDP and these two approaches to splenic preservation demonstrated that the rate of successful spleen preservation was significantly improved following the splenic vessel preservation technique (96.4% vs 84.7%, P = 0.03) [16].

Splenic preservation at the time of operation is influenced by tumor biology and surgeon preference. The magnification afforded by the laparoscopic approach can improve visualization of the resection bed, leading to a higher rate of splenic preservation [17]. Butturini et al. compared results of 116 DPs, of which 43 were performed laparoscopically. They demonstrated a higher incidence of splenic preservation in the laparoscopic group (44.2% vs 11%, P < 0.001) with comparable rates of morbidity (48.2% vs 45.2%, P = 0.71) [18]. Song et al. looked at perioperative outcomes in 359 LDP cases, 90%

of which were benign resections. Splenic preservation was successful 49.6% of the time and the overall complication rate was 12% [17]. In a retrospective analysis of 360 DPs that included 71 LDPs, DiNorcia et al. showed similar rates of postoperative morbidity (43.9% vs 39%, P = 0.56), POPF (14.6% vs 13.3%, P = 0.82), length of hospital stay (5 vs 6 days, P = 0.13), and mortality (2.4% vs 0.5%, P = 0.29) between the spleen-preserving group and DP with splenectomy [19]. The laparoscopic group in this study had a larger percentage of benign cases (87.3% vs 61.5%, P < 0.01) than the open group.

Other technical considerations include the method of gland transection and stump closure. Surgical staplers are the preferred method for both pancreatic gland transection and stump closure. Some surgeons advocate for staple line reinforcement with a variety of existing products [20]. Absorbable mesh reinforcement of a stapled pancreatic transection line reduces the leak rate with distal pancreatectomy [20], but no randomized data exist to support this maneuver [21]. Gland thickness and quality and staple height used may be more critical determinants of adequate stump closure [22]. Another option recently described is the use of radiofrequency

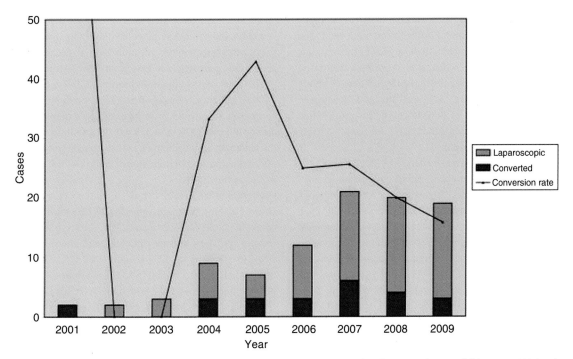

Figure 23.3 Conversion rate of laparoscopic distal pancreatectomy over time. Note that the conversion rate fell between 2006 and 2009 as the number of cases performed rose. Source: DiNorcia *et al.* [19]. Reproduced with permission of Springer.

ablation. The advantage of this approach is the efficacy of sealing the stump [23]. The limitations include damage to more of the neighboring gland and the expense of the current devices.

Conversions to the open approach through either an upper midline or left subcostal incision are most often indicated for bleeding, adhesions, or presence of malignancy that cannot be managed safely laparoscopically [6] (Figure 23.3). An intermediate option to consider is the use of a hand access port if the operation fails to progress or if there is increasing hemorrhage [7]. Existing data suggest that the hand access approach may be particularly useful in obese patients.

23.2.3 Outcomes

23.2.3.1 Operative

Meta-analyses of published literature on operative times comparing LDP and open distal pancreatectomy (ODP) have not demonstrated statistically significant differences [24–28]. In one analysis from Johns Hopkins of

18 studies involving 1814 patients, the laparoscopic approach added an average 19.71 minutes to the time for the open technique [24]. Song *et al.* demonstrated decreased mean operative time from 226 to 190 minutes for LDP in their center after 20 cases [17]. Several meta-analyses have shown that blood loss is significantly lower in LDP (263–354.98 mL less, 95% confidence interval [CI] −529.29 to −180.66, P < 0.001), as is transfusion rate (odds ratio [OR] 0.28, 95% CI 0.11–0.76, P = 0.01) [24,25]. Reported conversion rates for indications listed previously are 9.2–11.5% [6,28,29]. An important bias inherent in these reports is the lack of randomization, as some of the comparison ODP cases may not have been suited to a laparoscopic approach.

23.2.3.2 Complications

In their multicenter analysis of 637 DPs, including 159 LPD, the Central Pancreas Consortium (CPC) demonstrated significantly shorter hospital admission days in the LPD group (5.9 vs 9.0 days, P < 0.01) [30]. An important aspect of this work was that five of the eight participating centers were not using the laparoscopic approach, so the comparison is more likely to be valid. Other authors have shown a similar trend, with decreases of 2.7–5 days in hospital length of stay for LPD compared with OPD [24,26,31]. Venkat *et al.* reported a decreased time to oral intake for the LDP group by 1.5 days (95% CI −2.52–0.52, P = 0.003) [24] and Jin and colleagues showed reduced time to first flatus for this group after surgery (weighted mean difference 1.80 days, 95% CI 2.14–1.47, P < 0.001) [26].

Venkat *et al.*, in their meta-analysis of 18 studies of LDP vs ODP, showed the average rate of postoperative morbidity in the LDP group (780 cases) to be 33%, compared with 44% in the ODP cohort (1034 cases) [24]. Table 23.1 provides summary data for distal pancreatectomy morbidity ranging from 20% to as high as 50% for minimally invasive approaches, with the most common complications reported as intra-abdominal fluid collection (9.6%), surgical site infection (2.9%), and postoperative hemorrhage (3.5%), or intra-abdominal abscess (0.8%) [19,24,26,30,32,33]. LDP is a safe procedure with an overall perioperative mortality rate of 0.4% according to a recent analysis [24]. Thirty-day readmission rate and reoperation rates are 12.6% and 2.1%, respectively [24].

Pancreatic fistula is a common complication after distal pancreatectomy, including LDP, and it is defined according to the 2005 ISGPF definition as drain output of any measurable volume on or after postoperative day 3 with amylase level greater than three times the upper normal serum value [41]. Each fistula is classified as A, B, or C with most sources in the literature denoting B and C as "clinically relevant" fistulas. A recent meta-analysis of LDP has demonstrated a 19.1% overall incidence of fistulas with 9.5–12.5% being grades B/C [24,31]. Predictive risk factors for complications from LDP, including pancreatic fistula, are body mass index (BMI) >27, pancreatic specimen length >8 cm, and estimated blood loss (EBL) >150 mL [42]. Either way, the authors feel that compared with ODP, LDP may not reduce fistula formation but likely will not increase it either.

23.2.3.3 Pathology

Laparoscopic distal pancreatectomy has been used generally for smaller, benign tumors or indolent malignancies. In an analysis of 360 DPs, DiNorcia reported shorter average length of pancreas resected (7.7 ± 3.2 cm vs

10.0 ± 3.6 cm, P < 0.01) and smaller median tumor size (2.5 cm, interquartile range [IQR] 1.5–4.0 cm vs 3.6 cm, IQR 2.0–6.0 cm; P < 0.01) for LDP cases than for ODP resection, indicating a surgeon bias for minimally invasive procedures targeted towards more benign disease. In this series, the laparoscopic approach was less likely to be used in patients with adenocarcinoma (4.2% vs 30.2%, P < 0.01). A review by Jusoh and Ammori demonstrated comparable numbers of malignant cases between LDP and ODP series (320 vs 463, P = 0.271) with the majority of malignant lesions being cystic neoplasms and neuro-endocrine tumors. Of note, tumor grade was not reported in this review [28].

In another large, multicenter study, the CPC compared short- and long-term outcomes for 23 LDP and 189 ODP cases in patients with pancreatic ductal adenocarcinoma [37]. There was no significant difference in tumor size (4.5 ± 2.8 cm vs 3.5 ± 1.3 cm, P = 0.10), total node retrieval (12.5 ± 8.5 nodes vs 13.8 ± 8.4 nodes, P = 0.47), positive nodes (1.4 ± 1.9 positive nodes vs 1.0 ± 1.8 positive nodes, P = 0.36), and positive margin percentage (27% vs 26%, P = 0.98) between LDP and ODP, although the LDP cohort had shorter hospital stay (10.7 ± 6.3 days vs 7.4 ± 3.4 days, P = 0.03). The meta-analysis by Venkat *et al.* included four studies on positive margin status, and they found no significant difference between the LDP (15 of 331, 4.5%) and ODP (45 of 514, 8.8%) groups [24]. Median lymph node extraction via LDP was found to be significantly lower in one series comparing LDP with ODP (5.2 vs 9.4, P = 0.04) [36]. Waters *et al.* showed a similar trend (14 for LDP vs 11 in ODP) in their analysis of 40 cases [43]. DiNorcia reported that median lymph node dissection was similar in both the LDP and ODP groups (6, IQR 2.5–12.0 vs 8, IQR 3.0–13.0, P = 0.29) [19]. These studies contain heterogeneous pathology and should be interpreted with caution.

23.2.3.4 Survival

In their 2010 multi-institutional study of 212 patients undergoing DP for adenocarcinoma, the CPC reported that, at a median follow-up of 10 months, median actuarial survival was 16 months (range 0–82 months) for all patients [37]. Method of resection (LDP vs ODP) did not affect overall survival on multivariate analysis in that study, leading the authors to conclude that LDP is an acceptable approach for resection of pancreatic ductal adenocarcinoma (PDAC) of the left pancreas in selected patients [37]. Smaller series have described median

Table 23.1 Summary of selected laparoscopic and open distal pancreatectomy in the literature.

Author (year)	Conversion rate (%)	No. of patients		Mean blood loss (mL)		Mean length of stay (days)		Postoperative morbidity rate (%)		Pancreatic fistula rate (%)		Mortality (%)		Tumor Size (cm)		Malignant Histology (%)		Positive Margins (%)****		Mean nodes procured (range)		Median Follow-up (months)		Recurrence ***** (%)	
		LDP	ODP	LDP	ODP	LDP	ODP	LDP	ODP	LDP	ODP	LDP	ODP	LDP	ODP	LDP	ODP	LDP	ODP	LDP	ODP	LDP	ODP	LDP	ODP
Velanovich (2006) [32]	20	15	15	NR	NR	5*	8*	20	27	13	13	0	0	NR	NR	20	32	NR	NR	NR	NR	NR	NR	0	0
Eom et al. (2008) [34]	NR	31	62	NR	NR	11.5	13.5	36	24	9.7	6.5	0	0	3.95	6.15	9.7	6.5	NR	NR	NR	NR	17.3	46.8	0	1.6
Kooby et al. (2008) [30]	13	142	200	357	588	5.9	9	40	57	11	18	0	1	3.2	3.3	36	49	8	7	NR	NR	NR	NR	NR	NR
Finan et al. (2009) [35]	12	44	98	157	719	5.9	8.6	NR	NR	50	46	0	4.8	3.3	7.7	25	42.3	0	0	9.4	5.2	NR	NR	NR	NR
Baker et al. (2009) [36]	3.6	27	85	219	612	4	8	37	35.1	22	14	0	2	3.78	4.03	29	30.1	NR	NR	6	7	NR	NR	NR	NR
Jayaraman et al. (2010) [8]	30	107	236	175*	300*	5*	6*	26	33	15	13	0	0.8	3	3	17	47	3	4	6	7	NR	NR	NR	NR
Kooby et al. (2010) [37]	17	212	189	422	790	7.4	10.7	NR	NR	NR	NR	0	0.9	3.6	3.5	100	100	27	26	14	12.3	10	10	NR	NR
Vijan et al. (2010) [38]	4	100	100	171	519	6.1	8.6	34	29	17	17	0	1	3.3	4	23	23	0	0	NR	NR	NR	NR	NR	NR
DiNorcia et al. (2010) [19]	25.3	71	168	150*	900*	5	6	28.2	43.8	11.3	14.1	0	1	2.5	3.6	12.7	38.5	2.8	13	6	8	NR	NR	NR	NR
Abu Hilal et al. (2011) [39]	0	35	16	200*	394*	7*	11*	40	69	29	44	0	6.3	3.3	3.4	19	11	25	33	NR	NR	NR	NR	NR	NR
Limongelli et al. (2012) [40]	6	16	29	160	365	6.4	8.8	25	41	18	20	0	3	3.2	4.3	36	45	6	7	NR	NR	NR	NR	NR	NR
Mehta et al. (2012) [33]	NR	30	30	294	726	8.7	12.6	50	43.3	16.7	13.3	0	3.3	3.8	4.3	23.3	23.3	NR	NR	8.4	13.8	NR	NR	NR	NR
Totals		830	1228																						
Means	13.09			254.29	617.00	6.77	9.53	33.62	40.22	19.34	19.90	0.00	2.01	3.36	4.30	29.23	37.31	8.98	11.25	8.76	9.26	13.65	28.40	0.00	0.80

LDP, laparoscopic distal pancreatectomy; ODP, open distal pancreatectomy; NR, not reported.

*, median reported.

****, median reported malignancy.

survival of 14–19 months for adenocarcinoma after LDP [44,45].

23.3 Pancreatic enucleation

Laparoscopic pancreatic enucleations (Lap EN) involve removal of a lesion from the surrounding pancreatic parenchyma without formal pancreatic gland resection (Figure 23.4).

First described by Amikura *et al.* in 1995, Lap EN is typically performed for small, benign tumors or those exhibiting low-grade malignant behavior [46]. These procedures do not require dissection of the major abdominal vasculature or the creation of surgical anastomoses. Literature on Lap EN is confined to case reports, small series, and a few retrospective reviews [44,45,47–49]. While Lap EN is associated with low mortality, this procedure has high morbidity and relatively high incidence of POPF.

As with formal laparoscopic pancreatic resections, patient selection for Lap EN is critical to performing the procedure safely. The literature suggests that the Lap EN approach is best suited for patients with well-localized, small (<4 cm in diameter), benign-appearing lesions on the anterior surface of the pancreas, located at least 2–3 mm away from the main pancreatic duct [50]. The latter point is important to avoid iatrogenic injury to the duct during surgery and subsequent pancreatic leak. Intraoperative ultrasound is a useful adjunct for tumor characterization and localization in this procedure [50]. The procedure is most commonly used to treat insulinomas; other pathology includes nonfunctioning pancreatic neuroendocrine tumors, serous and mucinous cystadenomas, solid pseudopapillary tumors, and intraductal papillary mucinous neoplasms (IPMNs) [51].

Owing to heterogeneity in the literature, operative and postoperative parameters vary widely. Operating room (OR) times range from 50 to 405 minutes, conversion rates to open are 0–75%, and POPF incidences 0–78% [52]. Costi *et al.* retrospectively examined 29 Lap EN cases performed during a 15-year period at a single institution, stratifying procedures as *simple* (enucleation without any other accompanying surgery) or *complex* (associated with major accompanying procedure) [49]. In the *simple* cohort (22 patients), mean operating time was 144 minutes, average blood loss 112 mL, conversion rate 9%. Overall morbidity was 63%; eight patients (36%) developed POPF and mortality was 0% [49]. The high morbidity and rate of POPF, even in *simple* Lap EN as defined by Costi, are echoed in other published reports with less homogeneity of analysis.

(a)   (b)

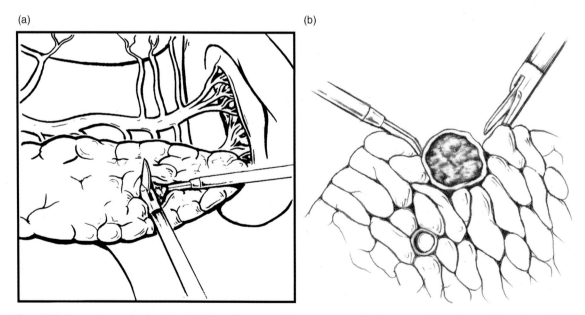

Figure 23.4 Pancreatic enucleation. Panel (a) shows laparoscopic instruments enucleating a tumor from the anterior surface of the pancreatic tail. Panel (b) demonstrates how the tumor is away from the main pancreatic duct.

Fernandez-Cruz *et al.* reported a 35% incidence of POPF in Lap EN compared with both spleen-preserving LDP (7.7%) and LDP with splenectomy (10%) [45]. Other series report morbidity and POPF of 17–42% and 13–35%, respectively, but these studies are hindered by various definitions of POPF and use of the Clavien–Dindo classification of morbidity [44,45,48,53]. Furthermore, drain placement, use of somatostatin analogues, and postoperative imaging varies as well, indicating that morbidity and fistula rates may be underreported in these studies.

With regard to oncological parameters and long-term outcomes, Lap EN data are sparse. Crippa *et al.* suggested lymph node sampling during Lap EN procedures with conversion to pancreatectomy if nodal involvement is confirmed at the time of surgery [51]. Other authors have endorsed traditional resection over Lap EN for any neuroendocrine pathology other than insulinoma [54]. In the Costi series, nine patients had malignant pathology at the time of operation and the authors followed patients for an average of 81 months. There was no local recurrence in any of the patients with malignant pathology, but the authors found three patients (33%) with regional recurrence of malignancy in the follow-up period [49]. Lap EN appears safe and feasible for well-selected benign tumors, but the literature supports more formal surgical approaches for larger benign disease and frank malignancy.

23.4 Laparoscopic pancreaticoduodenectomy

Laparoscopic pancreaticoduodenectomy (LPD) was first described in 1994 by Gagner and Pomp in an advanced laparoscopic surgical trial to reduce postoperative morbidity [55]. This was followed by a series of 10 patients three years later that demonstrated a high conversion rate (40%) and long operating time (510 min) [56]. The complicated procedure demands careful dissection near the portal vein confluence during resection and then creation of three reconstructive anastomoses (biliary, intestinal, pancreatic) requiring laparoscopic suturing. In the nearly 20 years since it was introduced, a handful of case reports and retrospective series from high-volume institutions have been published on LPD, showing it to be both safe and feasible [56–61]. Some surgeons have reported favorable operative outcomes of LPD over OPD, but selection and reporting bias are possible confounding factors to be considered [57,62,63]. In the

literature, oncological parameters, including margin status and nodal retrieval, are similar between LPD and OPD in comparison series, but again selection bias appears towards small, right-sided malignancies in the laparoscopic cohorts [64].

Given the technical challenges of LPD, stringent patient selection guidelines have been followed by surgeons conducting the operation. Nonobese patients are more amenable to laparoscopic resection as the presence of excessive adiposity in the omentum makes the procedure more difficult. The following selection parameters are typically adhered to for eligible patients:

- pancreatic head tumors <3 cm in diameter without evidence of vascular invasion
- well-differentiated or moderate-grade ampullary tumors restricted to the second part of the duodenum
- lower common bile duct tumors without extrabiliary involvement [57].

Preoperative imaging using helical computed tomography (CT) or endoscopic ultrasound (US) is a useful adjunct to carefully defining tumor extension. The technical details of LPD have been given previously in the literature [55,57,58]. While no standard procedure exists, some centers favor a hand-assist approach for reconstruction while others undertake the procedure completely laparoscopically (Figure 23.5) [57,65].

Conversions to the open approach are typically for tumor adhesion to the portal vein, uncontrolled bleeding, and failure to progress [58,64]. While earlier series showed a preference for resection of benign disease, recent publications demonstrate that more malignant cases are selected, however carefully, for laparoscopic resection. With regard to malignancy, some authors prefer resecting ampullary adenocarcinoma laparoscopically because of its further distance from the SMA and SMV while other centers have selected pancreatic adenocarcinoma for resection with adequate margin status [4,29,57,59].

While the last four years have seen a rise in the number of published analyses of LPD, to date only seven papers feature 25 or more patients [57–59,64,66–68]. Average mean operating time is 440 minutes. Kim *et al.* noted a stepwise decrease in their median operative time with greater surgeon experience. Compared with their first 30 cases, where median operative time was 588 minutes, subsequent breakdown of an additional 70 cases showed OR time decreased to 474 and then 396 minutes [67].

Along with decreased operative times, published conversion rates in high-volume series have seen a decline,

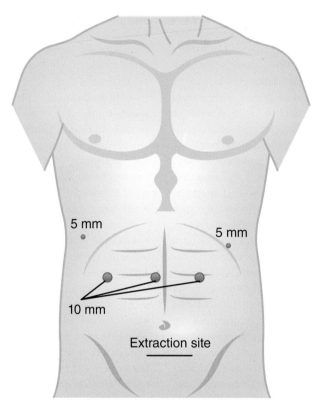

Figure 23.5 Typical port positions for LPD. Source: Kim *et al.* [67]. Reproduced with permission of Springer.

from 40% reported by Gagner *et al.* down to an average of 6.8% in the last three years [29,63,64,67,68]. Several centers are reporting 0% conversions [59,66,68]. Similar trends are evident in estimated blood loss, mean length of hospital stay, and morbidity, all likely attributable to greater surgeon proficiency and refined technique (Figure 23.6). Complication rate for LDP varies from 0 to as high as 60%. Incidence of pancreatic fistula, regardless of definition used, also has a wide range of 0–36% [59,64,66,67,69]. Mortality is low in LPD, with most series reporting 0–3 total deaths in the perioperative period (Table 23.2).

A few studies have directly compared LPD with the open procedure [4,60,64,69]. Chalikonda *et al.* noted similar morbidity (30% vs 44%, P = 0.14) in an analysis of 30 cases of minimally invasive LPD compared with open PD [69]. The minimally invasive cohort had decreased length of stay (9.79 days vs 13.26 days, P = 0.043) and a longer operating time (476.2 min vs 366.4 min P = 0.0005) as well [69]. Pugliese *et al.* found no significant differences in morbidity (45% in LPD vs

44% in OPD), incidence of POPF (27% for both LPD and OPD) or hospital length of stay (18 days in LPD vs 18 days in OPD) in a comparison of 13 LPD with 41 open cases [60]. Cho retrospectively compared 15 LPD and 15 OPD and found no statistically significant differences in morbidity (27% vs 26%), blood loss (445 ± 384 mL vs 552 ± 336 mL), or hospital stay (16.4 ± 3.7 days vs 15.6 ± 1.3 days) [4]. Kendrick reported decreased blood loss (400 vs 600 mL, P < 0.001) and hospital length of stay (6 vs 10 days, P < 0.001) in his center's comparison series of 52 LPD and 129 OPD [68]. Asbun *et al.* compared 53 LPD vs 215 OPD over a six-year period at the Mayo Clinic Florida which demonstrated a significant decrease in EBL (195 vs 1032 mL, P < 0.001), transfusion requirement (0.6 vs 4.7 units, P < 0.001), intensive care unit (ICU) stay (1 vs 3 days, P < 0.001) and hospital length of stay (8 vs 12.4 days, P < 0.001) in the LPD cohort [64]. Morbidity rates were equal (24.5% vs 24.7%) as well as the proportion of clinically significant (grade B/C) fistula (11% vs 15.3%) [64]. These are all unmatched,

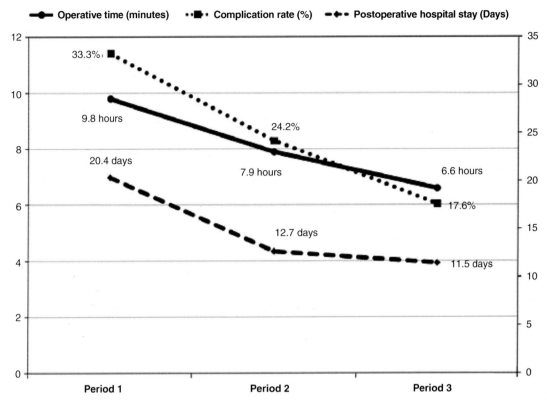

Figure 23.6 Decreased OR time, hospital stay, and morbidity with increased surgeon experience [67].

retrospective studies with relatively small sample sizes but they demonstrate a trend toward beneficial perioperative outcomes for LPD in well-selected patients.

With regard to oncological considerations, there is a greater proportion of malignant cases in the LPD literature than in other laparoscopic pancreatic publications. Of the papers reporting tumor size, the average is 2.6 cm which corresponds to the trend of selecting small, circumscribed lesions for laparoscopic resection [57–59,64]. Mean nodal retrieval is 17, with ranges of 3–34 procured, and authors have achieved R0 margins in over 97% of LPD resections of malignancy. Kendrick reported equivocal outcomes for tumor size (3.2 vs 3.4 cm), margin-negative resection (83% vs 83%), and number of lymph nodes harvested (17 vs 18) in a recent analysis of 52 laparoscopic resections of PDAC compared with 129 open resections of the same pathology [68]. In their comparison of LPD vs OPD at the Mayo Clinic Florida, Asbun *et al.* reported superior nodal retrieval in the LPD cohort (23.44 vs 16.84 nodes, $P < 0.001$). This translated to lower lymph node ratio for those patients with node-positive disease undergoing the laparoscopic approach (0.159 vs 0.241, $P = 0.0072$). Furthermore, they achieved R0 margins in 94.9% of laparoscopic cases versus only 83% in the open cohort, although this difference was not statistically significant [64].

Substantial long-term oncological outcomes for LPD are not readily available owing to the paucity of literature published to date. Median follow-up is 17 months and, for papers reporting recurrences rates, these average 17.5% (range 7.5–38%) [57,58,60,67]. In their first series, Palanivelu *et al.* showed median survival of 49 months with a five-year actuarial survival rate of 32% among the 40 patients with malignancy [57]. However, there was selection bias for early malignant lesions to be resected laparoscopically. Additional data on long-term survival will likely come with further patient surveillance.

This review demonstrates that LPD is a safe, feasible, and noninferior approach to resection of right-sided pancreatic lesions, both benign and malignant, in well-selected patients at high-volume centers. Randomized

Table 23.2 Summary of laparoscopic pancreaticoduodenectomy in the literature

Author (year)	No. of patients	Benign	Malignant	Pathology	Conversion Rate (%)	Hand assist (%)	Mean operative time (min)	Mean blood loss (mL)	Mean Length of Stay (days)	Postoperative Morbidity rate (%)	Pancreatic Fistula rate (%)	Mortality (%)	Tumor Size (cm)****	Mean nodes procured (range)	Positive Margins (%)****	Median Follow-up (months)	Recurrence**** (%)
Gagner et al. (1997) [56]	10	2	8	4 PDAC, 3 AMP, 2 pancreatitis, 1 cholangiocarcinoma	40	33	510	NR	22.3	50	17	0	NR	7 (3–14)	0	19	NR
Staudacher et al. (2005) [65]	7	2	2	2 PNET, 1 PDAC, 1 MM, 3 not recorded	43	100	416	325	12	0	0	0	NR	26 (16–47)	0	4.5	NR
Lu et al. (2006) [61]	5	0	5	4 duodenal adenocarcinoma, 1 PNET	0	0	528	770	NR	60	20	20	NR	NR	NR	NR	NR
Dulucq et al. (2006) [58]	25	3	19	11 PDAC, 4 AMP, 2 DA, 1 PNET, 2 CP, 1 RCC, 1 SCA	12	41	287	107	16.2	32	4.5	4.5	2	18 (––)	0	19.2	11
Palanivelu et al. (2007) [57]	42	2	40	24 AMP, 9 PDAC, 4MCA, 3 CC 2 pancreatitis	0	0	370	65	10.2	NR	7.1	2.4	2.9	13 (18–21)	0	36.5	7.5
Pugliese et al. (2008) [60]	19	1	18	11 PDAC, 4 AMP, 3 CC, 1 mesenchymal tumor	32	54	461	180	18	37	23	0	2.5	12 (4–22)	0	32	33
Cho et al. (2009) [4]	15	7	8	6 mucinous adenoma, 3 MCA, 2 PNET, 1 AMP, 1 PDAC, 1 duodenal plasmacytoma, 1 pancreatic trauma	0	100	338	445	16.4	27	13	0	NR	18.5 (––)	0	NR	NR
Palanivelu et al. (2009) [66]	75	3	72	29 AMP, 23 PDAC, 10MCA, 10 CC, 3 CP	0	0	357	74	8.2	26	7	1.33	NR	14 (8–22)	2.6	NR	NR
Asbun et al. (2012) [64]	53	14	39	22 PDAC, 8 IPMN, 6 PNET, 8 AMP, 2 SCA, 3 CC, 1 solid pseudopapillary neoplasm, 1 GIST, 2 CP	15	5.6	541	195	8	45.3	16.7	5.7	2.7	23 (––)	5.1	3.33	NR
Kendrick and Cusati (2010) [59]	65	19	46	32 PDAC, 12 IPMN, 8 AMP, 4 NET, 3 CP, 1 CC, 1 RCC, 1 cystadenoma, 1 duodenal adenoma	4.6	0	368*	240*	7*	42	18	1.6	3	15 (6–31)*	11	7.2	16

Study				Tumor type													
Suzuki et al. (2011)[70]	6	1	5	4 AMP, 1 PDAC, 1 IPMN	0	100	581*	471*	23*	33.3	33.3	0	NR	18 (16–27)*	0	36	NR
Ammori and Ayiomamitis (2011)[29]	7	0	7	5 PDAC, 2 AMP	0***	14.3	628	350	11.11	28.6	28.6	0	NR	20.8 (11–32)**	NR	5	NR
Zureikat et al. (2011)[71]	14	2	12	8 PDAC, 2 CC, 1 duodenal adenocarcinoma, 1 GIST, 1 IPMN, 1 CP	14	0	456*	300*	8*	62	36	7.1	2.2	18.5 (–)	0	9.5	8.3
Kendrick (2012)[68]	52	0	52	52 PDAC	0	0	370	400	6	NR	NR	NR	3.2	17	17	24	38
Kim et al. (2013)[67]	100	88	12	37 IPMN, 17 solid pseudopapillary tumors, 15 PNET, 7 SCA, 7 PDAC, 2 MCA, 5 AMP, 5 duodenal GIST, 1 CP, 1 RCC, 1 CC, 2 benign cyst	4.7*****	0	474	NR	15	25	6	1	2.8	13 (7–34)	0	10.2	9.1
Totals	495	142	343														
Means	24.5	10.1			12.4	29.9	440.0	291.1	13.0	36.0	16.4	3.1	2.7	17	2.7	17.2	17.6

AMP, ampullary adenocarcinoma; CC, cholangiocarcinoma; CP, chronic pancreatitis; DA, duodenal adenocarcinoma; GIST, gastrointestinal stromal tumor; IPMN, intraductal papillary mucinous neoplasm; MCA, mucinous cystadenoma; MM, malignant melanoma; NET, neuroendocrine tumor; PDAC, pancreatic ductal adenocarcinoma; PNET, pancreatic neuroendocrine tumor; RCC, renal cell carcinoma; SCA, serous cystadenoma.

trials of LPD and open procedures are necessary to strengthen the assessments that can be made when comparing the two groups. With further experience and more follow-up data on long-term patient outcomes, LPD can be better utilized for malignancy.

23.5 Conclusion

Through improved technology and growing experience, laparoscopic pancreatic resections are being performed more commonly. Laparoscopic distal pancreatectomy is suited best for patients with contained tumors in the body and tail of the pancreas, and it appears to provide similar outcomes to open resection, with fewer complications, lower blood loss, and shorter hospital stays for cases of similar difficulty. Laparoscopic enucleations are less commonly performed but have a role in the management of indolent small tumors away from the main pancreatic duct. The paucity of cases means that randomized evaluation of the laparoscopic approach and the open approach is not feasible. Experience with laparoscopic pancreaticoduodenectomy is growing, but more data are necessary to prove the value of this approach against the open procedure.

KEY POINTS

- Distal pancreatectomy can provide comparable oncological outcomes with fewer complications, lower blood loss, and shorter hospital stay when compared with open surgery.

- Laparoscopic enucleation has an important role in the management of indolent small tumors not involving or approaching the main pancreatic duct.

- Outcomes of laparoscopic versus open pancreas surgery are difficult to assess because of differences in technique, perioperative chemotherapy and chemoradiation, patient selection, surgeon and patient bias, and availability of experienced laparoscopic surgeons.

- Laparoscopic pancreaticoduodenectomy is still in the developmental phase and practiced by a limited number of surgeons in selected centers.

References

1 Litynski G. Erich Mühe and the rejection of laparoscopic cholecystectomy (1985): a surgeon ahead of his time. J Soc Laparoendosc Surg 1998; 2:341–346.

2 Tiwari MM, Reynoso JF, High R, Tsang AW, Oleynikov D. Safety, efficacy, and cost-effectiveness of common laparoscopic procedures. Surg Endosc 2011; 25(4):1127–1135.

3 Hartley JE, Mehigan BJ, Monson JR. Alterations in the immune system and tumor growth in laparoscopy. Surg Endosc 2001; 15(3):305–313.

4 Cho A, Yamamoto H, Nagata M, et al. Comparison of laparoscopy-assisted and open pylorus-preserving pancreaticoduodenectomy for periampullary disease. Am J Surg 2009; 198 (3):445–449.

5 Kudsi OY, Gagner M, Jones DB. Laparoscopic distal pancreatectomy. Surg Oncol Clin North Am 2013; 22(1): 59–73.

6 Borja-Cacho D, Al-Refaie WB, Vickers SM, Tuttle TM, Jensen EH. Laparoscopic distal pancreatectomy. J Am Coll Surg 2009; 209(6):758–765; quiz 800.

7 Kneuertz PJ, Patel S, Chu C, et al. Laparoscopic distal pancreatectomy: trends and lessons learned through an 11-year experience. J Am Coll Surg 2012; 215(2):167–176.

8 Jayaraman S, Gonen M, Brennan MF, et al. Laparoscopic distal pancreatectomy: evolution of a technique at a single institution. J Am Coll Surg 2010; 211(4):503–509.

9 Shatz DV, Schinsky M, Pais LB, et al. Immune responses of splenectomized trauma patients to the 23-valent pneumococcal polysaccharide vaccine at 1 versus 7 versus 14 days after splenectomy. J Trauma 1998; 44(5):760–765.

10 Fisichella PM, Shankaran V, Shoup M. Laparoscopic distal pancreatectomy with or without splenectomy: how i do it. J Gastrointest Surg 2011; 1(15):215–218.

11 Robinson S, Saif R, Charnley RM, French JJ, White SA. Surgical adjuncts to laparoscopic distal pancreatectomy. MITAT 2011; 20(6):369–373.

12 Kang CM, Kim DH, Lee WJ. Ten years of experience with resection of left-sided pancreatic ductal adenocarcinoma: evolution and initial experience to a laparoscopic approach. Surg Endosc 2010; 24(7):1533–1541.

13 Kooby DA. Laparoscopic pancreatic resection for cancer. Expert Rev Anticancer Ther 2008; 8(10):1597–1609.

14 Warshaw AL. Conservation of the spleen with distal pancreatectomy. Arch Surg 1988; 123(5):550–553.

15 Fernandez-Cruz L, Blanco L, Cosa R, Rendón H. Is laparoscopic resection adequate in patients with neuroendocrine pancreatic tumors? World J Surg 2008; 32(5):904–917.

16 Jean-Philippe A, Jacquin A, Laurent C, *et al.* Laparoscopic spleen-preserving distal pancreatectomy: splenic vessel preservation compared with the Warshaw technique. JAMA Surg 2013; 148(3):246–252.

17 Song KB, Kim SC, Park JB, *et al.* Single-center experience of laparoscopic left pancreatic resection in 359 consecutive patients: changing the surgical paradigm of left pancreatic resection. Surg Endosc 2011; 25(10):3364–3372.

18 Butturini G, Partelli S, Crippa S, *et al.* Perioperative and long-term results after left pancreatectomy: a single-institution, non-randomized, comparative study bettween open and laparoscopic approach. Surg Endosc 2011; 25:2871–2878.

19 DiNorcia J, Schrope BA, Lee MK, *et al.* Laparoscopic distal pancreatectomy offers shorter hospital stays with fewer complications. J Gastrointest Surg 2010; 14(11):1804–1812.

20 Thaker RI, Matthews BD, Linehan DC, *et al.* Absorbable mesh reinforcement of a stapled pancreatic transection line reduces the leak rate with distal pancreatectomy. J Gastrointest Surg 2007; 11(1):59–65.

21 Jensen EH, Portschy PR, Chowaniec J, Teng M. Meta-analysis of bioabsorbable staple line reinforcement and risk of fistula following pancreatic resection. J Gastrointest Surg 2013; 17(2):267–272.

22 Subhedar PD, Patel SH, Kneuertz PJ, *et al.* Risk factors for pancreatic fistula after stapled gland transection. Am Surg 2011; 77(8):965–970.

23 Rostas JW, Richards W, Thompson LW. Improved rate of pancreatic fistual after distal pancreatectomy: parenchymal division with the use of saline-coupled radiofrequency ablation. HPB (Oxford) 2012; 14 (Aug):560–564.

24 Venkat R, Edil B, Schulick RD, *et al.* Laparoscopic distal pancreatectomy is associated with significantly less overall morbidity compared to the open technique: a systematic review and meta-analysis. Ann Surg 2012; 255 (Jun):1048–1059.

25 Nigri GR, Rosman AS, Petrucciani N, *et al.* Metaanalysis of trials comparing minimally invasive and open distal pancreatectomies. Surg Endosc 2011; 25(5):1642–1651.

26 Jin T, Altaf K, Xiong JJ, *et al.* A systematic review and meta-analysis of studies comparing laparoscopic and open distal pancreatectomy. HPB (Oxford) 2012; 14(11):711–724.

27 Nakamura M, Nakashima H. Laparoscopic distal pancreatectomy and pancreatoduodenectomy: is it worthwhile? J Hepatobiliary Pancreat Sci 2013; 20 (Apr):421–428.

28 Jusoh AC, Ammori BJ. Laparoscopic versus open distal pancreatectomy: a systematic review of comparative studies. Surg Endosc 2012; 26(4):904–913.

29 Ammori BJ, Ayiomamitis G. Laparoscopic pancreaticoduodenectomy and distal pancreatectomy: a UK experience and a systematic review of the literature. Surg Endosc 2011; 25(7):2084–2099.

30 Kooby DA, Gillespie T, Bentrem D, *et al.* Left-sided pancreatectomy: a multicenter comparison of laparoscopic and open approaches. Ann Surg 2008; 248(3):438–446.

31 Sui CJ, Li B, Yang JM, Wang SJ, Zhou YM. Laparoscopic versus open distal pancreatectomy: a meta-analysis. Asian J Surg 2012; 35(1):1–8.

32 Velanovich V. Case–control comparison of laparoscopic versus open distal pancreatectomy. J Gastrointest Surg 2006; 10 (1):95–98.

33 Mehta SS, Doumane G, Mura T, Nocca D, Fabre JM. Laparoscopic versus open distal pancreatectomy: a single-institution case–control study. Surg Endosc 2012; 26(2):402–407.

34 Eom BW, Jang JY, Lee SE, *et al.* Clinical outcomes compared between laparoscopic and open distal pancreatectomy. Surg Endosc 2008; 22(5):1334–1338.

35 Finan KR, Cannon EE, Kim EJ, *et al.* Laparoscopic and open distal pancreatectomy: a comparison of outcomes. Am Surg 2009; 75(8):671–679; discussion 679–680.

36 Baker MS, Bentrem DJ, Ujiki MB, Stocker S, Talamonti MS. A prospective single institution comparison of peri-operative outcomes for laparoscopic and open distal pancreatectomy. Surgery 2009; 146(4):635–643; discussion 643–645.

37 Kooby DA, Hawkins WG, Schmidt CM, *et al.* A multicenter analysis of distal pancreatectomy for adenocarcinoma: is laparoscopic resection appropriate? J Am Coll Surg 2010; 210(5):779–785, 786–787.

38 Vijan SS, Ahmed KA, Harmsen WS, *et al.* Laparoscopic vs open distal pancreatectomy: a single-institution comparative study. Arch Surg 2010; 145(7):616–621.

39 Abu Hilal M, Hamdan M, di Fabio F, *et al.* Laparoscopic versus open distal pancreatectomy: a clinical and cost-effectiveness study. Surg Endosc 2012; 26(6):1670–1674.

40 Limongelli P, Belli A, Russo G, *et al.* Laparoscopic and open surgical treatment of left-sided pancreatic lesions: clinical outcomes and cost-effectiveness analysis. Surg Endosc 2012; 26(7):1830–1836.

41 Bassi C, Dervenis C, Butturini G, *et al.* Postoperative pancreatic fistula: an international study group (ISGPF) definition. Surgery 2005; 138(1):8–13.

42 Weber SM, Cho CS, Merchant N, *et al.* Laparoscopic left pancreatectomy: complication risk score correlates with morbidity and risk for pancreatic fistula. Ann Surg Oncol 2009; 16 (10):2825–2833.

43 Waters JA, Canal DF, Wiebke EA, *et al.* Robotic distal pancreatectomy: cost effective? Surgery 2010; 148(4):814–823.

44 Marangos IP, Buanes T, Røsok BI, *et al.* Laparoscopic resection of exocrine carcinoma in central and distal pancreas results in a high rate of radical resections and long postoperative survival. Surgery 2012; 151(5):717–723.

45 Fernandez-Cruz L, Cosa R, Blanco L, *et al.* Curative laparoscopic resection for pancreatic neoplasms: a critical analysis from a single institution. J Gastrointest Surg 2007; 11(12): 1607–1621; discussion 1621–1622.

46 Amikura K, Alexandar HR, Norton JA, *et al.* Role of surgery in management of adrenocorticotropic hormone-producing islet cell tumors of the pancreas. Surgery 1995; 118(6): 1125–1130.

47 Ayav A, Bresler L, Brunaud L, *et al.* Laparoscopic approach for solitary insulinoma: a multicentre study. Langenbeck's Arch Surg 2005; 390(2):134–140.

48 Dedieu A, Rault A, Collet D, Masson B, Sa Cunha A. Laparoscopic enucleation of pancreatic neoplasm. Surg Endosc 2011; 25(2):572–576.

49 Costi R, Randone B, Mal F, *et al*. Laparoscopic minor pancreatic resections (enucleations/atypical resections). A long-term appraisal of a supposed mini-invasive approach. Wideochir Inne Tech Malo Inwazyjne 2013; 8(2):117–129.

50 Zhang T, Du X, Zhao Y. Laparoscopic surgery for pancreatic lesions: current status and future. Front Med 2011; 5(3):277–282.

51 Crippa S, Boninsegna L, Partelli S, Falconi M. Parenchyma-sparing resections for pancreatic neoplasms. J Hepato-Biliary-Pancreat Sci 2010; 17(6):782–787.

52 Sweet MP, Izumisato Y, Way LW, *et al*. Laparoscopic enucleation of insulinomas. Arch Surg 2007; 142(12):1202–1204; discussion 1205.

53 Mabrut JY, Fernandez-Cruz L, Azagra JS, *et al*. Laparoscopic pancreatic resection: results of a multicenter European study of 127 patients. Surgery 2005; 137(6):597–605.

54 Burns WR, Edil BH. Neuroendocrine pancreatic tumors: guidelines for management and update. Curr Treat Options Oncol 2012; 13(1):24–34.

55 Gagner M, Pomp A. Laparoscopic pylorus-preserving pancreatoduodenectomy. Surg Endosc 1994; 8(5):408–410.

56 Gagner M, Pomp A. Laparoscopic pancreatic resection: is it worthwhile? J Gastrointest Surg 1997; 1(1):20–25; discussion 25–26.

57 Palanivelu C, Jani K, Senthilnathan P, *et al*. Laparoscopic pancreaticoduodenectomy: technique and outcomes. J Am Coll Surg 2007; 205(2):222–230.

58 Dulucq JL, Wintringer P, Mahajna A. Laparoscopic pancreaticoduodenectomy for benign and malignant diseases. Surg Endosc 2006; 20(7):1045–1050.

59 Kendrick ML, Cusati D. Total laparoscopic pancreaticoduodenectomy: feasibility and outcome in an early experience. Arch Surg 2010; 145(1):19–23.

60 Pugliese R, Scandroglio I, Sansonna F, *et al*. Laparoscopic pancreaticoduodenectomy: a retrospective review of 19 cases. Surg Laparosc Endosc Percutan Techn 2008; 18(1):13–18.

61 Lu B, Cai X, Lu W, Huang Y, Jin X. Laparoscopic pancreaticoduodenectomy to treat cancer of the ampulla of Vater. J Soc Laparoendosc Surg 2006; 10(1):97–100.

62 Dulucq JL, Wintriger P, Stabilini C, *et al*. Are major laparoscopic pancreatic resections worthwhile? A prospective study of 32 patients in a single institution. Surg Endosc 2005; 19(8):1028–1034.

63 Zureikat AH, Breaux J, Steel J, Hughes S. Can laparoscopic pancreaticoduodenectomy be safely implemented? J Gastrointest Surg 2011; 15(7):1151–1157.

64 Asbun HJ, Stauffer J. Laparoscopic vs open pancreaticoduodenectomy: overall outcomes and severity of complications using the Accordion Severity Grading System. J Am Coll Surg 2012; 215(6):810–819.

65 Staudacher C, Orsenigo E, Baccari P, di Palo S, Crippa S. Laparoscopic assisted duodenopancreatectomy. Surg Endosc 2005; 19(3):352–356.

66 Palanivelu C, Rajan PS, Rangarajan M, *et al*. Evolution in techniques of laparoscopic pancreaticoduodenectomy: a decade long experience from a tertiary center. J Hepatobiliary Pancreat Surg 2009; 16(6):731–740.

67 Kim SC, Song K, Jung YS, *et al*. Short-term clinical outcomes for 100 consecutive cases of laparoscopic pylorus-preserving pancreatoduodenectomy: improvement with surgical experience. Surg Endosc 2013; 27(1):95–103.

68 Kendrick ML. Laparoscopic and robotic resection for pancreatic cancer. Cancer 2012; 18(Nov–Dec):571–576. *et al*.

69 Chalikonda S, Aguilar-Saavedra JR, Walsh RM. Laparoscopic robotic-assisted pancreaticoduodenectomy: a case-matched comparison with open resection. Surg Endosc 2012; 26(9):2397–2402.

70 Suzuki O, Kondo S, Hirano S, *et al*. Laparoscopic pancreaticoduodenectomy combined with minilaparotomy. Surg Today 2012; 42(5):509–513.

71 Zureikat AH, Nguyen KT, Bartlett DL, Zeh MJ, Moser AJ. Robotic-assisted major pancreatic resection and reconstruction. Arch Surg 2011; 146(3):256–261.

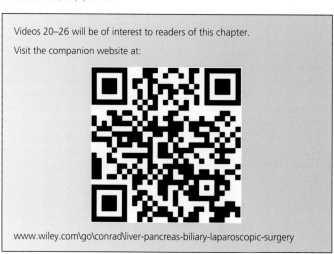

Videos 20–26 will be of interest to readers of this chapter.

Visit the companion website at:

www.wiley.com\go\conrad\liver-pancreas-biliary-laparoscopic-surgery

CHAPTER 24

Indications and contraindications for laparoscopic pancreas surgery

Hanno Niess and Jens Werner

Department of General, Visceral, Transplantation, Vascular and Thoracic Surgery, Hospital of the University of Munich, Munich, Germany

EDITOR COMMENT

It is important to us that we provide a balanced view on the advantages of laparoscopic surgery in this book. This is especially true for laparoscopic pancreas surgery, an approach that is in its developmental stages. For this chapter we have elicited the opinion of experts to provide a critical discussion of the advantages and short-comings of laparoscopic pancreas surgery. The lack of randomized and prospective data regarding the advantages of a minimally invasive approach over an open one, as well as some of the technical challenges of laparoscopic pancreaticoduodenectomy, are highlighted. Nonetheless, the promising available retrospective data on laparoscopic distal pancreatectomy and pancreatic enucleation are discussed. This chapter concludes with an excellent section on the minimally invasive management of pancreatitis, focusing on indications for intervention, timing, and approaches. This balanced and sometimes critical view on minimally invasive pancreas surgery by expert pancreatic surgeons reminds the community of the overall goals of surgery, which is excellence in outcomes.

Keywords: laparoscopic distal pancreatectomy, laparoscopic enucleation, laparoscopic pancreatectomy, laparoscopic pancreatico-duodenectomy, minimally invasive management of pancreatitis

24.1 Introduction

In a number of abdominal operations, minimally invasive approaches have yielded favorable outcomes regarding postoperative pain, blood loss, recovery time, and functional convalescence compared with open surgery. Moreover, the use of laparoscopic surgery, particularly in patients with colon cancer, has shown that the benefits of laparoscopy can be achieved without compromises on oncological outcomes [1].

The benefits of laparoscopic approaches are mainly due to reduced access trauma and minimal mechanical abdominal wall and organ retraction. The laparoscopic approach has therefore become the standard approach for a majority of abdominal surgeries performed today and an important pillar of fast-track programs for colorectal surgery. The downsides of a laparoscopic approach include difficulties in achieving adequate exposure,

resulting in a narrow working space, limited orientation in a three-dimensional space, fewer degrees of freedom with instrumentation as well as decreased haptic feedback. In 2014, at our institution, a minimally invasive approach was selected for surgeries of the colon, rectum, appendix, gallbladder, esophagus, and spleen in 50%, 50%, 86%, 76%, 17%, and 43% of cases, respectively. These case distributions might be reflective of the use of laparoscopy at referral centers with obligations to complex patient care as well as student and resident training.

Gagner and Cuschieri first successfully used minimally invasive approaches for major pancreatic resections in 1994 [2,3]. However, the rapid development of this technique to become the widely accepted standard approach in pancreatic surgery has been limited by several factors, including the pancreas' retroperitoneal location and fragility of the gland, the complexity of the surrounding anatomical structures, the proximity to major blood vessels and the proneness of these procedures to postoperative complications. Laparoscopic surgery in patients with pancreatic diseases was therefore mainly limited to diagnostic or palliative purposes. With the development of novel energy devices such as ultrasound dissectors and staplers, more widespread use of laparoscopic techniques for pancreatic resections occurred. The resulting case series and studies indicate promising results of the minimal invasive approach in selected cases.

The development of laparoscopic pancreas resection mirrors the advancements in laparoscopic colon surgery: in colon surgery, the indications evolved from benign, such as diverticulosis, towards malignant tumors over time. In pancreas surgery, lesions included small endocrine tumors or in some cases cystadenomas located in the distal pancreas, where no reconstruction following resection is needed. With increasing experience with the technique, some surgeons have expanded the indications to small malignant lesions in the pancreas. However, obtaining a negative resection margin and performing adequate lymph node dissection are nonetheless pivotal for oncological

outcome and only sparse data exist indicating equivalence of open and laparoscopic techniques for pancreas surgery. Therefore, most surgeons still do not use laparoscopy for pancreatic surgery or limit the laparoscopic approach to benign and low-grade malignant lesions confined to the pancreas. In our experience, because of the aggressive biology of pancreatic cancer, few patients present with malignant lesions that are eligible for a laparoscopic approach, which makes these indications at our institution relatively rare. This in turn reduces the case volume available to ascend the steep learning curve that exists for these difficult laparoscopic procedures.

Despite the observed overall reduction in the operative morbidity of pancreatic surgery over the last decades, these operations are still associated with a high rate of severe complications and perioperative mortality compared with nonpancreatic procedures. Although the extent of the access trauma (i.e. laparotomy vs laparoscopy) accounts for some of the overall morbidity, in large pancreatic resections the procedural trauma may far exceed the access trauma [4] (Figure 24.3). Proper

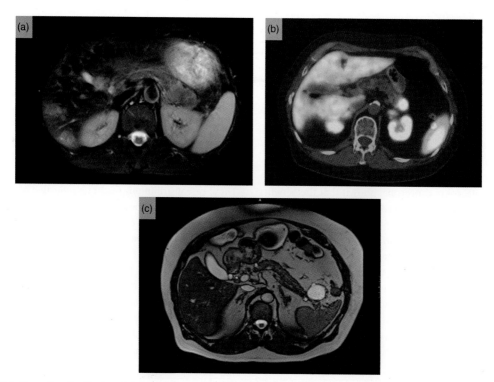

Figure 24.1 Examples of indications for the laparoscopic approach in distal pancreatectomy. Representative MR/DOTA-TATE PET CT images of patients operated on laparoscopically at our institution. Indications were: (a,b) neuroendocrine tumor, (c) mucinous cystic neoplasia.

healing of the anastomoses created during the reconstruction phase of pancreatic resections represents the main determinant of postoperative morbidity and mortality. In cases of ductal adenocarcinoma of the pancreas, overall and disease-free survival rates are positively influenced by adjuvant chemotherapy protocols. Complications in the postoperative course can delay the timely initiation of adjuvant treatment and thus may negatively influence survival rates. In our opinion, anastomoses during pancreatic surgery should be created under optimal conditions, as they are the key determinant for postoperative complications. A completely laparoscopic approach by surgeons with limited laparoscopic experience may potentially impact negatively on the reconstruction as a result of the drawbacks in exposure and lack of haptic feedback as well as the limitations of instruments available today.

When no pancreatic anastomosis has to be created, the benefits of the laparoscopic approach may outweigh these technical challenges even for surgeons with intermediate laparoscopic experience. These procedures include distal pancreatectomy with or without splenectomy, enucleation, and pancreatic necrosectomy.

24.2 Indications, contraindications, and outcomes

24.2.1 Laparoscopic distal pancreatectomy (LDP)

Distal pancreatectomy (DP) is the most commonly performed laparoscopic pancreatic operation. Data from a population-based study in the United States, which analyzed almost 9000 distal pancreatectomies, indicate that the proportion of laparoscopic procedures tripled in the preceding 10 years, to 7.3% of cases in 2009. On a national level, the projected number of LDP was 1908 per year [5]. In Figure 24.2 and Figure 24.3, common indications for the laparoscopic approach as well as important steps of the procedure are shown.

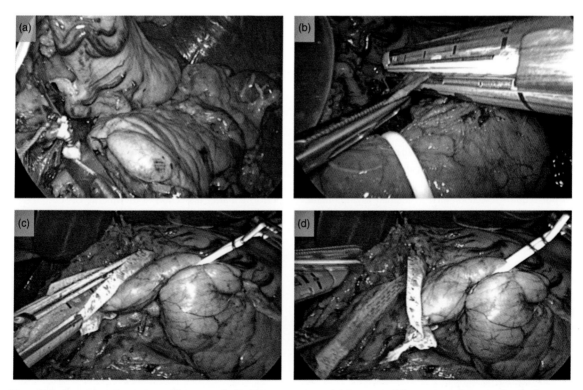

Figure 24.2 Screenshots from stages of laparoscopic distal pancreatectomy. (a) Exposure of the pancreas after accessing the lesser sac. (b) Division of the splenic vein using stapling device. (c,d) Division of the pancreatic parenchyma using Gore Seamguard covered staple line reinforcement.

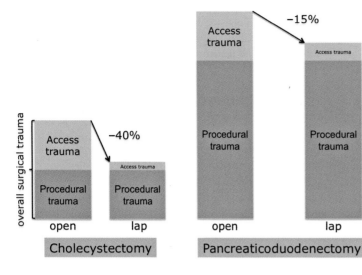

Figure 24.3 Estimated proportion of access trauma in relation overall surgical trauma. When equal procedural traumata, i.e. the actual resection and for PD also the reconstruction phases, are assumed, the proportion of access trauma in relation to overall surgical trauma is much higher for smaller procedures such as cholecystectomy. Hence, it is essential to minimize dissection trauma and postoperative complications in a laparoscopic Whipple procedure to preserve a potential benefit of the minimally invasive approach. If both cannot be ensured, an open approach is safer.

Indications for LDP range from neuroendocrine tumor other than gastrinoma, mucinous cystic neoplasia, large serous cystadenoma, intraductal papillary mucinous neoplasms (IPMNs), chronic pancreatitis, solid pseudopapillary tumors, pancreatic pseudocysts to pancreatic adenocarcinoma, metastasis, or other malignant lesions [6,7]. With the increasing sensitivity of modern abdominal imaging, a higher number of small, asymptomatic benign or premalignant lesions are discovered. For benign to low-grade malignant lesion, performing LDP with preservation of the spleen is an important option. The advantages include prevention of the very rare but potentially life-threatening overwhelming postsplenectomy sepsis with encapsulated bacteria and the reduction in left-sided portal hypertension. Nevertheless, the availability of laparoscopy should not be seen as an indication to resect benign lesions that typically do not require resection, such as a small asymptomatic serous cystadenoma.

Splenic salvage can be achieved by sparing both the splenic vein and the artery, as described by Mallet-Guy and Vachon in 1943 [8]. Alternatively, the Warshaw technique can be performed, in which the splenic vessels are both divided. This results in the spleen being perfused via the short gastric vessels [9]. The question of whether to perform en bloc splenectomy or to salvage the spleen, and if so, by which technique, is a matter of debate. For open distal pancreatic resection, retrospective studies have shown data both supporting and refuting splenic preservation. Some investigators found a lower rate of pancreatic complications such as fistulas or subphrenic abscesses in the splenic resection

group [10]. Others have shown higher rates of postoperative infectious and severe complications in patients who underwent splenic resection [11].

In cases of malignant neoplasms, most surgeons would advocate performing en bloc splenectomy along with distal pancreatectomy in order to achieve a negative retroperitoneal margin and complete lymph node dissection [12]. Some authors, however, describe positive effects of splenic preservation even in cases of pancreatic adenocarcinoma as long as no direct tumor infiltration of the spleen is present [13]. It has been hypothesized that the putative immune surveillance mechanism of the preserved spleen may even improve long-term survival following resection of pancreatic cancer [14]. By using the Warshaw technique for salvage of the spleen, the important extended retroperitoneal lymphadenectomy can be performed after dissection of the splenic vessels.

It remains unclear if splenic function following spleen-preserving distal pancreatectomy can still be considered normal, especially following separation of the splenic vessels. In a large study by Beane et al., the authors concluded that no short-term advantage can be achieved by preserving the spleen using the Warshaw technique rather than splenic resection [15]. Even in LDPs performed with the intention of sparing the splenic vessels, a small retrospective study revealed postoperative occlusion of the splenic artery and vein in 14% and 59% of cases, respectively. This phenomenon occurs at higher frequency with the laparoscopic approach. Thus the authors concluded that laparoscopic instruments used for pancreatic dissection from the splenic vessels and the laparoscopically available methods of hemostasis are a main cause for this high rate of postoperative splenic vein occlusion [16,17]. Thus, further development of laparoscopic instruments and optimization of surgical technique are needed.

So far, no randomized, controlled prospective studies comparing open and laparoscopic distal pancreatectomy have been published. However, more than 20 retrospective comparative studies exist in the literature on this topic to date (Table 24.1). Conclusions from most of these reports, however, are limited by the selection bias involved in these uncontrolled retrospective studies: several of these studies, for example, limit the laparoscopic approach to benign diseases, spleen-preserving procedures or to patients without prior operations. Furthermore, in many studies conversion rates to open procedures are not reported or even excluded from the studies. Numerous studies comparing open distal pancreatectomy (ODP) and LDP differ significantly in baseline characteristics such as lesion size or rate of malignant lesions, with larger and more malignant tumors preferentially operated on via an open approach.

Nigri *et al.* performed a meta-analysis on the first 10 studies on this topic [18]. The results of this analysis indicate a reduction of blood loss, overall complications, shorter time to oral intake and shorter hospital stay in patients who underwent LDP, with no significant differences in operative time. In a more recent meta-analysis from Venkat *et al.* that comprised 18 retrospective studies with over 1800 patients, findings were similar but the analyses were more detailed [19]. In addition to the meta-analysis by Nigri *et al.*, the authors assessed the quality of the included studies and conducted sensitivity and subgroup analyses. The overall findings of the analysis indicate superiority of the laparoscopic approach with respect to lower blood loss, lower overall complication and wound infection rates, and shorter length of hospital stay, while no difference in operating time was noted.

A subgroup meta-analysis was performed on the 10 available studies with matched clinicopathological findings in order to overcome, at least in part, the strong selection bias of these studies. In our opinion, selection bias is the main barrier for drawing final conclusions from these retrospective comparative studies. Nevertheless, LDP in most of these studies has shown less blood loss, faster recovery, and fewer surgical site infections while no difference in overall postoperative complications and even significantly longer operation times for LDP were observed.

To further support evidence for the benefits of LDP, a multicenter study from the Central Pancreas Consortium using matched-pair analysis of age, ASA score, tumor size, resected pancreas length, and diagnosis indicates significantly reduced overall complication rates, reduced blood loss, and shorter hospital stay in the laparoscopic group, while achieving the same negative margin rates [20]. In another retrospective multicenter study from the same group of patients who underwent LDP for ductal adenocarcinoma focusing on oncological outcome, the authors were not able to observe a difference in number of lymph nodes harvested, rate of positive resection margins, or overall survival rates between ODP and LDP. A limitation is, however, that the latter group consisted of 23 patients only [21]. In our opinion, these findings should be confirmed in prospective, multicenter, randomized trials before LDP can be considered an oncologically equivalent alternative to ODP for treatment of pancreatic cancer.

Postoperative pancreatic fistula following DP is one of the most concerning complications. It seems that the risk for pancreatic fistulas is independent of the selected operative approach, as the vast majority of studies report no difference between ODP and LDP in rate or severity of fistulas. Risk factors that are regarded as more relevant for the development of pancreatic fistulas following distal pancreatectomy than the choice of operative approach are surgical technique and a soft gland. Accordingly, the randomized, controlled DISPACT trial, which compared hand-sewn (rarely used in LDP) with stapled closure of the pancreatic remnant, was unable to identify specific risk factors for the development of pancreatic fistula [22].

We believe that obese patients, who are at an increased risk for postoperative atelectasis and pneumonia, may particularly benefit from the smaller access trauma and reduced postoperative pain of LDP. Besides body habitus, other patient factors such as cardiopulmonary comorbidities or a history of previous abdominal operations might make the surgeon decide on the conventional open approach.

Although it has been hypothesized from retrospective data that LDP and ODP may be equally effective in achieving negative margins and optimal oncological outcome in a selected patient group, it is our practice to limit the laparoscopic approach to benign, premalignant, and low-grade malignant lesions, while laparoscopic surgery for malignant disease should be entered in registries or included in randomized controlled trials (RCTs). In particular, laparoscopic resection of locally advanced

Table **24.1** Comparative series of laparoscopic distal pancreatectomies with >50 patients.

Reference	LDP/ODP	OR time (min)	Blood loss (mL)	Mortality	Morbidity	Pancreatic fistula	Tumor size (cm)	% malignancy	Conversion rate	Lymph node harvest
Cho [31]	254 lap	NS	>300 cc: 24%	0.5%	12%	23%	>3.5 cm: 40%	9%	9.4%	n/a
	439 open		>300 cc: 54%*	1%	15%	27%	58%	29%		
DiNorcia [47]	71 lap	250	150	0%	28.2%	11.3%	2.5/3.6	12.7%	25.3%	6/8
	92 open	270*	900*	1%	43.8%	14.1%		38.5%		
Jayaraman [48]	107 lap	194	150	0%	27%	15%	3	17%	30%	6/7
	236 open	163*	350*	0.8%	40%*	13%	3*	47%		
Vijan [49]	100 lap	214	171	3%	34%	17%	3.3	23%	4%	NS
	100 open	208	519*	1%	29%	17%	4*	23%		
Kim [50]	93 lap	195	NS	0%	24.7%	8.6%	3	0%	n/a	n/a
	35 open	190		0%	29%	14.3%	3	0%		

LDP, laparoscopic distal pancreatectomy; ODP, open distal pancreatectomy; NS, no significant difference; OR, operating room.
*P < 0.05; n/a: data not available.

malignancies or tumors located close to the pancreatic neck and major blood vessels bears significant technical challenges.

24.2.2 Laparoscopic pancreas enucleation (LPE)

Pancreatic enucleation is a technique that allows for parenchyma-sparing resection of tumors. Thus, the chances of preserving a sufficient degree of the exo- and endocrine function of the pancreas are higher than under extended pancreatic resection such as PD or DP. Enucleation of the pancreas does not fulfill the criteria of an adequate oncological resection, although lymphadenectomy can be performed. However, safety margins are not sufficient for malignant disease. Therefore, the potential presence of malignancy of the lesion to be resected should be very carefully considered prior to performing an enucleation.

In our opinion, diagnoses that allow for this limited pancreatic resection include insulinoma and other neuroendocrine tumors not exceeding 2 cm in size, and potentially side-branch IPMNs outside the Sendai criteria [23]. We believe that for mucinous cystic neoplasms and nonfunctioning neuroendocrine tumors (NF–NET) exceeding 2 cm in diameter, the risk of inadequate treatment with enucleation may be too high. We believe that these patients should rather be treated by extended pancreatic resection including lymphadenectomy. NF–NETs smaller than 2 cm show malignancy when discovered incidentally in 6% of cases only. However, this proportion rises exponentially with increasing tumor size [24]. In the rare case of isolated pancreatic metastases, some authors advocate enucleation as the treatment of choice. However, the recurrence rate of metastases to the pancreas is higher following enucleation than following pancreatectomy [25].

In conclusion, to be eligible for laparoscopic enucleation, any lesion should be benign, not be in excess of 3 cm in size (in NF–NET <2 cm), and be distant from the main pancreatic duct (2–3 mm) [6,23]. Enucleation of any lesion closer to the duct than 2–3 mm leads to an increased risk of local duct necrosis and postoperative pancreatic fistula [26]. We think that lesions closer than 2–3 mm to the pancreatic duct should be resected rather than enucleated.

Amikura *et al.* published the first report of a laparoscopically performed enucleation of an islet cell tumor of the pancreas in 1995 [27]. As with any laparoscopic pancreatic procedure, no RCTs and, in the case of LPE, not even large comparative studies assessing the benefits

of laparoscopic over open access exist in the literature. However, it is generally accepted that the indications for open pancreatic enucleation can be applied to LPE, when the lesion is located superficially in the pancreatic body or tail, distant from the splenic vessels and main pancreatic duct, thus allowing a safe preparation. A thorough preoperative diagnostic imaging work-up and the use of intraoperative ultrasound are crucial for the successful localization of the lesion. Failure to identify the tumor intraoperatively represents a common cause for conversion to laparotomy [28].

As for distal pancreatectomy, postoperative pancreatic fistulas are the most important complication following enucleation. The existing case series indicate that the safety of LPE may be similar to that of open enucleation [26]. Rates reported from comparatively large case series (with the largest comprising 24 patients) for postoperative pancreatic fistulas, morbidity, and mortality following LPE range from 13% to 38%, 17% to 48.2%, and 0% to 4%, respectively [29,30].

In our experience, there is a significant difference between the open and laparoscopic approach in haptic feedback from tissues with surgical instruments available for dissection of the pancreatic parenchyma during enucleation. We think that there is room for improvement of surgical instrumentation available today for the laparoscopic approach. This might improve safety and allow for an even more widespread diffusion of the laparoscopic method of enucleation into surgical practice.

24.2.3 Laparoscopic pancreaticoduodenectomy (LPD)

Pancreaticoduodenectomy (PD) induces the greatest operative trauma from pancreatic resections and involves a considerable rate of severe postoperative complications. The procedure consists of extensive retroperitoneal dissection as well as the creation of three anastomoses, including that of the pancreatic remnant to reconstruct the upper gastrointestinal tract. Complete healing of these anastomoses is a key factor in avoiding significant complications that would, if they occur in cases of pancreatic cancer, significantly delay the initiation of adjuvant chemotherapy. Because of the complexity of LPD, many experienced pancreas surgeons hesitate to adopt the technique and LPD has thus been very slow to evolve since its first description in 1994.

Two main methods of conducting LPD have been described: (i) a total laparoscopic approach (TLPD), where all anastomoses are performed laparoscopically; and (ii) a laparoscopic-assisted hybrid approach (LAPD), in which the dissection is performed laparoscopically but the reconstruction is mainly conducted via a small laparotomy, which is also used to extract the specimen [31,32].

In early reported case series, most authors limited the use of LPD to resection of benign to low-grade tumors that were small in size and located close to the duodenal ampulla and distal common bile duct without any vascular or extrabiliary involvement. Thus, indications for LPD mainly included mucinous cystic neoplasms and IPMNs of the pancreatic head as well as other small ampullary and periampullary tumors [23]. Yet, there are also case series that included patients who underwent LPD for pancreatic ductal adenocarcinoma [32].

There are some retrospective studies in the literature that compare outcomes of open PD with one of the laparoscopic approaches (Table 24.2). A meta-analysis of six comparative studies analyzed 169 pooled patients who were treated only with TLPD, including robotic operations, compared with 372 patients who underwent open PD as control [33]. The pooled analysis indicated a decreased hospital stay and a higher number of lymph nodes retrieved in the LPD group. Other significant factors of the analysis were a higher rate of R0 resections and lower operative blood loss in the LPD group. The findings of this meta-analysis may be attributable to an underlying selection bias of the mostly unmatched retrospective studies. An indication of selection bias is the significantly higher rate of larger tumors in the open PD group. On the other hand, despite the smaller tumor size in these patients, operative time was significantly longer in the LPD group. Most of the studies were not analyzed in an intention-to-treat manner, i.e. cases of unexpected vascular involvement or any other cause for conversion to open PD (such as hemorrhage) excluded these patients from the LPD arm and instead were counted as open PD in several studies. It is also noteworthy that many of the retrospective comparative studies comprise open control groups with high complication rates, operative time, and blood loss as well as low number of harvested lymph nodes (see Table 24.2). One should bear in mind that even large case series of open surgery from unselected patient cohorts report a mean operation time of less than 350 minutes and a median number of harvested lymph nodes of 24 [34,35].

Despite the limitations of existing data, LPD may be technically feasible in selected cases. Although small case series may indicate adequate oncological safety, registries or controlled trials with long-term follow-up are necessary to prove equivalence in oncological outcome between open and laparoscopic PD. Therefore, it is important to emphasize that laparoscopic and open PD must be conducted by the same oncological principles with the same technique and operational steps.

24.2.4 Laparoscopic pancreatic necrosectomy

Acute pancreatitis is one of the most common gastrointestinal diseases causing hospitalization in the industrialized world. About 15% of patients with acute pancreatitis develop pancreatic necrosis and about a third of those patients suffer from secondary infection of the necrosis. The development of necrosis increases the risk for death in these patients to 15%, and in cases of secondary infection, this risk increases to 30% [36].

There is consensus among international experts that even severe necrotizing pancreatitis is best managed conservatively in the early phase of disease [37]. Sterile acute necrotic collections almost never require interventional treatment in the first weeks of disease. Later in the course, intervention is indicated only when significant symptoms exist. Any intervention should be delayed for about 4–6 weeks until the infected necrosis is walled off and demarcated with at least partial liquefaction. There is clear evidence from a RCT that early open surgical necrosectomy within the first 2–3 days after onset of acute pancreatitis, which was the treatment of choice a decade ago, results in higher morbidity and mortality than delayed intervention after at least 12 days [38]. Early open surgical intervention has been identified as an independent predictor of poor outcome in patients with necrotizing pancreatitis [39].

However, patients with infected necrosis, which usually does not occur until the second or third week following onset of symptoms, are required to undergo interventional treatment. The diagnosis of infected necrosis, and thus indication for intervention, may be proved by fine needle aspiration (FNA) of necrotic tissue/fluid and positive culture results. However, the use of FNA is reduced owing to today's possibilities of percutaneous and endoscopic drainage placement. Infection should be strongly suspected in patients who develop systemic inflammatory response syndrome (SIRS) or organ failure later in the course of necrotizing pancreatitis (>7 days). In particular, this includes those patients who were

Table 24.2 Comparative studies of laparoscopic pancreaticoduodenectomies (LPD).

Reference	LPD/OPD	OR time (min)	Blood loss (mL)	Mortality	Morbidity	Pancreatic fistula	Tumor size (cm)	% PDAC	Conversion rate	Lymph node harvest
Asbun [51]	53 TLPD	541	195	5.7%	NS	16.7%	2.74	41.5%	15%	23.44
	215 OPD	401*	1032*	8.8%	NS	17.3%	3.14	46.5%		16.84*
Kuroki [52]	20 LAPD	656.6	376.6	n/a	NS	45%	n/a	0%	0%	n/a
	31 OPD	554.6*	1509.5*	n/a	NS	39%	n/a	12.9%		n/a
Zureikat [53]	14 TLPD	456	300	7%	62%	36%	2.2	57%	14%	18.5
	14 OPD	372*	400	0%	42.8%*	42.8%	3.6*	57%		19.1
Cho [31]	15 LAPD	338	445	0%	27%	13%	n/a	6.7%	0%	18.5
	15 OPD	287	552	0%	27%	13%	n/a	13.3%		20

LAPD, laparoscopically assisted pancreaticoduodenectomy; OPD, open pancreaticoduodenectomy; PDAC, pancreatic ductal adenocarcinoma; TLPD, total laparoscopic pancreaticoduodenectomy.
*P < 0.05.
In our opinion, the open control groups of some of these studies show unaccceptable results.

previously clinically stable or even improving [37]. The use of antibiotics to prevent occurrence of infected necrosis has been extensively studied, but double-blinded, placebo-controlled studies failed to show a positive effect of this treatment [40].

Optimal timing of interventions and using an approach of gradual increase in invasiveness of these interventions are pivotal and have a strong impact on several outcome parameters in the treatment of patients with necrotizing pancreatitis. There is strong evidence suggesting that, compared with less invasive approaches, the physiological stress of open necrosectomy is more detrimental to the already severely ill patient.

Several minimally invasive approaches to pancreatic necrosis have been described. These can be classified according to the access route (peritoneal, retroperitoneal, transoral) and the method used for visualization (laparoscopic, rigid nephroscopic, flexible endoscopic) [41]. The transperitoneal laparoscopic approach includes laparoscopic visualization of the pancreas followed by hand-assisted or laparoscopic debridement of infected necrosis. The advantage of this approach is the good accessibility of all abdominal compartments but most surgeons fear the intra-abdominal dissemination of an extra-abdominal septic focus and thus avoid a transperitoneal laparoscopic approach. The more commonly performed techniques, however, use the retroperitoneal access route that is usually established under radiological image guidance. Through dilation of the tract or minimal incision, a rigid nephroscope, laparoscope, or flexible endoscope can be inserted into the cavity for direct visualization, debridement, and irrigation. These techniques have been termed "sinus tract endoscopy" and "video-assisted retroperitoneal debridement (VARD)." In the former, a nephroscope is inserted through the dilated drain tract and debridement is carried out using forceps followed by jet irrigation of the cavity [42]. The procedure is repeated if the patient fails to recover. The authors report a median of 3–5 procedures per patient until sufficient control of the septic focus is achieved. In a large but unmatched, and thus potentially biased, comparative retrospective study of the open approach, significant differences favoring sinus tract endoscopy concerning mortality rate, complication rate, organ failure rate, and required postoperative intensive care unit (ICU) support were reported [43].

The VARD technique involves a subcostal incision along a preoperatively placed drain followed by limited direct debridement. Then video-assisted debridement with use of gas insufflation of the retroperitoneum and a 0° camera is performed. Continuous lavage is started postoperatively via two large drains. In contrast to sinus tract endoscopy for pancreatic necrosectomy, VARD allows vigorous debridement, thus resulting in a median number of only one procedure per patient [44].

The prospective, randomized PANTER trial compared the effects of open necrosectomy as described by Beger [45] against a step-up approach of interventional drainage placement (either percutaneous or endoscopic) followed by minimally invasive VARD if there was no clinical improvement after drain placement [46]. The study population consisted of patients with confirmed or suspected infected necrosis, and the study interventions were performed at a median time of about 30 days after onset of symptoms, which was similar in both groups. Although the study did not directly compare the two operation methods of open necrosectomy with VARD, but rather compared it with a less invasive treatment scheme, and thus one cannot conclude from this trial that one operation method is superior to the other, the results of the study show a clear benefit from the less invasive treatment approach. Thirty-five percent of patients were sufficiently treated by interventional drain placement and did not need surgery at all. Patients in the minimally invasive group had significantly fewer major complications such as multiple organ failure, fewer incisional hernias, fewer cases of new-onset diabetes and exocrine insufficiency, and fewer ICU admissions. Mortality rate and length of ICU as well as hospital stay did not differ significantly.

KEY POINTS

- Minimally invasive pancreatic surgery is in a developmental stage and prospective data comparing it with open surgery are lacking. The benefits of laparoscopic pancreas surgery from reduced access and retraction trauma will be offset if significant complications occur.

- Oncological principles are key in performing laparoscopic pancreas surgery for cancer. Benign and borderline malignant lesions are good indications for a minimally invasive approach.

- Distal pancreatectomy has demonstrated good outcomes compared with open surgery for selected patients.

> - Laparoscopic enucleation, mainly performed for neuroendocrine tumors of the pancreas, is an organ-sparing approach with limited morbidity. The main pancreatic duct needs to be protected.
>
> - Minimally invasive management of pancreatitis needing intervention is an important innovation, but the principles of open pancreatitis management regarding indication, timing, and extent of debridement apply.

References

1 Clinical Outcomes of Surgical Therapy Study Group. A comparison of laparoscopically assisted and open colectomy for colon cancer. N Engl J Med 2004; 350:2050–2059.

2 Cuschieri A. Laparoscopic surgery of the pancreas. J Roy Coll Surg Edinburgh 1994; 39:178–184.

3 Gagner M, Pomp A. Laparoscopic pylorus-preserving pancreatoduodenectomy. Surg Endosc 1994; 8:408–410.

4 Cuschieri SA, Jakimowicz JJ. Laparoscopic pancreatic resections. Semin Laparosc Surg 1998; 5:168–179.

5 Tran Cao HS, Lopez N, Chang DC, et al. Improved perioperative outcomes with minimally invasive distal pancreatectomy: results from a population-based analysis. JAMA Surg 2014; 149:237–243.

6 Siech M, Bartsch D, Beger HG, et al. [Indications for laparoscopic pancreas operations: results of a consensus conference and the previous laparoscopic pancreas register]. Der Chirurg 2012; 83:247–253.

7 Niess H, Conrad C, Kleespies A, et al. Surgery for metastasis to the pancreas: is it safe and effective? J Surg Oncol 2013; 107:859–864.

8 Mallet-Guy P, Vachon A. Pancréatites Chroniques Gauches. Paris: Masson, 1943.

9 Warshaw AL. Conservation of the spleen with distal pancreatectomy. Arch Surg 1988; 123:550–553.

10 Benoist S, Dugue L, Sauvanet A, et al. Is there a role of preservation of the spleen in distal pancreatectomy? J Am Coll Surg 1999; 188:255–260.

11 Shoup M, Brennan MF, McWhite K, et al. The value of splenic preservation with distal pancreatectomy. Arch Surg 2002; 137:164–168.

12 Strasberg SM, Linehan DC, Hawkins WG. Radical antegrade modular pancreatosplenectomy procedure for adenocarcinoma of the body and tail of the pancreas: ability to obtain negative tangential margins. J Am Coll Surg 2007; 204: 244–249.

13 Balcom JHt, Rattner DW, Warshaw AL, et al. Ten–year experience with 733 pancreatic resections: changing indications, older patients, and decreasing length of hospitalization. Arch Surg 2001; 136:391–398.

14 Schwarz RE, Harrison LE, Conlon KC, et al. The impact of splenectomy on outcomes after resection of pancreatic adenocarcinoma. J Am Coll Surg 1999; 188:516–521.

15 Beane JD, Pitt HA, Nakeeb A, et al. Splenic preserving distal pancreatectomy: does vessel preservation matter? J Am Coll Surg 2011; 212:651–657; discussion 657–658.

16 Yoon YS, Lee KH, Han HS, et al. Patency of splenic vessels after laparoscopic spleen and splenic vessel-preserving distal pancreatectomy. Br J Surg 2009; 96:633–640.

17 Yoon YS, Lee KH, Han HS, et al. Effects of laparoscopic versus open surgery on splenic vessel patency after spleen and splenic vessel-preserving distal pancreatectomy: a retrospective multicenter study. Surg Endosc 2015; 29(3):583–588.

18 Nigri GR, Rosman AS, Petrucciani N, et al. Metaanalysis of trials comparing minimally invasive and open distal pancreatectomies. Surg Endosc 2011; 25:1642–1651.

19 Venkat R, Edil BH, Schulick RD, et al. Laparoscopic distal pancreatectomy is associated with significantly less overall morbidity compared to the open technique: a systematic review and meta-analysis. Ann Surg 2012; 255:1048–1059.

20 Kooby DA, Gillespie T, Bentrem D, et al. Left-sided pancreatectomy: a multicenter comparison of laparoscopic and open approaches. Ann Surg 2008; 248:438–446.

21 Kooby DA, Hawkins WG, Schmidt CM, et al. A multicenter analysis of distal pancreatectomy for adenocarcinoma: is laparoscopic resection appropriate? J Am Coll Surg 2010; 210:779–785, 786–777.

22 Diener MK, Seiler CM, Rossion I, et al. Efficacy of stapler versus hand-sewn closure after distal pancreatectomy (DISPACT): a randomised, controlled multicentre trial. Lancet 2011; 377:1514–1522.

23 Subar D, Gobardhan PD, Gayet B. Laparoscopic pancreatic surgery: an overview of the literature and experiences of a single center. Best Pract Res Clin Gastroenterol 2014; 28:123–132.

24 Bettini R, Partelli S, Boninsegna L, et al. Tumor size correlates with malignancy in nonfunctioning pancreatic endocrine tumor. Surgery 2011; 150:75–82.

25 Bassi C, Butturini G, Falconi M, et al. High recurrence rate after atypical resection for pancreatic metastases from renal cell carcinoma. Br J Surg 2003; 90:555–559.

26 Crippa S, Bassi C, Salvia R, et al. Enucleation of pancreatic neoplasms. Br J Surg 2007; 94:1254–1259.

27 Amikura K, Alexander HR, Norton JA, et al. Role of surgery in management of adrenocorticotropic hormone-producing islet cell tumors of the pancreas. Surgery 1995; 118:1125–1130.

28 Ayav A, Bresler L, Brunaud L, et al. Laparoscopic approach for solitary insulinoma: a multicentre study. Langenbeck's Arch Surg 2005; 390:134–140.

29 Mabrut JY, Fernandez-Cruz L, Azagra JS, et al. Laparoscopic pancreatic resection: results of a multicenter European study of 127 patients. Surgery 2005; 137:597–605.

30 Fernandez-Cruz L, Cosa R, Blanco L, et al. Curative laparoscopic resection for pancreatic neoplasms: a critical analysis

from a single institution. J Gastrointest Surg 2007; 11:1607–1621; discussion 1621–1602.

31 Cho A, Yamamoto H, Nagata M, *et al.* Comparison of laparoscopy-assisted and open pylorus-preserving pancreaticoduodenectomy for periampullary disease. Am J Surg 2009; 198:445–449.

32 Kendrick ML, Cusati D. Total laparoscopic pancreaticoduodenectomy: feasibility and outcome in an early experience. Arch Surg 2010; 145:19–23.

33 Correa-Gallego C, Dinkelspiel HE, Sulimanoff I, *et al.* Minimally-invasive vs open pancreaticoduodenectomy: systematic review and meta-analysis. J Am Coll Surg 2014; 218:129–139.

34 Fernandez-del Castillo C, Morales-Oyarvide V, McGrath D, *et al.* Evolution of the Whipple procedure at the Massachusetts General Hospital. Surgery 2012; 152:S56–63.

35 Strobel O, Hinz U, Gluth A, *et al.* Pancreatic adenocarcinoma: number of positive nodes allows to distinguish several n categories. Ann Surg 2015; 261(5):961–969.

36 Petrov MS, Shanbhag S, Chakraborty M, *et al.* Organ failure and infection of pancreatic necrosis as determinants of mortality in patients with acute pancreatitis. Gastroenterology 2010; 139:813–820.

37 Freeman ML, Werner J, van Santvoort HC, *et al.* Interventions for necrotizing pancreatitis: summary of a multidisciplinary consensus conference. Pancreas 2012; 41:1176–1194.

38 Mier J, Leon EL, Castillo A, *et al.* Early versus late necrosectomy in severe necrotizing pancreatitis. Am J Surg 1997; 173:71–75.

39 Van Santvoort HC, Bakker OJ, Bollen TL, *et al.* A conservative and minimally invasive approach to necrotizing pancreatitis improves outcome. Gastroenterology 2011; 141:1254–1263.

40 Da Costa DW, Boerma D, van Santvoort HC, *et al.* Staged multidisciplinary step-up management for necrotizing pancreatitis. Br J Surg 2014; 101:e65–79.

41 Werner J, Feuerbach S, Uhl W, Buchler MW. Management of acute pancreatitis: from surgery to interventional intensive care. Gut 2005; 54:426–436.

42 Carter CR, McKay CJ, Imrie CW. Percutaneous necrosectomy and sinus tract endoscopy in the management of infected pancreatic necrosis: an initial experience. Ann Surg 2000; 232:175–180.

43 Raraty MG, Halloran CM, Dodd S, *et al.* Minimal access retroperitoneal pancreatic necrosectomy: improvement in morbidity and mortality with a less invasive approach. Ann Surg 2010; 251:787–793.

44 Horvath K, Freeny P, Escallon J, *et al.* Safety and efficacy of video-assisted retroperitoneal debridement for infected pancreatic collections: a multicenter, prospective, single-arm phase 2 study. Arch Surg 2010; 145:817–825.

45 Beger HG, Buchler M, Bittner R, *et al.* Necrosectomy and postoperative local lavage in necrotizing pancreatitis. Br J Surg 1988; 75:207–212.

46 Van Santvoort HC, Besselink MG, Bakker OJ, *et al.* A step-up approach or open necrosectomy for necrotizing pancreatitis. N Engl J Med 2010; 362:1491–1502.

47 DiNorcia J, Schrope BA, Lee MK, *et al.* Laparoscopic distal pancreatectomy offers shorter hospital stays with fewer complications. J Gastrointest Surg 2010; 14(11):1804–1812.

48 Jayaraman S, Gonen M, Brennan MF, *et al.* Laparoscopic distal pancreatectomy: evolution of a technique at a single institution. J Am Coll Surg 2010; 211(4):503–509.

49 Vijan SS, Ahmed KA, Harmsen WS, *et al.* Laparoscopic vs open distal pancreatectomy: a single-institution comparative study. Arch Surg 2010; 145(7):616–621.

50 Kim SC, Park KT, Hwang JW, *et al.* Comparative analysis of clinical outcomes for laparoscopic distal pancreatic resection and open distal pancreatic resection at a single institution. Surg Endosc 2008; 22(10):2261–2268.

51 Asbun HJ, Stauffer JA. Laparoscopic vs open pancreaticoduodenectomy: overall outcomes and severity of complications using the Accordion Severity Grading System. J Am Coll Surg 2012; 215(6):810–819.

52 Kuroki T, Adachi T, Okamoto T, Kanematsu T. A non-randomized comparative study of laparoscopy-assisted pancreaticoduodenectomy and open pancreaticoduodenectomy. Hepatogastroenterology 2012; 59(114):570–573.

53 Zureikat AH, Breaux JA, Steel JL, Hughes SJ. Can laparoscopic pancreaticoduodenectomy be safely implemented? J Gastrointest Surg 2011; 15(7):1151–1157.

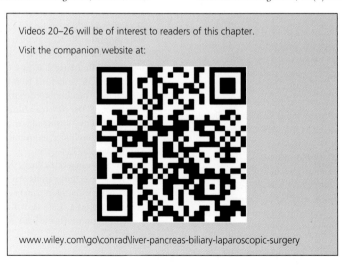

Videos 20–26 will be of interest to readers of this chapter.

Visit the companion website at:

www.wiley.com\go\conrad\liver-pancreas-biliary-laparoscopic-surgery

PART II
Video Atlas

The procedures carried out in the videos are designed to be viewed in conjunction with the text, images, and anatomic schemes shown in this section.

Video and Figure Abbreviations

BD	bile duct
HA	hepatic artery
IRHV	inferior right hepatic vein
IVC	inferior vena cava
LHA	left hepatic artery
LHV	left hepatic vein
LPP	left portal pedicle
LPV	left portal vein
MHV	middle hepatic vein
P	portal branch
PP	portal pedicle
PV	portal vein
RAHA	right anterior hepatic artery
RAPP	right anterior portal pedicle
RHA	right hepatic artery
RHV	right hepatic vein
RIHV	right inferior hepatic vein
RPHA	right posterior hepatic artery
RPHV	right posterior hepatic vein
RPP	right portal pedicle
RPPP	right posterior portal pedicle
V	venous branch

VIDEO 1

Intraoperative ultrasonography for safe laparoscopic livery surgery

Video duration 9 minutes 42 seconds

In this video, we will show you intraoperative ultrasonography for safe laparoscopic liver surgery.

Left lateral sectionectomy

The first section will show you the key structures that should be identified for left lateral sectionectomy. The first two structures that should be identified are the drainage of the left and the middle hepatic veins; in particular, the drainage of the middle hepatic vein into the IVC is important to identify. Identifying the left hepatic vein a little bit more lateral will allow for safe staple division at the end of the case. Moving the probe inferiorly, we identify the portal branches of segments II and III. Identifying the portal branches of segment II and its relationship to the left hepatic vein can be helpful in identifying the left hepatic vein inside the parenchyma. Here, we open up the parenchyma which will facilitate staple division of the portal branch of segment III. Now, we will staple divide the portal branch of segment II. We know from the ultrasound that the left hepatic vein will be quite close to it. The transmitted respiratory variation into the left hepatic vein seen on the parenchymal transection margin gives you a hint where the left hepatic vein will be found. Because we know from the ultrasound the relationship between the middle hepatic vein and the left hepatic vein, we can progress with the parenchymal transection and finally staple divide the left hepatic vein. At the end of the case, we have divided the portal branches to segments II and III, as well as the left hepatic vein.

Right hepatectomy

In this section, we will discuss which landmark structure should be identified on intraoperative ultrasound for a right hepatectomy. The landmark structure that will guide the parenchymal transection is the middle hepatic vein. At the end of the case, the right hepatic vein will be divided. It is crucial to identify the drainage anatomy on intraoperative ultrasound. In every laparoscopic right hepatectomy, the hepatic venous drainage of segment VIII must be checked on preoperative imaging. Not knowing where the drainage of segment VIII is and injuring it can lead to significant bleeding at the end of the case. In this patient, the segment VIII branch drains into the middle of the hepatic vein but it can also drain directly into the IVC. Other important branches are V4 and V5. They can be identified by positioning the probe along the axis of the middle hepatic vein. We try to identify the middle hepatic vein very early after opening up the parenchyma. The first branch of the middle hepatic vein we will encounter is also identified on ultrasound as the V5 branch. This branch is clipped and divided. As mentioned, the middle hepatic vein guides our parenchymal transection. We recommend identifying the hepatic venous drainage of segment VIII for each right hepatectomy because when we know from

Laparoscopic Liver, Pancreas, and Biliary Surgery, First Edition.
Edited by Claudius Conrad and Brice Gayet.
© 2017 John Wiley & Sons, Ltd. Published 2017 by John Wiley & Sons, Ltd.

intraoperative ultrasound where this branch is, we can safely identify and transect it. The final image shows you the anatomy at the end of the case.

Segmentectomy of segment VIII

Next, we will show you the critical structures to be identified on ultrasound for an anatomical segmentectomy of segment VIII. The critical structures here are the V8 drainage vein and the middle hepatic vein with its relationship to the tumor. Placing the probe horizontally, we identify the relationship between the tumor and the portal branch to segment VIII. The right hepatic vein will determine the lateral resection margin. We recommend using the ultrasound and the energy device at the same time to mark the resection margin on the liver surface. The next section will show you how to identify the portal pedicle to segment VIII that is involved with the tumor. The use of Doppler flow imaging can be helpful at this step. A hemostatic agent made of oxidized regenerated cellulose can be used as a fixed point which can be identified on intraoperative ultrasound. Here, we see the portal branch of segment VIII in the resection margin. The right posterior portal pedicle should be identified and injury to it avoided. The clamp on

the P8 branch can be identified on the ultrasound and can be useful for orientation. The resection line itself can also be identified on the ultrasound. Next, we place a clip on the P8 branch. Intact vascularization of the future liver remnant should be confirmed with ultrasound. Here, we confirm drainage of segment IVa. Next, we confirm drainage of segment IVb.

Posterior superior sectionectomy

The next section will cover identification of the drainage of the right hepatic vein for posterior superior segmentectomy. For this case, we place cuff ports transthoracically. While performing inferior traction on the liver, we identify the drainage of the right hepatic vein with intraoperative ultrasound. Again, the drainage of V8 should be identified. Here, we open up the parenchyma to control the right hepatic vein. We know from the ultrasound that the drainage vein of segment VIII will be close. It is clipped and divided with scissors. Now the drainage of the right hepatic vein is completely exposed. On this image, the important structures that we identified on intraoperative ultrasound (the right hepatic vein, middle hepatic vein, and P8 branch) can be seen. The clip marks the drainage vein of segment VIII.

Anatomy figures

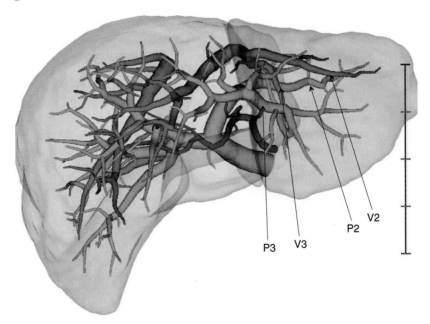

Figure v1.1 Relevant anatomy for laparoscopic left lateral sectionectomy. The operation begins by opening the umbilical fissure. The key is to avoid injury to the main LPP or the P4b pedicle. The MHV can be surprisingly close to the falciform ligament. Undercutting the falciform ligament should be avoided. Care must be taken during the dissection of the drainage of the LHV into the IVC. An MHV injury at a common drainage with the MHV can lead to significant injury.

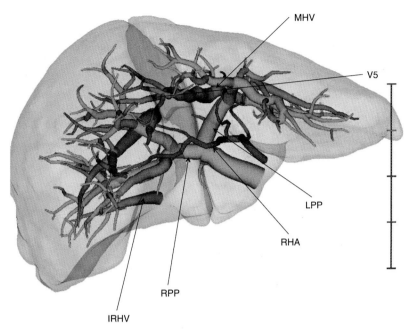

Figure v1.2 Critical anatomy for a right hepatectomy. The RPP as well as the RHA are exposed. The key is to avoid injury to the LPP. This patient has a common RPP but also a trifurcation and staged division is frequently seen.

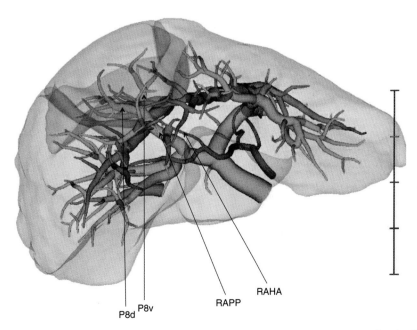

Figure v1.3 Critical anatomy for a resection of segment VIII. The typical portal branching of segment VIII is a dominant P8 ventral and P8 dorsal PP coming off the RAPP.

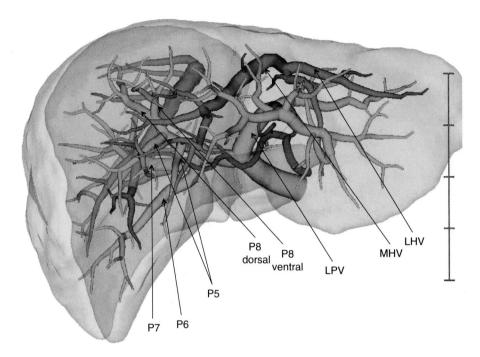

Figure v1.4 Critical anatomy for a posterior sectionectomy. During the dissection, the RAPP is preserved while P6 and P7 are taken. In this case, the patient has a trifurcation and therefore P6 and P7 should be taken individually.

VIDEO 2

Left lateral sectionectomy

Video duration 7 minutes 17 seconds

In this video, we will show a left lateral sectionectomy. A left lateral sectionectomy is a good starting case for a laparoscopic liver surgery experience. Nevertheless, the approach needs to be very structured.

OUTLINE

The video has the following outline:
- Port positioning
- Division of segment III portal branch
- Division of segment II portal branch
- Division of the left hepatic vein and specimen mobilization
- Important points.

This scheme demonstrates the port positioning (Figure v2.1). Make sure to place the ports far enough to the left that the round ligament does not obstruct your view (but far enough medial to have a view along the parenchymal transection line).

With ultrasound, we identify the drainage of the left hepatic vein (Figure v2.2). At this step, check the common drainage with the middle hepatic vein as this can be injured during the staple division of the left hepatic vein. Next, we check for the segment II portal branch as well as the segment III portal pedicle (Figure v2.3 and Figure v2.4).

Next, we will dissect out and divide the segment III portal branch. The segment III portal branch runs in the umbilical fissure. In order to facilitate staple division, we open the parenchyma above and below the segment III portal branch.

Here, the Glissonian sheath to the segment III portal branch comes into view. Now the segment III portal

Port Positioning

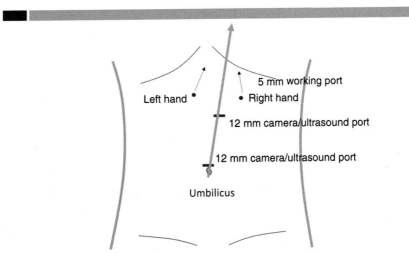

Figure v2.1 Port positioning for a left lateral sectionectomy. Place the ports far enough to the left so that the round ligament does not obstruct your view. The ports should nevertheless be far enough medial to have a view along the parenchymal transection plane.

Laparoscopic Liver, Pancreas, and Biliary Surgery, First Edition.
Edited by Claudius Conrad and Brice Gayet.
© 2017 John Wiley & Sons, Ltd. Published 2017 by John Wiley & Sons, Ltd.

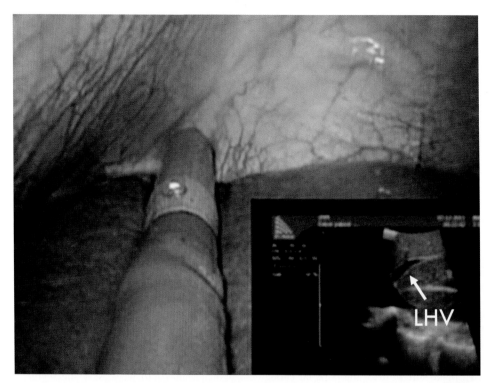

Figure v2.2 With intraoperative ultrasound determine the drainage of the LHV into the IVC.

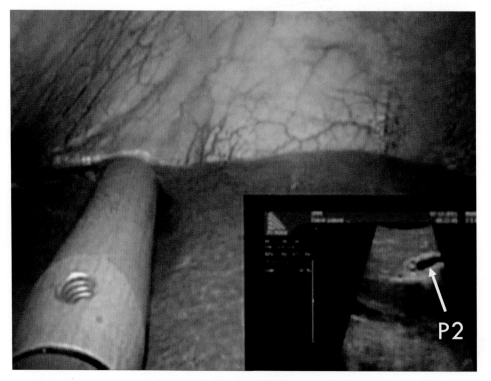

Figure v2.3 Use intraoperative ultrasound to determine the location of the P2.

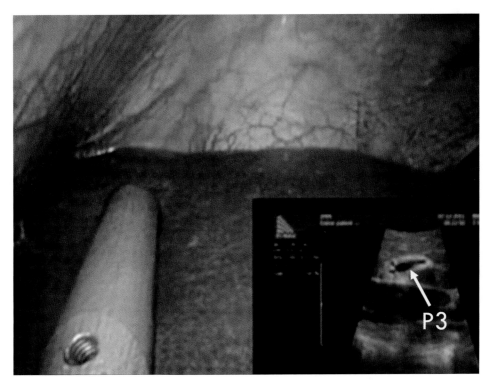

Figure v2.4 Shortly after P2 is controlled P3 is divided.

branch can be easily divided with a stapler. As we carry on with the parenchymal transection, we encounter the segment II portal branch. Here, the segment II portal branch has been dissected out and can be divided with a stapler. The last step is the division of the left hepatic vein and specimen mobilization.

Undercutting the falciform ligament can lead to injury of the middle hepatic vein. Using ultrasound, identify its location as well as its drainage either in the left hepatic vein or in the IVC. Also watch out for a prominent umbilical fissure vein.

In order to avoid injury to the extraparenchymal portion of the left hepatic vein, we carry on the dissection using scissors. Here, you can see how we open up the parenchyma above the left hepatic vein with an energy device. Now we have identified the precise location of the left hepatic vein. We completely isolate the left hepatic vein before the staple division. As we staple, we divide the left

hepatic vein. We always have a vascular clamp ready in case of stapler misfiring. The final step is specimen mobilization, for which we divide the left triangular ligament. Finally, we confirm hemostasis at the parenchymal transection margin. The specimen is placed into an endoscopic retriever bag and removed from the abdomen.

IMPORTANT POINTS

- Ports are placed more medially for inline working.
- Use ultrasound to identify the portal branch to segments II and III as well as the middle hepatic vein.
- Control the portal branch to segment III early.
- Leave the falciform ligament attached: it can guide the transection plane and can also be used for retraction.
- Do not undercut the falciform ligament as this can lead to middle hepatic vein injury. Use ultrasound to understand the anatomy of the middle hepatic vein.

Anatomy figures

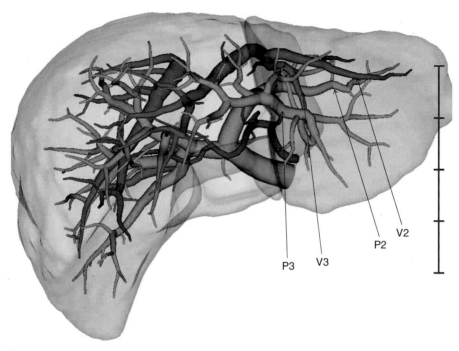

Figure v2.5 Relevant anatomy for laparoscopic left lateral sectionectomy. The operation begins with opening the umbilical fissure. The key is to avoid injury to the main LPP or the P4b pedicle. The MHV can be surprisingly close to the falciform ligament. Undercutting the falciform ligament should be avoided. Care must be taken during dissection of the drainage of the LHV into the IVC. An MHV injury at a common drainage with the MHV can lead to significant injury.

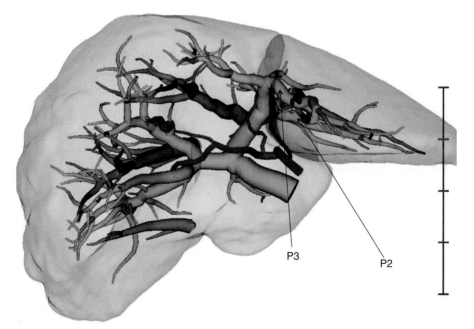

Figure v2.6 Initial view for laparoscopic left lateral sectionectomy. After opening the umbilical fissure, the PP to segment III and, shortly thereafter, the pedicle to segment III are controlled. Notice the closeness of these two pedicles (P3 and P2).

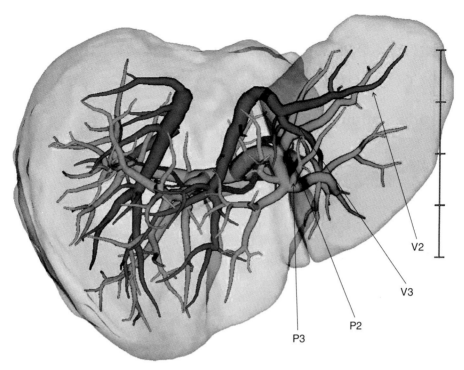

V2

V3

P2

P3

Figure v2.7 Cranial to caudal view. Notice again the closeness of P3 and P2, which are usually controlled with a stapler.

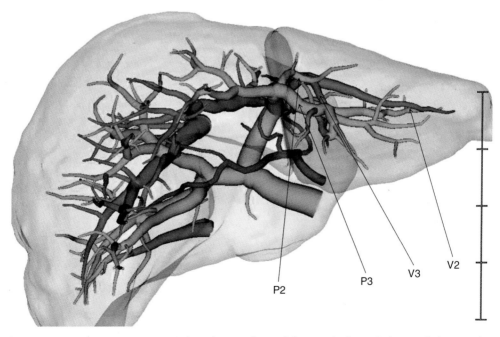

V2

V3

P3

P2

Figure v2.8 Operative view. Here we can see again how the P2 and P3 pedicles curve back anteriorly towards the operative surgeon. Injury to the main LPP needs to be avoided when opening the umbilical fissure.

VIDEO 3

Left lateral sectionectomy using a laparoscopic single access device

Video duration 6 minutes 49 seconds

In this video, we will show a left lateral sectionectomy using a laparoscopic single access device.

> **OUTLINE**
>
> The video will cover
> - Port positioning
> - Parenchymal transection
> - Suturing
> - Important points.

It is very important to determine the positioning of the single access device on preoperative imaging before the case. Owing to the lack of triangulation, inline working along the axis of parenchymal transection is very important (Figure v3.1). We begin the case with intraoperative ultrasound. The relationship between the lesion and the vascular structures is determined and lesions in the future liver remnant are excluded. Using an endoclosure device, we place a suture around the ligamentum teres. This can be used to retract the liver superiorly. Next, we open up the parenchyma to expose the portal pedicle to segment III. For this, we divide the bridge between segments III and IVb. This uncovers the umbilical fissure bearing the portal pedicle to segment III. Next, we open up the

Port positioning

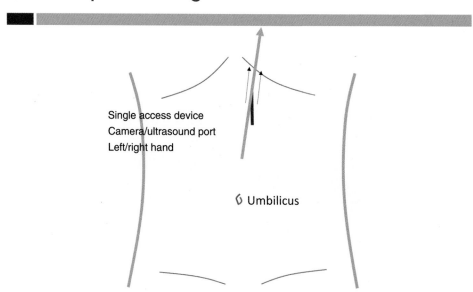

Single access device
Camera/ultrasound port
Left/right hand

◊ Umbilicus

Figure v3.1 Determine the positioning of the single access device on preoperative imaging before the case.

parenchyma along the falciform ligament. Then we determine the relationship between portal pedicle segment II and the lesion.

We are now ready to staple divide the portal pedicle to segment III. Because of the size of the stapler handle, it is difficult for the assistant to help at this step. Nevertheless, we always try to bring in a vascular clamp along the axis of the stapler in case of stapler misfiring. We can now continue the parenchymal division along the falciform ligament. With an additional staple firing, we open up the parenchyma. At this point, we are ready to staple divide the portal pedicle to segment II. We are now uncovering the intraparenchymal portion of the left hepatic vein. The left hepatic vein is now staple divided as well. Despite the limitation of working with a single access device, it is very important to bring in a vascular clamp at this step. In case of stapler misfiring, having a vascular clamp ready is crucial. With division of the left triangular ligament, the specimen is completely detached.

At the end of the case, we notice a minor bile leak from the portal pedicle to segment III. We will suture this bile leak closed. Suturing while using a single access device can be very difficult owing to the lack of triangulation. Therefore, we are using an automated needle driver that can be angled along the axis. You can see here oversewing of the staple line. The picture in the top right-hand corner shows the outside view. Rotation of the needle driver is activated with the thumb. The further away the suture target is, the more difficult it gets. A clip at the end of the suture can provide additional security.

> **IMPORTANT POINTS**
>
> - Safety first – the use of the single access device should not compromise the safety of the surgery in any way.
> - The single access device should be placed in line with the parenchymal transection line. This should be determined from preoperative imaging.
> - Articulating instruments can facilitate the surgery, for example the suturing process.
> - New devices will make this surgery easier and safer in the future.

Anatomy figures

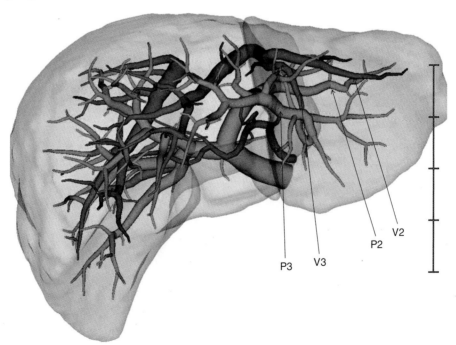

Figure v3.2 Relevant anatomy for laparoscopic left lateral sectionectomy. The operation begins with opening the umbilical fissure. The key is to avoid injury to the main LPP or the P4b pedicle. The MHV can be surprisingly close to the falciform ligament. Undercutting the falciform ligament should be avoided. Care must be taken during dissection of the drainage of the LHV into the IVC. An MHV injury at a common drainage with the MHV can lead to significant injury.

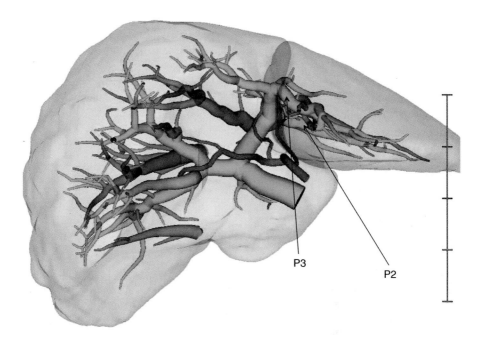

Figure v3.3 Initial view for laparoscopic left lateral sectionectomy. After opening the umbilical fissure, the PP to segment III and, shortly thereafter, the pedicle to segment III are controlled. Notice the closeness of these two pedicles (P3 and P2).

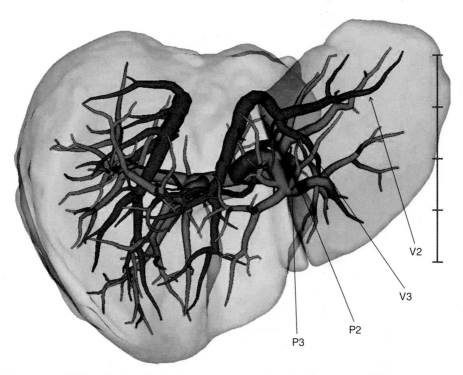

Figure v3.4 Cranial to caudal view. Notice again the closeness of P3 and P2, which are usually controlled with a stapler.

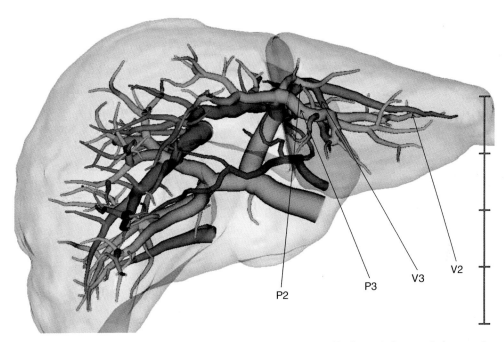

P2   P3   V3   V2

Figure v3.5 Operative view. Here we can see again how the P2 and P3 pedicles curve back anteriorly towards the operative surgeon. Injury to the main LPP needs to be avoided when opening the umbilical fissure.

Segmentectomy I with resection of inferior vena cava

Video duration 19 minutes 21 seconds

In this video, we show you a caudate lobectomy with resection of the inferior vena cava (IVC).

The port positioning is similar to a left hepatectomy (Figure v4.1). The ports at the costal margin are used for retraction and the vascular clamp.

The first step is the intraoperative ultrasound. On this ultrasound image, the tumor invading the IVC can be seen.

We are also looking out for the caudate veins which will be controlled during the parenchymal transection (Figure v4.2).

Good spatial understanding of the tumor relationship to the liver and IVC is crucial for this case (Figure v4.3). After the intraoperative ultrasound, we mobilize the liver. This is the view with superior traction of the left lateral segment. Next, we open up the hepatocaval ligament.

Port positioning

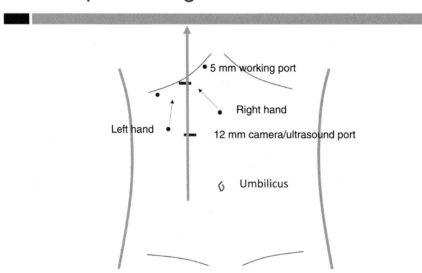

5 mm working port

Right hand

Left hand

12 mm camera/ultrasound port

Umbilicus

Figure v4.1 The set-up is similar to a left hepatectomy with the ports placed slightly further to the patient's left. The ports at the costal margin are used for retraction and the vascular clamp.

Laparoscopic Liver, Pancreas, and Biliary Surgery, First Edition.
Edited by Claudius Conrad and Brice Gayet.
© 2017 John Wiley & Sons, Ltd. Published 2017 by John Wiley & Sons, Ltd.

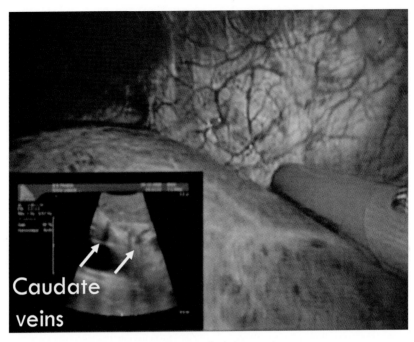

Figure v4.2 The caudate veins will be controlled during the parenchymal transection.

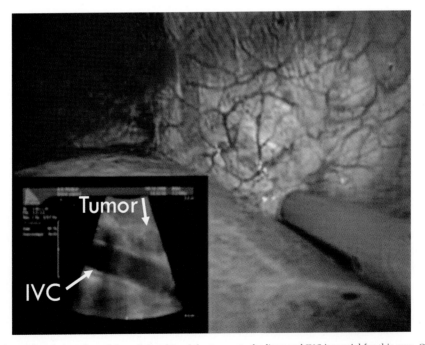

Figure v4.3 Good spatial understanding of the relationship of the tumor to the liver and IVC is crucial for this case. On ultrasound, the close relationship between tumor and IVC is determined.

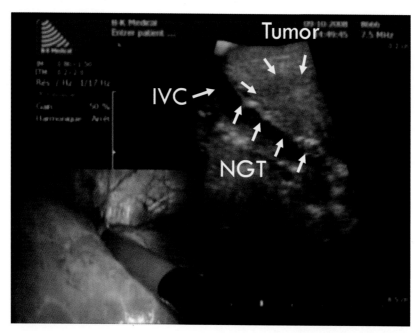

Figure v4.4 The hepatocaval space is dissected out and a nasogastric tube (NGT) fed into this space ventral to the IVC. It is identified on ultrasound.

Here, we are following the ligament of Arantius in the cephalad direction. Of note, this patient has a replaced left hepatic artery which we need to preserve for this case. Here, we are opening up the ligament of Arantius further. Wide mobilization is necessary for this case. Here, we are dissecting the intrahepatic IVC.

Now we are continuing our dissection at the epiploic foramen. Porta and duodenum are retracted with the suction. Short hepatic veins are controlled with clips. Here, we are continuing our dissection along the hepatocaval ligament. Here, we are beginning the dissection of the hepatocaval space. Complete mobilization of the liver on the right side is crucial, and here we are dissecting the right triangular ligament. We are also dissecting the hepatocaval ligament on the right side. For later dissection of the hepatocaval space, we are also taking down the falciform as well as the coronary ligament. Here, the suprahepatic IVC comes into view. At this point, the landing zone of the dissection of the hepatocaval space has been completely dissected out.

Next, we would like to show you the dissection of the hepatocaval space. The nasogastric tube (NGT) can be useful in this dissection. It is crucial to be very gentle at this step to avoid injury to the IVC. After the outlet of the hepatocaval space has been dissected, we begin the

dissection of the inlet. We are very gentle at this step to avoid any injury. Using ultrasound, we control the path of the nasogastric tube through the hepatocaval space. Here, the air artifacts of the nasogastric space can be seen next to the lesion.

The next step is the parenchymal transection (Figure v4.4). The liver is retracted superiorly. We are beginning the parenchymal transection and identifying caudate veins. After opening the parenchyma a little bit, we are opening out one of the caudate veins. The caudate vein is cut and divided. Additional caudate veins are dissected out. They are also controlled with clips and divided. Here, another caudate lobe branch is dissected out; it will be clipped and divided. Now the superior portion of the caudate lobe is completely dissected out. Here at the dissection of the superior part of the caudate lobe, we are controlling a caudate vein. At this step, we are deepening the transection along the paracaval portion of the caudate lobe. Here, an additional caudate vein is identified and it will be dissected out, clipped, and divided. In this image, we can see the lesion inferiorly. We are deepening our transection line down to the IVC. We are reaching a point at our dissection where the caudate lobe has been entirely freed and only the lesion is adherent to the IVC. Here, we are ensuring the hepatocaval space has been completely dissected out. Here, we are dissecting between the left and middle hepatic veins. In order to ensure a bloodless field, a hemostatic agent is placed in that space.

The last step of the operation is the partial IVC resection. The caudate lobe has been entirely freed, and it is only adherent to the IVC at the level of the metastasis. We are ensuring good mobility of the IVC for the later reconstruction. In order to ensure enough mobility after clamping for the partial resection of the IVC, we are dissecting some of the hepatocaval ligament fibers. Now we are placing a vascular clamp along the IVC where a metastasis is invading it. Here, the clamped part of the IVC is dissected off. At this step, the specimen is completely detached. We are placing the specimen in an endoscopic retrieval bag. We are proceeding to suture close the IVC. We are now ready to slowly open the vascular clamp. Finally, we confirm that we have excellent hemostasis.

> **IMPORTANT POINTS**
>
> - Caudate lobe resection requires an optimal liver mobilization.
> - The laparoscopic view along the IVC facilitates the dissection.
> - Avoid bleeding during dissection of the hepatocaval space in order to maintain excellent working conditions.
> - Be aware of caudate veins.
> - A laparoscopic IVC resection is a very challenging case. In addition to laparoscopic skills, it requires careful preparation to manage significant blood loss.

Anatomy figures

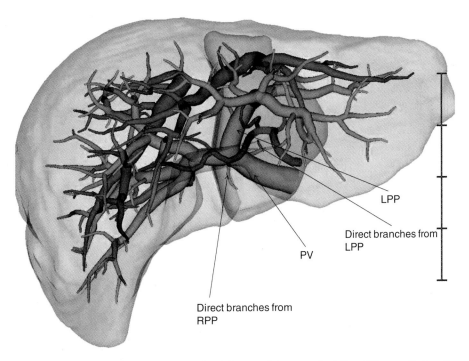

Figure v4.5 Critical anatomy of the caudate lobe. The caudate lobe extends between the IVC and PP up to the hepatic venous confluence. Venous drainage is from direct branches from IVC. Direct branches from left and RPP supply segment I.

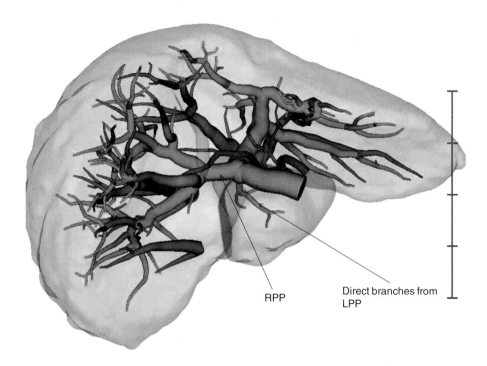

RPP

Direct branches from
LPP

Figure v4.6 Relationship of portal structures to segment I. The direct branches from the left and right portal pedicles can cause significant bleeding. They are relevant not only when performing a caudate lobectomy but also when dissecting out the main PP for other types of liver resection.

VIDEO 5

Segmentectomy IV

Video duration 14 minutes 14 seconds

In this video, we demonstrate an anatomical resection of segment IV.

The port positioning is similar to a left hepatectomy (Figure v5.1). As we make progress during the parenchy-mal transection, we will move from position 1 to position 2 (Figure v5.2). A good understanding of the anatomy from the preoperative imaging and intraoperative ultrasound is essential.

This is a CT 3D reconstruction with the tumors indicated in purple. Notice the tumor close to the drainage of the middle hepatic vein into the IVC. Therefore, this segment IV resection will encompass the middle hepatic vein.

This is an overview of the anatomy. The first step is thorough examination of the liver to understand the anatomy and rule out metastases in the future liver remnant. In addition to the superficial metastases you can see on the surface, we need to account for two more. This is the metastasis located at the drainage of the middle hepatic vein to the IVC (Figure v5.3). It is important to have a good understanding of the drainage of the middle hepatic vein and right hepatic vein into the IVC (Figure v5.4). The last

Port positioning

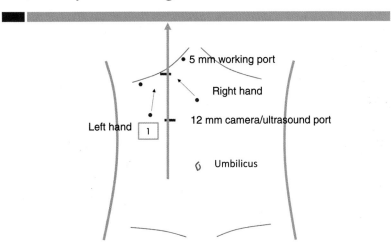

Figure v5.1 The port positioning for a segmentectomy IV is similar to a left hepatectomy. As we make progress during the parenchymal transection, we will move from position 1 to position 2.

Laparoscopic Liver, Pancreas, and Biliary Surgery, First Edition.
Edited by Claudius Conrad and Brice Gayet.
© 2017 John Wiley & Sons, Ltd. Published 2017 by John Wiley & Sons, Ltd.

Port positioning

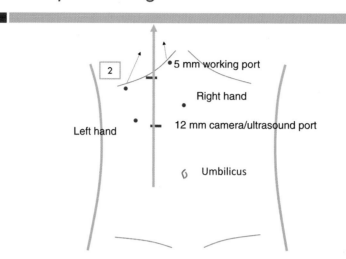

Figure v5.2 As we make progress during the parenchymal transection, we will move from position 1 to position 2. Position 2 is used for the dissection at the level of the hepatic venous confluence.

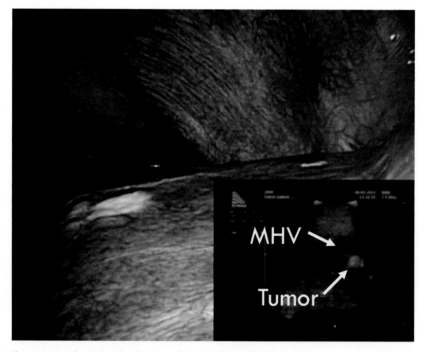

Figure v5.3 This is the metastasis located at the drainage of the MHV to the IVC.

metastasis we need to account for is the one abutting the middle hepatic vein between segments IVb and V (Figure v5.5). For correlation, this is an image from the 3D reconstruction shown earlier (Figure v5.6).

In the next section, we show you the optimization of working conditions for the parenchymal transection, which includes mobilization and retraction of the liver as well as preparation to perform a Pringle maneuver. In the first step,

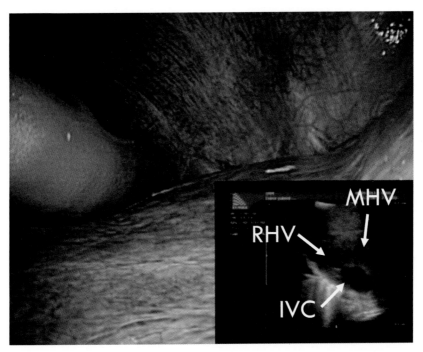

Figure v5.4 It is important to have a good understanding of the drainage of the MHV and RHV into the IVC.

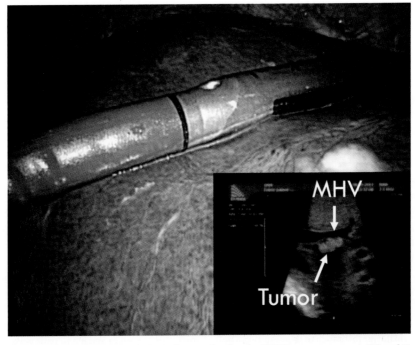

Figure v5.5 The last metastasis we need to account for is the one abutting the MHV between segments IVb and V.

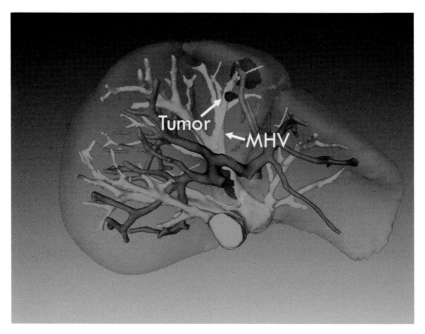

Figure v5.6 Three-dimensional vascular reconstruction of the patient's anatomy with tumor location. Notice the tumor abutting the MHV at its drainage into the IVC.

we divide the cystic duct, leaving the gallbladder attached to the liver. We will use it for retraction. Using an endoclosure device, we pass an Ethibond suture around the ligamentum teres for retraction. The falciform ligament, however, is left attached which also helps with retraction. For possible later Pringle maneuver, we pass an umbilical tape around the porta. Next, we divide the parenchymal bridge between segments III and IVb. This will facilitate exposure of the portal structures.

Once the parenchymal bridge has been entirely opened, we approach the left portal pedicle. Therefore, we switch to scissors for more careful dissection. Next, we lower the hilar plate. Using scissors, we open the most medial part of the hepatoduodenal ligament. Careful dissection is necessary to avoid injury to the portal structures going to the left of the liver. While lowering the hilar plate, we expose the drainage vein to segment V. Placing a hemostatic agent into the crevice will give us excellent visualization of the portal structures during our dissection.

The next step is parenchymal transection between the left lateral and left medial sectors. We continue our dissection past the ligamentum teres along the falciform ligament. At this point, we control the portal branch to segment IVb. The portal branch is clipped and divided. The portal branches to segment IVa will be controlled later once the parenchymal line has been deepened. Next, we control the drainage vein to segment IVb; after dissecting it out fully, it will be cut and

divided. In order to gain more mobility for retraction, we open up the coronary ligament further. With this added mobility, we can expose our transection line further and continue our dissection. Now that we have good exposure to the main left portal pedicle, we can clip and divide the portal pedicle to segment IVa. The portal branches are dissected out, clipped, and divided.

As mentioned earlier, the portal branches to segment IVb have already been controlled. However, we know from preoperative imaging, as well as intraoperative ultrasound, that there is an additional portal branch to segment IVa. By opening up the liver further, we are exposing that branch. Now the portal branch to segment IVa is fully exposed. We confirm on ultrasound that this is indeed a branch to segment IVa. Placing a clamp on the branch helps to identify it on ultrasound; shaking the clamp is helpful. Also clamping and unclamping the branch on Doppler flow mode helps to identify the branch. After we confirm that this is the branch to segment IVa, it can be divided using thermofusion. The left border of segment IV is divided by the left hepatic vein. It is exposed here and we follow its drainage into the IVC. This dissection here is critical. We expose the confluence of the middle hepatic vein and left hepatic vein and their drainage into the IVC. The middle hepatic vein defines the border of segment IV. We dissect out the coronary ligament further to get better exposure of the middle hepatic vein drainage in the IVC. This will help us at the completion of the dissection at the middle hepatic vein. After completion of the dissection between the left lateral segment and the medial sector, we have excellent demarcation of segment IV.

The next step is parenchymal transection along the middle hepatic vein. The gallbladder is used for retraction. Here, we are exposing the drainage vein to segment V which is clipped and divided. With superior traction on the specimen, we start to draw in the two transection lines. We continue the transection between segment IV and VIII. With this mobility of the specimen, we can proceed with dividing the middle hepatic vein. We confirm with the laparoscopic DeBakey clamp that we have good access in case of stapler misfiring. Now the middle hepatic vein can be staple divided.

We continue our parenchymal transection along the middle hepatic vein between segments IVa and VIII. However, we need to identify the drainage vein to segment VIII prior to completing our dissection. Now we have identified the drainage vein to segment VIII, from which we have some bleeding. The bleeding is controlled with a compress. As we have better exposure of the branch, we can place a vascular clamp. We expose the drainage vein to segment VIII further for later staple division. The segment VIII drainage vein is staple divided. Now the specimen is completely mobile and can be removed using an endoscopic retriever bag.

We complete the case by placing a collagenous sponge coated with fibrinogen and thrombin on the transection surface. Prior to completing the case, we inspect the middle hepatic vein staple line.

IMPORTANT POINTS

- Ensure that you have an optimal set-up prior to the parenchymal transection. This includes a set-up for retraction and Pringle maneuver.
- Intraoperative ultrasound is crucial.
- Leaving the falciform ligament as well as the gallbladder attached will help with retraction.
- Use anatomical landmarks so that you do not get lost during the parenchymal transection. Also, have an alternative resection plan in mind.

Anatomy figures

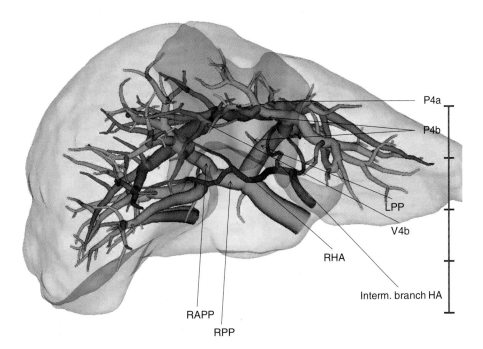

Figure v5.7 Critical anatomy for a resection of segment IV. The resection follows the main left and right PP. The key is that all short branches off the main PP are controlled to prevent bile leaks and injuries to the main PP. P4b and P4a often have a variable anatomy, with several portal branches feeding each segment. The intermediate branch of the HA is also controlled early. It can come off the LHA, the RHA, or between the RHA and LHA.

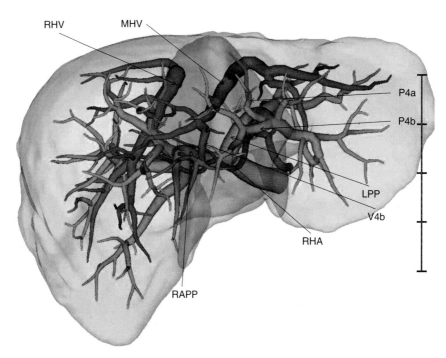

Figure v5.8 Relationship of portal structures and RHV and MHV. Dominant branches, especially those off the MHV, need to be controlled at the beginning of the parenchymal transection.

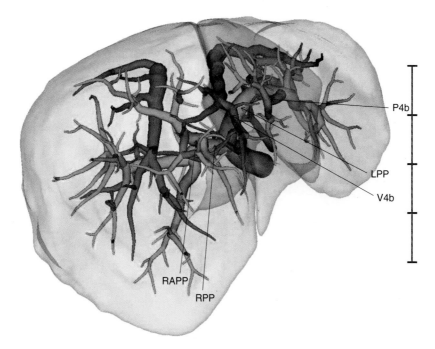

Figure v5.9 View along the parenchymal transection plane. If the MHV is included in the specimen, it is typically exposed during the parenchymal transection. Care needs to be taken to avoid injury to the LHV when dividing the MHV at its common drainage with the LHV into the IVC.

Segmentectomy IVa

Video duration 8 minutes 33 seconds

In this video, we will show you a resection of segment IVa.

Figure v6.1 demonstrates the port positioning which is slightly higher than during resection of segment IVb. Next, we will show the transection of the medial border between segments IVa and II. The umbilical fissure has been opened (see Video 7) and we are dissecting between segments III and IVb. The aim of this dissection is to expose the main left portal pedicle which gives out branches to segments IVa and b. In order to avoid an injury to the main portal pedicle, this dissection is carried out with scissors.

Here the left main portal pedicle has been exposed with its branches to segment IVa, II, and III (Figure v6.2). One of the branches to segment IVa is dissected out, clipped, and divided. We now continue our transection along the falciform ligament which has been divided earlier; this defines the border between segments IVa and II. We are now approaching the IVC where we will expose the drainage of the middle hepatic vein into the IVC. This

Port positioning

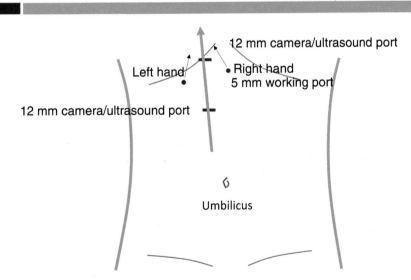

12 mm camera/ultrasound port

Left hand

Right hand
5 mm working port

12 mm camera/ultrasound port

Umbilicus

Figure v6.1 The port positioning for a segmentectomy 4a is slightly higher than that for a resection of segment IVb.

Laparoscopic Liver, Pancreas, and Biliary Surgery, First Edition.
Edited by Claudius Conrad and Brice Gayet.
© 2017 John Wiley & Sons, Ltd. Published 2017 by John Wiley & Sons, Ltd.

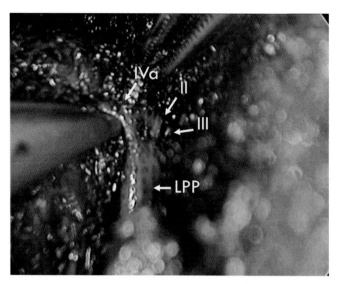

Figure v6.2 Here the left main PP has been exposed with its branches to segment IVa, II, and III.

dissection is carried out with a blunt suction tip or with scissors. Here, the drainage of the middle hepatic vein into the IVC has been exposed (Figure v6.3).

Next, we will show the transection between segments IVa and b. We divide the liver capsule along the line of the main left portal pedicle. At the bottom of the parenchymal transection line, you can see the main left portal pedicle. It is critical not to injure it. The main left portal pedicle is a good landmark to define the inferior border of segment IVa (Figure v6.4). Slightly more proximal to the portal branch of segment IVa, that has already been controlled, is an additional one that will be controlled with a clip and divided.

Next, we will dissect out and follow the middle hepatic vein which defines the lateral border of our dissection. Here, we are approaching the distal part of the middle hepatic vein. The middle hepatic vein comes into view (Figure v6.5).

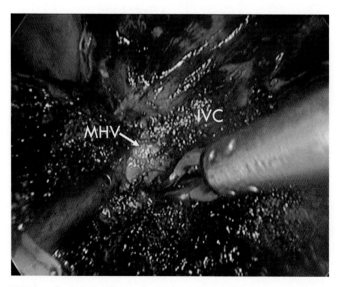

Figure v6.3 Drainage of the MHV into the IVC. Avoidance of a venous injury at this step is critical.

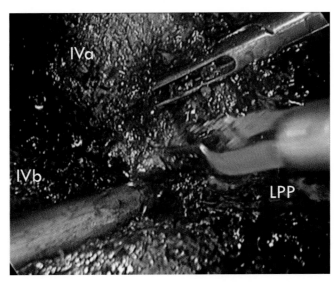

Figure v6.4 The main LPP is a good landmark to define the inferior border of segment IVa.

Using ultrasound, we identify the course of the middle hepatic vein between segments IVa and VIII. We open the capsule along the course of the middle hepatic vein. This parenchymal transection line will join with the earlier parenchymal transection between segments II and IVa. This will occur at the level of the hepatic venous confluence.

We deepen the transection until the middle hepatic vein is reached. With superior traction on the specimen, we join the parenchymal transection along the left portal pedicle, seen in the inferior part of the picture, and the middle hepatic vein. As you can see, we are completely exposing the medial aspect of the middle hepatic vein. Minor bleeding from small holes in the middle hepatic vein is controlled with bipolar forceps. At the confluence of the left and middle hepatic veins, the drainage vein to segment IVa is controlled (Figure v6.6). At this step, segment IVa is completely detached. This shows the resection cavity at the completion of the case with an exposed middle hepatic vein.

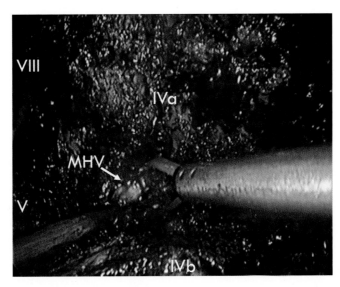

Figure v6.5 Here the distal part of the MHV has been exposed.

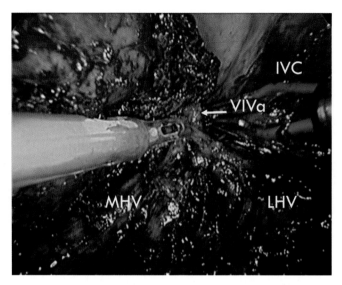

Figure v6.6 At the confluence of the LHV and MHV the drainage vein to segment IVa (VIVa) is controlled.

IMPORTANT POINTS

- Resection of segment IVa begins with opening the umbilical fissure.
- Be familiar the anatomical variants of the segment IV portal pedicle.
- Avoid injury to the left main portal pedicle and follow the middle hepatic vein to its drainage into the IVC.

Anatomy figures

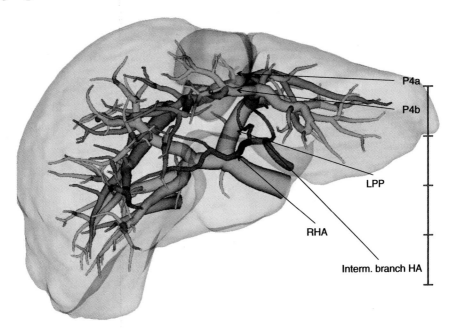

Figure v6.7 Critical anatomy for a resection of segment IVa. After opening the umbilical fissure, the first PP branch encountered is usually P4b. This needs to be preserved. As the parenchymal transection deepens, P4a will be encountered and needs to be controlled.

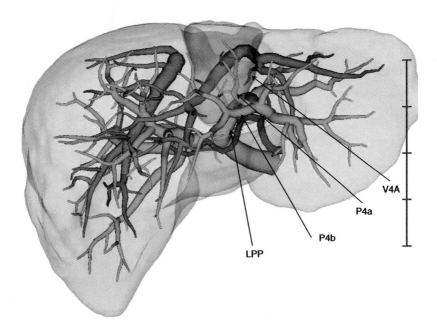

Figure v6.8 Relationship of portal structures and LHV and MHV. The parenchymal transection follows LHV and MHV. V4a branches need to be controlled.

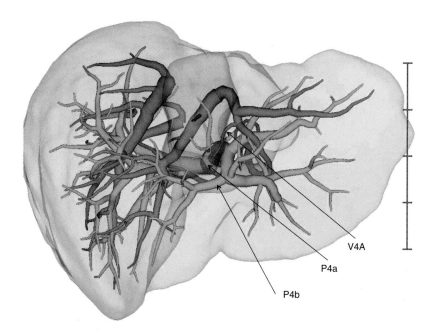

V4A

P4a

P4b

Figure v6.9 View from superior to inferior. The dorsal border of segment IVa is the IVC and the confluence of LHV and MHV. The confluence is usually several centimeters below the liver capsule but can also be very close.

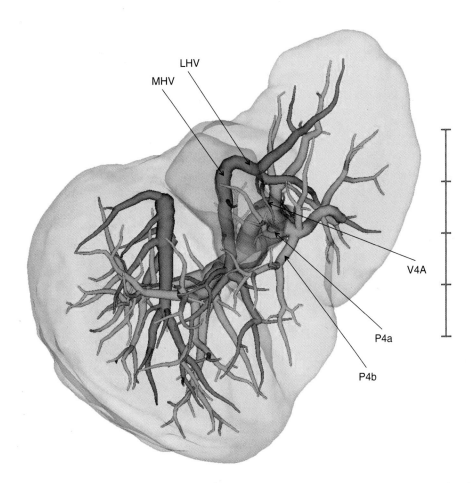

Figure v6.10 View from superior to inferior. The confluence (if present) of the LHV and MHV forms the dorsal border of segment IVb and is usually dissected last.

VIDEO 7

Segmentectomy IVb

Video duration 10 minutes 27 seconds

In this video, we demonstrate a IVb segmentectomy.

> **OUTLINE**
>
> The video is divided into the following parts:
> - Port positioning
> - Opening the umbilical fissure
> - Controlling the segment IVb pedicle
> - Dissection along the main left portal pedicle
> - Transection between segments IVb and V
> - Transection between segments IVa and IVb
> - Important points.

Figure v7.1 demonstrates the port positioning. The first step is opening the umbilical fissure. Here you see the large lesion in segment IVb. We place an umbilical tape around the porta in case a Pringle maneuver becomes necessary. While leaving the ligamentum teres and falciform ligament intact, we are opening the umbilical fissure. Injury to the portal structures in the left lateral sector at this step needs to be avoided. The parenchymal bridge between the left lateral and medial sectors is divided. This helps with opening the umbilical fissure. We are now further opening the umbilical fissure along the falciform ligament. By deepening this parenchymal transection line, we will approach the portal pedicles to segments IVa and b (Figure v7.2).

Next, we will control the portal pedicle to segment IVb. Here you can see the segment IVb portal pedicle above the

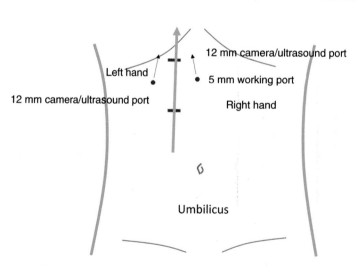

Figure v7.1 Port positioning for a segmentectomy IVb.

Laparoscopic Liver, Pancreas, and Biliary Surgery, First Edition.
Edited by Claudius Conrad and Brice Gayet.
© 2017 John Wiley & Sons, Ltd. Published 2017 by John Wiley & Sons, Ltd.

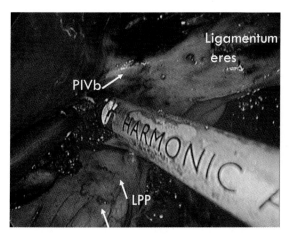

Figure v7.2 By deepening this parenchymal transection line, we will approach the portal pedicles to segments IVa and b.

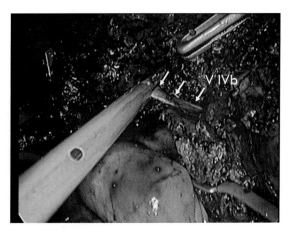

Figure v7.4 The segmental drainage vein to IVb is completely dissected out.

bipolar forceps (Figure v7.2). The IVb portal pedicle is completely dissected out. In order to avoid a thermal injury to the left portal pedicle, we are using scissors at this step. Once the IVb portal pedicle is completely dissected out, it is clipped and divided. Here we are continuing to deepen the transection lie between segments III and IVb.

Next, we perform the dissection along the left main portal pedicle. The first step of this dissection is lowering the hilar plate. You can see the gallbladder at the left side

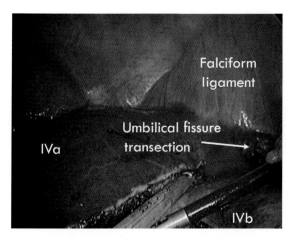

Figure v7.3 This parenchymal transection line will ultimately join the earlier parenchymal transection line along the umbilical fissure.

of the image. Here we are dissecting the left main portal pedicle superiorly. This parenchymal transection line will ultimately join the earlier parenchymal transection line along the umbilical fissure (Figure v7.3). Next, we will transect the liver between segments IVb and V. We can see a good demarcation of segment IVb. We recommend leaving the gallbladder attached as a handle. It is important to avoid injury to the middle hepatic vein at this step. Here, the drainage vein of segment IVb comes into view which drains into the middle hepatic vein; we will control it later in the case.

The final step is transection between segments IVa and IVb. The parenchymal transection line between IVa and IVb will join the earlier transection line along the umbilical fissure. Here, we are dissecting out the drainage vein to segment IVb. The segmental drainage vein to IVb is completely dissected out (Figure v7.4). It is clipped and divided. Here the two parenchymal transection lines are joining. Now the specimen is completely detached from the rest of the liver.

IMPORTANT POINTS

- Avoid bile leaks from IVb portal pedicle variants.
- Do not injure the portal pedicle to segment IVa.
- Leave the gallbladder and falciform ligament attached for retraction.
- Avoid injury to the main left portal pedicle.

Anatomy figures

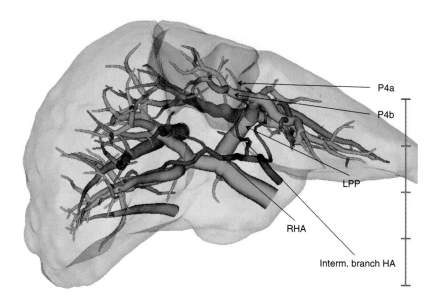

Figure v7.5 Critical anatomy for a resection of segment IVa. After opening the umbilical fissure, the first PP branch encountered is usually P4b. This needs to be preserved. As the parenchymal transection deepens, P4a will be encountered and needs to be controlled.

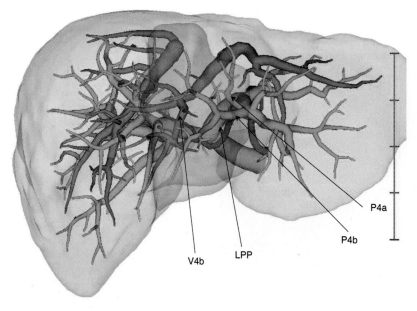

Figure v7.6 Relationship of portal structures and LHV and MHV. The parenchymal transection follows the LHV and MHV. V4a branches need to be controlled.

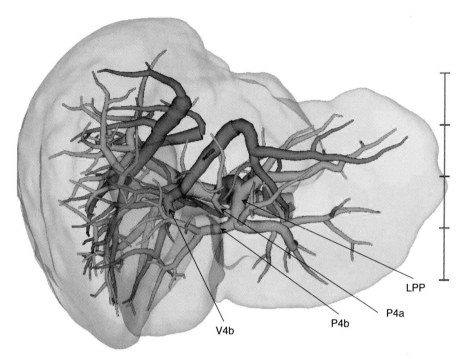

LPP

P4a

P4b

V4b

Figure v7.7 View from superior to inferior. It is difficult to define the precise border between segments IVb and IVa if there is no good demarcation after taking P4b. Note also that the border usually does not follow a straight line.

VIDEO 8

Bisegmentectomy IVb and V

Video duration 9 minutes 0 seconds

In this video we demonstrate a bisegmentectomy of segments IVb and V.

Figure v8.1 demonstrates the port positioning. Segments IVb and V are centrally located and a good understanding of the anatomy is important, which we will gain from the intraoperative ultrasound.

First, we open up the liver between segments III and IVb. This will be the landing zone of our dissection and will help us orient during intraoperative ultrasound. In Figure v8.2, we can see the relationship between the tumor, the ventral branch of segment VIII, and the anterior portal pedicle. The portal branch to segment V goes into the tumor. The border between segments V and VI is defined by the right hepatic vein which we identify here (Figure v8.3). This will be our lateral border of transection. With ultrasound, we identify the inferior border of our transection which is the anterior portal pedicle (Figure v8.4. With ultrasound control, we begin our parenchymal transection between the borders of segment V and segment VI defined by the right hepatic vein.

Next, we would like to show you the parenchymal transection. We deepen our parenchymal transection which we have begun using ultrasound control. We open up the liver

Port positioning

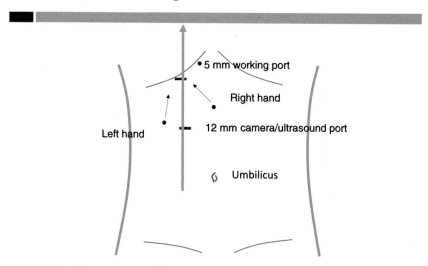

Figure v8.1 Port Positioning for a bisegmentectomy IVb/V.

Laparoscopic Liver, Pancreas, and Biliary Surgery, First Edition.
Edited by Claudius Conrad and Brice Gayet.
© 2017 John Wiley & Sons, Ltd. Published 2017 by John Wiley & Sons, Ltd.

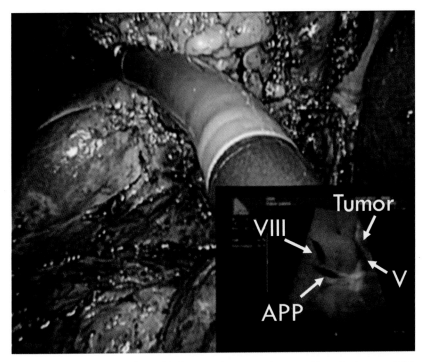

Figure v8.2 This ultrasound image shows the relationship between the tumor, the ventral branch of segment VIII, segment V pedicle, and the APP.

capsule to the inferior portion of our parenchymal transection defined by the anterior portal pedicle. Using ultrasound again, we confirm the location of the portal branch of segment V going into the tumor. From the air artifacts, we can see that the transection line is close to the anterior portal pedicle, the inferior border of our parenchymal transection line (Figure v8.5). Dissection at the anterior portal pedicle is done with scissors. We are now dissecting the border between segments V and VIII. This dissection will join the earlier transection line at the border between segments III and IVb.

Now that the parenchymal transection line has been defined, we can deepen our dissection. Here we are dissecting at the border between segments IVb and IVa. The most distal drainage of the middle hepatic vein is controlled using bipolar forceps. Using ultrasound control, we dissect out the portal branch to segment V going into the tumor. At this step, the dissection of the portal branch of segment V has been completed and we can proceed to the portal pedicle dissection. The suction tip aids in the dissection of the portal

pedicle. At this step, we are dissecting the cystic duct and the cystic artery for better exposure of the portal pedicle. Next, we separate the hilar plate from the portal structures, using laparoscopic scissors. With the Doppler flow mode on the ultrasound, we confirm excellent flow to segment VIII.

After we have confirmed that the portal pedicle to segment V is isolated and there is good flow to the rest of the portal pedicle, we can proceed with transecting it. We transect the portal branch to segment V using scissors. At this step, the specimen is completely detached and we are confirming excellent hemostasis.

By injecting air through the cystic duct we confirm that (1) there is no bile leak, and (2) there is excellent biliary drainage to the anterior sector. The white air artifacts confirm the presence of excellent biliary drainage. Also, the lack of air bubbles at the parenchymal transection surface confirms the absence of a bile leak. The cystic duct is controlled using an Endoloop; this is the final operative site.

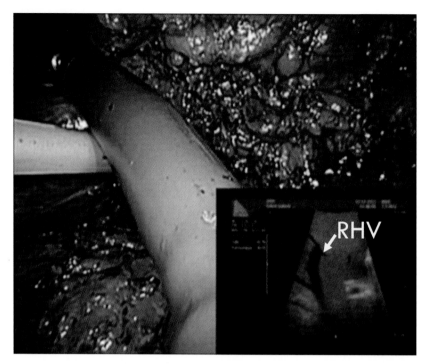

Figure v8.3 The border between segments V and VI is defined by the RHV.

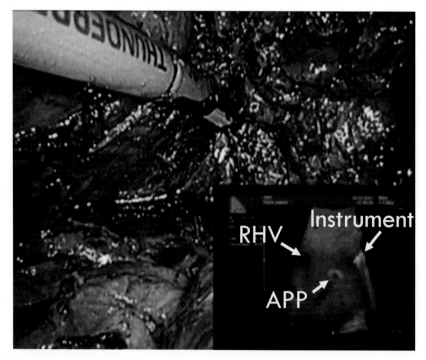

Figure v8.4 With ultrasound, we identify the inferior border of our transection which is the APP.

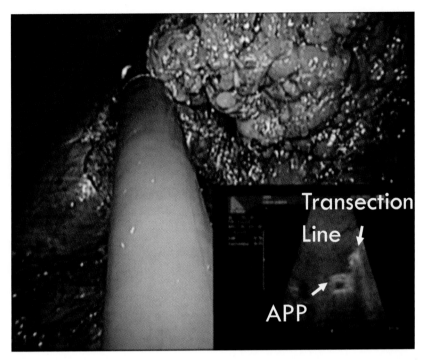

Figure v8.5 The air artifacts demonstrate that the transection line is close to the APP, the inferior border of our parenchymal transection line.

IMPORTANT POINTS

- Have a good preoperative understanding of the portal branching.
- Use ultrasound to anticipate anatomical landmarks.
- Spend time on the hemostasis during the parenchymal transection for excellent working conditions.
- Confirm drainage to the remaining segments using ultrasound.

Anatomy figures

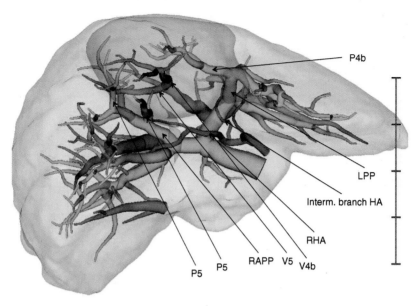

Figure v8.6 Critical anatomy for resection of segments IVb and V. After opening the umbilical fissure, the first PP branch encountered is P4b which is controlled. P4a can be close behind P4b. Also, there can be (most commonly) more than one P4b branches. If an intermediate branch of the HA is present, it should be taken. There are usually several PPs to segment V coming off the RAPP.

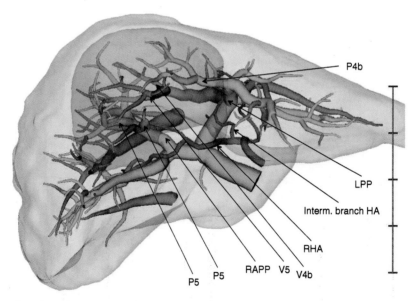

Figure v8.7 Relationship of portal structures and V4b and V5 drainage veins. The MHV bisects segments IVb and V. It gives off drainage veins to segments IVb and V. Injury to the RAPP during dissection of the inferior border of segment V should be avoided.

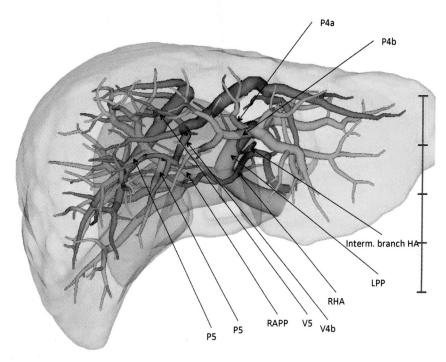

Figure v8.8 View from ventral to dorsal. Segment V is especially rich in portal pedicles and drainage veins that need to be controlled during parenchymal transection.

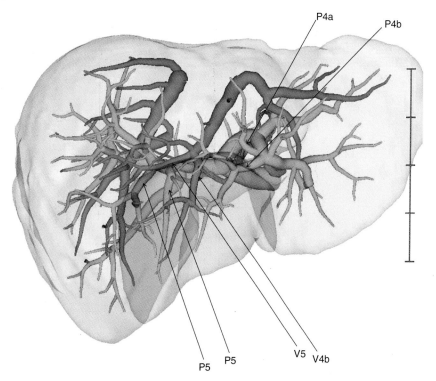

Figure v8.9 View from superior to inferior. The RHV is the lateral border of the transection. RHV can give off prominent drainage veins to segment V. V5 and V4b drainage veins from the MHV will be encountered when performing the superior aspect of the parenchymal transection.

VIDEO 9

Segmentectomy VI

Video duration 9 minutes 44 seconds

In this video, we present an anatomical resection of segment VI.

> **OUTLINE**
>
> The outline of this video is as follows:
> - Port positioning
> - Distinction between P6 and P7 on ultrasound
> - Dissection of the hepatocaval ligament
> - Dissection of Rouviere's sulcus
> - Parenchymal transection
> - Important points.

The port portioning for resection of segment VI is more variable than for other segmentectomies. In general, the ports are placed more laterally (Figure v9.1). An effective approach might be to place an umbilical port first and then to place the rest of the ports depending upon the relative location of the liver.

Next, we identify important structures for resection of segment VI. One important landmark structure is the right hepatic vein (Figure v9.2), which defines the medial border of segment VI. Very important is the branching of the right posterior portal pedicle (RPPP) into P6 and P7 you will learn more about this later in the video.

We will begin the dissection at the hepatocaval ligament; the dissection of Rouviere's sulcus will end up at the hepatocaval ligament. Performing this dissection early in the case gives us a safe landing zone. This is the view along the IVC and segment VI can be seen on the left side with the lesion. Short hepatic vein branches are controlled using thermofusion. In addition, we transect the right triangular

Port positioning

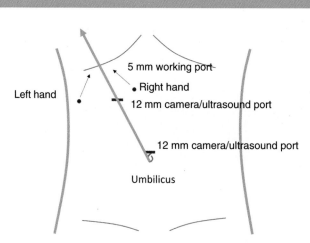

Figure v9.1 The port portioning for resection of segment VI is more variable than for other segmentectomies. In general, the ports are placed more laterally and placing the patient in left decubitus position can improve degree of freedom of the instruments.

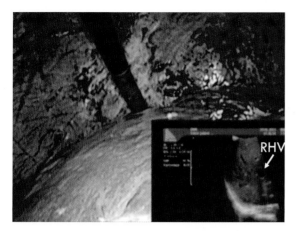

Figure v9.2 The RHV constitutes the medial border of segment 6 and should be identified at the beginning of the case.

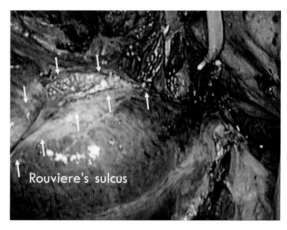

Figure v9.4 We achieve control of the portal branch to segment VI through opening up Rouviere's sulcus. Notice that the RPP is very close to the surface of Rouviere's sulcus.

ligament in order to mobilize the liver. We achieve control of the portal branch to segment VI through opening up Rouviere's sulcus (Figure v9.3). Here, we can see the dissection of the hepatoduodenal ligament which is located on the right side of the image. Please bear in mind that the portal branches to the caudate lobe can be found at this location and must be controlled early, prior to beginning the parenchymal transection.

We will control the portal branch to segment VI through opening up Rouviere's sulcus (Figure v9.4). Please be careful when you open up this capsule as the portal structures can be found very close. Opening up Rouviere's sulcus will help in performing intraoperative

ultrasound. The air artifacts can help identify the right posterior portal pedicle. Pushing with forceps in the sulcus on the right posterior portal pedicle ensures that we are distal to the location where the segment VII portal pedicle arises (Figure v9.5, Figure v9.6).

As mentioned earlier, our landmark structure is the right hepatic vein which defines the medial border of segment VI. It can be seen here in the middle of the image. Here we are controlling a portal branch going into segment VI. Here we are connecting the dissection of Rouviere's sulcus with the earlier dissection of the hepatocaval ligament. Indocyanine green counterstaining can be helpful

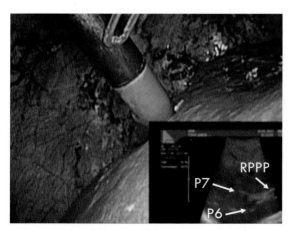

Figure v9.3 Opening up Rouviere's sulcus will help in performing intraoperative ultrasound. RPPP divides on the ultrasound image into P6 and P7.

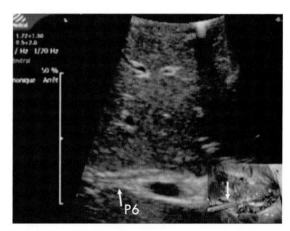

Figure v9.5 Pushing with forceps in the sulcus on the RPPP ensures that we are distal to the take-off of the segment VII portal pedicle.

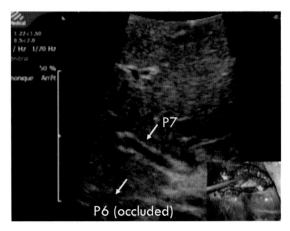

Figure v9.6 On this image P6 has been occluded while P7 is preserved.

to define the border to neighboring segments. Here you can see the border between segments V and VI. Here we have connected the dissection of Rouviere's sulcus to the dissection of the hepatocaval ligament.

The final step is the dissection along the right hepatic vein. Ultrasound is crucial in identifying the right hepatic vein in its intraparenchymal location. After opening the parenchyma along the right hepatic vein, we confirm that we have a good flow to the portal branch of segment VII.

Finally, we control the drainage vein of segment VI into the right hepatic vein. We detach the specimen and remove it from the abdomen using an endoscopic retriever bag.

IMPORTANT POINTS

- In general, the ports are placed more lateral than for a right hepatectomy.
- Early dissection of the hepatocaval ligament allows for safe opening of Rouviere's sulcus to dissect out the segment VI portal branch.
- Use ultrasound to identify the branching between segments VI and VII of the right posterior portal pedicle.
- The right hepatic vein defines the medial border of segment VI and should guide your parenchymal transection.

Anatomy figures

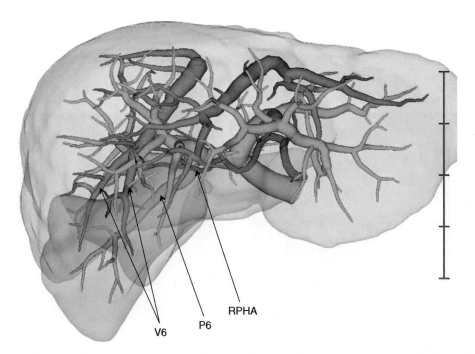

Figure v9.7 Critical anatomy for resection of segment VI. This patient has a prominent PP to segment VI. V6 drainage veins come off the RHV.

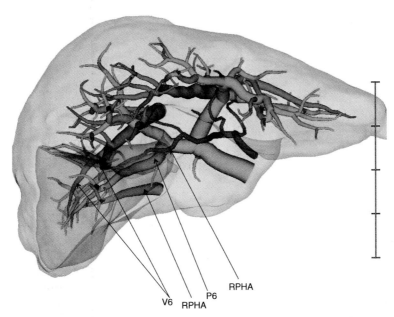

Figure v9.8 Relationship of portal structures and V6 drainage veins. Notice the relationship between the PP to segment VI and the RIHV and the V6 drainage veins into the RHV.

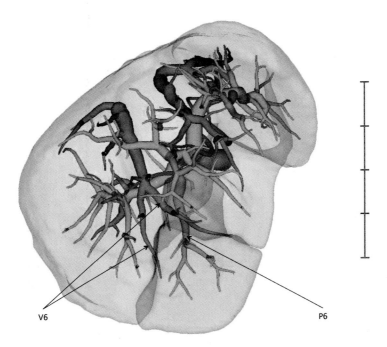

Figure v9.9 View from superior to inferior. Notice the close relationship between the P6 and the two V6 drainage veins.

VIDEO 10
Segmentectomy VII

Video duration 8 minutes 23 seconds

In this video, we will demonstrate a resection of segment VII.

The patient is positioned in a modified French position. The legs are in stirrups, the left side is down and the right side is up, and the right arm is positioned above the patient's head. The surgeon stands either on the right side or between the legs of the patient. The ports are positioned as shown in Figure v10.1. The 12 mm port for the camera has to be positioned high enough to enable a good view of the drainage of the right hepatic vein into the IVC.

In this patient, the left lateral sector has already been removed. Here you can see placement of the two 12 mm ports. A balloon port for the high 12 mm port ensures opposition of the diaphragm. Next we perform an intra-operative ultrasound. A key structure to identify is the

Port positioning

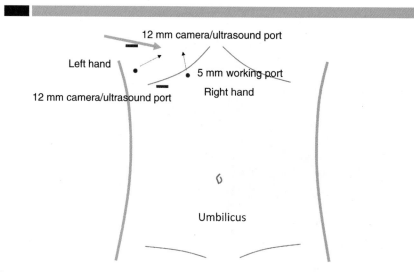

Figure v10.1 The patient is positioned in a modified French position. The legs are in stirrups, the left side is down and the right side is up, and the right arm is positioned above the patient's head. The surgeon stands either on the right side or between the legs of the patient.

Laparoscopic Liver, Pancreas, and Biliary Surgery, First Edition.
Edited by Claudius Conrad and Brice Gayet.
© 2017 John Wiley & Sons, Ltd. Published 2017 by John Wiley & Sons, Ltd.

right hepatic vein and its drainage into the IVC. The right hepatic vein constitutes the medial border of segment VII. Here we open the parenchyma right above the drainage of the right hepatic vein into the IVC. It is important to avoid the injury of the right hepatic vein at this step. Here we continue to deepen the parenchymal transection plane in order to expose the drainage of the right hepatic vein into the IVC.

Next, we will show the dissection along the IVC. For this part, we are using scissors. A small hole in the IVC or the right hepatic vein made by scissors can be more easily repaired than a hole made with an energy device. Blunt dissection with the suction tip at this step can also be very helpful.

Next, we show the exposure of the right hepatic vein along the medial border of segment VII. Using the blunt suction tip for dissection, we are exposing the lateral wall of the right hepatic vein. The next step would be controlling the venous branches draining segment VII into the right hepatic vein. Here the dominant drainage vein of segment VII comes into view. Using ultrasound with Doppler flow and the laparoscopic vascular clamp, we confirm that we have indeed exposed the drainage vein of segment VII. On this image, we can see two drainage veins of segment VII (Figure v10.2). On this Doppler image, the right hepatic vein is demonstrated.

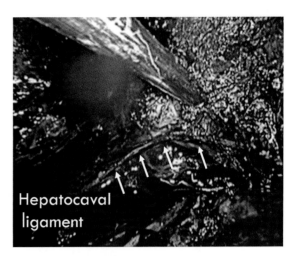

Figure v10.3 Finally the hepatocaval ligament is transected.

We can now proceed to clipping and dividing the drainage vein of segment VII. The second drainage vein to segment VII is exposed, clipped, and divided. We have identified it previously using ultrasound with Doppler flow. Next, we will dissect the border between segments VI and VII and control the pedicle to segment VII. The liver is elevated with the liver retractor and we are deepening our parenchymal transection line between segments VI and VII. Here, we have identified the portal pedicle to segment VII which we will control using the bipolar forceps.

The final steps are mobilizing the specimen off the IVC. Some blunt dissection with the suction tip can be helpful at this step. Finally we will transect the hepatocaval ligament (Figure v10.3).

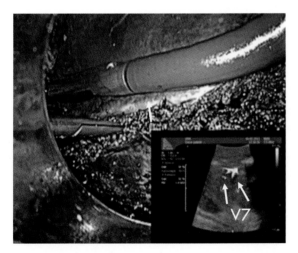

Figure v10.2 Using ultrasound with Doppler flow and the laparoscopic vascular clamp, we confirm that we have indeed exposed the drainage vein of segment VII. The two drainage veins of segment VII can be seen.

IMPORTANT POINTS

- It is important to position the trocars high transdiaphragmatically.
- The right hepatic vein serves as a landmark.
- Dissection at the IVC is carried out with scissors.
- The segment VII portal pedicle is best identified using ultrasound.
- It is critical to avoid injury to the segment VI portal pedicle.

Anatomy figures

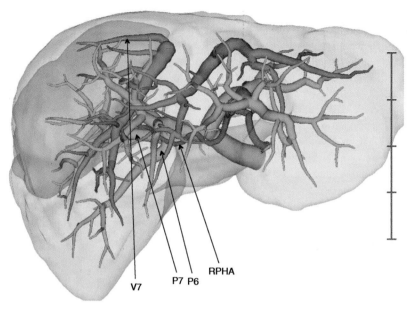

Figure v10.4 Critical anatomy for resection of segment VII. The patient has a trifuction of P6, P7, and RAPP. Several drainage veins constitute the RHV.

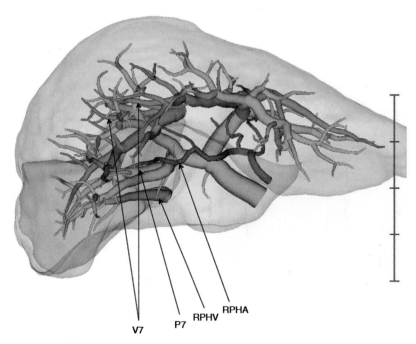

Figure v10.5 Relationship of PP P7 and V7 drainage veins. P7 can come off a common RPPP or form a trifurcation, as is seen in this patient. Usually P7 is superior and posterior to P6. When controlling P7, injury to P6 has to be avoided.

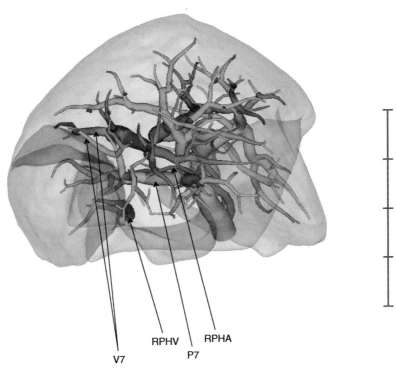

Figure v10.6 View from lateral to medial. An RPHV, in addition to several drainage veins off the RHV, drains segment VII in this patient.

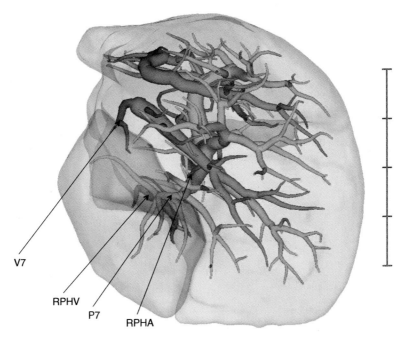

Figure v10.7 View from lateral to medial. Injury to the RHV, especially at its drainage into the IVC, needs to be avoided during the parenchymal transection of the superior border.

VIDEO 11

Segmentectomy VIII (transthoracic access)

Video duration 6 minutes 41 seconds

In this video, we demonstrate a segmentectomy of segment VIII using a transthoracic access.

> **OUTLINE**
>
> The video is divided into the following parts:
> - Transthoracic port placement
> - Determining the borders of segment VIII
> - Parenchymal transection and dissection
> - Management of bleeding
> - Important points.

Let's start with port placement (Figure v11.1). The scheme demonstrates the port positioning. Here we show port positioning under the costal margin, and in the 10th and 11th intercostal space. For the intercostal trocars, we use cuffed ports. This will help to keep the diaphragm out of the field.

The next step of the operation is determining the anatomical borders of segment VIII. The scar indicates the lesion in segment VIII. Using ultrasound, we identify the portal branch to segment VIII (Figure v11.2). The tumor is superior to it and can be seen as well. We are now injecting indocyanine green to this branch to stain segment VIII. This is done with ultrasound guidance. An ultrasound head that facilitates the cannula greatly helps with this process. Although the medial border stains nicely, the inferior and lateral margins are not well demarcated. We therefore revert to ultrasound guidance to stain the inferior and lateral margins. Here we use the right hepatic vein as a landmark. This determines the lateral border of segment VIII.

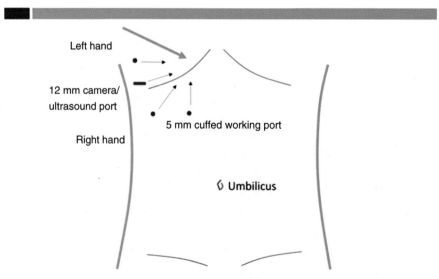

Figure v11.1 Ports are placed just under the costal margin and the 10th and 11th intercostal space.

Laparoscopic Liver, Pancreas, and Biliary Surgery, First Edition.
Edited by Claudius Conrad and Brice Gayet.
© 2017 John Wiley & Sons, Ltd. Published 2017 by John Wiley & Sons, Ltd.

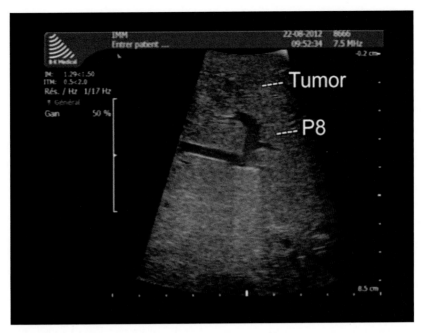

Figure v11.2 Using ultrasound, we identify the portal branch to segment VIII. The tumor is superior to it and can also be seen.

The next step covers parenchymal transection and dissection. Hemostasis is facilitated with the fenestrated bipolar forceps. Here you can see the dissection of the medial border of segment VIII (Figure v11.3). The dissection of the coronary ligament bearing the suprahepatic part of the IVC is performed using scissors. Scissors allow

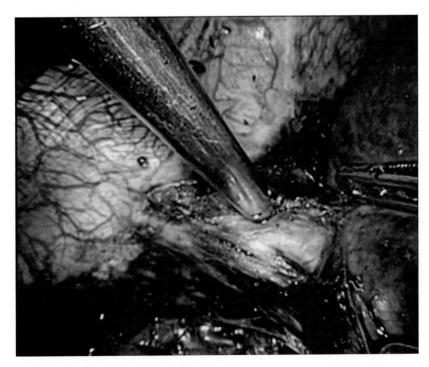

Figure v11.3 The suprahepatic IVC has been dissected out using scissors.

more tactile feedback than the harmonic cutting device. Also, an injury with the scissors can be more easily repaired than one caused by a harmonic cutting device.

At this step, the superior border of segment VIII has been entirely dissected out. We now continue the dissection at the inferior border of segment VIII, approaching the portal branch feeding the segment. We now clip the portal branch to segment VIII and divide it with scissors. Now the posterior border of segment VIII is dissected off the middle hepatic vein. In this last step, we encounter some significant bleeding and we will show you some of our techniques in managing this bleeding. At this step, we encounter bleeding from the middle hepatic vein. We apply bipolar coagulation directly to major hepatic veins which can be very helpful. In order to determine the exact location of the bleeding, we are improving exposure. This unfortunately leads to more bleeding. The bleeding is temporarily controlled with the bipolar forceps until a vascular clamp can be applied. As there is still some bleeding, we introduce gauze into the abdomen which can be applied to the bleeding site with compression. In addition, parenchymal compression can be applied which can stop bleeding temporarily. As the hole in the middle hepatic vein has been clearly identified, we suture close the hole. Now that the bleeding has been controlled, we

continue the parenchymal transection along the superior border of segment VIII.

Segment VIII is now almost completely mobile and superior traction helps to detach the segment from the rest of the liver. The exposed MHV, as well as the portal branch, confirms the anatomical resection of segment VIII. Before completing the case, we go back to inspect the bleeding from the middle hepatic vein. As this is continuing, we apply a patch soaked in human thrombin and fibrinogen to the bleeding site. Wrapping the patch in gauze helps with the laparoscopic application.

IMPORTANT POINTS

- Transthoracic access provides an excellent view of segment VIII.
- Laparoscopic ultrasound is essential for anatomical resection of segment VIII.
- Using scissors for the dissection of critical structures adds safety.
- The laparoscopic liver surgeon needs to be well versed in the various techniques of controlling bleeding laparoscopically. This is especially true when attacking a challenging case such as an anatomical resection of segment VIII.

Anatomy figures

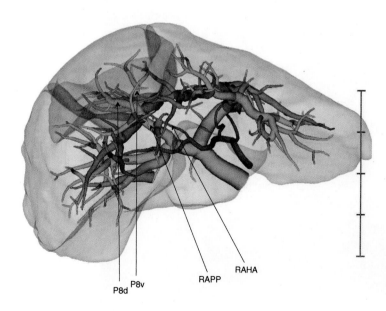

Figure v11.4 Critical anatomy for resection of segment VIII. The typical portal branching of segment VIII is a dominant P8 ventral and P8 dorsal PP coming off the RAPP.

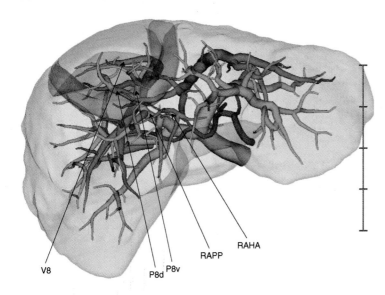

Figure v11.5 Portal pedicle to segment VIII. At the distal end of the RAPP is P8v and P8d. The V8 drainage vein can be a dominant branch close to the drainage of the RHV into the IVC (as in this patient). Injury to this branch during either a laparoscopic right hepatectomy or a segmentectomy VIII can lead to significant bleeding. Therefore we recommend identifying this branch on preoperative imaging and during the dissection.

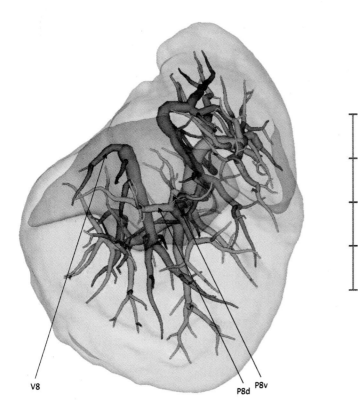

Figure v11.6 View from superior to inferior. Segment VIII drains into the RHV and MHV. This patient has prominent V8 drainage veins of the RHV. A prominent V8 drainage vein (not this patient) can come off the MHV which can be easily injured near the end of the parenchymal transection for a right hepatectomy.

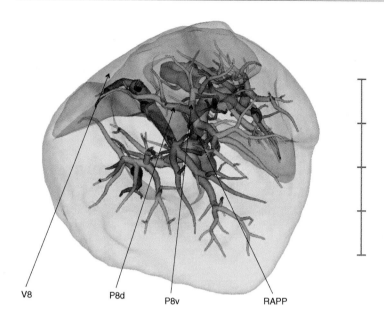

V8   P8d   P8v   RAPP

Figure v11.7 View from lateral to medial. Notice the relationship of P8 ventral and P8 dorsal and the RHV and MHV.

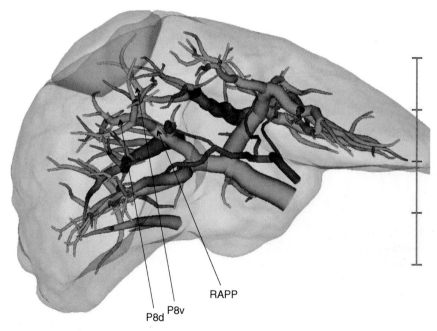

RAPP

P8d   P8v

Figure v11.8 Sub-segmentectomy segment VIII ventral. With the knowledge of portal branching into P8 ventral and dorsal, anatomical resection of the sub-segments of segment VIII can be performed. Since segment VIII is a large segment, knowledge of this branching allows for parenchyma-sparing surgery.

VIDEO 12
Left hepatectomy

Video duration 13 minutes 24 seconds

In this video we will demonstrate a left hepatectomy.

OUTLINE

The video is divided into the following parts:

- Port positioning
- Mobilization of the left liver
- Ultrasound
- Portal dissection
- Parenchymal transection
- Division of the left hepatic vein
- Important points.

First, we would like to show you the port positioning (Figure v12.1). The port positioning of the right and left hepatectomy is similar. However, for a left hepatectomy, the line of transection is more towards the left and more in a craniocaudal direction. This is the port positioning for the portal dissection. As the parenchymal transection progresses, we move to this port positioning (Figure v12.2).

Next, we will show you mobilization of the left liver. We begin by taking down the falciform ligament. Now that the coronary and triangular ligaments have been dissected, the left lobe of the liver is mobile. A very important component of this operation is the intraoperative ultrasound. Identification of the middle hepatic vein is crucial for the parenchymal transection (Figure v12.3). Having an accurate understanding of the precise location of the middle hepatic vein will help you to avoid getting lost with the two-dimensional view of

the laparoscopic camera. The other important structure is drainage of the left hepatic vein into the IVC (Figure v12.4). Identifying the presence of an umbilical fissure vein will avoid its injury and significant bleeding.

The next step is the portal dissection, which begins with transection of the cystic duct. The hilar plate is lowered and we leave the gallbladder attached as a handle. We now focus the dissection on the left portal pedicle. Here, the Glissonian sheath of the left portal pedicle is opened. Then we open up the hepatoduodenal ligament. We continue the dissection along the ligament of Arantius. This gives us more mobility of the liver and we can continue the dissection of the left portal pedicle. For dissection of the left portal pedicle, we open the hepatoduodenal ligament more widely. The first structure that has been dissected out is the left hepatic artery. The main left hepatic artery and the branch to segment IV are dissected out individually. In the background, the left portal vein comes into view. The left hepatic artery is clipped and divided. Back bleeding is controlled with thermofusion. Now the anterior branch to segment IV is divided using thermofusion. We continue to mobilize the left portal vein off the Glissonian sheath. Once the left portal vein is completely dissected out, it is clipped and divided.

The last step of portal dissection is dissecting out the left bile duct. Using a right-angled dissector, we dissect the left bile duct off the Glissonian sheath. We clip the distal part and we will divide proximally. After division of the bile duct, you can see the proximal lumen which we will

Laparoscopic Liver, Pancreas, and Biliary Surgery, First Edition.
Edited by Claudius Conrad and Brice Gayet.
© 2017 John Wiley & Sons, Ltd. Published 2017 by John Wiley & Sons, Ltd.

Port positioning

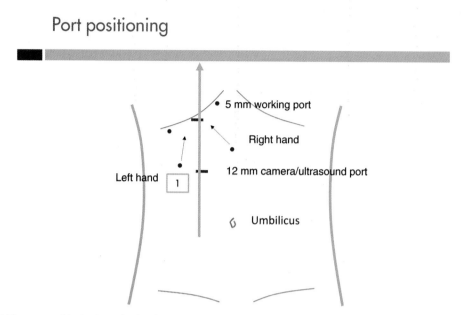

Figure v12.1 The port positioning is similar for the right and left hepatectomy. However, for a left hepatectomy, the line of transection is more towards the left and more in a craniocaudal direction.

suture close. When the bile duct is divided close to its take-off from the common bile duct, suture closing it will avoid stricturing of the remaining right bile duct.

Next we will show you the parenchymal transection. The landmarks for the parenchymal transection are the middle hepatic vein identified earlier on ultrasound as well as the

demarcation line. As we can see here, leaving the gallbladder attached after division of the cystic duct allows it to act as a handle. Here we are getting right on the middle hepatic vein and dividing the drainage vein of segment IVb.

The drainage vein to segment IVb is clipped and divided using thermofusion. We continue to divide the liver

Port positioning

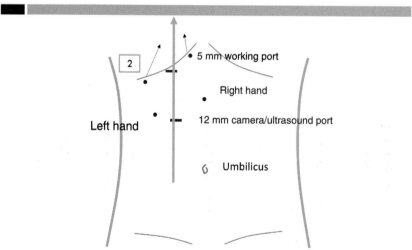

Figure v12.2 As the parenchymal transection progresses and we approach the hepatic venous confluence we move to this port positioning.

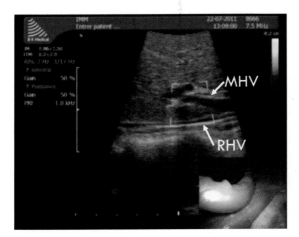

Figure v12.3 Identification of the MHV is crucial for the parenchymal transection.

capsule following the line of demarcation. Following the middle hepatic vein ensures an optimal line of parenchymal transection. Here we are identifying the drainage vein to segment IVa. The drainage vein is clipped and divided. As we continue the parenchymal transection, we reach the dome of the liver. Here we will find the drainage of the left hepatic vein and middle hepatic vein into the IVC. Here we can see the origin of the middle hepatic vein being dissected out.

The last step is division of the left hepatic vein. Prior to division, we always check whether we have a good angle to place a vascular clamp in case of stapler misfiring. Now the left hepatic vein is staple divided. Finally, we check for parenchymal bleeding at the resection surface and stop it using the bipolar forceps. Here we can see the exposed middle hepatic vein as well as the drainage veins to segments V and VIII. We go back and check the transected portal structures. We notice some bile leakage from the left bile duct which we control using suture closure.

The last step of the operation is removing the gallbladder. Finally, we would like to give you an overview of our dissection.

IMPORTANT POINTS

- Mobilize the left lobe early.
- Use ultrasound to identify the middle hepatic vein and left hepatic vein origin.
- Leave the gallbladder attached as a handle.
- Do not get lost during the parenchymal transection; let the middle hepatic vein guide you.
- Have a laparoscopic vascular clamp ready when staple dividing the left hepatic vein.

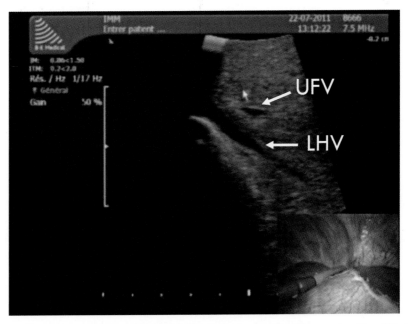

Figure v12.4 Drainage of the LHV into the IVC. Identifying the presence of an umbilical fissure vein will avoid its injury and significant bleeding.

Anatomy figures

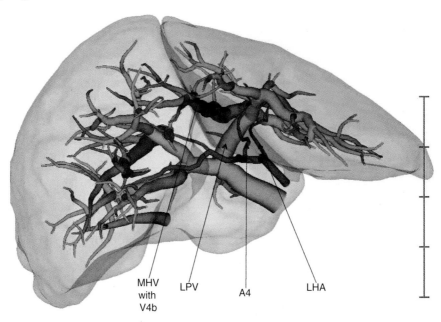

MHV with V4b   LPV   A4   LHA

Figure v12.5 Critical view during the portal dissection for a left hepatectomy. Usually, the A4 artery (intermediate branch of the LHA) is divided first. It is critical to identify the branching of the main portal vein into its left and right branch. This will avoid narrowing of the right portal vein. Once the parenchymal transection is begun at the border between S4b and 5, the horizontal crossing V4b drainage vein into the MHV will be identified.

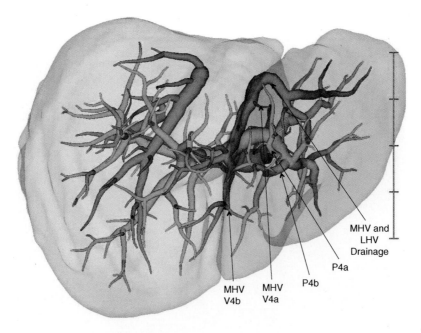

MHV and LHV Drainage   P4a   P4b   MHV V4b   MHV V4a

Figure v12.6 View at the beginning of the parenchymal transection. Once the portal structures have been controlled, the parenchymal transection follows the MHV. Two branches draining S4b are identified. As the transection progresses, the V4a drainage vein is identified. The MHV and LHV will often share a common drainage into the IVC.

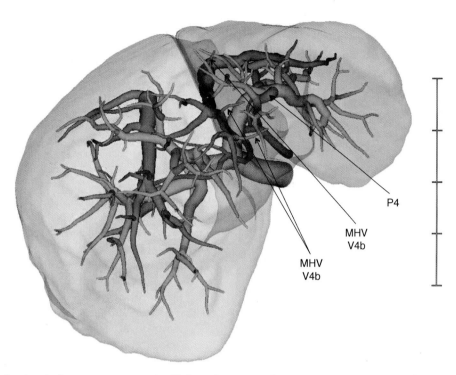

Figure v12.7 The view the laparoscopic surgeon should obtain during parenchymal transection. By orienting the camera along the axis of the MHV, the optimal view for the parenchymal transection is obtained. Small radicals of the P4a and b pedicle might reach to the parenchymal transection plane.

VIDEO 13
Right hepatectomy

Video duration 16 minutes 31 seconds

In this video, we demonstrate a laparoscopic right hepatectomy.

> **OUTLINE**
>
> The video is divided into the following parts:
> - Portal dissection
> - Parenchymal transection
> - Division of right hepatic vein
> - Specimen mobilization
> - Important points.

Figure v13.1 demonstrates the port positioning. The first 12 mm port is placed between the costal margin and the umbilicus. With this port and two 5 mm working ports, the portal dissection can be completed. Make sure not to place this port too low.

The second 12 mm port is placed to the right at the costal margin; this will allow completion of the parenchymal transection and dissection of the right hepatic vein. Here we show the 12 mm port coming into the right at the costal margin (Figure v13.2); notice the distance between this port and the liver.

The next step will be intraoperative ultrasound and identification of the middle hepatic vein. With the ultrasound, you are not only ruling out lesions in the future liver remnant – you are also identifying the middle hepatic vein as a landmark for the lateral parenchymal transection.

In order to lower the hilar plate, we divide the cystic duct and cystic artery. However, we recommend leaving

Port positioning

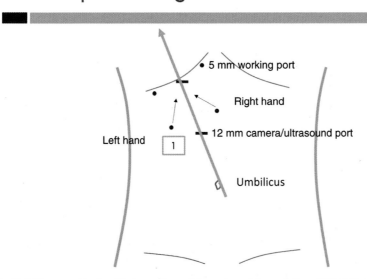

Figure v13.1 The first 12 mm port is placed between the costal margin and the umbilicus. With this port and two 5 mm working ports, the portal dissection can be completed. Make sure not to place this port too low.

Laparoscopic Liver, Pancreas, and Biliary Surgery, First Edition.
Edited by Claudius Conrad and Brice Gayet.
© 2017 John Wiley & Sons, Ltd. Published 2017 by John Wiley & Sons, Ltd.

Port positioning

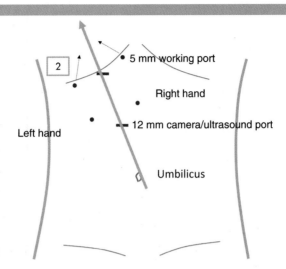

2

5 mm working port

Right hand

12 mm camera/ultrasound port

Left hand

Umbilicus

Figure v13.2 The second 12 mm port is placed to the right at the costal margin; this will allow completion of the parenchymal transection and dissection of the RHV.

the gallbladder itself attached to the liver to act as a handle. Here we can see the opening of the hilar plate itself which usually leads to minor bleeding. This step is necessary in order to be able to come easily around the bile duct later during the portal dissection. We place a hemostatic agent into the crevice after opening the hilar plate in order to avoid blood in the portal structures, to allow excellent visualization during the dissection later.

Here we open the hepatoduodenal ligament at its lateral portion. This will allow us to dissect out the right hepatic artery. Dividing the right hepatic artery at this step will open up the space and will help in dissecting out the right hepatic vein. The small right anterior and posterior right hepatic arteries will be controlled using thermofusion and later with a clip (Figure v13.3). The right hepatic artery is controlled using a locking clip.

The next step will be dissecting out the right portal vein branch. This is the dissection at the bifurcation between the right and left portal vein. Notice also the closeness of the left hepatic artery at this point of dissection (Figure v13.4). As we get closer to the portal vein, we switch to scissors for dissection. This allows for more tactile feedback and an injury with scissors can be much more easily controlled. Using scissors, the portal vein is now separated from the Glissonian sheath at the inferior portion. Using a 5 mm dissector, now the portal vein is completely mobilized, we

place a suture around the right portal vein in order to have traction which facilitates placing a locking clip. It is important to be careful with the branches of the right portal vein running directly into the caudate lobe. Injury to these branches can be difficult to control. Here we control these branches with thermofusion.

The next step is dissection of the retrocaval ligament and transection of the Spiegel lobe. This is the view along the IVC. You will encounter direct branches into the IVC which need to be controlled. In order to avoid any surprises, check on preoperative imaging for the right inferior hepatic vein. An additional short hepatic vein can be controlled using thermofusion.

The next step is transection of the paracaval portion of the caudate lobe, also known as Couinaud's segment IX. Because of the augmented view of the laparoscopic camera, this part may be performed more easily via a laparoscopic than an open procedure. Performing this step early in the operation will facilitate control of the bile duct (BD) (Figure v13.5). We are now placing a clamp behind the bile duct in the direction of the later stapling. The right bile duct is staple divided. It is important to make sure that you leave sufficient distance to the left bile duct to prevent postoperative stenosis.

At this point of the operation, all portal structures to the right side have been controlled and we are now moving

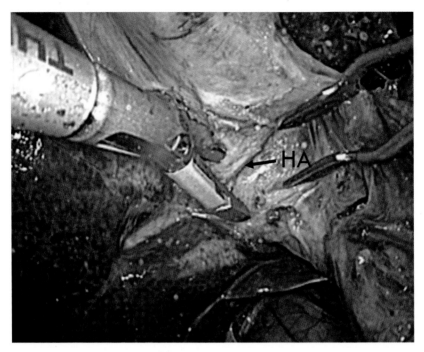

Figure v13.3 The small right anterior and posterior RHAs will be controlled using thermofusion and later with a clip.

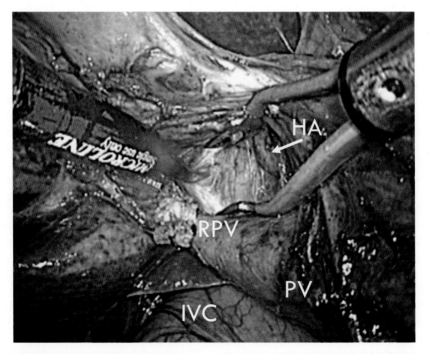

Figure v13.4 This is the dissection at the bifurcation between the right and left portal vein. Notice also the closeness of the LHA at this point of dissection.

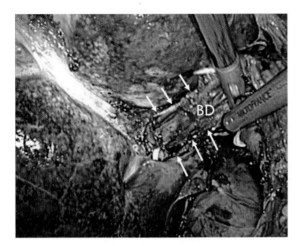

Figure v13.5 The next step is transection of the paracaval portion of the caudate lobe, also known as Couinaud's segment IX. Because of the augmented view of the laparoscopic camera, this part may be performed more easily via a laparoscopic than an open procedure. Performing this step early in the operation will facilitate control of the bile duct (BD).

on to the parenchymal transection. Our technique for the parenchymal transection is to activate the energy device outside the parenchyma and keep it activated while closing. At this location, we encounter the middle hepatic vein branch to segment V. It is easy to get lost with the transection plane in the two dimensions of the laparoscopic view. Having the IVC in view and keeping the falciform ligament attached can help to guide the parenchymal transection plane. Now the crucial landmark is

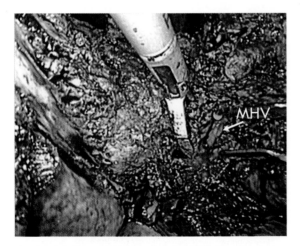

Figure v13.6 The crucial landmark is the middle hepatic vein that was identified using ultrasound at the beginning of the case.

the middle hepatic vein that was identified using ultrasound at the beginning of the case (Figure v13.6). This is very helpful if you are inside the parenchyma.

Because the paracaval portion of the caudate lobe was transected earlier, we can now connect the plane between the middle hepatic vein and the IVC. Once we get closer to the origin of the middle hepatic vein, we should look out for the segment VIII branch. We also strongly recommend identifying this branch during preoperative imaging. The flat IVC and the respiratory variations that can be seen are indicative of the low CVP.

Dissecting out the hepatic vein origin is always done using scissors. The last step of the operation is the staple division of the right hepatic vein and mobilization of the specimen. This is done with scissors because an injury with scissors can be much more easily controlled than an injury with an energy device. Now the right hepatic vein is completely dissected out and we will divide using a stapler. We recommend always having a vascular clamp ready in case of stapler misfiring, as seen here. The dissection of the hepatocaval ligament is now completed. Short hepatic veins are controlled using thermofusion.

With the division of hepatic vein branch VIII ventral, the specimen is now completely devascularized. The specimen needs to be detached from the triangular ligament; medial traction of the specimen with the help of the 30° camera aids in this process. Using Doppler, we confirm vascular inflow and outflow.

IMPORTANT POINTS

- Laparoscopic ultrasound is crucial during this operation. It is used to identify lesions in the future liver remnant and identify the MHV as a landmark for the parenchymal transection.
- After division of the cystic duct and cystic artery, we recommend leaving the gallbladder attached to the liver as it can be used for retraction.
- Complete the retrocaval ligament dissection as well as the paracaval portion of the Spiegel lobe transection early. This can help during division of the bile duct and during the parenchymal transection.
- Umbilical tape around the porta can be used as an emergent Pringle.
- Do not become lost because of the 2D laparoscopic view; let the MHV guide you.
- Have a vascular clamp ready when firing the stapler across the right hepatic vein.
- Finally, be prepared that specimen mobilization at the end may take time.

Anatomy figures

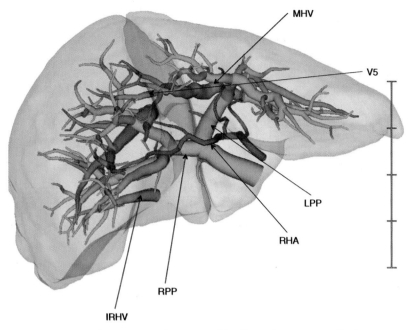

Figure v13.7 Critical anatomy for a right hepatectomy. The RPP as well as the RHA are exposed. The key is to avoid injury to the LPP. This patient has a common RPP but also a trifurcation is commonly seen.

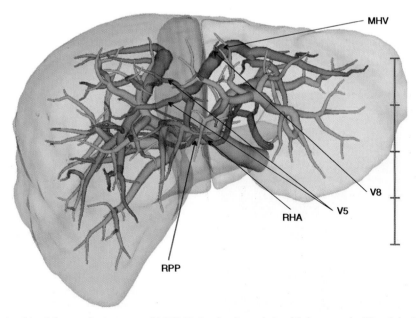

Figure v13.8 Relationship of the portal structures and MHV. Notice the close relationship between the PP and the MHV drainage veins to segment V (V5). During a cholecystectomy, the V5 branches can be close to the surface and cause significant bleeding. They need to be controlled at the beginning of the parenchymal transection.

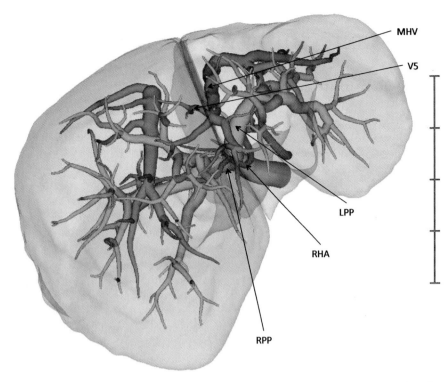

Figure v13.9 View along the parenchymal transection plane. After the RPP has been controlled and the V5 branches divided, we follow the MHV up to its drainage into the IVC. It is important to check preoperative imaging for a prominent V8 drainage vein (not present in this patient). Injury to a V8 drainage vein can lead to significant bleeding at near-completion of the case.

VIDEO 14

Left trisegmentectomy with caudate lobectomy

Video duration 16 minutes 12 seconds

In this video, we will show you a left trisegmentectomy with caudate lobectomy. The video is divided into the following parts:

The port positioning is similar to a left hepatectomy (Figure v14.1). After liver mobilization, portal pedicle dissection and the beginning of liver transection, we then move to position 2 (Figure v14.2).

The first step is to complete mobilization of the left liver. Here the falciform ligament is taken down and we are dissecting along the ligament of Arantius. We proceed to taking down the left triangular ligament. As full liver mobilization is necessary, we are now dividing the coronary ligament.

The next step is the left portal pedicle dissection. Here we are preparing for a potential Pringle maneuver should that become necessary during the parenchymal transection. We are now beginning to dissect the left portal

Port positioning

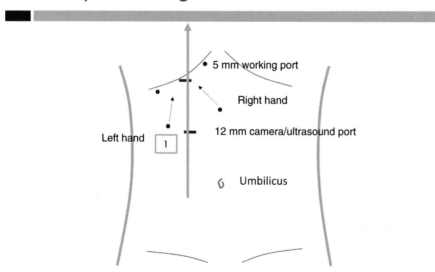

Figure v14.1 The port positioning is similar to a left hepatectomy.

Laparoscopic Liver, Pancreas, and Biliary Surgery, First Edition.
Edited by Claudius Conrad and Brice Gayet.
© 2017 John Wiley & Sons, Ltd. Published 2017 by John Wiley & Sons, Ltd.

Port positioning

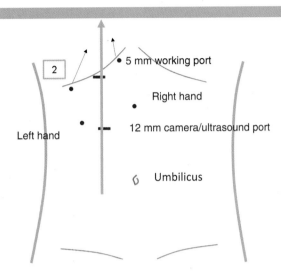

Figure v14.2 After liver mobilization, PP dissection and the beginning of liver transection, we then move to position 2.

structures. Here we are opening the hepatoduodenal ligament, and the left hepatic artery comes into view. At this step, the left hepatic artery and the medial branch of the segment IV artery, also known as the A4 branch, are dissected out (Figure v14.3). The arteries are clipped and divided. Here we are beginning to lower the hilar plate. To facilitate this step, the cystic duct is divided.

The next step is dissecting out the portal vein. After opening the Glissonian sheath, the portal vein comes

into view. The portal vein and right hepatic artery are separated (Figure v14.4). Next, the left hepatic duct is divided and then suture closed. We reopen the cystic duct and inject air into the biliary system. We are doing this with the right anterior portal pedicle clamped. The air artifacts in the ultrasound will help us delineate the posterior sector.

Now, the left portal vein is dissected out and divided and the left portal pedicle has been controlled, we dissect out and control the right anterior portal pedicle. Here, the right

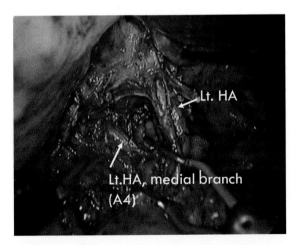

Figure v14.3 After liver mobilization, PP dissection, and the beginning of liver transection, we then move to position 2.

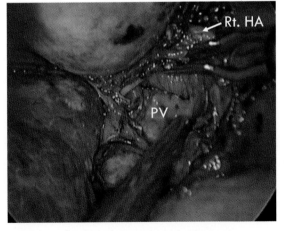

Figure v14.4 After opening the Glissonian sheath, the portal vein comes into view. The PV and RHA are separated.

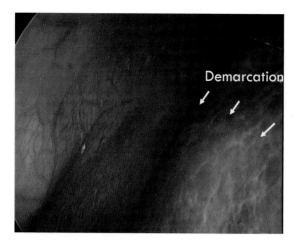

Figure v14.5 There is good demarcation between the RAPP and the RPPP.

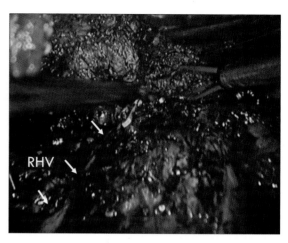

Figure v14.6 We continue the dissection directly on the RHV.

anterior sectoral artery comes into view. Here, the right anterior sectoral vein is dissected out and it will also be controlled and divided. Following the portal pedicle dissection, we will perform a caudate lobectomy. Here you can see us opening up the hepatocaval ligament. The ligament of Arantius is divided. Next, we will open up the hepatocaval space. Caudate veins are controlled and divided. Passing a suture behind those veins allows for some traction that facilitates clipping. The hepatocaval space is further opened.

The next crucial step is the parenchymal transection. Using ultrasound, we again confirm the location of the right hepatic vein. We can also see a nice demarcation line between the right anterior and right posterior sectors (Figure v14.5). Here we are beginning the parenchymal transection between segments V and VI. We are opening up the liver capsule along the demarcation line. Here we are making progress with the parenchymal transection between segments V and VI. Here, the segment V drainage vein into the right hepatic vein is controlled. We are encountering some minor bleeding of the right hepatic vein. As we make progress with the parenchymal transection, we encounter the drainage vein to segment VIII, also known as VIII ventral. We are continuing to follow the right hepatic vein. Minor bleeding from the right hepatic vein is controlled with the bipolar forceps. The dorsal drainage vein of segment VIII is dissected out and divided. We continue the dissection directly on the right hepatic vein (Figure v14.6). The drainage vein of segment VIII is dissected out, controlled, and divided. As we reach the origin of the right hepatic vein, we switch to scissors

for the dissection. Here, the anterior fissure vein is clipped and divided. Now, the right anterior and posterior sectors are completely separated. In the middle of the image, the IVC can be seen.

The last step of the operation is division of the left and middle hepatic veins. With inferior traction on the specimen, the middle and left hepatic veins are staple divided. Having a vascular clamp ready for stapler misfiring is crucial for this step. The exposed right hepatic vein confirms a true anatomical dissection (Figure v14.7). At the end of the case, we inspect the transection surface for any bleeding or bile leaks.

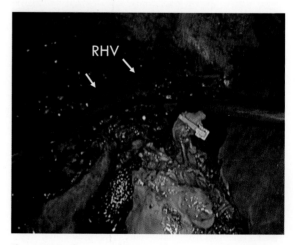

Figure v14.7 The exposed RHV confirms a true anatomical dissection.

IMPORTANT POINTS

- Start with the left portal pedicle and then proceed to the right anterior portal pedicle dissection.
- Be certain that the right posterior pedicle is intact to avoid damage to the future liver remnant.
- Use ultrasound to identify the right hepatic vein; it will guide your parenchymal transection.
- Have a laparoscopic vascular clamp ready when stapling the middle or left hepatic vein in case of stapler misfiring.

Anatomy figures

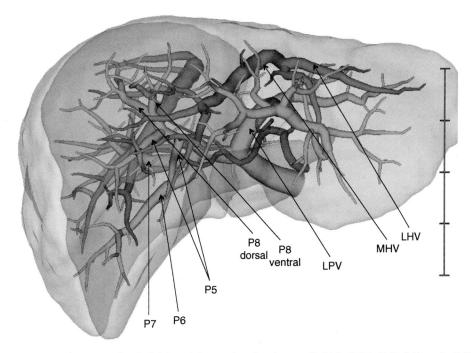

P8 dorsal P8 ventral LPV MHV LHV

P5

P7 P6

Figure v14.8 Relevant anatomy. Initially, the left liver inflow and outflow is controlled. The LPP is divided. Next, the RAPP is controlled. In this schema, there is a trifurcation of RAPP, P6, and P7.

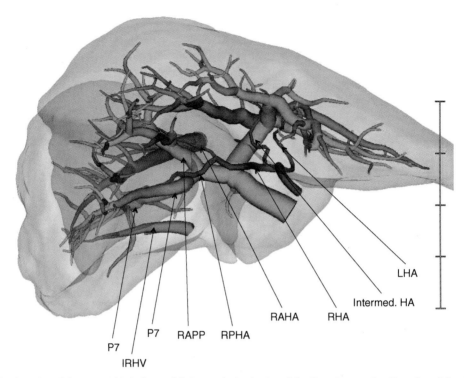

Figure v14.9 Dissection of the RAPP. This is the caudal view at the beginning of the dissection. During dissection of the RAPP, injury to the RPHA needs to be avoided. This patient has an IRHV which needs to be preserved or controlled.

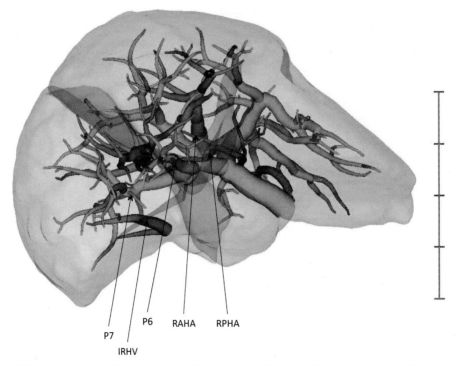

Figure v14.10 Additional view of portal structures. Preserving the RPHA while controlling the RAHA is critical.

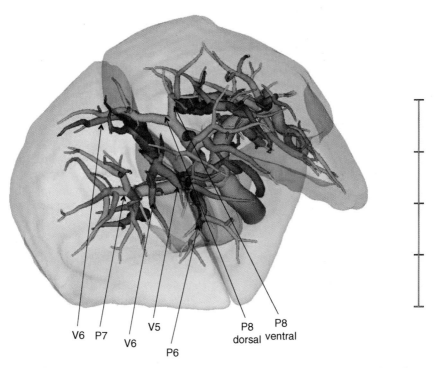

V6 P7   V6   V5   P8   P8
                          dorsal ventral
                  P6

Figure v14.11 Lateral view to the posterior section. Once the portal structures are controlled, the parenchymal transection is carried out along the RHV. V5 is taken first. P8 has a constant dorsal and ventral branch. The dorsal branch can reach into the parenchymal transection plane. At the end of the parenchymal transection, the MHV/LHV are divided.

VIDEO 15

Right trisegmentectomy

Video duration 19 minutes 30 seconds

In this video, we would like to show you a right trisegmentectomy.

The port position is similar to a left hepatectomy. We will move from position 1 (Figure v15.1) to position 2 (Figure v15.2) as we progress with the parenchymal transection.

The first step of the operation is controlling the right portal pedicle. Here we are taking down the falciform ligament and performing a complete liver ultrasound. Here we are determining the anatomical relation between the middle hepatic vein and the left portal pedicle (Figure v15.3). Here the lesion at segment IVa at the origin of the middle hepatic vein is seen, necessitating a right trisegmentectomy. Here we are beginning the dissection of the hepatoduodenal ligament. Area 12p lymph node station is dissected out and sent for frozen section analysis. Next, the cystic duct is clipped and divided.

The next step is lowering of the hilar plate. The right hepatic artery is dissected out, clipped, and divided. Here lymph node station 12p is dissected out. Now we are ready to clip and divide the right hepatic artery. Here the right

Port positioning

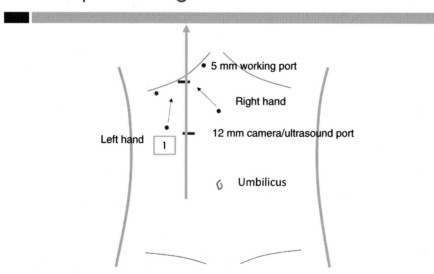

Figure v15.1 The port position is similar to a left hepatectomy.

Laparoscopic Liver, Pancreas, and Biliary Surgery, First Edition.
Edited by Claudius Conrad and Brice Gayet.
© 2017 John Wiley & Sons, Ltd. Published 2017 by John Wiley & Sons, Ltd.

Port positioning

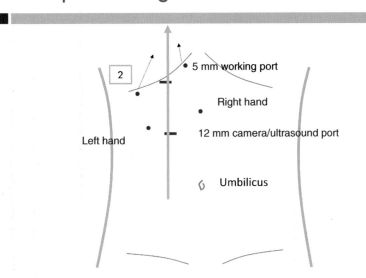

Figure v15.2 We will move to port position 2 once we progress with the parenchymal transection and to control the hepatic venous confluence.

anterior hepatic artery is clipped and divided. Next, the right posterior hepatic artery is controlled. We proceed to dissecting out the right portal vein. Using a right-angled dissector, we dissect the right portal vein off the Glissonian sheath. Once it is completely mobile, we can clip and divide it. The last structure of the right portal pedicle

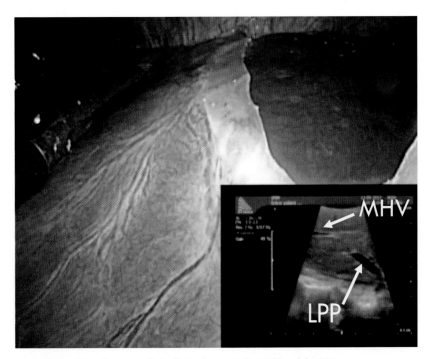

Figure v15.3 Here we are determining the anatomical relation between the MHV and the LPP.

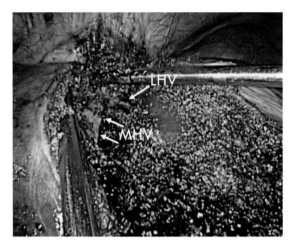

Figure v15.4 As we proceed with the parenchymal transection, the confluence between the MHV and LHV comes into view.

that needs to be controlled is the right bile duct. The right bile duct is divided with scissors. At this step, we are also beginning the division of the hepatocaval ligament.

The next step is controlling the portal pedicle to segments IVb and IVa. In order to control the portal pedicle to segment IV, we have to open the umbilical fissure. Opening the parenchyma here facilitates location of the portal pedicle to segment IVb. Using ultrasound, we are tracing our later parenchymal transection line. Injury to the left hepatic vein has to be avoided at all costs. Tracing out the parenchymal transection line at this step facilitates opening up the umbilical fissure.

With the parenchyma opened along the umbilical fissure, we are dissecting out the portal branch to segment IVb. The portal branch to segment IVb is usually located inside the parenchyma. Opening up the parenchyma widely above and below the portal pedicle facilitates controlling it. Using the gallbladder as a handle, we connect the earlier parenchymal transection line with the parenchymal transection line along the umbilical fissure. A key maneuver is ensuring that the portal pedicles to left lateral sectors are preserved. Here we are placing a vascular clamp on the portal pedicle to segment IVb while ensuring preserved flow to the left lateral sector. With this vascular clamp that fits through a 12 mm port, we confirm that we are all the way around the portal pedicle to segment IVb. The IVb pedicle is clipped and divided. Here the dissection is carried out along the paracaval portion of the caudate lobe. By opening up the paracaval portion of the caudate lobe,

the segment IVa branch is fully dissected out and clipped and divided. At this step, all the portal pedicles for our right trisegmentectomy have been taken and we can proceed to complete our parenchymal transection.

As we progress with the parenchymal transection, it is crucial to avoid injury to the left hepatic vein. We will come back to this part. Here we encounter minor bleeding from the left hepatic vein, which we stop using the bipolar forceps. Here, the coronary ligament is taken down. As we proceed with the parenchymal transection, the confluence between the middle hepatic vein and left hepatic vein comes into view (Figure v15.4). As mentioned before, it is crucial to avoid any injury to the left hepatic vein. At this step, the confluence between the middle and left hepatic veins is completely dissected out.

The last step is division of the right and middle hepatic veins. For later division of the middle hepatic vein, we have to ensure that its drainage into the IVC is completely dissected out. We use the suction tip and the blunt grasper below the middle hepatic vein to ensure that we can later control it without difficulty.

We are now ready to clip and divide the middle hepatic vein at its drainage into the IVC. Here the right trisegmentectomy specimen is completely dissected off the IVC. Now we are dividing the middle hepatic vein. The last structure that needs to be divided is the right hepatic vein which we can see in the background. The drainage of the right hepatic vein into the IVC is completely dissected out and we can proceed now to staple divide it. The right triangular ligament is divided in order to completely mobilize the specimen. We inspect the transection margin of the future liver remnant for any bleeding.

IMPORTANT POINTS

- Start by controlling the right portal pedicle and then proceed to dissecting out the portal pedicle to segments IVa and IVb.
- Dissecting out the segment IVa and IVb pedicle is greatly facilitated by opening up the parenchyma widely along the umbilical fissure.
- The left portal pedicle and left hepatic vein have to be protected at all costs.
- Frequent use of ultrasound during the parenchymal transection helps to identify and protect the left hepatic vein.
- Frequent use of ultrasound will also help to ensure that you do not become lost during the parenchymal transection.

Anatomy figures

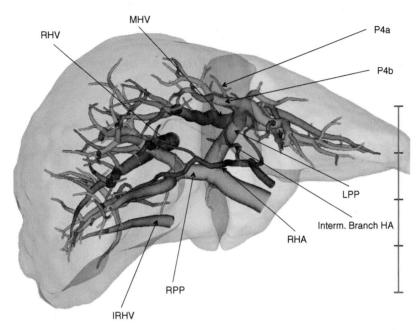

Figure v15.5 Critical anatomy for a right trisegmentectomy. After division of the RPP, including the RHA and the intermediate branch of the HA, P4b and P4a are divided. This is performed by opening up the umbilical fissure. The LPP must be protected.

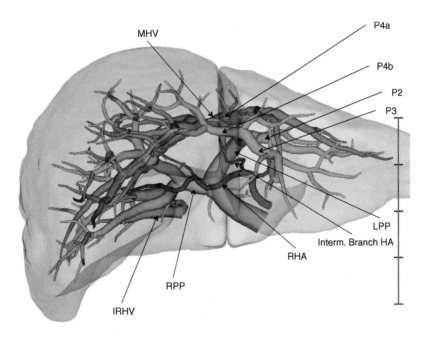

Figure v15.6 Relationship of portal structures and MHV. Notice the close relationship between the P4b and MHV.

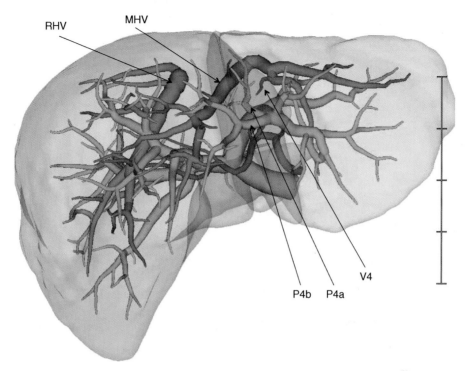

Figure v15.7 View along the parenchymal transection plane. After RPP, P4b and P4a have been controlled and the parenchymal transection plane follows the LHV. At completion of the parenchyma transection, the MHV and RHV are divided. Often, the MHV and LHV share a common drainage into the IVC. When dividing the MHV, the LHV drainage needs to be protected.

VIDEO 16

Posterior sectionectomy

Video duration 14 minutes 9 seconds

In this video, we will show you a posterior sectionectomy.

> **OUTLINE**
>
> The video is divided into the following parts:
> - Port positioning
> - Ultrasound
> - Dissection of the hepatocaval ligament
> - Preparation of the Pringle maneuver in case it is needed for controlled staged conversion
> - Dissection of the right posterior portal pedicle
> - Parenchymal transection
> - Important points.

This scheme demonstrates the port positioning (Figure v16.1). In addition, we recommend tilting the patient 45° to the left side.

A crucial step for this operation is intraoperative ultrasound. It is not only essential to rule out metastasis in the future remnant liver but also to identify the branching between right anterior and right posterior pedicles (Figure v16.2 and Figure v16.3). We strongly recommend identifying this image with the ultrasound in order to avoid injury to the right anterior portal pedicle. On this sequence, the hypoechoic lesion can be seen. Also, there is a cyst in the left top corner of the image which we will encounter during the parenchymal transection.

We perform the dissection of the hepatocaval ligament early in the case. This allows for safe completion of the parenchymal transection. For the dissection of the hepatocaval ligament, we displace the liver towards the left of the patient. The most lateral trocar can be used for retraction of the liver. Here the IVC comes into view and this

Port positioning

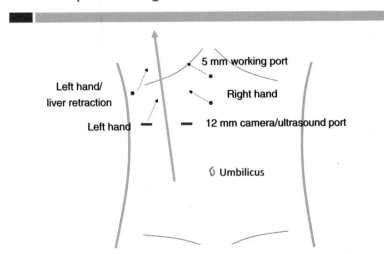

Figure v16.1 This scheme demonstrates the port positioning. In addition, we recommend tilting the patient more than 45° to the left side (so called modified French position).

Laparoscopic Liver, Pancreas, and Biliary Surgery, First Edition.
Edited by Claudius Conrad and Brice Gayet.
© 2017 John Wiley & Sons, Ltd. Published 2017 by John Wiley & Sons, Ltd.

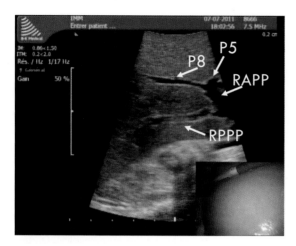

Figure v16.2 It is critical to identify the branching between RAPP and RPPP on ultrasound.

dissection is more safely done with scissors. Small short hepatic branches can be controlled using the bipolar forceps. As more of the hepatocaval ligament is transected, the liver becomes more mobile. This allows for safe transection of the superior and medial portion of the right triangular ligament. Laparoscopic posterior sectionectomy has a not insignificant risk for bleeding. Therefore, it is useful to be prepared to use the Pringle maneuver laparoscopically. This would allow for a safe and possibly staged conversion; by staged, we mean that another port or a hand port is placed to control the bleeding laparoscopically. If this cannot be done with minimal blood loss, immediate conversion is prudent. In order to

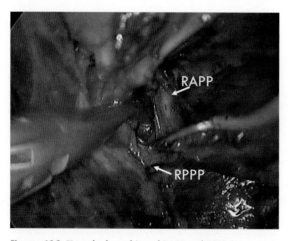

Figure v16.3 Here the branching of RAPP and RPPP is identified. It is critical to preserve the RAPP while dividing the RPPP.

have a good working condition in the porta, we retract the liver with an endo-closure device superiorly.

The next step is opening the hepatoduodenal ligament in order to expose the right posterior portal pedicle. Here you can see a Glissonian approach in exposing the right posterior portal pedicle. Gentle retraction on the non-tightened umbilical tape aids in exposure. At this step, we have dissected out the right posterior hepatic artery which opens up the space to dissect out the right posterior portal vein. We follow the right main portal pedicle until we find the initial branching of the right posterior portal pedicle. Here you can see the critical portion of the dissection between the right anterior and right posterior portal pedicle. You can see the right anterior portal pedicle appearing in the background of the dissection. We will pass a suture behind the right posterior portal pedicle with a 5 mm dissector in order to traction it for clip placement. Now the right posterior portal vein has been controlled. The next step is to control the bile duct.

With all the inflow to the posterior sector controlled, we can retract the liver more superiorly, which opens up the hepatocaval space. Performing this dissection early will allow for a safe landing zone of the parenchyma transection. Before beginning the parenchymal transection, we divide the paracaval portion of the caudate lobe.

The last step of this operation is the parenchymal transection. The right hepatic vein defines the medial border of the right posterior sectionectomy. We can also see the nice demarcation line between right anterior and posterior sectors. Using the gallbladder as a handle aids in the parenchymal transection. The drainage vein of segment VI is controlled using thermofusion. Here, we can safely connect the parenchymal transection with the dissection of the hepatocaval ligament. Using ultrasound as a guide, we define the border between segments VII and VIII. At this step, we identify a small simple cyst which we have seen earlier on ultrasound. Here we continue the parenchymal transection plane along the line defined by the right hepatic vein. Here, we expose the right hepatic vein between segments V and VI and follow it superiorly. The drainage vein to segment VI is controlled using the bipolar forceps as well as thermofusion. Once we reach the top portion of our transection, we identify the drainage of the right hepatic vein into the IVC using ultrasound. The bipolar forceps is used for hemostasis along the transection margin. Now the specimen is completely detached. At the end, we perform a cholecystectomy and remove both the specimen and the gallbladder using a retriever bag.

IMPORTANT POINTS

- It is important to have a good understanding of the branching between the right anterior and right posterior portal pedicles from preoperative imaging and intraoperative ultrasound.
- Perform the dissection of the hepatocaval ligament early.
- Umbilical tape around the porta can be used for a laparoscopic Pringle maneuver.
- The parenchymal transection should be guided by the right hepatic vein.

Anatomy figures

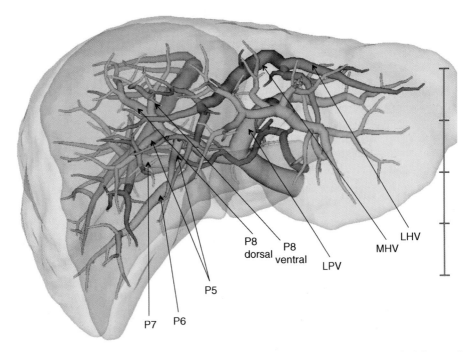

Figure v16.4 Critical anatomy for a posterior sectionectomy. During the dissection, the RAPP is preserved while P6 and P7 are taken. In this case, the patient has a trifurcation and therefore P6 and P7 should be taken individually.

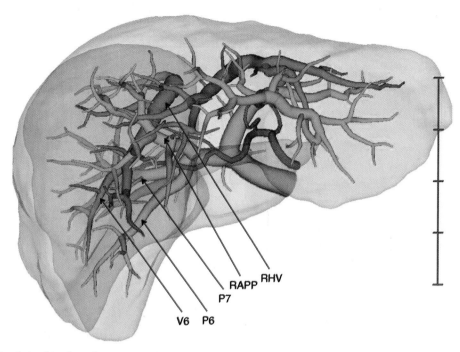

Figure v16.5 Relationship of portal structures and RHV. After controlling P6 and P7, the parenchymal transection follows the RHV. Notice its closeness to the RAPP, which should be preserved.

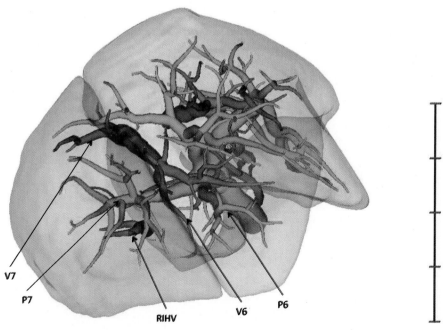

Figure v16.6 View along the right anterior fissure. V6 can be followed to the drainage into the RHV to find its intraparenchymal location. While the RHV guides the parenchymal transection, injury to V7 at the completion of the parenchymal transection must be avoided. An RIHV should be identified on preoperative imaging to avoid injury.

VIDEO 17

Hilar lymphadenectomy (with right hepatectomy and caudate lobectomy for Klatskin tumor)

Video duration 17 minutes 3 seconds

In this video, we demonstrate a hilar lymphadenectomy with right hepatectomy and caudate lobectomy for Klatskin tumor.

> **OUTLINE**
>
> The video is divided into the following parts:
> - Port positioning
> - Hilar lymph node dissection
> - Right hepatectomy with resection of segment I
> - Hepaticoduodenostomy
> - Important points.

The port positioning is similar to right hepatectomy and we choose position 1 for the portal dissection and position 2 later for the parenchymal transection phase (Figure v17.1 and Figure v17.2).

Next, we would like to show you the hilar lymph node dissection. This is an overview of the lower 12 mm port site. We begin by dissecting out the left portal structures in order to secure them to avoid injury. The first structure we dissect out is the left hepatic artery which is located close to lymph node station 12a. We secure the left hepatic artery with a vessel loop. After the left hepatic artery has been secured, we dissect out the left portal vein

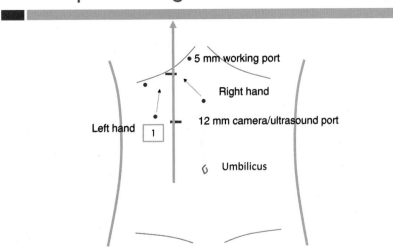

Figure v17.1 The port positioning is similar to right hepatectomy and we choose position 1 for the portal dissection.

Laparoscopic Liver, Pancreas, and Biliary Surgery, First Edition.
Edited by Claudius Conrad and Brice Gayet.
© 2017 John Wiley & Sons, Ltd. Published 2017 by John Wiley & Sons, Ltd.

Port positioning

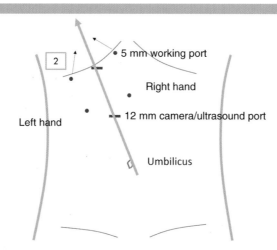

Figure v17.2 This port positioning is used later in the parenchymal transection and for controlling the hepatic venous confluence.

branch. After securing the left hepatic artery and vein, we can begin the lymph node dissection.

As mentioned earlier, lymph node station 12a is located close to the left hepatic artery (Figure v17.3). We are following the hepatic artery proximally in order to dissect lymph node station 12a. After opening up the hepato-duodenal ligament, we aim to dissect the common bile duct. Using indocyanine green and an infrared camera

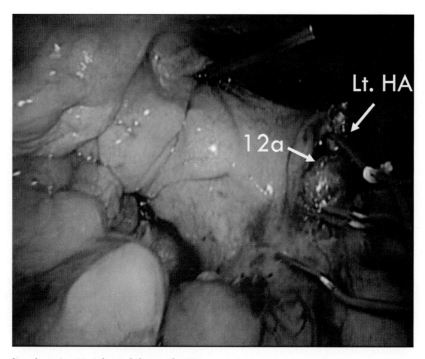

Figure v17.3 Lymph node station 12a is located close to the LHA.

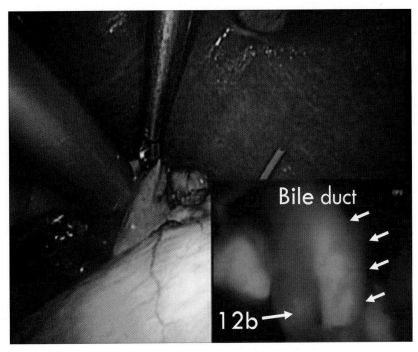

Figure v17.4 Using indocyanine green and an infrared camera helps us to identify the bile duct in the porta. You can see the bile duct and lymph node station 12b, which is right lateral to the common bile duct.

helps us to identify the bile duct in the porta. You can see the bile duct and lymph node station 12b which is right lateral to the common bile duct (Figure v17.4).

Ventral to the common bile duct, between the border of the duodenum and the common bile duct, is lymph node station 5. In order to gain more mobility for our dissection, we are kocherizing the first portion of the duodenum. As we continue our kocherization, the IVC comes into view (Figure v17.5). Next we dissect lymph node stations 12b and 5.

The next step is dissecting the bile duct off the portal vein. Now we are proceeding to transect the bile duct. As we open up the common bile duct, the plastic stent comes into view. Next we remove the plastic stent; at this step we routinely perform cultures. The proximal bile duct is sent for frozen section analysis. The proximal bile duct is closed with a 4.0 PDS suture. Now we are mobilizing the common bile duct off the main portal vein. As we proceed with the portal dissection, the right hepatic artery comes into view which will be clipped and divided. We are proceeding with our lymph node dissection and are now dissecting lymph node station 12p (Figure v17.6). Stripping all the lymph node tissue of the porta will facilitate exposure of the bifurcation of the portal vein.

Now that all lymphatic tissue has been stripped off the porta and the bifurcation of the portal vein has been exposed, we can proceed to performing the right hepatectomy with caudate lobectomy.

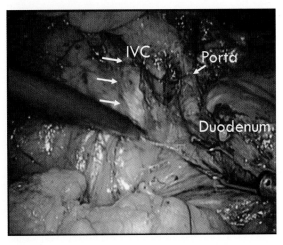

Figure v17.5 As we continue our kocherization, the IVC comes into view.

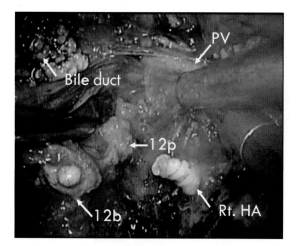

Figure v17.6 We are proceeding with our lymph node dissection and are now dissecting lymph node station 12p.

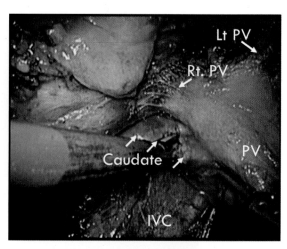

Figure v17.8 Here we are beginning the parenchymal transection of the caudate lobe.

The first step will be lowering the hilar plate; this usually leads to some minor bleeding. In order to maintain excellent working conditions in the porta, we will stop this bleeding with bipolar forceps and a hemostatic agent containing regenerated oxidized cellulose. This hemostatic agent is placed into the crevice. Lowering the hilar plate will help us to expose the left bile duct which we can see here. At this step we are opening up the left bile duct (Figure v17.7). We are exposing the left portal vein a bit more. Here we are beginning the parenchymal transection of the caudate lobe (Figure v17.8).

Beginning the parenchymal transection of the caudate lobe at this step will aid with mobility and transecting the right portal structures.

Now that the right portal vein has been completely dissected out, it can be clipped and divided. At this step, the left bile duct can be transected completely. The bile duct margin is sent for frozen section analysis. Now we can deepen our parenchymal transection along the middle hepatic vein. At this step, we are exposing the drainage vein to segment V and we will later use the middle hepatic vein as a landmark for our parenchymal transection (Figure v17.9).

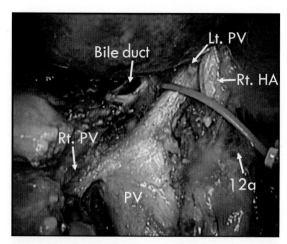

Figure v17.7 Lowering the hilar plate will help us to expose the left bile duct, which we can see here. At this step we are opening up the left bile duct.

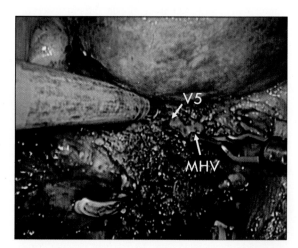

Figure v17.9 At this step, we are exposing the drainage vein to segment V and we will later use the MHV as a landmark for our parenchymal transection.

We are now following the demarcation line between segments IVb and V; the gallbladder helps with retraction. Having connected the two parenchymal transection lines, we can clip and divide the drainage vein to segment V and continue to follow the middle hepatic vein. Here we have followed the middle hepatic vein all the way towards its drainage into the IVC. As the right hepatic vein is completely exposed, it can be staple divided. As always, we have a vascular clamp ready in case of stapler misfiring. The specimen is completely removed by detaching it from the triangular ligament. It will be removed from the abdomen using an endoscopic retrieval bag.

The last step of the operation is the bilioenteric anastomosis. We will be using a hepaticoduodenostomy. The advantage of hepaticoduodenostomy is continued access to the anastomosis via an endoscopic route. The first step is a small enterotomy in the duodenum. After the enterotomy has been made, we perform a continuously running anastomosis using a monofilament suture. If there is any concern about the tension at the anastomosis at this step, the kocherization maneuver should be widened. After initial anchoring stiches, the back wall is constructed first. It is important to avoid back walling the anastomosis, so good visualization into the lumen of the small bile duct is crucial. The magnified view of the laparoscopic camera aids in constructing the small anastomosis. After constructing the back wall, the anterior wall is constructed. After final inspection of the operating site, we complete the case.

> **IMPORTANT POINTS**
>
> - Be sure you know the lymph node station to dissect.
> - Early division of the bile duct facilitates exposure.
> - Ensure that there is only minimal bleeding at the porta for optimal dissection and visualization.
> - Remove the caudate lobe for oncological purposes and optimize the trocar position for suturing the hepaticoduodenostomy.

Anatomy figures

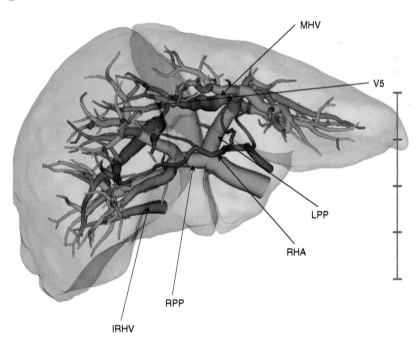

Figure v17.10 Critical anatomy for a right hepatectomy. The RPP as well as the RHA are exposed. The key is to avoid injury to the LPP. This patient has a common RPP but also a trifurcation is commonly seen.

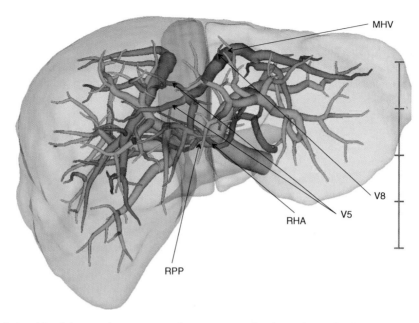

Figure v17.11 Relationship of the portal structures and MHV. Notice the close relationship between the PP and the MHV drainage veins to segment V (V5). During a cholecystectomy, the V5 branches can be close to the surface and cause significant bleeding. They need to be controlled at the beginning of the parenchymal transection.

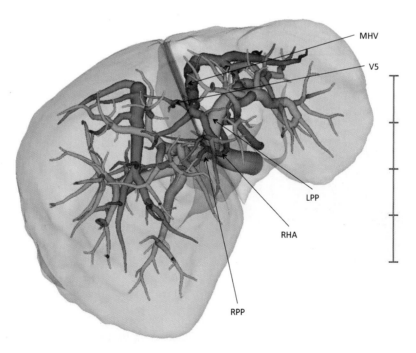

Figure v17.12 View along the parenchymal transection plane. After the RPP has been controlled and the V5 branches divided, we follow the MHV up to its drainage into the IVC. It is important to check preoperative imaging for a prominent V8 drainage vein (not present in this patient). Injury to a V8 drainage vein can lead to significant bleeding at near-completion of the case.

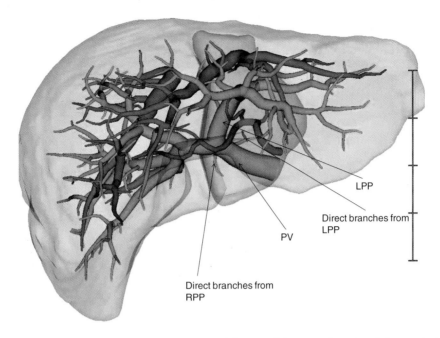

Figure v17.13 Critical anatomy of the caudate lobe. The caudate lobe extends between the IVC and PP up to the hepatic venous confluence. Venous drainage is from direct branches from IVC. Direct branches from left and RPP supply segment I.

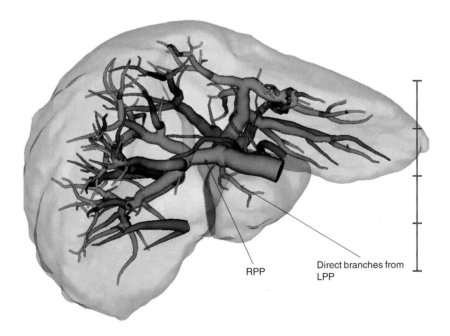

Figure v17.14 Relationship of portal structures to segment I. The direct branches from the LPP and RPP can cause significant bleeding. They are relevant not only when performing a caudate lobectomy but also when dissecting out the main PP for other types of liver resection.

VIDEO 18

Mesohepatectomy

Video duration 5 minutes 48 seconds

In this video we will demonstrate a total laparoscopic mesohepatectomy.

OUTLINE

The operative tactics are as follows:
- Dissection of the coronary ligament
- Parenchymal dissection along the falciform ligament
- Division of the right anterior sectoral pedicle
- Parenchymal dissection along the right portal fissure
- Division of the middle hepatic vein.

At completion of the case, the remaining liver segments will be I, II, III, VI, and VII. At the end of the case, we will have divided hepatic and portal venous branches to segments IVb and IVa, including the medial segmental branch of the left hepatic artery. We will have stapled off the right anterior sectoral branch of the right portal pedicle and we will divide portal and hepatic venous branches to segments V and VIII, including the middle hepatic vein at the end.

This scheme demonstrates the anatomy after a mesohepatectomy. The numbering indicates the operative tactics.

Let's start with dissection of the coronary ligament. The falciform ligament leading up to the coronary ligament is divided. As we approach the suprahepatic IVC, we will switch to dissection with laparoscopic scissors. Next, we demonstrate parenchymal dissection between the left lateral and the left medial sector along the falciform ligament. The dissection is begun to the right of the ligamentum teres. As we go deeper into the parenchyma, the first branches we encounter are the portal branches to segment IVb. These branches will be controlled with locking clips and divided. The parenchymal dissection is continued along the left border of segment IVa. This is continued until the anterior surface of the IVC is reached. Again, as we are approaching the IVC, laparoscopic scissors will be used for the dissection.

So far, we have completely defined the left border of our laparoscopic mesohepatectomy. We will move back now to the porta and staple and divide the right anterior sectoral pedicle. For the division of the right anterior sectoral pedicle, we elevate the liver using the gallbladder as a handle. This is the view of the porta along the hepatoduodenum ligament. The next step will be a Glissonian approach through dissection of the anterior sectoral branch of the right porta pedicle. After completion of the dissection, a vascular clamp is placed on the anterior sectoral pedicle. The resulting ischemia helps to define the border between segments V and VI. Using ultrasound, we confirm that the posterior sectoral pedicle is intact. We now staple and divide the anterior sectoral pedicle.

The next step of the operation is parenchymal dissection along the right portal fissure. Using systemically administered indocyanine green and a laparoscopic near infrared camera, we confirm the border between V and VI and preservation of the posterior sectoral branch. The parenchymal dissection is now continued along the right portal fissure. We are now reaching the border between segments VIII and VI and we are again using ultrasound to define the right hepatic vein as a landmark. With this information, the border between segments VII and VIII can be safely divided.

The final step of the operation is division of the middle hepatic vein. On this image, the central liver segments IV,

Laparoscopic Liver, Pancreas, and Biliary Surgery, First Edition.
Edited by Claudius Conrad and Brice Gayet.
© 2017 John Wiley & Sons, Ltd. Published 2017 by John Wiley & Sons, Ltd.

V, and VIII are almost completely mobile and the middle hepatic vein has already been clipped. The middle hepatic vein is now divided with scissors. Towards the end of the dissection, a branch from the middle hepatic vein to segment VIII is clipped and divided. The central liver is now detached completely from the remaining liver. On this view of the completed dissection, the respiratory variations of the right hepatic vein indicate the exact anatomical border to segment VI.

Open or laparoscopic, a total mesohepatectomy is technically a very challenging procedure. We have shown that a total laparoscopic approach is technically feasible and the dissection at the dome of the liver might be aided by a laparoscopic view. Intraoperative ultrasound or indocyanine green staining is helpful in defining the anatomical landmarks of this operation. In order to complete this operation safely, advanced laparoscopic skills and an excellent understanding of the hepatic anatomy are essential.

Acknowledgments

Laparoscopic parenchymal-sparing liver resection of lesions in the central segments: feasible, safe, and effective, Claudius Conrad. *Surg Endosc. 2015 Aug;29(8):2410-7. doi: 10.1007/s00464-014-3924-9. Epub 2014 Nov 13*. Source: Conrad 2014. Reproduced with permission of Springer.

Anatomy figures

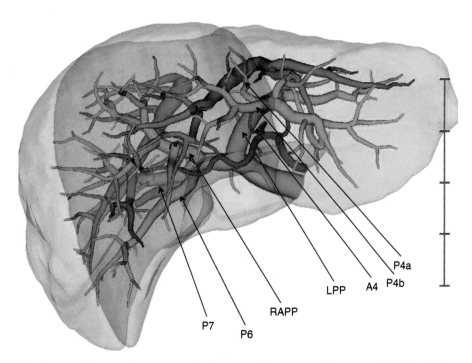

Figure v18.1 Critical anatomy for a mesohepatectomy. During a central hepatectomy, liver segments IV, V, and VIII are removed. The MHV is removed with the specimen. The lateral border is RHV and LPP. The medial border is LHV and LPP. A critical portal structure is the RAAP, which is removed at the time of surgery. It is important to protect the RPPP or P6 and P7. This patient has a trifurcation of RAPP, P6, and P7. On the left side, the intermediate branch of the left hepatic artery (A4) is taken as well as portal branches to segment IV.

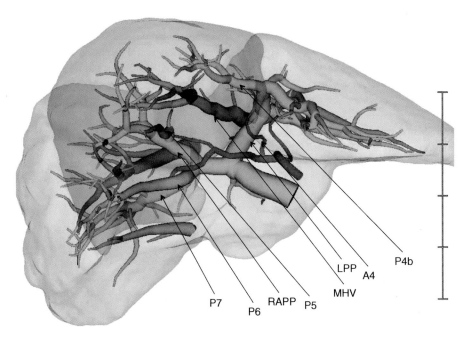

Figure v18.2 Caudal view for a mesohepatectomy. A critical structure to identify during the surgery is the RPP and its division into RAPP and RPPP. This patient has a trifurcation of RAPP, P6, and P7. The PP to segment IV usually consists of several branches that need to be controlled.

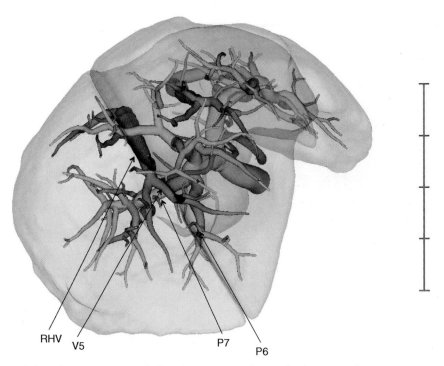

Figure v18.3 Lateral view. The RHV constitutes the lateral margin. P6 and P7 need to be preserved.

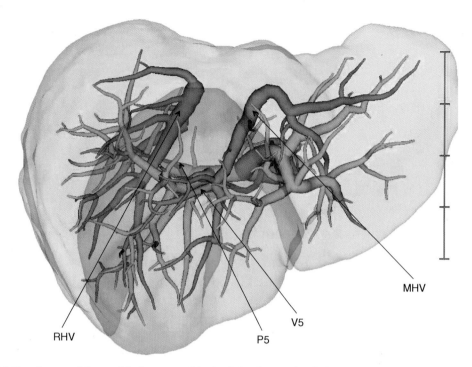

MHV

V5

RHV   P5

Figure v18.4 View from cranial to caudal. The MHV will be divided and resected with the specimen.

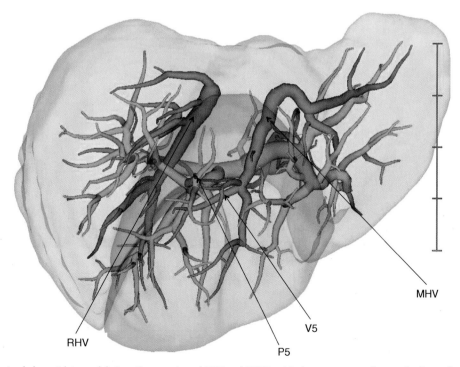

MHV

V5

RHV   P5

Figure v18.5 Angled cranial to caudal view. Preservation of RHV and LHV is critical to preserve outflow to the future liver remnant.

VIDEO 19

Living donor left lateral sectionectomy

Video duration 8 minutes 17 seconds

In this video, we demonstrate a living donor left lateral sectionectomy. Living donor liver transplantation in general is high-risk surgery. Laparoscopic graft harvest adds a significant level of complexity to the case. Only an expert transplant team with significant experience in living donor liver transplantation, parenchymal transection, and laparoscopic liver surgery should attempt such a case in patients who have been very well selected.

case of nonprogression and will minimize warm ischemia time in case of urgent conversion.

The falciform, coronary, and left triangular ligaments and ligament of Arantius are taken down and the hilar fissure opened. The parenchymal bridge between segments II and IV is divided.

The next step is the portal dissection. The porta is approached from the left side. First, the hepatic artery

> **OUTLINE**
>
> The video has the following outline:
> - Donor information
> - Port positioning
> - Liver mobilization
> - Portal dissection
> - Left bile duct division and parenchymal transection
> - Graft extraction
> - Important points.

The living donor is a 32-year-old man. He does not have any vascular variations. However, segments II and III drain independently from segment IV into the common bile duct (Figure v19.1). This scheme demonstrates the port positioning (Figure v19.2). It is advisable to mobilize the liver early (Figure v19.3). This can limit the incision in

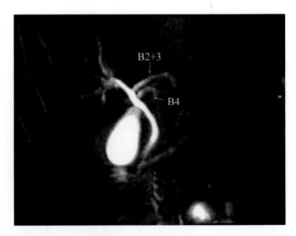

Figure v19.1 It is critical to have an excellent understanding of the vascular and biliary anatomy. Segments II and III drain independently from segment IV into the common bile duct.

Laparoscopic Liver, Pancreas, and Biliary Surgery, First Edition.
Edited by Claudius Conrad and Brice Gayet.

Port positioning

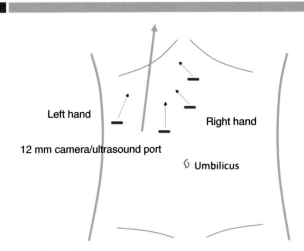

Figure v19.2 This scheme demonstrates the port positioning for a living donor left lateral sectionectomy graft harvest.

and then the portal vein are dissected out. Once the hepatic artery has been encircled, the left portal vein is dissected out. Here, the portal vein is being dissected out (Figure v19.4). A caudate branch is dissected out and controlled with a locking clip (Figure v19.5). The portal vein is dissected out and encircled with umbilical tape. The left branch of the portal vein is dissected out and encircled with scissors.

The next step is division of the left bile duct and the parenchymal transection. The liver capsule is opened along the falciform ligament (Figure v19.6). Then the transection is deepened and, in an open book approach, the left bile duct is approached. Portal branches to segment IV are controlled with locking clips (Figure v19.7). The V4 drainage vein is dissected out, clipped, and divided. The left lateral bile duct is exposed with an

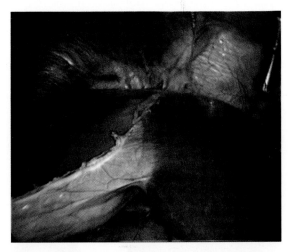

Figure v19.3 It is advisable to mobilize the liver at an early stage of the operation. In case of nonprogression or a complication, graft harvest can be expedited.

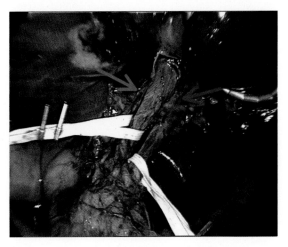

Figure v19.4 Once the HA has been encircled, the LPV is dissected out.

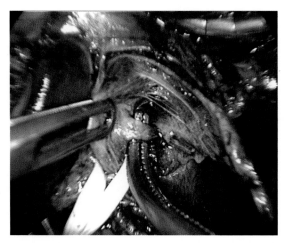

Figure v19.5 A caudate branch is dissected out and controlled with a locking clip.

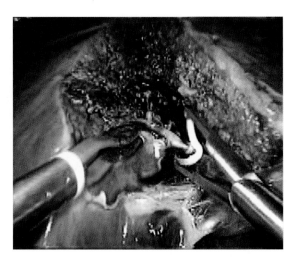

Figure v19.7 Portal branches to segment IV are controlled with locking clips.

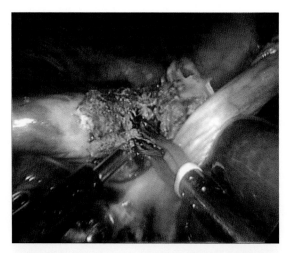

Figure v19.6 The liver capsule is opened along the falciform ligament.

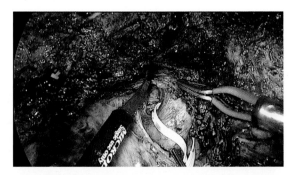

Figure v19.8 The bile duct is divided with laparoscopic scissors.

ultrasonic aspirator device (Figure v19.8). The bile duct is divided with laparoscopic scissors. The staying side of the bile duct is clipped (Figure v19.9).

We then proceed with the parenchymal transection. Bile duct division facilitates the parenchymal division, opening the transection plane further. As we approach the IVC, the left hepatic vein is dissected out and will be encircled with umbilical tape. This is the final step prior to graft extraction (Figure v19.10). Before division of inflow and outflow, we perform a Pfannenstiel incision through

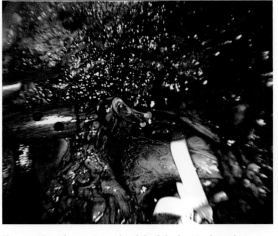

Figure v19.9 The staying side of the bile duct is clipped.

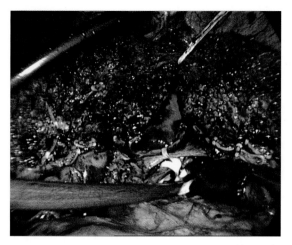

which we bring in an endoscopic retrieval bag. With division of the left hepatic artery and portal vein, the warm ischemia time begins. After stapling off the left portal vein, it is divided with scissors. The left hepatic vein is staple divided. The specimen is brought out through the Pfannenstiel incision.

Figure v19.10 This is the final step prior to graft extraction. Before division of inflow and outflow, a Pfannenstiel incision is performed through which we bring in an endoscopic retrieval bag.

> **IMPORTANT POINTS**
>
> - Only experienced liver transplant surgeons and laparoscopists should perform this operation.
> - Excellent understanding of donor portal and liver anatomy, especially biliary variations, is crucial.
> - Mobilize the liver early.
> - Protect remaining portal structures.
> - Prepare for graft extraction early to minimize warm ischemia time.

Anatomy figures

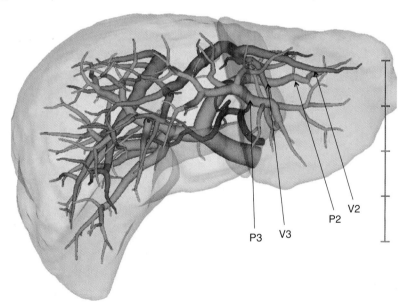

Figure v19.11 Relevant anatomy for laparoscopic living donor left lateral sectionectomy. For living donor liver transplantation, it is crucial to have an excellent understanding of donor anatomy. In addition to vascular anomalies, variations of the biliary system need to be identified preoperatively and anticipated during the operation to avoid injury.

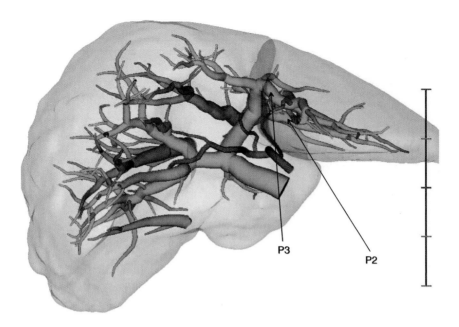

Figure v19.12 Initial view for laparoscopic living donor left lateral sectionectomy. It is key to avoid injury to the remaining structures in the porta. In the video, the parenchymal transection is performed medial to the branching of P3 and P2.

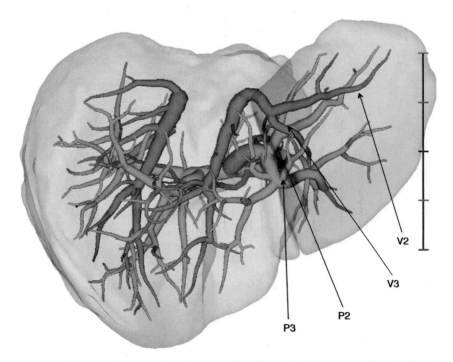

Figure v19.13 Cranial to caudal view. The LHV needs to be protected until the end of the surgery. It is staple divided at the drainage into the IVC.

Laparoscopic splenic resection

VIDEO 20

Total splenectomy

Video duration 7 minutes 10 seconds

In this video, we will show you a total splenectomy.

> **OUTLINE**
>
> The video is divided into the following parts:
> - Port positioning
> - Controlling the hilar vessels and short gastric vessels
> - Splenic mobilization
> - Specimen extraction
> - Important points.

Figure v20.1 demonstrates the port positioning. The positioning might have to be modified depending on the size of the specimen. The first step, particularly when removing a very large spleen, should be controlling the hilar vessels.

We gently retract the spleen laterally, and open up the splenorenal ligament. At this step, the tail of the pancreas can be easily damaged. Once the splenic hilar vessels have been completely uncovered, we clip the individual branches using locking clips. Adhesions to the spleen can cause capsular tears during mobiliza-

Port positioning

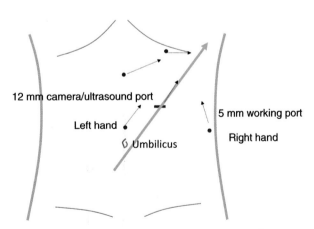

12 mm camera/ultrasound port

Left hand

Umbilicus

5 mm working port

Right hand

Figure v20.1 The patient is in the French position with slight left decubitus positioning. The port placement might have to be modified depending on the size of the specimen.

Laparoscopic Liver, Pancreas, and Biliary Surgery, First Edition.
Edited by Claudius Conrad and Brice Gayet.

tion; therefore, any adhesions should be divided early with gentle traction on the specimen. The splenic artery and venous branches of the middle portion of the spleen are controlled here. The next step is to control and divide the short gastric vessels. The left lateral section of the liver is retracted superiorly. Here you can see the division of adhesions between the spleen and stomach. Next, we open up the gastro-splenic ligament and control and divide the short gastric vessels.

After the initial step of the dissection of gastrosplenic ligament, the superior pole vessels can be identified and dissected out. Note the closeness of the pancreas to the superior pole vessels on this image. Now all of the hilar vessels have been controlled. With gentle traction superiorly, adhesions to the retroperitoneum are divided. The next step of the operation is splenic mobilization. Especially during inferior mobilization of the spleen, we need to be careful not to injure the splenic flexure of the colon.

The last step is specimen extraction. It is possible to avoid using an additional port by placing an endoscopic retrieval bag directly through the abdominal wall. We need to be careful not to rupture the spleen when placing it in the endoscopic retrieval bag

---

IMPORTANT POINTS

- Place the ports high enough in the left upper quadrant and far enough to the left. However, the final port position should be determined depending on the size of the specimen.
- Avoid minor tears in the splenic parenchyma or capsule, which can easily happen during retraction when the spleen is fixed as a result of adhesions.
- Avoid a pancreatic tail injury when dissecting out the hilar vessels.
- Gentle retraction avoids rupturing the spleen or bleeding at the end of the case.
- Consider placing the retrieval bag directly through the abdominal wall through a Pfannenstiel incision, for example, in order to avoid an additional port.

Partial splenectomy

Video duration 8 minutes 40 seconds

In this video, we will demonstrate a partial splenectomy.

OUTLINE

The video is divided into the following parts:
- Port positioning
- Division of the short gastric vessels and superior pole vessels
- Ultrasound
- Parenchymal transection
- Important points.

Figure v21.1 demonstrates the port positioning. It is important to place the ports high enough in the left upper quadrant and far enough to the left of the patient. To exemplify how high up in the upper quadrant and how far over to the left we place the ports, we show you here positioning of one of the 12 mm ports and two of the 5 mm ports.

The first step in devascularizing the superior pole of the spleen is division of the short gastric vessels. In order to expose the short gastric vessels, we need to lyze some adhesions between the left lateral section of the liver and the superior pole of the spleen. In order to fully mobilize the superior pole of the spleen, we need to mobilize the left lateral section of the liver. This is not a routine step for our partial splenectomy, but necessary here because of the abnormal size of the spleen. We can see here the left lateral section of the liver mobilized towards the right side of the patient. An Endoloop placed at the very tip of the

Port positioning

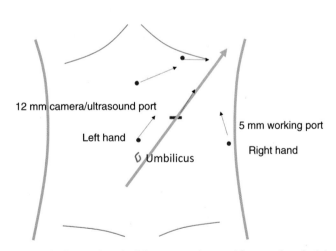

12 mm camera/ultrasound port

Left hand

◊ Umbilicus

5 mm working port

Right hand

Figure v21.1 It is important to place the ports high enough in the left upper quadrant and far enough to the left of the patient.

---

left triangular ligament facilitates this step. Beginning the division of the phrenicolienal ligament at this step facilitates the mobilization process. The gastrolienal ligament is now nicely exposed. With this exposure, we can now begin to divide the short gastric vessels.

This section demonstrates the division of the superior pole vessels. We continue our dissection inferiorly to expose the superior pole vessels. The superior pole artery is clipped and divided. The next step is to expose the superior pole vein. In the background, you can see the superior pole vein and we are switching to scissors for the dissection. In order to facilitate clip application, we are preshrinking the vein with bipolar forceps. Here you can see the application of the locking clips. Bleeding from a capsular tear can be stopped with a hemostatic agent made of oxidized regenerated cellulose.

Before we begin the parenchymal transection, we use ultrasound to confirm that the devascularization of the superior pole is complete. Using intraoperative ultrasound, we can see that the devascularization of the superior pole is not complete. We therefore expose the hilar vessels in the retroperitoneum to control additional branches to the superior pole. Clamping the vessels and confirming flow to the superior pole via ultrasound allows us to confirm complete isolation of the superior pole of the spleen.

The last step of the operation is parenchymal transection. A similar parenchymal transection technique as for the liver can be used here. Thanks to the vascular isolation, parenchymal back bleeding is minimal. The superior pole is now completely detached from the rest of the spleen. Minor bleeding can be stopped with the bipolar forceps.

IMPORTANT POINTS

- For total or partial splenectomies, place the ports high enough in the left quadrant.
- Avoid minor tears in the splenic parenchyma.
- Use ultrasound to define the zone of ischemia.
- Use gentle retraction during the splenic mobilization.
- Be mentally prepared to convert to a total splenectomy or an open procedure.

VIDEO 22

Pancreatic enucleation

Video duration 8 minutes 44 seconds

In this video, we will show you a pancreatic enucleation.

OUTLINE

The video is divided into the following parts:
- Port positioning
- Pancreatic exposure
- Ultrasound
- Enucleation
- Important points.

For port positioning, the pancreatic exposure, enucleation, and use of ultrasound need to be considered (Figure v22.1).

The first step is exposing the pancreas and locating the lesion, which in this case is located in the pancreatic body. We are exposing the pancreas by entering the lesser sac. Next, we will take the omentum off the transverse colon. Here the splenic flexure is taken down. Now the inferior border of the pancreas is mobilized. With superior traction on the pancreas, the retroperitoneal attachments are taken down. Be careful not to injure the splenic vein which

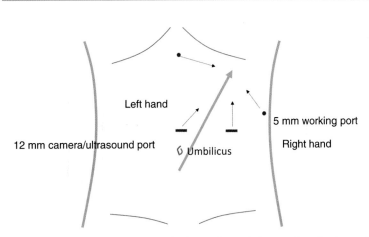

Port positioning

- Left hand
- 12 mm camera/ultrasound port
- Umbilicus
- 5 mm working port
- Right hand

Figure v22.1 For port positioning, the pancreatic exposure, enucleation, and use of ultrasound need to be considered.

Laparoscopic Liver, Pancreas, and Biliary Surgery, First Edition.
Edited by Claudius Conrad and Brice Gayet.
© 2017 John Wiley & Sons, Ltd. Published 2017 by John Wiley & Sons, Ltd.

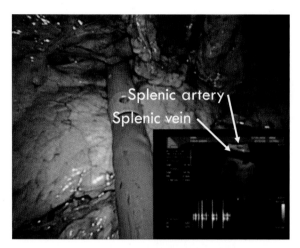

Figure v22.2 Ultrasound can be helpful in determining the relationship between the pancreatic duct and the lesion.

comes into view here. We continue our dissection along the inferior border of the pancreas towards the spleen.

Once the pancreatic body has been completely mobilized, we proceed with intraoperative ultrasound. It is important to identify the splenic artery and splenic vein in relationship to the lesion. Doppler mode can be helpful in identifying the artery and vein. On this Doppler flow image, the artery is superior and the

vein inferior. Here the cystic lesion to be enucleated comes into view. Ultrasound can also be helpful in determining the relationship between the pancreatic duct and the lesion (Figure v22.2).

The next step is the enucleation. Here the cystic lesion at the inferior border of the body of the pancreas comes into view. For retraction of the lesion, we are holding onto the fibrous tissue attached to the lesion rather than the lesion itself. At this step of the operation, we should be careful not to injure the pancreatic duct which we know from the intraoperative ultrasound is close to this location. A small duct of the main pancreatic duct is clipped and divided. Now the lesion is completely detached and we place it in an endoscopic retrieval bag for later removal. We now proceed to approximate the walls of the cavity in order to minimize a pancreatic fistula. Finally, a drain is placed in one of the port sites.

IMPORTANT POINTS

- Determine preoperatively that the pancreatic duct is not involved when you are planning an enucleation.
- Optimize port positioning for both exposure and enucleation.
- Use ultrasound to locate smaller lesions and parenchyma approximation that might potentially reduce the fistula rate.

Cystgastrostomy

Video duration 8 minutes 4 seconds

This video demonstrates a cystgastrostomy.

Figure v23.1 demonstrates the port positioning.

First, we will show you exposure of the cyst in the lesser sac. First, we separate the greater omentum from the transverse colon and transverse mesocolon; this step can be difficult in patients with recurrent episodes of pancreatitis or infections. One might consider an endogastric laparoscopic approach in such cases. Separating the greater omentum from the transverse colon and transverse mesocolon at a length of about 10–15 cm is enough for exposure. Here the posterior wall of the stomach comes into view. Grabbing the stomach at the lesser curvature and using superior traction aids exposure of the pancreas. As we are dividing the adhesions between the stomach and the pancreas, the cyst comes into view (Figure v23.2). We carefully uncover the cyst from the capsular and overlying pancreatic parenchyma. Once the inferior part of the cyst has been completely mobilized, we focus our dissection on the superior part.

The first step in creating a cystgastrostomy is the cystotomy. The ideal location for the cystotomy is best

Port positioning

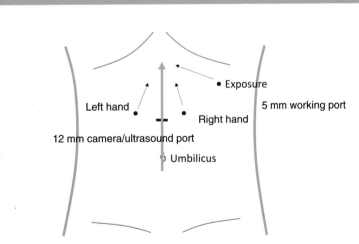

Figure v23.1 The scheme demonstrates the port positioning for a cystgastrostomy.

Laparoscopic Liver, Pancreas, and Biliary Surgery, First Edition.
Edited by Claudius Conrad and Brice Gayet.
© 2017 John Wiley & Sons, Ltd. Published 2017 by John Wiley & Sons, Ltd.

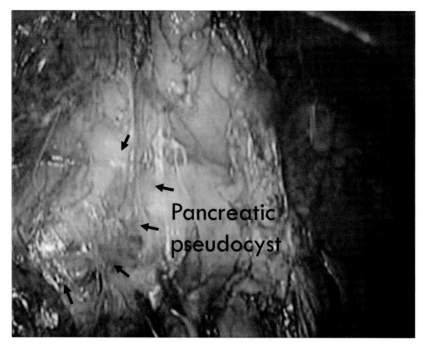

Figure v23.2 We are dividing adhesions between the stomach and the pancreas, and the cyst comes into view.

chosen with ultrasound. Factors that affect the choice of an ideal location for the cystotomy are safety but also ease of creating the anastomosis. Here, you see the amylase-rich pancreatic fluid leaking from the cyst. The next step is enlarging the cystotomy. Bleeding can be easily stopped with the bipolar forceps. The next step is the posterior wall anastomosis. We have shown here one technique of anchoring the suture with a large knot at the end of the suture. It is important to take large bites in order to incorporate the entire wall of the stomach as well as the entire wall of the cyst. The further we progress with the anastomosis, the easier it becomes.

Once the posterior wall has been completed, we perform a gastrotomy. Performing the gastrotomy at this step helps in choosing an ideal location. It is important not to make a false lumen but rather make a full-thickness gastrotomy.

The last step is anterior wall anastomosis. Here we show anchoring the suture with a slip knot; achieving good exposure while suturing the anastomosis can be difficult.

In order to avoid leaks, we reconstruct the anterior walls from both corners. As mentioned, full-thickness bites that also incorporate the mucosa are important. This will prevent the mucosa from obstructing the anastomosis. By including the entire wall of the cyst, we prevent postoperative bleeding. We perform the anastomosis of the anterior wall from both corners as we achieve better visualization that way.

IMPORTANT POINTS

- Optimal port positioning depends on the cyst location.
- Consider a laparoscopic endogastric approach for large cysts and the presence of adhesions.
- Use ultrasound to determine an optimal location for the cystotomy.
- Use generous bites when suturing.
- Tack down the gastric mucosa to avoid obstruction of the anastomosis.

VIDEO 24

Distal pancreaticosplenectomy

Video duration 11 minutes 12 seconds

In this video, we demonstrate a distal pancreaticosplenectomy.

> **OUTLINE**
>
> The video is divided into the following parts:
> - Port positioning
> - Pancreatic exposure
> - Dissection of the splenic vessels
> - Division of the short gastric vessels
> - Pancreatic transection
> - Splenic mobilization
> - Important points.

It is important to place the ports high enough in the left upper quadrant (Figure v24.1). The camera port should not only be high enough in the left upper quadrant but also far enough over to the left for good visualization. The working ports and the ports for retraction are placed to the left of the midline.

We are now beginning with the pancreatic exposure. One of the first steps is to deflect the colon downwards in order to avoid injury during the pancreatic exposure. All adhesions to the spleen are divided because traction can lead to capsular tears. The splenic flexure is deflected downwards for safe mobilization of the spleen. Here we are dividing the gastrosplenic ligament in order to expose the tail of the pancreas. Now that we have exposed the distal pancreas, we are placing an additional 12 mm port for later stapling. The ideal angle to the distal pancreas can be chosen once it has been exposed.

Port positioning

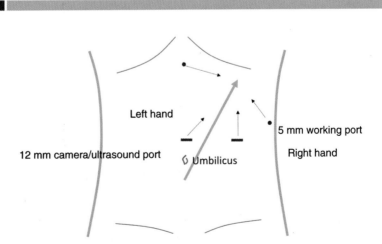

Left hand

5 mm working port

12 mm camera/ultrasound port   Umbilicus   Right hand

Figure v24.1 It is important to place the ports high enough in the left upper quadrant.

Laparoscopic Liver, Pancreas, and Biliary Surgery, First Edition.
Edited by Claudius Conrad and Brice Gayet.
© 2017 John Wiley & Sons, Ltd. Published 2017 by John Wiley & Sons, Ltd.

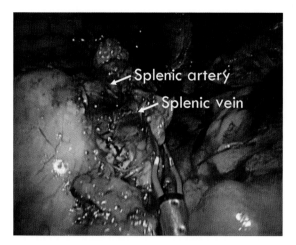

Figure v24.2 On this image the clipped splenic artery and the splenic vein are exposed.

We are now dissecting out the splenic artery; the splenic artery is located at the superior border of the pancreas and in order to expose it, we are opening the capsule of the pancreas. Here the splenic artery comes into view. The splenic artery is clipped and divided. We are now continuing our dissection distally along the gastrosplenic ligament. Next we are dividing additional short gastric vessels. Take time for hemostasis at this step in order to achieve good working conditions. Here we can see the adhesions between the stomach and the tumor. In order to avoid a positive margin, we would perform a sleeve gastrectomy to keep the adhesions with the specimen. This step is obviously specific to this case and not routinely performed during a distal pancreaticosplenectomy.

Next is the pancreatic transection. For safe staple division of the pancreas, the tissue should not be too thick. Therefore we are dissecting out the pancreas some more. Here we are dissecting out the pancreas off the retroperitoneum. Be careful to avoid a splenic vein injury. Now the clipped splenic artery and the splenic vein are exposed (Figure v24.2). We are continuing to thin out the pancreas in order to avoid having too much tissue to staple through. Now that the pancreas is thinned out enough, we are ready to staple. As we are also stapling across the splenic vein, we have a vascular clamp ready in case of stapler misfiring. Now the splenic artery can be easily divided.

The last step of the operation is splenic mobilization. Additional retroperitoneal attachments to the pancreas are divided. Adhesions to the lateral abdominal wall and the phrenicosplenic ligament are divided. Be careful to avoid a colonic injury at this step. With ventral traction on the spleen, the inferior portion of the phrenicosplenic ligament is divided. At this step, the specimen is completely mobile and can be removed from the abdomen.

IMPORTANT POINTS

- Ensure you place the ports high enough and far enough to the left.
- Take time for hemostasis in order to achieve excellent working conditions.
- Avoid bleeding from the splenic vasculature and use only gentle retraction on the spleen to avoid capsular tears.

VIDEO 25

Spleen-preserving pancreatectomy of the body and tail

Video duration 12 minutes 56 seconds

In this video, we will show you a spleen-preserving pancreatectomy of the body and tail.

> **OUTLINE**
>
> The video is divided into the following parts:
> - Port positioning
> - Pancreatic exposure
> - Pancreatic mobilization
> - Controlling the hilar vessels
> - Splenic artery division
> - Division of the pancreas
> - Splenic vein division
> - Important points.

Figure v25.1 demonstrates the port positioning; the two 12 mm ports accommodate the camera and ultrasound. The port positioning might have to be modified depending on the location of the lesion in the pancreas.

In this first step, we expose the body and tail of the pancreas. In order to do this, we open up the lesser sac below the gastroepiploic arcade. Ventral traction on the stomach facilitates this process. As we continue our dissection distally, we should be careful not to injure the splenic flexure.

The next step will be pancreatic mobilization. We begin our dissection at the inferior border of the pancreas. At this step, we are careful not to go through the colonic mesentery. We continue our dissection very close to the inferior border of the pancreas. During this dissection,

Port positioning

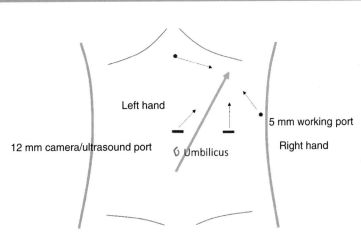

Figure v25.1 The figure demonstrates the port positioning. The two 12 mm ports accommodate the camera and ultrasound. The port positioning might have to be modified depending on the location of the lesion in the pancreas.

Laparoscopic Liver, Pancreas, and Biliary Surgery, First Edition.
Edited by Claudius Conrad and Brice Gayet.
© 2017 John Wiley & Sons, Ltd. Published 2017 by John Wiley & Sons, Ltd.

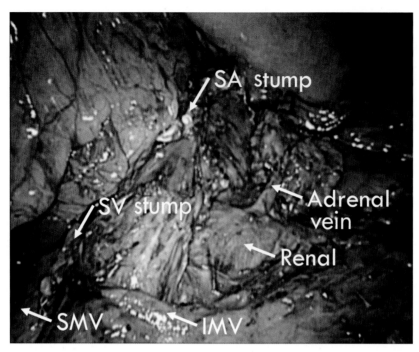

Figure v25.2 In this image, the splenic artery stump, splenic vein stump, adrenal vein, renal vein, IMV, and SMV can be seen.

the splenic vein comes into view. Be careful not to cause injury to the duodenum at this step. We follow the splenic vein towards the tail of the pancreas. As we follow the Gerota's fascia, the anterior kidney comes into view. Here we complete the division of the lienocolic ligament. At this step of the operation, the inferior and distal part of the pancreas is completely mobile.

We now continue our dissection more proximally towards the body of the pancreas. Here you can see the portal venous confluence coming into view. Using ultrasound, we confirm the location of the lesion within the pancreas and its location relative to the splenic vein and artery. On this ultrasound image, you can see the lesion and the splenic vein at 5 o'clock in relationship to the lesion. We will now continue our dissection of the retroperitoneum, staying ventral to the renal vessels. Here you can see the left renal vein and left kidney coming into view. At this step, we need to be careful not to injure the left adrenal gland or its vessels. Here you can see the left adrenal vein draining into the left renal vein. In contrast to the original description of radical anterior modular pancreatosplenectomy, we do not resect the left adrenal gland with the retroperitoneum. At this step, the aorta

comes into view. We proceed to sampling the left celiac plexus. The celiac trunk is just a little bit more superior and injury should be avoided. Here, all the retroperitoneal tissue lateral to the adrenal gland is resected.

We now focus our attention on mobilizing the superior and the distal part of the pancreas. For this, we continue to open up the gastrosplenic ligament and divide one or two short gastric vessels. As we are planning on dividing splenic vessels later, more short gastrics should not be taken. This avoids left-sided portal venous hypertension. As we are dissecting the superior aspect of the pancreatic tail, we need to be careful not to injure the splenic vessels. Here the splenic artery and splenic vein can be seen. With superior traction on the specimen, the inferior aspect of the pancreatic tail is dissected out. Here we are dividing the inferior aspect of the splenorenal ligament. We are now ready to divide the hilar vessels. We are planning on preserving the spleen with the Warhsaw technique. This means the spleen will be perfused via the short gastrics, while the splenic vessels are taken. Here the splenic artery is dissected out and divided. We will now dissect out, clip, and divide the splenic artery proximal to the lesion. For this, we need to completely expose the dorsal side of the pancreas. With ventral traction on the pancreas, the attachments to the retroperitoneum are divided.

At this step, we begin dissection of the origin of the splenic artery. We now move to the superior border of the pancreas to continue our dissection of the splenic artery. Here you can see the bifurcation between the splenic artery and hepatic artery. Now that the splenic artery is completely dissected at its origin, it can be clipped and divided.

The next step of the operation is pancreatic division at its neck. Here we begin the parenchymal transection just above the portal venous confluence. Here you can see the portal vein appearing in the background.

The last step of the operation is division of the splenic vein. The specimen is completely detached from the retroperitoneum. On this image, the splenic artery stump, splenic vein stump, adrenal vein, renal vein, IMV, and SMV can be seen (Figure v25.2). The specimen is placed in the endoscopic retrieval bag for later removal. We are

planning on suture closing the transection surface of the pancreas. We are suture closing the pancreatic remnant, ensuring the pancreatic duct is well incooperated in the running suture. At completion of the case, we place a drain.

IMPORTANT POINTS

- Take time for hemostasis in order to achieve excellent working conditions.
- Avoid bleeding from the splenic vasculature, including the hilum when controlling the splenic vessels more proximally.
- Avoid injury to the retroperitoneal vessels such as the renal vein or adrenal gland.
- When taking the splenic vessels, inspect the spleen at the end of the case to ensure you have good perfusion.
- Should you have a splenic vein injury and need to take the splenic vein, you should also clip the splenic artery. This will avoid left-sided portal venous hypertension.

VIDEO 26

Pancreaticoduodenectomy

Video duration 20 minutes 9 seconds

In this video, we will show you a laparoscopic pancreaticoduodenectomy (Whipple procedure).

For the colonic mobilization and the beginning of the Kocher maneuver, the operative surgeon stands at the left side of the patient (Figure v26.1). The rest of the surgery is performed from this position (Figure v26.2).

Performing the Whipple procedure laparoscopically should not compromise the oncological soundness of the operation. Therefore, an adequate lymph node dissection should be performed. Several adhesions to the gallbladder are lyzed. We are following the cystic duct on to the portal structures and we will strip the porta of all lymphatic tissue. Here lymph node stations 5, 12, and 8a are removed. A hepatic artery injury should be avoided at this step. Here we are following the hepatic artery towards lymph node stations 8p and 9. The dissection directly at the hepatic artery should be performed using scissors. The cystic duct and cystic artery are divided and the gallbladder removed.

Before we can begin the Kocher maneuver, the colon is deflected downwards. The deflection of the colon

Port positioning

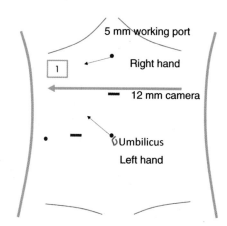

Figure v26.1 For the colonic mobilization and the beginning of the Kocher maneuver, the operative surgeon stands at the left side of the patient.

Laparoscopic Liver, Pancreas, and Biliary Surgery, First Edition.
Edited by Claudius Conrad and Brice Gayet.
© 2017 John Wiley & Sons, Ltd. Published 2017 by John Wiley & Sons, Ltd.

Port positioning

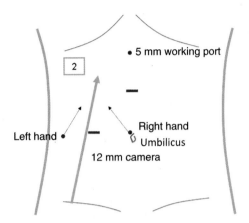

Figure v26.2 The remainder of the operation following colonic mobilization and Kocher maneuver is performed from this position.

downwards follows our operative approach for right colectomy. We have to mobilize the colon just enough in order to begin the kocherization comfortably. For the Kocher maneuver, we ensure gentle traction on the duodenum; as we see here, the IVC is exposed. It is important to be gentle during duodenal retraction with the laparoscopic instruments in order to avoid perforation. We recommend doing as much as possible of the Kocher maneuver above the transverse mesocolon because the exposure is easier.

We are performing an aortocaval lymph node dissection before transecting the intestine, stomach or pancreas. Only in very selective circumstances do we complete a Whipple if the aortocaval lymph nodes are positive. In order to avoid postoperative lymph leak, we are applying a clip to the lymphatic vessel. The lymph nodes are sent for frozen section analysis. At this step, we will terminate the procedure if the lymph node(s) turn out to be positive.

This is the view along the IVC with the drainage of the left renal vein (Figure v26.3). Here we are removing the right celiac plexus which we are also sending for frozen section. Watch out for the celiac trunk at this step of the operation. We would discourage you from harvesting both the celiac plexi as this can lead to diarrhea that is difficult to manage (Figure v26.4).

We are now proceeding to the portal venous confluence dissection. As in open surgery, injury to the portal venous confluence should be avoided at all costs. We are beginning our dissection at the inferior border of the pancreas and follow the jejunal branches towards the portal venous confluence. Here the portal vein comes into view. Here we are following the gastrocolic trunk to its drainage into the portal vein. The gastrocolic trunk will be

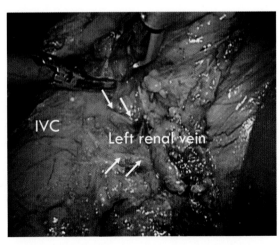

Figure v26.3 This is the view along the IVC with the drainage of the left renal vein.

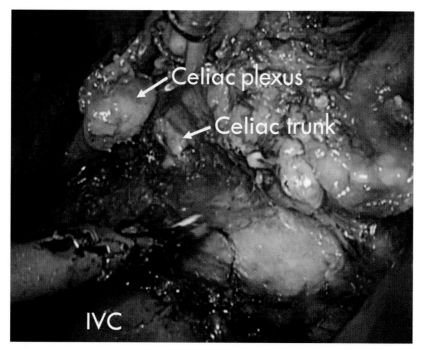

Figure v26.4 We would discourage you from harvesting both the celiac plexi as this can lead to diarrhea that is difficult to manage.

divided using the energy device. Now the portal venous confluence has been dissected out.

The next stage is gastric and jejunal transection. Here you can see the division of the ligament of Treitz. In open surgery, creation of an anastomosis at the level of the ligament of Treitz is difficult but it is much easier in laparoscopic surgery. Creation of the anastomoses at the level of the ligament of Treitz prevents having to mobilize a lot of the duodenum. An additional port is now placed to accommodate the stapler. Next we proceed to dividing the distal stomach. The omentum and the gastroepiploic arcade are divided. The stomach is staple divided. Before transecting the pancreas, we will control the gastroduodenal artery (Figure v26.5).

The gastroduodenal artery is dissected out using scissors. As in open surgery, the gastroduodenal artery should be ligated with enough distance to the hepatic artery. The gastroduodenal artery is divided using thermofusion. Now the portal vein is exposed at the superior border of the pancreas.

We can now proceed to transect the pancreas. Pancreatic transection is performed with the energy device.

The inferior pancreaticoduodenal arcade is controlled with stitches. Now the pancreas is completely transected. Next is the retroperitoneal dissection. The jejunum is pulled through from the ligament of Treitz. We are now transecting the retroperitoneum along the

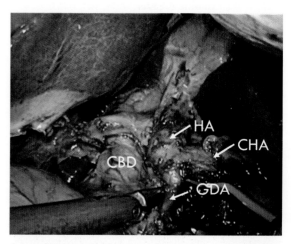

Figure v26.5 Before transecting the pancreas, we will control the gastroduodenal artery.

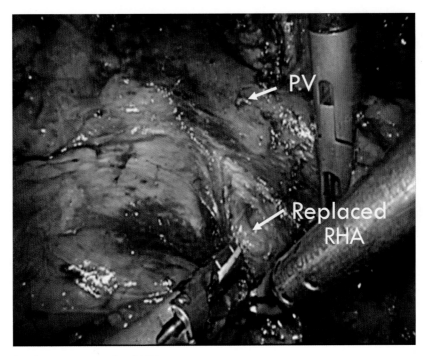

Figure v26.6 This view demonstrates a replaced RHA.

SMA. Here, a replaced right hepatic artery comes into view (Figure v26.6). With blunt dissection and the bipolar forceps, the portal vein is detached from the retroperitoneum. The posterior pancreaticoduodenal vein will be dissected out and divided. Here we are dividing the retroperitoneal attachments along the replaced right hepatic artery. Here the replaced right hepatic artery, superior mesenteric artery, and portal vein can be seen (Figure v26.7). The last ridge of peritoneal attachments is divided.

Finally, we will divide the bile duct and determine the perfusion of the pancreatic margin using ICG staining. Here we are dividing the bile duct using scissors. Prior to constructing a pancreaticoenteric anastomosis, we are controlling the perfusion of the pancreatic margin using systemic ICG administration with the near infrared laparoscopic camera (Figure v26.8). Using this technique, we are identifying an area of hypoperfusion. We resect this pancreatic area in the hope of reducing the pancreatic leak rate. Finally, we are mobilizing the pancreatic remnant stump for easier construction of the pancreaticoenteric anastomosis.

We have had mixed experiences with laparoscopically performed pancreaticogastrostomies and pancreaticojejunostomies. At the beginning of the laparoscopic Whipple experience, we recommend a mini-laparotomy at this step and reconstructing via an open technique.

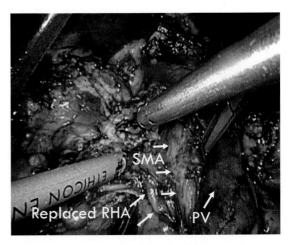

Figure v26.7 Here we can see the replaced RHA, superior mesenteric artery, and PV.

Afterword

Minimal invasive surgery has a firm place in many surgical fields. Open cholecystectomy and appendectomy have been almost completely replaced by laparoscopic procedures and inguinal hernias are also commonly performed through minimal invasive accesses. The low mortality and reduced morbidity of today's bariatric surgery would not be possible with open surgery. Oncological procedures such as colectomies and rectal resections can be safely performed using minimal access surgery with comparable outcomes to traditional surgery in experienced centers. The benefits of laparoscopic surgery are the smaller abdominal incisions which result in reduced postoperative pain and faster recovery time as well as the lower rate of incisional hernias. Minimal invasive procedures also have reduced blood loss and therefore require fewer blood transfusions. All these factors together result in reduced activation of the systemic inflammatory response as assessed by cytokines, which may also contribute to the overall faster recovery. For many patients, the better cosmetic results of laparoscopic surgery are also important.

These benefits of minimal invasive surgery have been demonstrated in many large randomized controlled trials. However, they often come at the price of longer operating times, more expensive equipment, and longer learning curves because of the loss of three-dimensional view, loss of tactile feedback, and the fulcrum effect. These problems of laparoscopic surgery are paramount for operations in complex anatomical areas such as the hepatopancreatobiliary tract. It is noteworthy that the widened indications for laparoscopic procedures usually corresponded with advancements in instruments and devices that made more complex minimal invasive procedures possible.

As the authors of the previous chapters have highlighted, pancreatic surgery poses special problems for the adoption of minimal invasive procedures. The complex anatomical position of the pancreas in the retroperitoneal space, surrounded by vital organs and vessels, requires highly experienced surgeons with detailed knowledge of the anatomical situation to perform safe operations and avoid potentially life-threatening complications. Besides expertise in pancreatic surgery, surgeons performing minimal invasive pancreatic procedures need profound training in advanced laparoscopy. Aside from surgeon factors, the technical setting must be appropriate. Laparoscopic devices, for example for the transection of the pancreas, should be improved to avoid pancreatic fistulas and other technical complications. Furthermore, laparoscopic intracorporeal suturing is a challenging and time-consuming process, mainly responsible for the complications and long duration of minimal invasive pancreaticoduodenectomy. Thus, it is quite possible to perform resection but not reconstruction.

These ramifications of minimal invasive surgery currently limit a wider application of laparoscopy to distal pancreatectomy and maybe enucleation of small benign lesions. However, before routine clinical implementation, well-designed and stringently conducted randomized controlled trials must be performed in experienced centers to evaluate the safety and oncological outcome. As Rutz and Kooby nicely demonstrate in Chapter 23, the current evidence for minimal invasive distal pancreatectomy stems mainly from retrospective case series, with significant differences regarding type of tumor, clearly favoring benign and cystic lesions as well as smaller tumor sizes in the case of laparoscopic procedures. Ductal adenocarcinomas of the pancreas were only marginally investigated in the currently available studies. In our opinion, there is currently a limited role for minimal invasive approaches in pancreaticoduodenectomy, mainly owing to the difficulties of performing the pancreaticojejunostomy and biliodigestive anastomosis. The long duration of this operation and the associated morbidity currently outweigh its potential benefits. The very limited numbers of reports about these procedures in the 20 years since their first description indicate that there are many obstacles to a wider application. If these challenges can be diminished and the duration of laparoscopic pancreaticoduodenectomy can be shortened, the validity of this operation should be re-evaluated in randomized trials.

In summary, the promises of minimal invasive surgery make it likely that laparoscopic pancreatic surgery will have benefits for patients. Laparoscopic pancreatic surgery should be evaluated in randomized controlled trials to establish its true benefit. If the promises hold up, it will be a viable alternative to open procedures in selected patients.

Beat Müller-Stich, Adrian T. Billeter,
and Markus W. Büchler
Department of General, Visceral,
and Transplantation Surgery,
University of Heidelberg Hospital,
Heidelberg, Germany

Afterword

Since the establishment of laparoscopic cholecystectomy, appendectomy or colorectal surgery, there has been growing evidence that well-selected patients with liver or pancreas tumors may have a greater benefit from laparoscopic surgery compared to an open approach. In particular, cirrhotic patients with well-preserved liver function might have the greatest benefit from a laparoscopic approach. This new textbook on laparoscopic hepatopancreatobiliary (HPB) surgery illustrates the most current laparoscopic technologies used for resection of liver and pancreas tumors. The chapters are authored by well-known experts in HPB surgery and summarize the rapid developments in this area. The 24 comprehensive chapters cover the presented topics in depth and are illustrated by many color images. The book provides the latest information not only on minimally invasive surgery but also on anatomical, imaging, and anesthesia aspects. It also covers cutting-edge surgical approaches such as robotic surgery and laparoscopic living donor hepatectomy. This book should become one of the classic references for those who are interested in laparoscopic HPB surgery.

Prof. Dr. med. Pierre-Alain Clavien, PhD
UniversitätsSpital Zürich
Klinik für Viszeral- und Transplantationschirurgie
Zürich, Switzerland

Index

Page numbers in *italics* indicate figures; page numbers in **bold** indicate tables

Laparoscopic Liver, Pancreas, and Biliary Surgery, First Edition.
Edited by Claudius Conrad and Brice Gayet.
© 2017 John Wiley & Sons, Ltd. Published 2017 by John Wiley & Sons, Ltd.